Pharmacology

Reviews & Rationales

Mary Ann Hogan, RN, CS, MSN

Clinical Assistant Professor
University of Massachusetts, Amherst
Amherst, Massachusetts

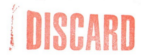

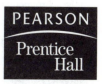
PEARSON

Prentice
Hall

Upper Saddle River, New Jersey 07458

Library of Congress Cataloging-in-Publication Data

Pharmacology : reviews and rationales / [edited by] Mary Ann Hogan.
    p. ; cm. — (Prentice Hall nursing reviews & rationales)
  Includes bibliographical references and index.
  ISBN 0-13-030462-X
  1. Pharmacology—Examinations, questions, etc. 2. Nursing—
  Examinations, questions, etc.
  [DNLM: 1. Pharmaceutical Preparations—Examination Questions. 2.
  Pharmaceutical Preparations—Nurses' Instruction. QV 18.2 P5356 2005]
  I. Hogan, Mary Ann, MSN. II. Series.

  RM301.13.P476 2005
  615'.1'076—dc22
                                                    2004005934

Notice: Care has been taken to confirm the accuracy of the information presented in this book. The author, editors, and the publisher, however, cannot accept any responsibility for errors or omissions or for the consequences for application of the information in this book and make no warranty, express or implied, with respect to its contents.

The author and the publisher have exerted every effort to ensure that drug selections and dosages set forth in this text are in accord with current recommendations and practice at time of publication. However, in view of ongoing research, changes in government regulations, and the constant flow of information relating to drug therapy and drug reactions, the reader is urged to check the package inserts of all drugs for any change in indications of dosage and for added warnings and precautions. This is particularly important when the recommended agent is a new and/or infrequently employed drug.

The author and publisher disclaim all responsibility for any liability, loss, injury, or damage incurred as a consequence, directly or indirectly, of the use and application of any of the contents of this volume.

Publisher: Julie Levin Alexander
Assistant to Publisher: Regina Bruno
Editor-in-chief: Maura Connor
Managing Development Editor: Marilyn Meserve
Development Editor: Jeanne Allison
Director of Production and Manufacturing:
   Bruce Johnson
Managing Production Editor: Patrick Walsh
Production Liaison: Danielle Newhouse
Production Editor: Jessica Balch,
   Pine Tree Composition
Manufacturing Manager: Ilene Sanford
Manufacturing Buyer: Pat Brown

Design Director: Cheryl Asherman
Design Coordinator: Maria Guglielmo
Interior Designer: Jill Little
Cover Designer: Joseph DePinho
Director of Marketing: Karen Allman
Marketing Manager: Nicole Benson
Editorial Assistant: Bonnie Bennett-Walker
Channel Marketing Manager: Rachele Strober
Manager of Media Production: Amy Peltier
New Media Project Manager: Stephen Hartner
Composition: Pine Tree Composition, Inc.
Printer/Binder: Courier/Westford
Cover Printer: Phoenix Color

Pearson Education Ltd., *London*
Pearson Education Australia Pty. Limited, *Sydney*
Pearson Education Singapore, Pte. Ltd.
Pearson Education North Asia Ltd., *Hong Kong*
Pearson Education Canada, Ltd., *Toronto*
Pearson Educaión de Mexico, S.A. de C.V.
Pearson Education—Japan, *Tokyo*
Pearson Education Malaysia, Pte. Ltd.
Pearson Education, Upper Saddle River, New Jersey

DISCARD

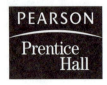

PEARSON
Prentice
Hall

10 9 8 7 6 5 4 3 2 1
ISBN 0-13-030462-X

Contents

Preface

INTRODUCTION

Welcome to the new Prentice Hall Reviews and Rationales Series! This 9-book series has been specifically designed to provide a clear and concentrated review of important nursing knowledge in the following content areas:

- Child Health Nursing
- Maternal-Newborn Nursing
- Mental Health Nursing
- Medical-Surgical Nursing
- Pathophysiology
- Pharmacology
- Fundamentals and Skills
- Nutrition and Diet Therapy
- Fluids, Electrolytes, & Acid-Base Balance

The books in this series have been designed for use either by current nursing students as a study aid for nursing course work or NCLEX-RN licensing exam preparation, or by practicing nurses seeking a comprehensive yet concise review of a nursing specialty or subject area.

This series is truly unique. One of its most special features is that it has been authored by a large team of nurse educators from across the United States and Canada to ensure that each chapter is written by a nurse expert in the content area under study. Prentice Hall Health representatives from across North America submitted names of nurse educators and/or clinicians who excel in their respective fields, and these authors were then invited to write a chapter in one or more books. The consulting editor for each book, who is also an expert in that specialty area, then reviewed all chapters submitted for comprehensiveness and accuracy. The series editor designed the overall series in collaboration with a core Prentice Hall team to take full advantage of Prentice Hall's cutting edge technology, and also reviewed the chapters in each book.

All books in the series are identical in their overall design for the reader's ease and convenience (further details follow at the end of this section). As an added value, each book comes with a comprehensive support package, including free CD-ROM, free companion website access, and a Nursing Notes card for quick clinical reference.

STUDY TIPS

Use of this review book should help simplify your study. To make the most of your valuable study time, also follow these simple but important suggestions:

- Use a weekly calendar to schedule study sessions.
  - Outline the timeframes for all of your activities (home, school, appointments, etc.) on a weekly calendar.
  - Find the "holes" in your calendar, which are the times in which you can plan to study. Add study sessions to the calendar at times when you can expect to be mentally alert and follow it!
- Create the optimal study environment.
  - Eliminate external sources of distraction, such as television, telephone, etc.
  - Eliminate internal sources of distraction, such as hunger, thirst, or dwelling on items or problems that cannot be worked on at the moment.
  - Take a break for 10 minutes or so after each hour of concentrated study both as a reward and an incentive to keep studying.
- Use pre-reading strategies to increase comprehension of chapter material.
  - Skim the headings in the chapter (because they identify chapter content).
  - Read the definitions of key terms, which will help you learn new words to comprehend chapter information.
  - Review all graphic aids (figures, tables, boxes) because they are often used to explain important points in the chapter.
- Read the chapter thoroughly but at a reasonable speed.
  - Comprehension and retention are actually enhanced by not reading too slowly.
  - Do take the time to reread any section that is unclear to you.
- Summarize what you have learned.
  - Use questions supplied with this book, CD-ROM, and companion website to test your recall of chapter content.
  - Review again any sections that correspond to questions you answered incorrectly or incompletely.

TEST-TAKING STRATEGIES

Use the following strategies to increase your success on multiple-choice nursing tests or examinations:

- Get sufficient sleep and have something to eat before taking a test. Take deep breaths during the test as needed. Remember, the brain requires oxygen and glucose as fuel. Avoid concentrated sweets before a test, however, to avoid rapid upward and then downward surges in blood glucose levels.
- Read the question carefully, identifying the stem, the 4 options, and any key words or phrases in either the stem or options.
  - Key words in the stem such as "most important" indicate the need to set priorities, since more than 1 option is likely to contain a statement that is technically correct.
  - Remember that the presence of absolute words such as "never" or "only" in an answer option is more likely to make that option incorrect.
- Determine who is the client in the question; often this is the person with the health problem, but it may also be a significant other, relative, friend, or another nurse.

- Decide whether the stem is a true response stem or a false response stem. With a true response stem, the correct answer will be a true statement, and vice-versa.
- Determine what the question is really asking, sometimes referred to as the issue of the question. Evaluate all answer options in relation to this issue, and not strictly to the "correctness" of the statement in each individual option.
- Eliminate options that are obviously incorrect, then go back and reread the stem. Evaluate the remaining options against the stem once more.
- If two answers seem similar and correct, try to decide whether one of them is more global or comprehensive. If the global option includes the alternative option within it, it is likely that the more global response is the correct answer.

THE NCLEX-RN LICENSING EXAMINATION

The NCLEX-RN licensing examination is a Computer Adaptive Test (CAT) that ranges in length from 75 to 265 individual (stand-alone) test items, depending on individual performance during the examination. Upon graduation from a nursing program, successful completion of this exam is the gateway to your professional nursing practice. The blueprint for the exam is reviewed and revised every three years by the National Council of State Boards of Nursing according to the results of a job analysis study of new graduate nurses (practicing within the first six months after graduation). Each question on the exam is coded to one *Client Need Category* and one or more *Integrated Processes.*

Client Need Categories

There are 4 categories of client needs, and each exam will contain a minimum and maximum percent of questions from each category. Two categories have subcategories within them. The *Client Needs* categories according to the NCLEX-RN Test Plan effective April 1, 2004 are as follows:

- Safe, Effective Care Environment
  - Management of Care (13–19%)
  - Safety and Infection Control (8–14%)
- Health Promotion and Maintenance (6–12%)
- Psychosocial Integrity (6–12%)
- Physiological Integrity
  - Basic Care and Comfort (6–12%)
  - Pharmacological and Parenteral Therapies (13–19%)
  - Reduction of Risk Potential (13–19%)
  - Physiological Adaptation (11–17%)

Integrated Processes

The integrated processes identified on the NCLEX-RN Test Plan effective April 1, 2004, with condensed definitions, are as follows:

- Nursing Process: a scientific problem-solving approach used in nursing practice; consisting of assessment, analysis, planning, implementation, and evaluation.
- Caring: client-nurse interaction(s) characterized by mutual respect and trust and that are directed toward achieving desired client outcomes.
- Communication and Documentation: verbal and/or nonverbal interactions between nurse and others (client, family, health care team); a written or electronic recording of activities or events that occur during client care.
- Teaching/Learning: facilitating client's acquisition of knowledge, skills, and attitudes that lead to behavior change.

More detailed information about this examination may be obtained by visiting the National Council of State Boards of Nursing website at http://www.ncsbn.org and viewing the *NCLEX-RN Examination Test Plan for the National Council Licensure Examination for Registered Nurses*.

How to Get the Most Out of this Book

Chapter Organization

Each chapter has the following elements to guide you during review and study:

- Chapter Objectives: describe what you will be able to know or do after learning the material covered in the chapter.

Objectives

▮ Review basic principles of growth and development.

▮ Describe major physical expectations for each developmental age group.

▮ Identify developmental milestones for various age groups.

▮ Discuss the reactions to illness and hospitalization for children at various stages of development.

- Review at a Glance: contains a glossary of key terms used in the chapter, with definitions provided up-front and available at your fingertips, to help you stay focused and make the best use of your study time.

Review at a Glance

anticipatory guidance *the process of understanding upcoming developmental needs and then teaching caregivers to meet those needs*

cephalocaudal development *the process by which development proceeds from the head downward through the body and towards the feet*

chronological age *age in years*

critical periods *times when an individual is especially responsive to certain environmental effects, sometimes called sensitive periods*

development *an increase in capability or function; a more complex concept that*

is a continuous, orderly series of conditions that lead to activities, new motives for activities; and eventual patterns of behavior

developmental age *age based on functional behavior and ability to adapt to the environment; does not necessarily correspond to chronological age*

- Pretest: this 10-question multiple choice test provides a sample overview of content covered in the chapter and helps you decide what areas need the most—or the least—review.

Pretest

1 The nurse discusses dental care with the parents of a 3-year-old. The nurse explains that by the age of 3, their child should have:

(1) 5 "temporary" teeth.
(2) 10 "temporary" teeth.
(3) 15 "temporary" teeth.
(4) 20 "temporary" teeth.

2 The mother of a 6-month-old infant is concerned that the infant's anterior fontanel is still open. The nurse would inform the mother that further evaluation is needed if the anterior fontanel is open after:

(1) 6 months.
(2) 10 months.
(3) 18 months.
(4) 24 months.

- Practice to Pass questions: these are open-ended questions that stimulate critical thinking and reinforce mastery of the chapter content.

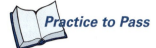

Practice to Pass

What would you explain as normal motor development for a 10-month old infant?

- NCLEX Alerts: the NCLEX icon identifies information or concepts that are likely to be tested on the NCLEX licensing examination. Be sure to learn the information flagged by this type of icon.

NCLEX!

- Case Study: found at the end of the chapter, it provides an opportunity for you to use your critical thinking and clinical reasoning skills to "put it all together;" it describes a true-to-life client case situation and asks you open-ended questions about how you would provide care for that client and/or family.

Case Study

> A 6-month-old female infant is brought into the pediatric clinic for a well-baby visit. You as the pediatric nurse will be assigned to care for this family.
>
> ❶ Identify the primary growth and development expectations for a 6-month-old.
>
> ❷ What type common behavior is expected of this 6-month-old towards the nurse?
>
> ❸ What immunization(s) are recommended at this age to maintain health and wellness?
>
> *For suggested responses, see page 406.*

- Posttest: a 10-question multiple-choice test at the end of the chapter provides new questions that are representative of chapter content, and provide you with feedback about mastery of that content following review and study. All pretest and posttest questions contain rationales for the correct answer, and are coded according to the phase of the nursing process used and the NCLEX category of client need (called the Test Plan). The Test plan codes are PHYS (Physiological Integrity), PSYC (Psychosocial Integrity), SECE (Safe Effective Care Environment), and HPM (Health Promotion and Maintenance).

Posttest

1   When using the otoscope to examine the ears of a 2-year-old child, the nurse should:

(1) Pull the pinna up and back.
(2) Pull the pinna down and back.
(3) Hold the pinna gently but firmly in its normal position.
(4) Hold the pinna against the skull.

2   To assess the height of an 18-month-old child who is brought to the clinic for routine examination, the nurse should:

(1) Measure arm span to estimate adult height.
(2) Use a tape measure.
(3) Use a horizontal measuring board.
(4) Have the child stand on an upright scale and use the measuring arm.

CD-ROM

For those who want to practice taking tests on a computer, the CD-ROM that accompanies the book contains the pretest and posttest questions found in all chapters of the book. In addition, it contains 10 NEW questions for each chapter to help you further evaluate your knowledge base and hone your test-taking skills. In several chapters, one of the questions will have imbedded art to use in answering the question. Some of the newly developed NCLEX test items are also designed in this way, so these items will give you valuable practice with this type of question.

Companion Website (CW)

The companion website is a "virtual" reference for virtually all your needs! The CW contains the following:

- 50 NCLEX-style questions: 10 pretest, 10 posttest, 10 CD-ROM, and 20 additional new questions
- Definitions of key terms: the glossary is also stored on the companion website for ease of reference
- In Depth With NCLEX: features art drawings or photos that are each accompanied by a one- to two-paragraph explanation. These are especially useful when describing something that is complex, technical (such as equipment), or difficult to mentally visualize.
- Suggested Answers to Practice to Pass and Case Study Questions: easily located on the website, these allow for timely feedback for those who answer chapter questions on the web.

Nursing Notes Clinical Reference Card

This laminated card provides a reference for frequently used facts and information related to the subject matter of the book. These are designed to be useful in the clinical setting, when quick and easy access to information is so important!

ABOUT THE PHARMACOLOGY BOOK

Chapters in this book cover "need-to-know" information about medications that belong to a wide variety of drug classes and associated nursing management. The first chapter reviews general principles of pharmacology with an emphasis on safety. Chapters 2 through 15 explore drug classes used to treat health problems that affect specific body systems. The final chapter explores the use of herbal agents as supplements and phytomedicines. Mastery of the information in this book and effective use of the test-taking strategies described will help the student be confident and successful in testing situations, including the NCLEX-RN, and in actual clinical practice.

Pharmacology is an ever-evolving field because drug therapy changes over time as new research evidence becomes available. Care has been taken to ensure that drug information in this book is accurate and current; however, this is a condensed review book, not a full pharmacology textbook or official drug reference. Before administering any medication, the reader should check the manufacturer's product literature to verify recommended dose, route, duration of therapy, and any contraindications. Neither the publisher nor the author assumes liability for any injury or damage arising from information contained in this condensed review book.

ACKNOWLEDGMENTS

This book is a monumental effort of collaboration. Without the contributions of many individuals, this first edition of *Pharmacology: Reviews and Rationales* would not have been possible. A grateful acknowledgement goes to all the contributors who devoted their time and talents to this book. Their chapters will surely assist both students and practicing nurses alike to extend their knowledge in the area of pharmacology. A special acknowledgement also goes to Mitra Sahebazemani, RN, BSN, who assisted me with the formatting and editing of a number of tables in this book. Your time, talents, and efforts are sure to benefit the readers of this book.

I owe a special debt of gratitude to the wonderful team at Prentice Hall Health for their enthusiasm for this project, as well as their good humor, expertise, and encouragement as the series developed. Maura Connor, Editor-in-Chief for Nursing books, was unending in her creativity, support, encouragement, and belief in the need for this series. Marilyn Meserve, Executive Development Editor for Nursing, devoted many long hours to coordinating different facets of this project, and tirelessly and cheerfully provided encouragement as well. Her high standards and attention to detail contributed greatly to the final "look" of this series. Jeanne Allison, Developmental Editor, actively kept in communication with the different writers in this book. Editorial assistant Bonnie Bennett-Walker helped to keep the project moving forward, and I am grateful for her efforts as well. A very special thank you goes to the designers of the book and the production team, led by Danielle Newhouse, who brought the ideas and manuscript into final form.

Thank you to the team at Pine Tree Composition, led by Project Coordinator Jessica Balch, for the detail-oriented work of creating this book. I greatly appreciate their hard work, attention to detail, and spirit of collaboration. Special thanks also go to Carlos Cooper, Lisa Donovan and staff at the Pearson Education Development Group for designing and producing the *Nursing Notes* clinical reference card that accompanies this book.

I would like to acknowledge and thank my husband Michael, and children Mike Jr., Katie, Kristen, and Billy, who sacrificed hours of time that would have been spent with them, to bring this book to publication. Your love and support kept me energized, motivated, and at times, even sane. I love you all! Finally, I would like to thank Patricia Miller, Director of the former Baystate Medical Center School of Nursing, who freely took the time and effort to mentor me during my early years in nursing education.

---

*Reference: National Council of State Boards of Nursing, Inc. *NCLEX Examination Test Plan for National Council Licensure Examination for Registered Nurses*. Effective April 1, 2004. Retrieved from the World Wide Web January 30, 2004 at http://www.ncsbn.org/public/resources/res/NCSBNRNTestPlan Booklet.pdf.

Reviewers

Skip Davis, PhD, MSN, BSN
Assistant Professor
San Francisco State University
San Francisco, California

Pattie Garrett Clark, RN, MSN
Associate Professor and Nursing Outreach
    Coordinator
Abraham Bladwin College
Tifton, Georgia

Janice Hausauer, MSN, BSN, ANCC-FNP
Adjunct Assistant Professor
Montana State University, Bozeman
Bozeman, Montana

Mercy Popoola, RN, CND, PhD
Assistant Professor
Georgia Southern University
Statesboro, Georgia

Anita K. Reed, BSN, MSN
Lecturer in Nursing
St. Joseph College
Rensselaer, Indiana

Contributors

Julie Adkins, RN, MSN, APRN-BC
Family Nurse Practitioner
West Frankfort, Illinois
Chapters 7 and *12*

Carolyn M. Burger, MSN, RN,C, OCN
Assistant Professor
Miami University
Middletown, Ohio
Chapter 2

Janet Courtney, RN, MSN
Professor, Department of Nursing
Holyoke Community College
Holyoke, Massachusetts
Chapter 1

Joseann Helmes DeWitt, RN, MSN, C, CLNC
Assistant Professor of Nursing
Department of Baccalaureate Nursing
Alcorn State University
Natchez, Mississippi
Chapter 15

Suzanne Kay Marnocha
Assistant Professor of Nursing
University of Wisconsin, Oshkosh
Oshkosh, Wisconsin
Chapter 5

Caron Martin, MSN, RN
Assistant Professor of Nursing
Northern Kentucky University
Highland Heights, Kentucky
Chapter 14

Lee Murray, MSN, RN, CS, CADAC
Assistant Professor of Nursing
Holyoke Community College
Holyoke, Massachusetts
Chapter 11

Lynn Wemett Nicholls, RN, MSN
Chapter 9

Donna Polverini, RN, MS
Assistant Professor
America International College
Springfield, Massachusetts
Chapter 16

Roni Ruhlandt, MSN, RN, CCRN, CNRN
Campus College Chair
College of Health Sciences and Nursing
University of Phoenix, Grand Rapids Campus
Grand Rapids, Michigan
Chapter 10

Susan K. Steele, MN, DNS, AOCN
Clinical Nurse Specialist: General Health
    System
Clinical Instructor: Southeastern Louisiana
    University College of Nursing
Chapter 3

Bethany Hawes Sykes, EdD, RN CEN
Assistant Professor, Department of Nursing
Salve Regina University
Newport, Rhode Island
Chapter 6

Geralyn M. Valleroy-Frandsen, Ed D, MSN, RN
Associate Professor of Nursing
Maryville University
St. Louis, Missouri
Chapter 8

Daryle Wane, MS, APRN, BC
Assistant Professor of Nursing
Pasco-Hernando Community College
New Port Richey, Florida
Chapter 4

Student Consultants

Alisa Beaulieu
Santa Fe Community College
Gainesville, Florida

Alison Cody
Germanna Community College
Locust Grove, Virginia

Daniel Dale
Valdosta State University
Valdosta, Georgia

Stephanie Hornby
George Mason University
Fairfax, Virgina

Amy Jeter
Ohio University-Chillicothe
Chillicothe, Ohio

Joan Lawrence
Auburn University
Auburn, Alabama

Lisa Marie Mays
Boise State University
Boise, Idaho

Shawn Shaughnessy
Santa Fe Community College
Gainesville, Florida

Phyllis Thieken
Ohio University-Chillicothe
Chillicothe, Ohio

Jenefer Thomas
Boise State University
Boise, Idaho

Gyleen Vickerman
Boise State University
Boise, Idaho

Carolyn Wilkinson
Auburn University
Auburn, Alabama

A Guide To
Prentice Hall's Reviews and Rationales Series

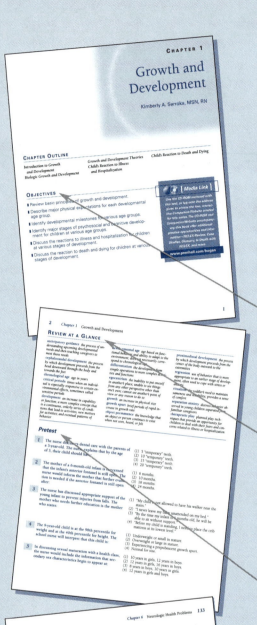

Each chapter has the following **feature elements** to guide you during review and study.

Chapter **Objectives** describe what you will be able to know or do after learning the material covered in the chapter.

Review at a Glance contains a glossary of key terms used in the chapter, with definitions provided up-front and available at your fingertips, to help you stay focused and make the best use of your study time.

The **Pretest** is a 10-question multiple choice test providing a sample overview of content covered in the chapter and helps you decide what areas need the most – or the least – review.

The **Practice to Pass** questions are open-ended questions that stimulate critical thinking and reinforce mastery of the chapter content.

NCLEX The NCLEX icon identifies information or concepts that are likely to be tested on the NCLEX licensing examination.

A detailed **Outline Review** of core content is given to provide both a comprehensive overview and review.

The **Case Study**, found at the end of the chapter, provides an opportunity for you to use your critical thinking and clinical reasoning skills to "put it all together." It describes a true-to-life client case situation and asks you open-ended questions about how you would provide care for that client and/or family.

The **Posttest** is a 10-question multiple-choice test at the end of the chapter providing new questions that are representative of chapter content. This posttest provides you with feedback about mastery of that content following review and study.

Answers and Rationales For all questions, answers and rationales for each correct answer are provided.

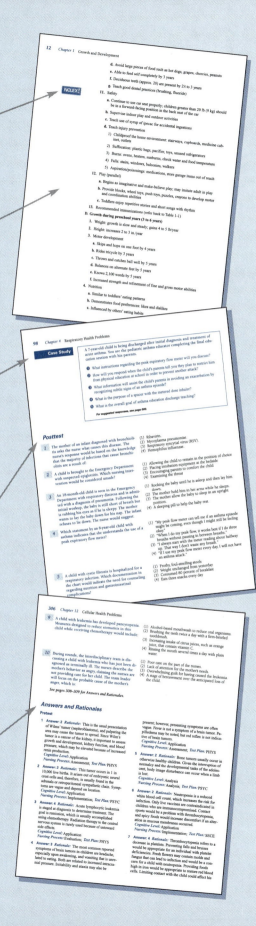

CHAPTER 1

Safety and Pharmacology

Janet Courtney, RN, MSN

CHAPTER OUTLINE

*Pharmacology and the Nursing
  Process*
Legal Regulation

*Prescription and Nonprescription
  Medications*
Medication Classification Systems

Terminology Related to Pharmacology
*Issues Related to Medication
  Administration*

OBJECTIVES

▮ Describe legal regulatory issues related to medication administration.

▮ Identify the difference between generic and trade names.

▮ Identify differences between prescription and over-the-counter medications.

▮ Define terms commonly used in pharmacology.

▮ Describe differences between a side effect and an adverse or toxic effect of a medication.

▮ Describe factors that affect medication absorption and response.

▮ List the six rights of medication administration.

▮ Calculate medication dosages accurately.

▮ Describe nurses' roles and responsibilities related to client education regarding medication therapy.

▮ Discuss cultural considerations related to client education regarding medication therapy.

 [Media Link]

Use the CD-ROM enclosed with this text, or log onto the address given to access the free, interactive Companion Website created for this series. The CD-ROM and Companion Website accompanying this book offer additional practice opportunities and information—NCLEX Review, Case Studies, Glossary, In Depth with NCLEX, and more.

www.prenhall.com/hogan

REVIEW AT A GLANCE

absorption *what happens to a drug from the time it is introduced into the body until it reaches the circulating fluids and tissues*

critical concentration *the amount of a drug needed to cause a therapeutic effect*

distribution *movement of a drug to the body's tissues*

drug *chemical that is introduced into the body to cause some sort of change; used interchangeably with the term medication*

drug abuse *use of a drug in a fashion inconsistent with medical or social norms*

drug metabolism *also known as biotransformation, is the enzymatic alteration of drug structure; most drug metabolism takes place in the liver*

excretion *removal of the drug from the body, such as via the skin, saliva, lungs, bile, kidneys, and feces*

first-pass effect *a phenomenon that occurs following ingestion of an oral drug, in which a large percentage of the drug is destroyed in the gastrointestinal system and never reaches the tissues*

half-life *the time it takes for the amount of drug in the body to decrease to one-half of the peak level it previously achieved*

negligence *failure to provide care that a reasonable person would use in a similar circumstance*

pharmacodynamics *how a drug affects the body*

pharmacokinetics *how the body acts on a drug*

pharmacology *the study of drugs and their interactions with living systems*

pharmacotherapeutics *also known as clinical pharmacology; the branch of pharmacology that involves the use of drugs to treat, prevent or diagnose disease*

selective toxicity *the ability of a drug, such as penicillin, to attack only those systems found in foreign cells*

Pretest

1 When the nurse is administering medication to a hospitalized client, which of the following is the most accurate way to assure that the right patient gets the medication?

(1) Ask the client, "Are you Dale Jones?"
(2) Check the client's identification band.
(3) Check the client's room number and bed assignment.
(4) Ask the client why he or she is getting the medication.

2 The mother of the pediatric client asks the nurse, "What's the difference between Advil and ibuprofen? I can buy ibuprofen at a cheaper price, but the instructions from the clinic says to use Children's Advil Liquid." The nurse responds to this question using which of the following statements?"

(1) "The instructions from the clinic should be followed exactly without substitutions."
(2) "There is no difference between Advil and ibuprofen."
(3) "Advil and ibuprofen are two different drugs with similar effects."
(4) "This question should be referred to the prescribing physician."

3 A pregnant client takes an over-the-counter (OTC) iron preparation. Drug data lists the drug as Pregnancy Category A. The nurse teaches the client which of the following pieces of information?

(1) To stop the medication during pregnancy
(2) To immediately report to the physician that she has taken the drug while pregnant
(3) That this medication is classified as safe to use during pregnancy
(4) There may be staining of the baby's first teeth from this medication

4 The client taking diltiazem hydrochloride (Cardizem) 30 mg PO qid is experiencing symptoms of toxicity of this calcium channel blocker medication. Which of the following assessments will be of highest priority for the nurse to make to assist in this situation?

(1) The client's body temperature, looking for elevation
(2) The rate, depth, and regularity of the client's respirations
(3) The client's daily weight, looking for weight loss
(4) The client's dietary intake of grapefruit juice

5 In addition to less efficient renal excretion, what other physical change in aging may lead to a need to reduce medication dosage in an elderly client?

(1) Increased rate of drug absorption
(2) Decreased total body fluid proportionate to body mass
(3) Decreased efficiency in drug distribution
(4) Increased rate of drug metabolism by the liver

6 A 3-year-old client weighing 33 pounds is to receive liquid Advil (ibuprofen) 150 mg PO q6 hrs prn for temperature above 101°F. How much drug will the nurse plan to give the client from a bottle labeled 100 mg/5 mL?

(1) 1 teaspoon
(2) 5 mL
(3) 7.5 mL
(4) The answer cannot be calculated from the data given

7 A client receiving nadolol (Corgard) for hypertension tells the nurse, "I get dizzy when I stand up." Which of the following is the most appropriate response by the nurse?

(1) "This is an expected side effect of the drug, and you should use caution and move slowly when standing up."
(2) "You may be experiencing a toxic effect of the drug, and I will notify the physician."
(3) "Dizziness is not related to the drug, but I will need to ask you a few more questions."
(4) "Episodes of dizziness when moving are common symptoms of high blood pressure."

8 An elderly client is given a prescription for celecoxib (Celebrex) for pain and stiffness of osteoarthritis of the hips and back. Which of the following is the best first step in teaching the client about the newly ordered drug?

(1) Doing a thorough medication assessment to see what other drugs the client is taking
(2) Giving the client a printed pamphlet describing the new drug
(3) Telling the client where a medication organizer can be purchased
(4) Giving a short, simple verbal explanation about the drug and its effects

9 The medication administration record shows that the client is to receive lisinopril (Zestril) 10 mg PO at 9:00 A.M. The client's drug supply has tablets labeled fosinopril (Monopril) 20 mg. Which action by the nurse ensures that the right drug and the right dose are administered?

(1) Give one tablet of Monopril from the drug supply.
(2) Given one-half tablet of Monopril from the drug supply.
(3) Ask the client if the 20 mg tablet looks familiar.
(4) Read the original physician order to verify the drug order.

10 The nurse is planning to instruct a Hispanic American client about the drug regimen prescribed for newly diagnosed hypertension. When developing the plan, the nurse is aware that individuals from this ethnic group may exhibit which of the following tendencies?

(1) Live in an extended family setting in which men are the decision makers
(2) Value education in all forms
(3) Prefer using written materials as a way of learning
(4) Dislike using medication to treat health problems

See pages 21–22 for Answers and Rationales.

I. Pharmacology and the Nursing Process

A. Assessment

1. Medication order

2. Client's history of allergies

3. Client's current condition

4. Purpose for the medication prescription

5. Client's understanding of the purpose of the medication

6. Need for conversion when preparing a dose of medication

B. Analysis/nursing diagnosis

1. Risk for injury

   a. Can occur if the client takes a medication that he or she is hypersensitive (allergic) to

   b. Can occur if the medication is taken incorrectly

      1) An insufficient dose will lead to development of signs and symptoms of original disorder

      2) An excessive dose can lead to signs and symptoms of toxicity or other adverse effects

2. Knowledge deficit

   a. Is often pertinent when a client is given a prescription for a new medication

   b. Should also be assessed with each client encounter to ensure ongoing knowledge

   c. Insufficient knowledge of medication therapy may lead to suboptimal results of therapy or other complications

C. Planning/goal setting

1. Client will remain free of injury

2. Client will verbalize purpose of medication

3. Client will respond appropriately to the medication

D. Implementation

1. Review medication order for completeness and accuracy

2. Determine client history of allergies

3. Review client's condition for which medication is ordered

4. Measure client's vital signs if indicated

5. Determine the need for conversion when calculating correct dose of medication

6. Prepare and administer the medication dose correctly

7. Determine client's understanding regarding the prescribed medication

8. Teach client about medication, including name, dose, route, frequency, purpose, any follow-up lab work, and side/adverse effects including when to notify prescriber

9. Document the administration of the medication and client's response to therapy

E. Evaluation

1. Client receives correct medication and dosage

2. Client's vital signs remain within normal limits

3. Client responds appropriately to medication; effectiveness is achieved

4. Client does not experience adverse effects of medication

II. Legal Regulation

A. Food and Drug Administration (FDA)

1. An agency of the United States Department of Health and Human Services (USDHHS) that regulates the development and sale of **drugs** (chemicals that exert an effect on the body) to assure safety and efficacy

2. Controls the process of scientific testing to evaluate therapeutic and toxic effects of a chemical that may potentially become a drug/medication

3. Phases of drug development

   a. A drug must pass through several stages of development before receiving final FDA approval to be marketed to the public

   b. Stages of development include Preclinical trials, Phase I studies, Phase II studies, Phase III studies, FDA approval, Phase IV studies (Box 1-1)

B. Controlled substances

1. Are substances that are considered to have potential for **drug abuse,** use of the substance in a manner inconsistent with medical or social norms

2. The Controlled Substance Act of 1970 regulates the manufacturing, distribution, and dispensing of drugs that are known to have abuse potential

3. The FDA studies a drug and determines its abuse potential

4. The Drug Enforcement Agency (DEA), a part of the Department of Justice, enforces the control of a drug

5. The DEA monitors the prescription, distribution, storage, and use of a controlled substance in an attempt to decrease substance abuse of prescribed medications

6. Controlled substances are assigned to one of five DEA schedules based on their potential for abuse and physical and psychological dependence (Box 1-2 and Box 1-3)

C. Pregnancy categories (Box 1-4, p. 7)

1. Are guidelines for the use of a particular drug during pregnancy

2. Indicate a drug's potential or actual teratogenic or adverse effects on the fetus

---

Box 1-1	
Phases of Drug Development	***Preclinical Trials:*** Testing on laboratory animals is done to determine whether the drug has the presumed effect in living tissue and to evaluate any adverse effects. ***Phase I Studies:*** A tightly controlled study is conducted that involves the use of healthy human volunteers to test the drug. ***Phase II Studies:*** The drug is administered to clients who have the disease that the drug was intended to treat. ***Phase III Studies:*** The drug is used in the clinical setting to determine any unanticipated effects or lack of effectiveness. ***Food and Drug Administration (FDA) Approval:*** Drugs that complete Phase III are evaluated by the FDA and if FDA approval is received, the drug may be marketed. ***Phase IV Study:*** A phase that involves continual evaluation of the drug following approval for marketing.

Box 1-2

DEA Schedules of Controlled Substances

Schedule I: High abuse potential and no accepted medical use
Schedule II: High abuse potential with severe dependence liability
Schedule III: Less abuse potential than Schedule II drugs and moderate dependence liability
Schedule IV: Less abuse potential than Schedule III drugs and limited dependence liability
Schedule V: Limited abuse potential

NCLEX!

3. The FDA requires that each new drug be assigned a pregnancy category

4. The FDA recommends that no drug be administered during pregnancy regardless of the pregnancy category, unless the benefit of the drug clearly outweighs the risks of use

D. Investigational medications and informed consent

NCLEX!

1. *Informed consent:* an autonomous decision made by a specific individual based on the nature of the condition, the treatment options, and the risks involved

2. The client must be competent to give consent for procedures and treatment

3. Informed consent should be in writing; it should include explanation of procedure, medication, or treatment, description of benefits and harmful results, and an opportunity for client to ask questions

4. Information should be written in language understandable to the client

5. Consent must be obtained by the medical practitioner ordering the medication, treatment, or procedure

NCLEX!

6. The nurse administering the medication explains the purpose of the drug and answers questions the client may have

7. A client has the right to decline information and waive the informed consent and undergo treatment; this decision must be documented in the medical record

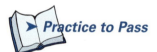

▶ Practice to Pass

A pregnant client experiences occasional headaches and backaches. She asks you what over-the-counter (OTC) medication she can take to relieve these discomforts. How will you respond?

8. During urgent medical or surgical intervention, such as severe bleeding, fractured skull, gunshot or stab wounds, an informed consent can be waived

9. When the client is a minor, unconscious, or incompetent, consent must be obtained from a responsible family member or legal guardian

10. When a nurse is involved in the informed consent process, in most states the nurse is only responsible for witnessing the signature of the client on the informed consent form

11. The most common concern in the use of investigational drugs is that all adverse effects have not been identified; the client is not able to be fully informed about these; therefore, the decision-making process is not ideal

Box 1-3

Examples of Controlled Substances by DEA Schedule

Schedule I: Heroine, marijuana, cocaine
Schedule II: Narcotics, amphetamines, barbiturates
Schedule III: Nonbarbiturate sedatives, nonamphetamine stimulants, limited amounts of certain narcotics
Schedule IV: Some sedatives, nonnarcotic analgesics, antianxiety agents
Schedule V: Drugs that may contain small amounts of narcotics such as codeine, used as antitussives or antidiarrheals

Category A: Adequate studies in pregnant women have not demonstrated a risk to the fetus in the first trimester of pregnancy, and there is no evidence of risk in later trimesters.

Category B: Animal studies have not demonstrated a risk to the fetus but there are no adequate studies in pregnant women. Or, animal studies have shown an adverse effect, but adequate studies in pregnant women have not demonstrated a risk to the fetus during the first trimester of pregnancy, and there is no evidence of risk in later trimesters.

Category C: Animal studies have shown an adverse effect on the fetus but there are no adequate studies in humans; the benefit from the use of the drug in pregnancy may be acceptable despite its potential risks. Or, there are no animal reproduction studies and no adequate studies in humans.

Category D: There is evidence of human fetal risk, but the potential benefits from the use of the drug in pregnant women may be acceptable despite its potential risks.

Category X: Studies in animals or humans demonstrate fetal abnormalities or adverse reactions and reports indicate evidence of fetal risk. The risk of use in a pregnant woman clearly outweighs any possible benefits.

E. Regulation of nursing practice related to medication therapy

1. Nurse Practice Act

    a. Is a series of statutes enacted by each state legislature to regulate the practice of health care providers including nurses in that state

    b. The Nurse Practice Act describes the role of the nurse in relation to medication administration

    c. Advanced practice nurses may have prescriptive privileges; check individual state statute to determine laws governing prescriptive authority in that state

2. Standards of care

    a. Some standards of care are global guidelines by which the nurse should practice, without a specific focus on medication therapy

    b. Other standards of care may be based on research of specific health problems and include recommendations for care including medication therapy

    c. An example is the stepped-care approach to treating hypertension; medication therapy is recommended in specific sequences based on client response

3. Professional misconduct: a violation of the Nurse Practice Act that can result in disciplinary action against a nurse; examples of professional misconduct are failing to wear an identification badge or sharing client's personal information with others without the client's consent; medication therapy as part of the plan of care can be construed to be personal information

4. Disciplinary action: denying or suspending any license to practice by boards of nursing because of unprofessional conduct; nurses who are involved in drug diversion are subject to disciplinary action

5. Malpractice: a form of **negligence** or professional misconduct; includes actions that are bad, wrong, or injudicious in the professional care of the client that result in injury, unnecessary suffering, or death to the client (such as a serious medication error); this may also occur through omission of a necessary act, that is, failure to give an ordered medication

F. Legal liability

1. The administration of medications by the nurse includes several aspects of legal liability

2. A legal order from a health care provider with prescription-writing authority, usually a physician, begins the process of medication delivery to a client; see Box 1-5 for a list of elements of a complete drug order

3. Nurses are responsible for their actions even when there is a written medication order

    NCLEX!

    a. If a drug order is incorrect, either the dose is inaccurate or the drug ordered is not indicated for the client's health condition, the nurse who administers the drug is liable for the error along with the prescriber

    b. The nurse must question any order that appears inappropriate and can refuse to give the drug until the order is clarified

4. Nurses, along with physicians and pharmacists, participate in the system to maintain medication safety that is used in the agency

    NCLEX!

    a. One important feature of such a system is the recording of allergy to medications that a client reports

    b. The nurse is the "last stop" in the system and has a crucial role in ensuring accuracy in medication administration

    c. The use of, storage, dispensing of, and documentation for drugs that are controlled substances is a highly regulated part of the medication administration system in a health care agency

5. The nurse acts to ensure that the *right client* receives the *right medication* in the *right dose* via the *right route* at the *right time;* the nurse then completes the *right documentation* (the time of medication administration and documents client's responses to the medication)

6. The nurse is responsible for assessing the client's condition in relation to the use of the ordered medication, the client's response to the medication, including any expected or unexpected responses to the medication

    NCLEX!

7. The nurse must have knowledge of the effects and potential effects of every drug that is given to a client

8. The nurse takes measures to protect the client from any safety hazards that may be expected from a medication's effects; this may include measures to protect the client from falling if the medication has a sedative effect

---

Box 1-5	The following points should be included in a complete drug order:
Elements of a Drug Order	• Full name of the client
	• Date and time the drug order is written
	• Name of the drug to be given to the client
	• Dosage of the drug
	• Frequency of drug administration
	• Route of drug administration
	• Signature of person writing the order

9. Professional liability insurance: nurses need their own liability insurance for protection against malpractice lawsuits, including those involving medication errors

III. Prescription and Nonprescription Medications

A. Generic, chemical, and trade names

1. Generic name: the original designation that is given to the drug when the drug company applies for the approval process; each drug has only one generic name such as acetaminophen

2. Chemical name: names that reflect the chemical structure of the drug; this is often long and complex; is of use to pharmacists and researchers

3. Trade name: also known as brand name, a name given to an approved drug by the pharmaceutical company that developed it; the number of trade names that a drug can have is large; for instance, acetaminophen has 31 trade names including Tylenol

B. Nonprescription or over-the-counter (OTC) medications

1. Are products that are available without a prescription for self-treatment of a variety of complaints

2. The regulation and evaluation of OTC drugs is under FDA supervision

3. Advantages of using OTC medications include reduced health care costs, less time lost from work, less travel, and fewer side effects

4. Potential problems with OTC drug use include improper use, lack of counseling, labeling concerns, and possible delay in obtaining needed treatment

IV. Medication Classification Systems

A. Two possible approaches

1. Medications with similar characteristics might be classified together based on clinical indication; an example is analgesic medications, which relieve pain

2. Medications can also be grouped together by the body system upon which they act; an example is central nervous system medications

B. Benefits of a classification system

1. Knowledge of a drug's classification helps the nurse to understand intended effects and common side effects of the medication being administered

2. It also assists the nurse to organize knowledge of thousands of drugs that are used for a wide variety of therapeutic indications

V. Terminology Related to Pharmacology

A. Critical concentration: the amount of a drug needed to cause a therapeutic effect

B. Distribution: the transport of a drug in body fluids from the bloodstream to various tissues of the body and then to its site of action

C. Drug: any substance used in the diagnosis, treatment, or prevention of a disease or condition; this term is used interchangeably with the word medication

D. First-pass effect: a phenomenon that occurs following ingestion of an oral drug, in which a large percentage of the drug is inactivated in the liver after being absorbed from the GI tract as the drug is carried from the GI circulation through the hepatic portal circulation; this explains why oral medication doses need to be larger than parenteral doses

E. **Half-life:** the time required to reduce to one-half that amount of unchanged drug that is in the body at the time equilibrium is established

F. **Pharmacodynamics:** what drugs do to the body and how drugs interact with body tissue

G. **Pharmacokinetics:** what the body does to a drug or how a drug is altered as it travels through the body

H. **Pharmacology:** the study of drugs and their interactions with living systems

I. **Pharmacotherapeutics:** also known as clinical pharmacology; the branch of pharmacology that involves using drugs to treat, prevent, or diagnose disease

J. **Selective toxicity:** the ability of a drug, such as penicillin, to attack only those systems found in foreign cells

VI. Issues Related to Medication Administration

A. **The six rights:** right medication, right dose, right client, right route, right time, and (recently) right documentation

B. **Factors affecting absorption and response**

1. **Absorption:** the movement of a drug from its site of administration into the blood

2. Physiological factors affecting drug absorption

   a. Weight: the recommended dosage of a drug is based on drug evaluation studies and is targeted at a 150-lb individual

   b. Age: a factor to be considered primarily in children and older adults

   c. Gender: males have more vascular muscles than a female; therefore, the effects of an intramuscular (IM) injection will be noted sooner in a male than in a female; females have more fat cells than males; therefore, drugs that deposit in fat may be slowly released in the female and cause effects for a more prolonged period of time than for males

3. Chemical and physical factors affecting drug absorption

   a. Lipid solubility: highly soluble drugs are absorbed more rapidly than drugs whose lipid solubility is low

   b. pH partitioning: the difference between the pH of plasma and the pH at the site of administration is such that drug molecules will have a greater tendency to be ionized in the plasma

   c. Range of dissolution: the faster the dissolution of medication, the more rapid the onset of drug absorption will be

   d. Blood flow: medications are absorbed most rapidly from sites where blood flow is high

   e. Routes of administration: the barriers to absorption associated with each route are different, so the patterns of absorption differ between routes

C. Unintended responses to drugs

1. Side effect: unavoidable secondary drug effect produced at therapeutic doses, e.g., gastric irritation caused by aspirin

NCLEX!

2. Adverse drug reaction: undesired response to a drug; may range from mild to life-threatening

    a. Toxicity: an adverse drug reaction caused by excessive dosing, e.g., coma from an overdose of morphine; some drugs have a small therapeutic index, that is, the dose required to produce a therapeutic effect is close to the toxic dose of that drug

    b. Allergic reaction: an adverse physiological reaction of immunologic origin; in order for an allergic reaction to occur there should be prior sensitization of the immune system; the drug dosage has no effect on the intensity of allergic reactions

    c. Idiosyncratic effect: an adverse drug reaction based on a client's genetic predisposition

3. Iatrogenic disease: a drug- or physician-induced disease

4. Teratogenic effect: a drug-induced birth defect

5. Carcinogenic effect: ability of a drug to cause cancer

D. Medications and children

1. Children metabolize drugs differently than adults in that they metabolize medications faster than adults

NCLEX!

2. Children have immature body systems for handling drugs

    a. Drug responses may be unusually intense and prolonged

    b. Absorption of intramuscular (IM) medications in neonates is slower than in adults; Figure 1-1 shows the vastus lateralis site for IM injection for a newborn and children up to three years of age

    c. Absorption of IM medications in infants is more rapid than in adults

Figure 1-1

The vastus lateralis muscle is used for IM injections in newborns, infants, and children up to 3 years of age.

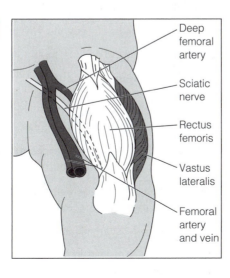

Deep femoral artery

Sciatic nerve

Rectus femoris

Vastus lateralis

Femoral artery and vein

d. Neonates are more sensitive to medications that affect the central nervous system (CNS) because the blood-brain barrier is not fully developed

e. In neonates, the medication metabolizing capacity of neonates is low

f. Renal **excretion** (a process whereby drugs and pharmacologically active or inactive metabolites are eliminated from the body) of medications is low in neonates

g. Most pharmacokinetic parameters in children 1 year and older are similar to those in adults

E. Medications and older adults

1. Older adults undergo physical changes as part of the aging process that affect the response to a drug that is administered

2. Altered response may be due to less effective absorption, less efficient **distribution** (the transport of a drug in body fluids from the bloodstream to various tissues of the body and then to its site of action), less efficient perfusion, altered metabolism, and less efficient excretion

3. The rate of drug absorption may be slowed in the elderly

4. Concentrations of water-soluble drugs may be high, and concentrations of lipid-soluble drugs may be low in the elderly

5. Reduced liver and/or renal function may prolong medications effects; this is because with reduced metabolism and/or excretion of a drug, the drug may work for a prolonged amount of time or toxic effects may become apparent

6. Adverse drug reactions are more common in the elderly than in younger adults

7. Noncompliance is more common among the elderly; the factors contributing to noncompliance include low income, forgetfulness, complex regimens, side effects, failure to follow instructions, inability to obtain medications

F. Calculating medication dosages

1. Calculation of medication dosage by body weight

   a. 1 kg = 2.2 lb

   b. To convert from pounds to kilograms, divide by 2.2

      • Example: a client weighs 154 pounds: $154 \div 2.2$ = the client weighs 70 kg

   c. To convert from kilograms to pounds, multiply by 2.2

      • Example: a client weighs 20 kg: 20×2.2 = the client weighs 44 lb

2. Calculating daily dosages

   a. Dosages are expressed in terms of mg/kg/day, or mg/lb/day

      • Example: the drug vancomycin (Vancocin) can be given to the pediatric client with pseudomembranous colitis in doses up to 40 mg/kg/day

      • The pediatric client above who weighs 20 kg (44 lb) can receive 40 mg $\times$ 20 kg/day; 40 mg $\times$ 20 kg = 800 mg/day in 3 to 4 divided doses

   b. The total daily dosage is usually administered in divided doses per day

      • Example: from above drug order for vancomycin: $800 \text{ mg} \div 4 = 200 \text{ mg}$ each dose; this dose is within the recommended range for this client

NCLEX!

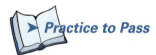

Practice to Pass

A client with chronic renal failure is taking medications to control hypertension and other health problems. What are the priority nursing considerations for this client in relation to the drug regimen?

c. The nurse is responsible for verifying that the drug order is within the recommended dosage range; if it is not, the order should be questioned and clarified

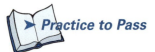

3. Intravenous fluid calculations

   a. First step: determine how many milliliters per hour (volume) needs to be given; this may be part of the original order or it may need to be calculated when the total volume and hours are given

      • Example: the physician orders 1000 mL IV solution to be given over 8 hours

      • $1000 \div 8 = 125$ mL per hour

   b. Second step: calculate the drops per minute; when the mL/hr is given, calculate the gtts/min

      • Example: the client's IV set delivers 10 gtt/mL;

      • 125 mL $\times 10$ gtts/mL $\div 60$ minutes $= 20.83$ gtts/min

      • Since a fractional drop cannot be counted, the nurse will set the IV drip rate at 21 gtts/min after rounding the decimal up or down appropriately

   c. The drop factor is the number of drops in 1 mL; drop factors of 10, 15, and 60 are the most common (the drop factor is determined by the manufacturer and is found on the IV tubing box)

G. Common routes of medication administration

   1. See Table 1-1 for a detailed description of routes for administering medications

   2. Enteral (via the GI tract): including oral administration as well as administration via a GI feeding tube; classic routes include the following

      a. PO: typical oral administration

      b. SL: sublingual, under the tongue

      c. Buccal: between the cheek and gum

      d. Via feeding tube

   3. Parenteral

      a. Intravenous (IV): through an IV catheter into a vein; is the fastest acting route

      b. Subcutaneous (SC): Figure 1-2 illustrates the angle of insertion for SC injections; typical volume is 0.5 to 1.0 mL per injection but should not exceed 1.5 mL; needle gauge is 25 to 29 and a 3/8- to 5/8-inch needle should be used

      c. Intramuscular (IM): Figure 1-3 illustrates the angle of insertion for IM injections using the Z-track method; total volume varies by age and injection site, commonly 1 to 2 mL in adults and 0.5 to 1 mL in children; needle size varies by age, commonly 21- to 23-gauge and 1 to 1.5 inches long

      d. Intradermal (ID): used for diagnostic testing, such as allergens or tuberculosis screening; uses a tuberculin syringe, usual dose is 0.01 mL to 0.1 mL using 25- to 27-gauge, 1/4 to 1/2-inch needle

   4. Topical: some medications may be given as a paste (e.g., nitroglycerin) or as a patch (e.g., nitroglycerin or scopolamine) to the skin, so medication is absorbed continually over time

▶ Practice to Pass

The physician orders morphine sulfate 15 mg SC for a client with pain. The medication is supplied as morphine sulfate 25 mg/mL. What volume of the drug will the nurse prepare to administer the right dose?

Table 1-1	Commonly Used Routes of Administration			
Routes	**Barriers to Absorption**	**Absorption Pattern**	**Advantages**	**Disadvantages**
Intravenous	No barriers	Instantaneous and complete	Rapid onset Control over levels of drug in the blood Use of large fluid volumes Use of chemically irritant drugs such as anticancer	High cost Difficulty and inconvenience Irreversibility Fluid overload Infection Embolism
Intramuscular and subcutaneous	Capillary wall	Rapidly or slowly depends the water solubility of the drug and blood flow to the site of the injection Intramuscular absorption faster than subcutaneous because of better blood flow to muscle tissue	Poorly soluble drugs in water Depot preparations (preparations from which medication is absorbed gradually over an extended time)	Discomfort and inconvenience Possible nerve damage
Oral	a. The layer of epithelial cells b. The capillary wall	Varies according to: a. Solubility and stability of the drug b. Gastric and intestinal pH c. Gastric emptying time, d. Food in the gut e. Co-administration of other drugs f. Special coatings on the preparation	Easy and convenient Inexpensive Safer than parenteral injection	Variability of absorption Inactivation Patient requirements i.e., cooperation, local irritation

H. Medication interactions

1. *Drug–food interaction* is important because it can result in toxicity or therapeutic failure

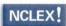

    a. Impact of food on drug absorption: may increase or decrease the rate of drug absorption and consequently increases or decreases the extent of absorption; if tetracyclines are administered with milk products or calcium supplements, absorption is reduced and antibacterial effects may be lost

    b. Impact of food on drug metabolism: may change the metabolism of the certain medications; grapefruit juice produces a 406% increase in blood levels of some calcium channel blockers used for hypertension

    c. Impact of food on drug toxicity: interaction between monoamine oxidase (MAO) inhibitors and foods rich in tyramine including yeasts extracts, aged cheese can result in a high blood pressure to a life-threatening level

    d. Impact of food on drug action: may have direct impact on drug action, such as foods rich in vitamin K (e.g., broccoli, cabbage) can reduce the effects of sodium warfarin (Coumadin)

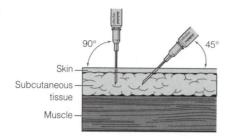

e. Timing of drug administration with respect to meals: may result in significant increase or decrease in medication absorption

2. *Drug–drug interaction* can occur whenever a client takes two or more medications; some interactions are intended and desired, but others are unintended

NCLEX!

a. Mechanisms of drug–drug interaction

1) Direct chemical or physical interaction: when drugs are combined in IV solutions and cause formation of a precipitate; the nurse inspects any solution that has been mixed with a drug carefully to detect crystals or cloudiness

2) Pharmacokinetic interaction: may alter the absorption, distribution, metabolism, and excretion; for example, heparin cannot cross the GI tract membrane so absorption via oral route is not possible; the drug must be given via parenteral route

3) Pharmacodynamic interaction: includes interactions at the same receptor or interactions at separate sites; naloxone (Narcan) is a drug that blocks access of opiate drugs to receptor sites so it used to reverse the action of opiates and is useful in the event of opiate overdose

b. Consequences of drug–drug interactions

1) Increased/decreased therapeutic effects

2) Increased/decreased adverse effects

3) Creation of a unique response

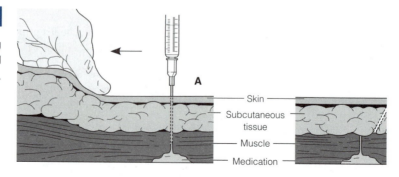

3. Incompatibility: the mixture of one medication or substance with another will result in an undesirable reaction

   a. These reactions could include chemical alteration, destruction, or pharmacologic effect

   b. An example is that diluting phenytoin (Dilantin) in Dextrose 5% will result in precipitating of solution, which can be fatal if administered to a client

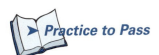

Practice to Pass

For a client with severe pain, which route of analgesic drug administration would provide the most rapid effect? Explain your answer.

I. Client education

1. Process of client education

   a. Assessment of need to learn

   b. Assessment of motivation

   c. Formulation of a nursing diagnostic statement and setting objective goals with client

   d. Teaching–learning activities aimed at the preferred learning style and general ability and educational level of the client

   e. Evaluation and reteaching if necessary depending on achievement of learning objectives

2. Nursing roles and responsibilities

   a. Applying the nursing process to client teaching

      1) Assessment: assess for the client's readiness for education; organize, analyze, and summarize the collected data

      2) Nursing diagnosis: formulating nursing diagnoses to address learning needs

      3) Planning and goals: assign priority to the nursing diagnoses; identify teaching strategies appropriate for goal; establish expected outcome

      4) Implementation: put the teaching plan into action; encourage the client to participate in learning

      5) Evaluation: evaluate the collected objective data; identify alterations that need to be made in the teaching plan; make referrals to appropriate sources

   b. Establish a good teacher–learner rapport

   c. Plan the best time for teaching and control the teaching environment for noise and other distractions

   d. Match the teaching methods to the client's primary learning style for optimum effectiveness, such as visual, auditory, tactile methods

   e. Use the teaching tools appropriate to the client's primary learning style such as lecture or verbal teaching, demonstration, written materials, videotapes or visual materials, physical models

   f. Identifying the barriers for learning such as disabilities, cultural or socioeconomic factors, communication, and excessive volume of learning materials

3. Client compliance

   a. The goal of client education is to encourage clients to adhere to their therapeutic regimen

    b. The teaching program should be directed toward stimulating client motivation to produce varying degrees of adherence

    c. Perform ongoing assessment of the variables that affect the client's ability to accept specific behaviors; these include variables such as age, gender, socioeconomic statues, education, severity of the illness, complexity of regimen, religious or cultural beliefs, and costs associated with a prescribed regimen

    d. Identify the problem of nonadherence to therapeutic regimens and plan counteractive strategies

    e. Establish comprehensive adherence-enhancing interventions

        1) Provide verbal instruction in small amounts, specific to activity

        2) Dispense optimal amounts of printed instructions

        3) Use material at client's comprehension level

        4) Dispense materials over time

        5) Assess level of client's understanding

        6) Encourage questions

        7) Augment verbal instructions with demonstrations

        8) Refer to community resources for additional skill development

        9) Goal setting: make goals attainable and very specific

        10) Reinforcement: provide feedback and praise for attempt

        11) Problem solving: identify problems and potential solutions for adherence

        12) Habit building: such as placing bedtime medication by clock radio

        13) Cueing: set up system of reminders to take medications, such as calendars or medication box

        14) Social support: involve others in behavior change plan

  4. Cultural considerations: cultural competence refers to a complex integration of attitudes, knowledge and skills that direct the nurse to provide care in a culturally sensitive manner (Table 1-2)

    a. Recognize special dietary needs for clients from selected cultural groups; sometimes foods preferred by clients may be those that interact with prescribed medications

    b. Review drug information to be aware of variations in individual response to medications based on ethnic and racial differences; some clients may require lower doses and some may have faster clearance rates of selected drugs based on cultural background

    c. Create an environment in which the traditional healing and practices of clients are respected; recognize that some clients may not value medication therapy as a primary mode of treatment for a health problem

    d. Establish effective communication by overcoming language barriers

        1) Greet client using the last or complete name

        2) Smile

Table 1-2	Comparative Characteristics of Culturally Diverse Clients			
Cultures	**Communication**	**Social Roles**	**Health Risks**	**Implementation**
African Americans	Direct eye contact is viewed as being rude, nonverbal communication is very important	Large extended family networks are important	Hypertension Coronary heart disease Sickle cell anemia Cancer	Be flexible and avoid rigidity in scheduling care Encourage involvement with family An herbalist may be consulted before an individual seeks medical treatment
Asian Americans	Silence is valued, eye contact considered rude, the word "no" considered disrespectful	Large extended family networks, devoted to tradition, education is highly valued	Hypertension Cancer Lactose intolerance Thalassemia	Limit eye contact Avoid gesturing with hands A healer may be consulted prior to medical treatment
European Americans	Eye contact is considered as trustworthiness	The nuclear family is the basic unit, the man is the dominant figure	Breast cancer Thalassemia Diabetes Heart disease	Eye contact indicates disrespect
Hispanic Americans	Eye contact indicates disrespect	The nuclear family is the basic unit, men are the decision makers, the extended family is highly valued	Diabetes Parasites Lactose intolerance	Protect privacy Offer to call priest or other clergy
Native Americans	Silence is valued, eye contact is avoided	Family oriented, elders are honored	Diabetes Tuberculosis Alcohol abuse Heart disease Gallbladder disease Accidents	Be attentive Clarify communication Obtain input from members of extended family May consult a medicine man

3) Pay attention to any effort by the client to communicate

4) Avoid talking loudly

5) Use short and simple sentences

6) Summarize and repeat frequently

7) Obtain and use the services of a qualified interpreter to ensure appropriate communication about the plan of care and prescribed medications; note that family members may not be the best choices for this task, depending on a number of variables, including age and sensitivity of information

8) Identify the cues that may signal lack of effective communication including absence of questions, efforts to change the subject, inappropriate laugher, and nonverbal cues

e. Establish flexible regulations pertaining to visitors such as length of visits

f. View each client as an individual and avoid stereotyping

g. Be aware of cultural preferences the client has in regards to space and distance, eye contact, time, touch, observance of holidays, diet

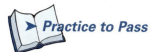

Practice to Pass

The client, who does not speak English, is being discharged with three prescriptions for medications. What strategies will the nurse use to meet responsibilities for client teaching in this situation?

    h. Maintain a broad and open attitude; expect the unexpected

    i. Try to understand the reasons for any behavior that you do not understand; ask for clarification

    j. Use any words you know in the client's language

  5. Health care beliefs

    a. Values are the beliefs and attitudes that may influence behavior and the process of decision making; they evolve from personal experiences

    b. Decisions about whether or not to use medications as therapy for health problems are often influenced by an individual's overall health care beliefs

    c. Ethical principles are codes that direct a person's actions

       1) They include the ability to make choices without external constraints, the need to maintain a balance between benefits and harms, and the obligation to tell the truth

       2) These are some areas in which ethical concerns arise for nurses and for clients related to treatment with drugs

    d. Ethical codes: provide broad principles for determining and evaluating client care

    e. American Nurses Association (ANA) Code of Ethics: an ideal framework for nurses to use in ethical decision-making

    f. Ethical dilemma: occurs when there is a conflict between two or more ethical principles including confidentiality, use of restraint, trust issues (not lying to the client, communicating to family and physician), refusing treatment or care, end-of life issues; drug therapy may play a role from time to time when issues arise in any of these areas, the nurse's role is to maintain ethical behavior in the course of administering medication therapy

---

Case Study

The nurse is visiting a 75-year-old client in the home. The client has type 1 diabetes mellitus, hypertension, and osteoarthritis in both knees. The client's sight is moderately impaired despite the use of eyeglasses. The client's medication regimen includes Humulin insulin 70/30 (combination insulins) 35 units subcutaneously in the morning, lisinopril (Prinivil) 5 mg by mouth daily, and celecoxib (Celebrex) 100 mg by mouth daily.

❶ What are two important medication administration safety issues that the nurse will assess in the client?

❷ What data will the nurse gather to evaluate the effects of the ordered medications?

❸ What measures can the nurse suggest to the client to ensure accuracy and compliance with the medication regimen?

❹ The client reports feeling "dizzy" at times. How will the nurse evaluate this concern?

❺ What criteria will the nurse use to select printed educational materials for this client's use?

For suggested responses, see page 636.

Posttest

1 The nurse is administering tetracycline hydrochloride (Tetracyn) 500 mg to a client with a gonorrhea infection. Which of the following nursing actions is indicated in this situation?

(1) Administer the drug with meals.
(2) Give the drug with a full glass of milk to prevent gastric irritation.
(3) Give the drug on an empty stomach with a full glass of water.
(4) Give the drug with a glass of orange juice or other source of vitamin C.

2 The client is being treated with phenelzine sulfate (Nardil), a monoamine oxidase inhibitor (MAOI) antidepressant. The nurse observes the client eating a lunch of yogurt, sliced bananas, and chocolate milk. In addition to notifying the MD, what action will the nurse take to monitor for a serious food–drug interaction?

(1) Monitor client's body temperature for elevation above normal.
(2) Observe client for respiratory depression.
(3) Test a urine specimen for glucose and ketones.
(4) Monitor client for elevated blood pressure.

3 A client who is taking several prescribed oral medications in treatment of congestive heart failure tells the nurse, "I'm going to take these at breakfast." Which response by the nurse is most appropriate?

(1) "Let's look at each medication to find out the best time to take the drug."
(2) "That depends on what you eat at breakfast."
(3) "That's a great idea."
(4) "What time do you usually have breakfast?"

4 The client received NPH insulin 30 units SC at 7:30 A.M. Which data will the nurse use to evaluate the client for the drug's therapeutic effectiveness?

(1) Client's blood pressure 2 hours after dose of drug.
(2) Client's appetite and food intake at lunch.
(3) Client's blood sugar level at 4:30 P.M.
(4) Client's oxygen saturation level before drug dose.

5 The client is taking theophylline (TheoDur) to treat asthma. The client complains of nausea and vomiting and headache; the laboratory data shows an elevated serum theophylline level at 22 mcg/mL. Which of the following is the most appropriate action for the nurse to take?

(1) Explain to the client that this is an expected side effect of the drug.
(2) Call the prescriber to report signs and symptoms of theophylline toxicity.
(3) Call the prescriber to get an order for antiemetic medication to reduce client's symptoms.
(4) Stop the ordered doses of TheoDur for 24 hours.

6 The nurse is preparing to administer an ordered dose of meperidine hydrochloride (Demerol) 100 mg PO to a client with postoperative pain. The drug data on Demerol indicates that this is a Schedule II controlled substance. The nurse takes which of the following actions based on this information?

(1) Uses special storage and documentation procedures for administering this drug
(2) Explains to the client that this drug has a low potential for abuse
(3) Has another licensed nurse witness the administration of the drug and co-sign the documentation of the drug
(4) Warns the client that the drug is highly addictive

7 The client taking warfarin (Coumadin) asks the nurse, "Why can't I eat broccoli and cabbage? I thought vegetables of all types are good nutritional sources." The nurse will utilize which of the following pieces of information in a response to the client?

(1) The client is correct; green leafy vegetables should be included in daily food intake.
(2) These food sources increase the effects of warfarin and may lead to dangerous bleeding problems.
(3) These food sources contain vitamin K, which decreases effects of the drug.
(4) These food sources contain vitamin C, which decreases effects of the drug.

8 The nurse administers the 4:00 P.M. dose of isophane insulin suspension (NPH) 10 units without monitoring the client's blood glucose level. The client has a hypoglycemic reaction at 6:00 P.M. involving seizure activity and a comatose state lasting several hours. Which of the following best describes the factors involved in this situation?

(1) The client experienced an idiosyncratic reaction to the drug.
(2) The client experienced an allergic reaction to the drug.
(3) The standard of care to assess the client's blood glucose before administering the drug was not followed.
(4) The nurse did not adhere to one or more of the "six rights" of medication administration.

9 The physician orders an IV solution of 1 liter of 5% dextrose in normal saline to be administered to a client over 6 hours. The nurse calculates the administration rate and sets the IV controller to which of the following rates?

(1) 50 mL per hour
(2) 100 mL per hour
(3) 166 mL per hour
(4) 200 mL per hour

10 A nurse is providing medication instruction to an elderly client with type 2 diabetes mellitus who takes glyburide (Micronase) 1.25 mg PO daily. Which statement, if made by the client, indicates that further instruction about the medication is needed?

(1) "I take the tablet before breakfast every day."
(2) "If I forget the dose on one day, I will take two tablets the next day."
(3) " I will avoid drinking alcohol while taking this drug."
(4) "I will visit the clinic every 2 weeks to have my blood glucose level checked."

See pages 22–23 for Answers and Rationales.

Answers and Rationales

Pretest

1 **Answer: 2** *Rationale:* The client's identification band is the most accurate way to verify a client's identity in the hospital; the client's medical record number is also on the band to further verify in the situation where two clients with same name are in the hospital. It is also acceptable to ask an oriented client to state his or her name and date of birth. Option 1 is incorrect because a confused client could answer inappropriately. Option 3 is incorrect because room and bed assignments can change. Option 4 is incorrect because it does not relate to client identification.
Cognitive Level: Analysis
Nursing Process: Implementation; *Test Plan:* SECE

2 **Answer: 2** *Rationale:* The drug has a generic name, ibuprofen, as well as several trade names. Advil and Motrin are examples of the trade names for this drug. The nurse will add a caution to the mother about reading the label carefully for dosage equivalency when changing brands of drug. The other responses are incorrect for this situation.
Cognitive Level: Application
Nursing Process: Implementation; *Test Plan:* PHYS

3 **Answer: 3** *Rationale:* Pregnancy Category A is assigned to drugs that have not shown to have adverse effects on fetal development. The other responses are factually incorrect (options 1 and 4) or unnecessary (option 2).
Cognitive Level: Application
Nursing Process: Implementation; *Test Plan:* SECE

4 **Answer: 4** *Rationale:* Grapefruit juice changes the metabolism of calcium channel blocker drugs and leads to an increase in serum drug levels. Of the responses presented, this one most directly assesses a known food–drug interaction and is the most specific response to the question posed. The assessment of a client's respiratory pattern is always important but is a general assessment that is made for every client at every interaction; it does not specifically target gaining information about the drug toxicity. Body temperature (option 1) and weight loss (option 3) are not directed at assessment related to drug toxicity.
Cognitive Level: Analysis
Nursing Process: Assessment; *Test Plan:* PHYS

5 **Answer: 2** *Rationale:* The decreased total body fluid proportion that accompanies physical aging increases

the concentration of water-soluble drugs and requires lower dosing in older adults. Elderly clients do not have an increased rate of drug absorption (option 1) or increased rate of drug metabolism (option 4). Decreased efficiency in drug distribution would not correlate with a need to lower the dosage (option 3).
Cognitive Level: Comprehension
Nursing Process: Analysis; *Test Plan:* PHYS

6 Answer: 3 *Rationale:* Use the following calculation formula:

$$\frac{100 \text{ mg}}{5 \text{ mL}} = \frac{150 \text{ mg}}{x \text{ mL}}; 100 \ x = 750; x = 7.5 \text{ mL}.$$

One teaspoon measures 5 mL (options 1 and 2). Option 4 is an incorrect statement.
Cognitive Level: Analysis
Nursing Process: Planning; *Test Plan:* SECE

7 Answer: 1 *Rationale:* Feeling dizzy when moving from lying or sitting to standing position is referred to as orthostatic hypotension and is a common side effect of the beta blocker drugs such as nadolol. The client should be taught to move slowly and to be careful until this effect diminishes after a few weeks of taking the drug. Dizziness is not a sign of toxicity (option 2), nor is it a common symptom of high blood pressure (option 4).
Cognitive Level: Analysis
Nursing Process: Implementation; *Test Plan:* PHYS

8 Answer: 1 *Rationale:* Older clients often take other prescribed drugs and this client may be currently using an over-the-counter (OTC) remedy for arthritis. The client may be also using herbs or other alternative remedies for arthritis. Because there is potential for drug–drug or drug–herb interaction, getting a thorough picture of the client's current drug regimen is the first step in planning for client education when a new drug is ordered. Option 2 is appropriate as a supplement after the nurse has taught the client about the medication. Option 3 may be unnecessary, given the information in the question. Option 4 is done after reviewing the client's medication profile to assess client's medication history.
Cognitive Level: Analysis
Nursing Process: Planning; *Test Plan:* HPM

9 Answer: 4 *Rationale:* This is an example of two different drugs with very similar names. The question of which drug is to be given to the client is answered by checking the original physician order and giving that drug. The other responses are incorrect because they

do not ensure that the correct dose and correct drug are given (Options 1 and 2) or are dangerous and inappropriate (option 3).
Cognitive Level: Analysis
Nursing Process: Implementation; *Test Plan:* SECE

10 Answer: 1 A client of Hispanic American culture often lives in the community with extended family who may visit often and want to be involved in care of a sick member. Men are typically decision makers. The nurse must be sensitive to the client's wishes regarding privacy when doing health teaching. The nurse should be aware that this cultural group cherishes its language, and teaching materials in the native language will be appreciated. The other responses are incorrect.
Cognitive Level: Comprehension
Nursing Process: Planning: *Test Plan:* HPM

Posttest

1 Answer: 3 *Rationale:* The drug tetracycline is absorbed best when given to the client on an empty stomach with a glass of water. Food (option 1), dairy products (option 2), iron, and antacids decrease the absorption of this drug. Option 3 is irrelevant to absorption of tetracycline.
Cognitive Level: Application
Nursing Process: Implementation; *Test Plan:* PHYS

2 Answer: 4 *Rationale:* The client is eating foods that contain tyramine, which interacts with the drug phenelzine and other MAOI drugs in a way that hypertensive crisis may occur. The actions in options 1, 2, and 3 will not detect this potentially life-threatening interaction.
Cognitive Level: Application
Nursing Process: Implementation; *Test Plan:* PHYS

3 Answer: 1 *Rationale:* The time of drug administration of oral drugs affects the relative speed with which they act. Drugs act more quickly when taken on an empty stomach. Some drugs irritate the gastrointestinal tract and need to be taken after a meal. Each drug should be reviewed to see what the drug manufacturer's recommendation is regarding timing of administration. The other responses do not address the issue of timing of medications.
Cognitive Level: Analysis
Nursing Process: Implementation; *Test Plan:* HPM

4 Answer: 3 *Rationale:* NPH insulin is used to therapeutically lower blood sugar level in clients with dia-

betes; the drug's effect peaks over 4 to 12 hours and lasts 24 hours. The other responses are incorrect.
Cognitive Level: Analysis
Nursing Process: Evaluation; *Test Plan:* PHYS

5 **Answer: 2** *Rationale:* The objective data (lab results) and the subjective data (nausea, headache) point to toxic levels of theophylline; this drug has a narrow therapeutic range, and the therapeutic level of the drug can quickly go to a toxic level. The prescriber should be notified of this situation to consider changing the dosage and/or frequency of the drug. Option 1 is false. Option 3 places the client at risk for harm. The action in option 4 is not within the legal scope of nursing practice
Cognitive Level: Analysis
Nursing Process: Implementation; *Test Plan:* SECE

6 **Answer: 1** *Rationale:* There are special procedures for prescribing, distributing, storing, and documenting the use of a controlled substance that every health care facility must follow. The nurse may retrieve, prepare, and administer the drug; in the event of a need to "waste" all or some of the drug for dosage or contamination reasons, the nurse must ask another licensed nurse to witness and co-sign that the drug was disposed of properly. The client in pain is not likely to become addicted to the drug and should be reassured about this. Fear of addiction is common among clients and leads to clients suffering with pain rather than accepting the drug.
Cognitive Level: Analysis
Nursing Process: Implementation; *Test Plan:* SECE

7 **Answer: 3** *Rationale:* Vitamin K is the antidote to Coumadin's effects; any food (such as broccoli or cabbage) or drug that contains vitamin K reduces the effects of the drug. Options 2 and 4 are false statements, while option 1 would be true if the client was not taking warfarin.
Cognitive Level: Application
Nursing Process: Planning; *Test Plan:* HPM

8 **Answer: 3** *Rationale:* The nurse is responsible for assessing the client's condition in relation to the use of the ordered medication and the client's response to the medication, including any expected or unexpected responses to the medication. In this situation, lowering of the client's blood glucose is an expected response to insulin, and the nurse did not follow the standards of care to monitor the blood glucose level. Options 1, 2, and 4 are incorrect conclusions about this situation. This was not an idiosyncratic or an allergic reaction to insulin (options 1 and 2). The nurse may have followed the six rights when administering the drug but was negligent in following the nursing process.
Cognitive Level: Analysis
Nursing Process: Evaluation; *Test Plan:* SECE

9 **Answer: 3** *Rationale:* The rate for administration is calculated by converting the 1L in the order to its equivalent: 1000 mL. For 1000 mL to be delivered in 6 hours, divide 1,000 by 6 = 166 mL. The IV controller delivers the rate set as the number of mL per 1 hour. The other responses are mathematically incorrect.
Cognitive Level: Application
Nursing Process: Implementation; *Test Plan:* SECE

10 **Answer: 2** *Rationale:* Because of the wording "further information is needed," the correct answer to this question is an incorrect statement on the part of the client. It is a general rule for any drug that doubling the dose after a missed dose is not recommended. This is particularly true for this medication, which has the effect of stimulating insulin release; a double dose may lower blood glucose level to an undesirable level. The other options indicate that the client does have an understanding about the medication.
Cognitive Level: Analysis
Nursing Process: Evaluation; *Test Plan:* HPM

References

Abrams, A. (2004). *Clinical drug therapy: Rationales for nursing practice* (7th ed.). Philadelphia: Lippincott Williams & Wilkins, pp. 1–69.

Agency for health care policy and research, http://www.ahcpr.gov.

Aschenbrenner, D., Cleveland, L., & Venable, S. (2002). *Drug therapy in nursing.* Philadelphia: Lippincott Williams & Wilkins, pp. 1–75.

Drug formulary, http://intmed.mcw.edu/drug.html.

Food and Drug Administration, http://www.fda.gov.

Harkreader, H., & Hogan, M. (2003). *Fundamentals of nursing: Caring and clinical judgment* (2nd ed.). St. Louis, MO: Elsevier Science, pp. 387–450.

Karch, A. (2003). *Focus on pharmacology* (2nd ed.). Philadelphia: Lippincott Williams & Wilkins, pp. 1–62.

Kee, J. (2002). *Laboratory diagnostic tests and nursing implications* (6th ed.). Upper Saddle River, NJ: Prentice Hall.

Kozier, B., Erb, G., Berman, A., & Snyder, S. (2004). *Fundamentals of nursing: Concepts, process and practice* (7th ed.). Upper Saddle River, NJ: Pearson Education.

Lehne, R. (2004). *Pharmacology for nursing care* (5th ed.). St. Louis, MO: Mosby, Inc., pp. 1–78.

McKenry, L., & Salerno, G. (2003). *Mosby's pharmacology in nursing* (21st ed. revised reprint). St. Louis, MO: Mosby, Inc., pp. 1–109.

Miller-Keane. (2003). *Encyclopedia & dictionary of medicine, nursing & allied health* (7th ed.). Philadelphia, PA: Saunders.

National Institutes of Safety and Health http://www.cdc.gov/niosh.homepage.html.

Pickar, G. (2004). *Dosage calculations* (7th ed.). Clifton Park, NY: Delmar Learning.

Smeltzer, S., & Bare, B. (2000). *Textbook of medical-surgical nursing* (9th ed.). Philadelphia: Lippincott Williams & Wilkins.

Stedman's medical dictionary (2000). (27th ed.). Philadelphia PA: Lippincott Williams & Wilkins.

Youngkin, E., Sawin, K., Kissinger, J., & Israel, D. (2001). *Pharmacotherapeutics: A primary care clinical guide.* Stamford, CT: Appleton & Lange.

CHAPTER 2

Anti-Infective Medications

Carolyn M. Burger, MSN, RN,C, OCN

CHAPTER OUTLINE

Antibiotics

Antimycobacterials

Antivirals

Antifungals

Antiprotozoals

Antihelminthics

OBJECTIVES

▐ Describe general goals of therapy when administering anti-infective medications.

▐ Discuss why antibiotics should not be discontinued until the prescribed therapy is complete.

▐ Identify actions and common side effects of various anti-infective medications.

▐ Describe most common adverse reactions to anti-infective medications.

▐ Discuss nursing considerations related to anti-infective medications prescribed to treat human immunodeficiency virus and acquired immunodeficiency syndrome.

▐ Describe why medication combinations are commonly used to treat tuberculosis and leprosy.

▐ Identify significant client education points related to the use of anti-infective medications.

 [Media Link]

Use the CD-ROM enclosed with this text, or log onto the address given to access the free, interactive Companion Website created for this series. The CD-ROM and Companion Website accompanying this book offer additional practice opportunities and information—NCLEX Review, Case Studies, Glossary, In Depth with NCLEX, and more.

www.prenhall.com/hogan

KEY TERMS

amebiasis *a protozoan infection of the colon usually transmitted in contaminated food or water; infection of the large intestine by the protozoan parasite called Entamoeba histolytica; transmitted through the fecal to oral route from contaminated food or water or from person to person contact; found throughout the world*

bactericidal *agent that destroys the causative microorganism*

bacteriostatic *agent that inhibits the growth of the causative microorganism and depends on the host's immune system to destroy the bacteria*

candidiasis *a fungal infection caused by Candida albicans transmitted by direct contact or as a superinfection; occurs in mucous membranes in warm, dark, moist areas as oral cavity (thrush), vagina, intestine, and cutaneously as beneath the breasts and diaper areas*

cross-sensitivity *a condition in which one class of drugs is chemically very similar to another class of drugs; allergy to one class may suggest allergy to the other class of drugs; cross-sensitivity occurrence between the penicillins and the cephalosporins has been reported to be 1 to 18%*

cytomegalovirus *a common virus that resides in the salivary glands; may cause cytomegalovirus pneumonia (potentially fatal) and CMV retinitis (with potential blindness) in the immunosuppressed clients; newborns are also at higher risk with infected mother; body fluid precautions required*

disulfiram-like reaction *also called antabuse effect; a reaction when certain medications are taken with even small amounts of alcohol; causes abdominal cramping, facial and upper body flushing, pulsating headache, weakness, uneasiness, vertigo, hypotension, palpitations,* shortness of breath, sweating, pruritic macular rash, tachycardia, nausea and vomiting; may occur within 10 to 30 minutes of alcohol ingestion and last 30 minutes to several hours

empiric therapy *drug therapy initiated based on clinical manifestations of a pathological or infectious process rather than on a scientifically defined etiology; selection of agent based on most common known cause of infection; drug may be adjusted after culture and sensitivity results are known if indicated*

giardiasis *most common protozoan intestinal, (usually duodenal,) infection transmitted by contaminated food or water or stool of infected clients; causes diarrhea, distention, and malodorous stools*

helminths *disease-producing parasites such as Nematoda (roundworms) and Platyhelminthes (flatworms) that include Cestodes (tapeworms), trematodes (flukes); parasite has to be identified because anthelminthics are specific; ova or larvae may be isolated in stool, urine, blood, sputum, or in host tissues*

herpes simplex *a viral infection classified as Type I (of facial areas including cold sore or fever blister) or Type II (genital herpes)*

herpes varicella *virus that causes chickenpox*

herpes zoster *the virus of chickenpox that has lain dormant in the nerves; eruptions of the infection occur along nerve routes, especially of the trunk; may be activated by immunosuppressed states or stress of disease*

peak drug level *serum blood level of antibiotic drawn 15 to 30 minutes after IV infusion is complete to determine that peak level is not at a toxic level*

pneumocystis carinii **pneumonia** *very serious protozoan infection of lungs occurring only in immunosuppressed clients*

pseudomembranous colitis *a type of superinfection that occurs when an antibiotic decreases or completely eliminates normal flora needed to maintain normal function in the GI tract; permits other bacteria or fungi or yeasts (unsusceptible to the antibiotic) to take over and cause infection*

Stevens-Johnson syndrome *an adverse reaction of the skin that resembles appearance of second degree burns with erythema multiforme, fever, and bullae (blister) lesions of mucous membranes of oropharynx, conjunctiva, vagina, and anus*

superinfection *a condition in which an antibiotic decreases or completely eliminates normal bacterial flora that consists of certain bacteria and fungi or yeasts needed to maintain normal function in various organs; permits other bacteria or fungi or yeasts (unsusceptible to the antibiotic) to take over and cause infection, e.g., vaginal yeast infection, pseudomembranous colitis, candidiasis*

tinea *fungal infections, called ringworm, caused by dermatophytes on foot (tinea pedis or "athlete's foot"), on scalp (tinea capitis), on body (tinea corporis), and in the groin (tinea cruris or "jock itch")*

toxoplasmosis *protozoan systemic infection transmitted by contact with oocysts in feces of domesticated animals, primarily in feline species*

trough drug level *blood specimen drawn just prior to the next scheduled IV dose of antibiotic to determine that the therapeutic level has been maintained between drug administration intervals*

Pretest

 1 **The client taking isoniazid (INH) reports paresthesia of the extremities. The nurse initially assesses the client for which of the following?**

(1) Hyperactive motor reflex responses
(2) Other clinical manifestations of hypercalcemia
(3) Concurrent self-administration of aluminum antacids
(4) Compliance with taking pyridoxine (vitamin B$_6$) supplement

2 Rifampin (Rifadin) is being initiated prophylactically for a client who lives with a family member who has *Haemophilus influenzae* meningitis. What client teaching would be most appropriate?

(1) Explain that Rifampin is being prescribed to treat meningitis.
(2) Adverse effects may be severe, such as convulsions and coma.
(3) Protect undergarments because rifampin (Rifadin) will cause the urine to become orange-red and will stain.
(4) Client will need to keep follow-up visits with health care provider, but it will not be necessary to continue blood test monitoring.

3 A client with benign prostatic hyperplasia (BPH) is receiving amantadine (Symmetrel) for influenza A. The nurse includes in the care plan to monitor the client for which of the following side effects?

(1) Increased risk for urinary retention
(2) Hypermotility of bowel
(3) Increased lacrimation
(4) Nephrotoxicity

4 A client with *herpes zoster* infection (shingles) has started therapy with acyclovir (Zovirax). The nurse performs what important intervention during the course of this treatment?

(1) Monitors for jaundice and elevated liver enzymes.
(2) Teaches the client to avoid sexual intercourse during therapy.
(3) Administers the dose early in the day, as it may cause insomnia.
(4) Encourages fluid intake of 2,500 to 3,000 mL daily since it is not contraindicated by other client conditions.

5 The nurse determines the client understands an important principle in self-administration of an oral antibiotic when the client makes which of the following statements?

(1) "I will continue to take the antibiotic as it is ordered, even though I no longer have a cough with yellow sputum."
(2) "When I missed a dose of my antibiotic this morning, I made up by taking two doses when it was time to take the next dose."
(3) "I am careful to take the antibiotic every day at breakfast, lunch, and dinner."
(4) "Even though the doctor prescribed amoxicillin (Amoxil) chewable tablets, I have no problem swallowing it whole."

6 A client has been on anti-infective therapy for 10 days and has developed diarrhea with 10 watery stools a day. The nurse should anticipate an order for which of the following?

(1) Monitor for clinical manifestations of metabolic alkalosis.
(2) Administer an anti-peristaltic agent as dicyclomine HCl (Bentyl).
(3) Administer an anti-diarrheal agent as kaolin and pectin (Kaopectolin).
(4) Collect stool specimen for cytotoxin assay to detect *Clostridium difficile*.

7 The client with pneumonia is being treated with amoxicillin (Amoxil). The nurse monitors for therapeutic effectiveness by noting which of the following?

(1) Normalization of fever beginning 96 hours after therapy starts
(2) No clinical manifestations of hypersensitivity
(3) Resolution of orthostatic hypotension
(4) Pulse oximetry of 98%

8 A client receiving penicillin (PCN) for several days complains of weakness, numbness, tingling in the extremities, and nausea. The nurse palpates a weak pulse and auscultates an irregular heart rate and decreased bowel sounds. The nurse further monitors the client for specific signs of which of the following imbalances?

(1) Hypokalemia
(2) Hypochloremia
(3) Hypercalcemia
(4) Hypophosphatemia

9 The prescriber ordered cefdinir (Omnicef), a third-generation cephalosporin for a client with a staphylococcal infection. The nurse collaborates with the prescriber about which of the following data related to the client?

(1) BUN 14 mg/dL
(2) Elevated granulocyte count
(3) Final culture and sensitivity (C & S) results not yet available
(4) History of type I hypersensitivity to penicillin

10 A client's white blood cell count differential shows a "shift to the left." The nurse recognizes that the client needs to be assessed for what type of infection?

(1) Bacterial
(2) Acute viral
(3) Parasitic
(4) Retroviral

See pages 95–96 for Answers and Rationales.

I. Antibiotics

A. Aminoglycosides

1. Action and use

   a. **Bactericidal:** aminoglycosides kill the bacteria cell

   b. Effective against aerobic gram-negative infections

   c. Used to sterilize bowel prior to surgery

   d. Used to destroy urease-producing bacteria to prevent absorption of ammonia in hepatic encephalopathy

   e. Toxicity limits use to serious gram-negative infections and specific conditions involving gram-positive cocci

   f. Used in infections caused by *Acinetobacter, Citrobacter, E. coli, Klebsiella pneumoniae, proteus, pseudomonas, Providencia, Salmonella, Serratia,* and *staphylococcus* organisms; also active against protozoal infections

2. Common medications (Table 2-1)

3. Administration considerations

   a. Intravenous (IV) route preferred for optimal distribution to tissues

   b. Used intramuscularly (IM) as well

   c. Oral route: poorly absorbed so effective orally only to sterilize bowel prior to surgery to (eliminate bacteria in bowel) or to prevent absorption of ammonia in hepatic encephalopathy

   d. Intrathecal or intraventricular injection: these routes used because of poor penetration of cerebral spinal fluid (CSF) by other routes

   e. Periocular instillations: because of poor penetration of eye fluids, direct instillations are used

4. Contraindications

   a. Allergy to the aminoglycosides

   b. Preexisting renal disease

Table 2-1	Generic/Trade Names	Usual Adult Dose	Administration Route
Aminoglycosides	Amikacin sulfate (Amikin)	7.5 mg/kg q12h	IM, IV
	Gentamicin sulfate (Garamycin)	3–5 mg/kg/d in 2–3 divided doses	IM, IV, topical
	Kanamycin sulfate (Kantrex)	PO 1 g q 1 h for 4 doses, then q 6 h for 36–72 h, IV/IM 15 mg/kg/d in equally divided doses q 8–12 h Inhalation: 250 mg diluted in 3 mL NS administered per nebulizer q 6–12 h	PO, IM, IV, irrigation intraperitoneal, inhalation
	Neomycin sulfate (Mycifradin)	PO 50 mg/kg in 4 divided doses for 2–3 days; IM 1.3–2.6 mg/kg q6h	PO, IM
	Netilmicin sulfate (Netromycin)	1.3–2.2 mg/kg q 8 h or 2–3.25 mg/kg q12h	IM, IV
	Paromomycin sulfate (Humatin)	25–35 mg/kg divided in 3 doses for 5–10 d	PO
	Streptomycin sulfate (Streptomycin)	Tuberculosis: 15 mg/kg up to 1 g/d as single dose; tularemia: 1–2 g/d in 1–2 divided doses for 7–10 d	IM
	Tobramycin sulfate (Nebcin)	IV/IM 3 mg/kg/d divided q 8 h up to 5 mg/kg/d; IV infused over 20–60 min	IM, IV, topical

   c. Receiving renal toxic agents as amphotericin B (Fungizone), vancomycin (Vancocin), loop diuretics as furosemide (Lasix)

   d. In myasthenia gravis

   e. Caution in pregnancy and lactation

  5. Significant drug interactions

   a. Aminoglycoside may be microbiologically inactivated with concurrently high concentration of penicillins greater than 200 mcg/mL

   b. Do not mix other medications in the same intravenous fluid

   c. With oral anticoagulant therapy, bleeding may increase because the aminoglycosides decrease synthesis of vitamin K in the intestinal tract

   d. Concurrent administration of dimenhydrinate (Dramamine) may mask signs of toxicity

  6. Significant food interactions: none reported

  7. Significant laboratory studies

   a. **Peak drug level:** blood specimen drawn 15 to 30 minutes after the intravenous (IV) infusion of aminoglycoside is completed to determine that toxic levels do not occur; dose may need to be decreased if peak too high

   b. **Trough drug level:** blood specimen drawn immediately prior to next IV infusion of aminoglycoside initiated to assure that therapeutic levels of drug are maintained between administrations; if therapeutic level is not sustained, increase in dose and/or in dosing frequency may be indicated

    c. White blood count (WBC) to monitor effectiveness of drug therapy

       1) Neutrophils and immature neutrophils called stabs or bands, are increased in acute bacterial infections

       2) Neutrophils and lymphocytes make up 75 to 90% of the leukocytes; when one part of the differential increases as in response to an acute infection, another part has to decrease; a "shift to the left" signifies an increase in neutrophils and, therefore, an acute bacterial infection

       3) This knowledge facilitates selection of an appropriate type of anti-infective drug

NCLEX!

    d. Serum creatinine and blood urea nitrogen (BUN) to monitor renal function; expected BUN to creatinine ratio is 20:1 or 15:1 depending on criteria of laboratory; creatinine is most specific test for renal function; if creatinine level rises 3 to 4 days into treatment, it indicates renal damage has occurred

8. Side effects: headache, paresthesia, skin rash, fever

9. Adverse effects/toxicity

NCLEX!

    a. Nephrotoxicity and ototoxicity are two common toxicities associated with therapy with the aminoglycosides

NCLEX!

    b. Nephrotoxicity: increased risk factors include advanced age (with associated declining renal function), hypotension, dehydration, preexisting renal disease, and coadministration of other nephrotoxic drugs

NCLEX!

    c. Ototoxicity: may be irreversible

       1) Auditory impairment and vestibular damage

       2) Possible damage to the 8th cranial nerve

       3) Risk increased with nephrotoxic drugs, prolonged treatment with aminoglycosides, impaired renal function, and other ototoxic drugs, such as furosemide (Lasix), vancomycin (Vancocin), amphotericin B, and certain antineoplastic agents

    d. Neuromuscular blockade: secondary to inhibition of acetylcholine release; may be seen in clients with myasthenia gravis or clients receiving neuromuscular blocking agents as pancuronium bromide (Pavulon) or succinylcholine (Anectine); use calcium salts to reverse the blockade

NCLEX!

    e. Superinfection: a secondary infection caused by eradication of normal flora

       1) **Candidiasis:** secondary infection usually of skin and mucous membranes caused by *Candida albicans*

         a) Often associated with immunosuppression

         b) Occurs on mucous membranes of the oropharynx (thrush), bronchi, vagina, and anus

         c) Appears as discrete white plaques; red, scaly, papular skin rash can occur in warm, moist, dark areas, such as in breast folds, axilla, groin

2) **Pseudomembranous colitis:** secondary infection of the bowel usually has *Clostridium difficile* as etiologic factor

 a) Manifested by 4 to 6 watery stools/day with blood and/or mucus, abdominal pain, and fever

 b) Antibiotic is discontinued and Vancocin orally (PO) or Flagyl IV or PO is prescribed

10. Nursing considerations

NCLEX!

a. Collect appropriate specimen for culture and sensitivity (C & S), if possible, prior to initiation of anti-infective therapy to ensure appropriate drug employed; **empiric therapy** (based on probable offending organism) is usually begun before test results available because of seriousness of infection

NCLEX!

b. Assess medications being taken that may result in a drug interaction

NCLEX!

c. Ensure client takes complete course of anti-infective for full beneficial effects, even if clinical manifestations of infection resolved; premature discontinuation can result in regrowth of microorganisms as well as development of drug resistance

NCLEX!

d. Monitor peak and trough aminoglycoside levels

NCLEX!

e. Monitor for nephrotoxicity

 1) Monitor serum creatinine, BUN, urine creatinine clearance and urinalysis results

 2) Nephrotoxicity manifestations include urinary casts and proteinuria

 3) Make certain the client is not taking other nephrotoxic drugs

 4) Keep accurate record of intake and output (I & O)

f. Monitor for ototoxicity

 1) Assess baseline hearing and monitor for hearing loss; may include audiometry testing

NCLEX!

 2) Clinical manifestations of ototoxicity include dizziness, light-headedness, tinnitus, fullness in ears, and hearing loss

 3) Monitor vestibular integrity: perform Romberg's test, if possible; have client stand alone with hands at sides and eyes open, then have client close eyes; minimum swaying of body is expected, but if unable to maintain standing position/balance, Romberg's test is positive indicating problem with balance

g. Arrange for dosage adjustment or medication change if indicated by results of above tests/assessments

NCLEX!

h. Maintain fluid hydration to protect the kidneys; intake should be 2,500 to 3,000 mL/day unless contraindicated by other conditions

NCLEX!

i. Observe for evidence that infection is resolving within 48 to 72 hours of therapy

NCLEX!

    j. Provide small frequent, nutritious meals with high quality proteins; drugs that may be taken with food may be associated with decreased gastrointestinal (GI) upset

    k. Assess for adverse reactions

    l. Evaluate effectiveness of teaching plan

  11. Client education

    a. Know drug name, dose, route, schedule regimen

NCLEX!

    b. Use around the clock dosing evenly spaced without disruption of sleep to maintain therapeutic blood level and enhance efficacy of drug

NCLEX!

    c. It is very important that full course of drug therapy be taken as prescribed to prevent repeat infection or development of drug resistance

    d. Keep premixed drug refrigerated as recommended

    e. Take safety precautions according to side effects that occur

    f. Take oral drug with food if not contraindicated to reduce risk of GI upset

    g. Eat small, frequent meals with at least 6 to 8 glasses of fluid a day

NCLEX!

    h. Report sore throat, watery stools greater than 4 to 6 per day, severe nausea or vomiting, indicating possible superinfection

NCLEX!

    i. Discard any outdated or unused drug to ensure against self-administration and drugs with decreased potency that could adversely affect future treatment and increase risk of development of drug resistance

NCLEX!

    j. Before taking any over-the-counter (OTC) drugs, check efficacy and possible adverse reactions with health care provider

B. Cephalosporins

  1. Action and use

NCLEX!

    a. Structurally and chemically related to the penicillins; practically identical to penicillin related to mechanism of action, drug effects, therapeutic effects, side effects, adverse effects, and drug interactions; **cross-sensitivity** may occur between the penicillins and the cephalosporins, meaning that allergy to one class may indicate hypersensitivity to the other in some clients

    b. Four generations of cephalosporins

      1) First through third generations: increased activity against gram-negative organisms and anaerobes; less activity against gram-positive organisms; first generation does not enter the cerebral spinal fluid (CSF) and has limited activity against aerobic gram-negative organisms as *E. coli, P. mirabilis, Klebsiella pneumoniae*

      2) Fourth generation: increased activity against gram-positive cocci and gram negative bacilli

    c. Usually bactericidal

    d. Sexually transmitted diseases (STDs)

      1) Third generation for cervicitis, urethritis, pharyngitis, and proctitis caused by *Neiserria gonorrhoeae*

2) Chlamydia is commonly associated with gonorrhea so may be given azithromycin (Zithromax) as a single dose or doxycycline (Vibramycin) concurrently

3) Ceftriaxone (Rocephin): treats chancroid, syphilis; add doxycycline (Vibramycin) to treat pelvic inflammatory disease (PID), epididymitis, or orchiditis

e. Used to treat respiratory infections as bronchitis, pharyngitis, otitis media, sinusitis, and pneumonia

f. Used to treat urinary tract infections (UTI), skin/tissue infections, Lyme disease

g. Used prophylactically and therapeutically in orthopedic disorders; cefazolin (Ancef) is drug of choice to prevent or treat bone infections associated with orthopedic surgery

h. Used for endocarditis prophylaxis prior to surgery for clients with history of rheumatic heart disease

i. Important to reserve use for appropriate clinical infections because bacterial resistance increasing

j. Most cephalosporins are excreted through urine except cefoperazone (Cefobid) and ceftriaxone (Rocephin), which are excreted in bile

2. Common medications (Table 2-2)

Table 2-2

Cephalosporins

Generic/Trade Names	Usual Adult Dose	Administration Route
Cefadroxil (Duricef)	1–2 g/d in 1–2 divided doses	PO
Cefazolin (Ancef, Kefzol)	250 mg–2 g q 8 h up to 2 g q 4 h (max 12 g/d)	IM, IV
Cephalexin (Keflex)	250–500 mg q 6 h	PO
Cephradine (Velosef)	PO: 250–500 mg q 6 h; IM/IV 2–4 g/d in 4 divided doses	PO, IM, IV
Cefaclor (Ceclor)	250–500 mg q 8 h	PO
Cefamandole Nafate (Mandol)	500 mg–1 g q 4–8 h up to 2 g q 4 h	IM, IV
Cefonicid (Monocid)	1 g q 24 h up to 2 g/24 h	IM, IV
Cefprozil (Cefzil)	250–500 mg q 12–24 h for 10–14 d	PO
Cefotetan (Cefotan)	1–2 g q 12 h	IM, IV
Cefuroxime axetil (Ceftin)	PO 250–500 mg q 12 h; IV/IM 750 mg–1.5 g q 6–8 h	PO, IM, IV
Cefuroxime sodium (Zinacef)	PO 250–500 mg q 12 h; IV/IM 750 mg–1.5 g q 6–8 h	PO, IM, IV
Loracarbef (Lorabid)	200–400 mg q 12 h taken 1 h a.c. or 2 h p.c.	PO
Cefdinir (Omnicef)	300 mg q 12 h for 10 d	PO
Cefixime (Suprax)	400 mg/d in 1–2 divided doses	PO
Cefoperazone (Cefobid)	1–2 g q 12 h, 16g/d in 2–4 divided doses	IM, IV
Cefotaxime (Claforan)	1–2 g q 8–12 h up to 2 g q 4 h (max 12 g/d)	IM, IV
Cefpodoxime proxetil (Vantin)	200 mg q 12h for 10 d	PO
Ceftibuten (Cedax)	400 mg QD for 10 d	PO
Ceftizoxime (Cefizox)	1–2 g q 8–12 h up to 2 g q 4 h	IM, IV
Ceftriaxone (Rocephin)	1–2 g q 12–24 h (max 4 g/d)	IM, IV
Cefoxitin (Mefoxin)	1–2 g q 6–8 h up to 12 g/d	IM, IV
Ceftazidime (Fortaz)	1–2 g q 8–12 h up to 2 g q 6 h	IM, IV

    a. First-generation cephalosporins: cefadroxil (Duricef), cefazolin (Ancef), cephalexin (Keflex), cephapirin (Cefadyl), and cephradine (Velosef)

    b. Second-generation cephalosporins: cefaclor (Ceclor), cefmetazole (Zefazone), cefonicid (Monocid), cefprozil (Cefzil), cefotetan (Cefotan), cefoxitin (Mefoxin), cefuroxime axetil (Ceftin), cefuroxime sodium (Zinacef), and loracarbef (Lorabid)

    c. Third-generation cephalosporins: cefdinir (Omnicef), cefixime (Suprax), cefoperazone (Cefobid), cefotaxime (Claforan), cefpodoxime proxetil (Vantin), ceftazidime (Fortaz), ceftibuten (Cedax), ceftizoxime (Cefizox), and ceftriaxone (Rocephin)

    d. Fourth-generation cephalosporins: cefipime (Maxipime), cefditoren (Spectracef)

3. Administration considerations

    a. Collect specimen for C & S from site of infection, if possible, prior to initiation of antibiotic; empiric therapy may be started if results not available to enhance effectiveness with early antibiotic administration

    b. Well absorbed from GI tract

      1) Absorption delayed with food but amount absorbed not affected

      2) Absorption not delayed with cefadroxil and cefprozil

    c. Do not readily enter CSF except for cefuroxime; third generation drugs readily enter CSF in presence of meningeal inflammation

    d. Check renal function prior to and during therapy to arrange for appropriate dosage adjustment; renal impairment significantly extends the half-life

    e. Crosses placenta

    f. Separate oral administration of antacids, histamine H_2 blockers, iron supplements and foods fortified with iron by 2 hours before and after oral administration of cephalosporins

    g. Separate oral administration of cefdinir from iron supplements and foods fortified with iron by 2 hours

    h. Intramuscular administration is painful and irritating; administer deep IM into large muscle; avoid repeated IM injections; IV is the preferred parenteral route

    i. Shake suspensions to disperse or dissolve particles of drug immediately before measurement

    j. Continue drug administration for at least 10 days to decrease risk of rheumatic fever in beta-hemolytic streptococcal bacterial infections such as "strep throat"; also acute glomerulonephritis can become a sequela of this infection if treatment is inadequate

4. Contraindications

    a. Cross-sensitivity with penicillins; not recommended for those who have had a Type I (anaphylactic) reaction to penicillin

    b. Use extreme caution if creatinine clearance is less than 50 mL/minute

NCLEX!

NCLEX!

NCLEX!

NCLEX!

NCLEX!

      c. Hepatotoxicity with cefoperazone and ceftriaxone

      d. Caution in pregnancy and lactation

5. Significant drug interactions

      a. Probenecid (Benemid): increases and prolongs half-life of cephalosporins

      b. Loop diuretics and aminoglycosides increase risk of nephrotoxicity

      c. Anticoagulants increase bleeding

      d. Use of ethanol with some cephalosporins such as cefoperazone and cefotetan can cause **disulfiram-like reaction** during therapy and up to 72 hours after drug discontinued; can occur within 30 minutes of alcohol ingestion; manifestations include weakness, pulsating headache, and abdominal cramps

      e. Antacids: concurrent use interferes with absorption of cefaclor, cefdinir, cefpodoxime

      f. Histamine H_2 antagonists: decrease the plasma concentration of cephalosporins

6. Significant food interactions

      a. Iron supplements and iron-fortified foods decrease absorption of cefdinir

      b. May take with food or milk if drug causes gastric irritation except ceftibuten, which is taken 1 hour before and 2 hours after meals

      c. Drug absorption enhanced with food with cefuroxime and cefpodoxime proxetil

7. Significant laboratory studies

      a. With parenteral administration and/or prolonged therapy, check urinalysis, BUN, serum creatinine to check renal function

      b. Monitor liver function tests when giving cefoperazone and ceftriaxone

      c. Monitor baseline and periodic prothrombin time (PT) and the international normalized ratio (INR) if taking oral anticoagulants and for increased bleeding, such as bleeding gums and easy bruising

         1) With long-term therapy of parenteral cefamandole, cefmetazole, cefoperazone, cefotetan, or moxalactam (Moxam)

         2) If PT prolonged, give exogenous vitamin K (Phytonadione) as prescribed

8. Side effects

      a. Central nervous system (CNS): lethargy, hallucinations, anxiety, depression, twitching, convulsions, coma

      b. GI: nausea, vomiting, mild diarrhea, abdominal cramps or distress, increased liver function tests such as aspartate aminotransferase (AST) and alanine aminotransferase (ALT), abdominal pain, colitis

      c. Hematologic: anemia, increased bleeding time, bone marrow depression, granulocytopenia

      d. Metabolic: hyperkalemia, hypokalemia, alkalosis

  e. Other: taste alteration, sore mouth; dark discolored or sore tongue; hives, pruritis, rash, edema

 9. Adverse effects/toxicity

  a. Hypersensitivity occurs in 5 to 16% of clients

  b. Cross-sensitivity with penicillins

  c. Serum-sickness–like illness

   1) Erythema multiform and other skin rashes, arthralgia, and fever

   2) Usually follows second course of treatment and may be delayed at least 10 days after initiation of drug

   3) Treat with antihistamines and corticosteroids

  d. Seizure activity

   1) Especially in renal impairment or in intraventricular administration

   2) Discontinue the cephalosporin to resolve activity

  e. In renal impairment, cancer, impaired vitamin K synthesis, malnutrition, low vitamin K stores, there is increased risk for the following:

   1) Coagulation disturbances with parenteral administration

   2) Disulfiram-like reaction in those who consume, or less frequently, inhale alcohol as in perfume, aftershave, alcohol swabs

  f. Immune hemolytic anemia: rare

  g. Pseudomembranous colitis: a superinfection in which the normal flora of the intestine has been altered and severe diarrhea develops; *Clostridium difficile* is usually the etiologic organism; clinical manifestations include watery stools greater than 4 to 6 per day, blood and mucus in stools, abdominal cramping, fever; the antibiotic is stopped and oral vancomycin (Vancocin) or metronidazole (Flagyl) is given

  h. Accumulation of biliary sludge or pseudolithiasis with ceftriaxone; clears after drug is discontinued

 10. Nursing considerations

  a. Monitor clinical therapeutic response

   1) Heat, redness, swelling, tenderness, or discharge abate after 48 to 72 hours

   2) Fever, malaise, leukocytosis improve

   3) Pulmonary infiltrates resolve and pulse oximetry normalizes in pneumonia

  b. Monitor site of infection throughout course of treatment; re-culture site if improvement is not observed in 48 hours

  c. Monitor injection sites for induration and tenderness; provide warm compresses and gentle massage to injection sites if painful or swollen; if phlebitis or redness at IV site develops, remove IV device and restart IV

  d. Monitor for renal toxicity: check serum creatinine, BUN, urine creatinine clearance, and keep accurate I & O

NCLEX!

NCLEX!

NCLEX!

NCLEX!

e. Monitor for unusual lethargy beginning after drug started; provide safety measures, including adequate lighting, use of side rails, and assistance with ambulation to protect client if CNS effects occur

f. For client with diabetes mellitus, use blood glucose monitoring or glucose enzymatic tests (Clinistix or TesTape) for urine glucose testing; false-positive urine glucose can occur with copper sulfate technique (Clinitest)

g. Offer small, frequent meals with quality protein as tolerated

h. Provide frequent oral care; offer ice chips or sugarless candy if stomatitis and sore mouth occur

i. Monitor for superinfections

1) Often subtle and nonspecific with clinical manifestations of oral or pharyngeal discomfort with oral candidiasis or perineal itching or discharge with vaginal candidiasis

2) Differentiate antibiotic diarrhea from pseudomembranous colitis; the latter is characterized by fever, abdominal cramping, at least 4 to 6 watery stools/day, stools with blood and/or mucus; send stool specimen culture for *Clostridium difficile*

j. Monitor for increased bleeding if taking anticoagulants

1) Assess for easy bruising or bleeding

2) If PT prolonged, give exogenous vitamin K

k. Monitor for hemolytic anemia (rare): check red blood cells (RBCs) with indices, tiredness or weakness, yellow skin or eyes; to observe for icterus in dark-skinned clients, check the hard palate

l. Monitor effectiveness of teaching plan/compliance and of comfort/safety measures

11. Client education

a. Know name, dose, purpose, take as prescribed with or without food, schedule regimen, possible side effects to ensure informed client and to promote compliance

b. Take safety precautions including changing position slowly and avoiding driving and hazardous tasks if CNS effects occur

c. Drink fluids and maintain nutrition, especially protein, to ensure adequate protein for drug binding and efficacy of action

d. Take complete course of treatment, which includes at least 2 days after resolution of clinical manifestations of infection, to enhance drug effectiveness and decrease risk of development of resistant strains of bacteria

e. Take around the clock at even intervals as possible without interrupting sleep in order to maintain therapeutic levels between doses

f. Discard any medication not taken after expiration date

g. Shake suspensions well to dispense or dissolve particles of drug immediately before measurement; use a measuring device for liquid/suspension and not a kitchen teaspoon (may vary from 2 to 10 mL/teaspoon)

NCLEX!

h. Report manifestations of hypersensitivity or superinfection to health care provider:

1) Difficulty breathing, severe rash, hives, severe headache, dizziness or weakness, aching joints

2) Severe diarrhea: call health care provider; mild diarrhea: may take absorbent anti-diarrheal agent; do not take anti-peristaltic agent that would promote retention of toxins, such as *C. difficile* in pseudomembranous colitis

3) Vaginal itching or discharge, sore mouth/throat, white patches on oral mucous membranes

i. Report side effects to the health care provider: anorexia, epigastric pain, nausea/vomiting indicating biliary sludge or pseudolithiasis if on ceftriaxone; discontinue drug and manifestations will resolve

NCLEX!

j. Refrain from alcohol during therapy and for 72 hours after drug discontinued to avoid disulfiram-like reaction

C. **Fluoroquinolones**

1. Action and use

a. Newest class of broad-spectrum bactericidal antibiotics

b. Used against gram-negative and selected gram-positive organisms; used in various bacterial infections depending on bacteria and site: lower respiratory tract infections, sinusitis, bone and joint infections, infectious diarrhea, UTIs, skin and soft tissue infections, intra-abdominal infections and sexually transmitted diseases

c. Many of the oral formulations are as effective as the parenteral forms

2. Common medications (Table 2-3)

3. Administration considerations

a. Administer around the clock evenly spaced and do not interrupt sleep, if possible, to maintain therapeutic blood level

b. Oral drug is tolerated better with food

Table 2-3	Generic/Trade Names	Usual Adult Dose	Administration Route
Fluoroquinolones	Ciprofloxacin (Cipro)	PO 250 mg q 12 h; IV 200 mg q 12 h infused over 60 min	PO, IV, Ophthalmic
	Enoxacin (Penetrex)	200–400 mg q 12 h for 7–14 d	PO
	Gatifloxacin (Tequin)	400 mg qd for 7–10 d	PO, IV
	Levofloxacin (Levaquin)	PO 500 mg q 24 h for 10 d; IV 500 mg infused over 60 min q 24 h for 7–14 d	PO, IV
	Lomefloxacin (Maxaquin)	400 mg qd for 10 d	PO
	Moxifloxacin (Avelox)	400 mg qd for 5–10 d	PO
	Norfloxacin (Noroxin)	400 mg bid	PO, Ophthalmic
	Ofloxacin (Floxin)	PO 200–400 mg q 12 h for 7–10 d; IV 400 mg q 12 h for 7 d	PO, IV, Otic, Ophthalmic
	Sparfloxacin (Zagam)	400 mg day 1 then 200 mg qd days 2–10	PO

4. Contraindications

    a. Known hypersensitivity to fluoroquinolones

    b. Caution in clients with renal dysfunction including those with advanced age, children, pregnant or lactating women; those with history of seizures

5. Significant drug interactions

    a. Oral antacids, iron, zinc preparations, and sucralfate reduce absorption

    b. Probenecid (Benemid) prolongs the half-life of fluoroquinolones

    c. The beta agonist effects of theophylline (TheoDur) may be increased; monitor clients with hypertension, ischemic heart disease, coronary insufficiency, congestive heart failure (CHF), or history of cerebrovascular accident (CVA or stroke)

    d. Cimetidine (Tagamet) may prolong half-life

    e. Cyclosporine (Sandimmune) increases risk of nephrotoxicity

    f. Glucocorticosteroids may increase risk for rupture of tendon

    g. Caffeine elimination with ciprofloxacin (Cipro), enoxacin (Penetrex), and norfloxacin (Noroxin) is decreased

    h. Use of ciprofloxacin with phenytoin (Dilantin) may lower levels of phenytoin

    i. Digoxin levels may increase with enoxacin

    j. Nitrofurantoin (Furadantin) may reduce the efficacy of norfloxacin

    k. Use of non-steroidal anti-inflammatory drugs (NSAIDs) with levofloxacin (Levaquin) increases CNS stimulation including seizures; levofloxacin may also increase or decrease blood glucose in conjunction with oral antidiabetic agents

    l. Risk of significant cardiovascular side effects may occur with use of certain cardiovascular agents and sparfloxacin (Zagam) or moxifloxacin (Avelox)

    m. Increased bleeding risk may occur with oral anticoagulants because the antibiotic alters intestinal flora and interferes with synthesis of vitamin K

6. Significant food interactions

    a. Limit alkaline foods that can alter pH of stomach and absorption

    b. Alkaline foods include dairy products, vegetables, and legumes

7. Significant laboratory studies

    a. Monitor ALT (SGPT), AST (SGOT), alkaline phosphatase, and bilirubin for elevation in liver toxicity

    b. Monitor for normalization of the WBC and other appropriate laboratory findings, such as cultures of infectious site, to evaluate therapy effectiveness

    c. Monitor PT and INR if on warfarin (Coumadin)

8. Side effects

    a. Headache, dizziness, fatigue, lethargy, insomnia, depression, restlessness, confusion, and convulsions

    b. Nausea, vomiting, diarrhea, constipation, flatulence, epigastric distress, oral candidiasis, dysphagia, pseudomembranous colitis; and elevated liver function tests, such as ALT, AST, bilirubin, and alkaline phosphatase

    c. Rash, pruritus, urticaria, photosensitivity, flushing

    d. Fever, chills, piloerection, blurred vision, tinnitus

9. Adverse effects/toxicity

    a. Superinfections: more common in prolonged therapy

    b. Hypersensitivity reaction

10. Nursing considerations

    a. Assure appropriate specimens have been sent for C & S prior to initiation of antibiotic therapy

    b. Check current medications for possible drug interactions

    c. Separate drug from oral antacids, iron and zinc salts, or sucralfate by 2 hours

    d. Monitor PT, INR, and manifestations of increased bleeding/bruising if also on oral anticoagulants

    e. Monitor renal function

    f. Provide more frequent meals with complete or complementary proteins to better ensure adequate albumin levels for drug efficacy

    g. Monitor for increased CNS irritability if client has history of epilepsy, ethanol abuse, or is concurrently taking theophylline

    h. Maintain hydration with 3 L fluid/day, if not contraindicated

11. Client education

    a. Know name, dose, schedule regimen, possible side effects to ensure knowledge about drug therapy and to promote compliance

    b. Take full course of antibiotic therapy to better ensure no regrowth of bacteria or evolution of resistance to the fluoroquinolones

    c. Take safety precautions including changing position slowly and avoiding driving and hazardous tasks if CNS effects occur

    d. Drink fluids and maintain nutrition, especially protein, to provide adequate protein for drug-binding and drug efficacy

    e. Report difficulty breathing, severe headache, dizziness, or weakness to health care provider

    f. May obtain baseline electrocardiogram if sparfloxacin or moxifloxacin given

    g. Do not take drugs with expired date; discard drug not used

    h. Teach to wear sunglasses, long-sleeves and long-legged garments, and hat to protect from direct sunlight; sunscreen or sunblock may not prevent photosensitivity reaction; avoid ultraviolet lights, tanning beds, and direct sunlight

D. Macrolides and lincosamides

1. Action and use

    a. Bacteriostatic (inhibiting the growth of bacteria) but can be bactericidal in high doses with some bacteria

b. Is highly protein-bound

c. Action is similar to other antibiotics

d. Is used in upper and lower respiratory tract infections, skin and soft tissue infections caused by *Streptococcus* or *Haemophilus* organisms

e. Used to treat syphilis, gonorrhea, chlamydia, Lyme disease, and *mycoplasma, listeria* and *corynebacterium* infections

f. Clarithromycin (Biaxin) is used with omeprazole (Prilosec) to treat *Helicobacter pylori* associated with peptic ulcers

g. Lincosamides may be bactericidal and bacteriostatic; used to treat chronic bone infections, genitourinary (GU) infections, intra-abdominal infections, pneumonia, and streptococcal or staphylococcal septicemia

2. Common medications (Table 2-4)

3. Administration considerations

NCLEX!

a. If erythromycin form has bitter taste, give with juice or applesauce

b. Give clindamycin (Cleocin) and lincomycin (Lincocin) with at least 8 ounces of fluid or on an empty stomach

c. If clindamycin (Cleocin) given IV, do not give by intravenous push (IVP) method; instead give by IV infusion

d. Zithromax: longer half-life with less frequent dosing, shorter term of therapy and has fewer or less intense GI side effects than others (may contribute to better compliance)

4. Contraindications

a. Hypersensitivity

b. Use caution with liver or renal dysfunction, GI disorders, the elderly, and pregnant or lactating women

c. Lincosamides are also contraindicated in ulcerative colitis/enteritis and children less 1 year of age

5. Significant drug interactions

a. Clindamycin and lincomycin: many drugs may be antagonistic, such as muscle relaxants, chloramphenicol (Chloromycetin), erythromycin, theophylline, antihistamines, penicillins, and oral anticoagulants

Table 2-4	Generic/Trade Names	Usual Adult Dose	Administration Route
Macrolides and Lincosamides	Azithromycin (Zithromax)	PO 500 mg on day 1 then 250 mg q 24 h for 4 more; IV 500 mg qd at least 2 d	PO, IV
	Clarithromycin (Biaxin)	250–500 mg bid for 10–14 d	PO
	Dirithromycin (Dynabac)	500 mg qd	PO
	Erythromycin (Erythrocin)	250–500 mg q 6 h; 333 mg q 8 h	PO, topical
	Troleandomycin (Tao)	250–500 mg q 6 h	PO
	Clindamycin (Cleocin)	PO 150–450 mg q 6 h; IM/IV 300–900 mg q 6–8 h (max 2,700 mg/d)	PO, IM, IV, topical
	Lincomycin (Lincocin)	500 mg q 6–8 h (max 8 g/d); IM 600 mg q 12–24 h; IV 600 mg–1 g q 8–12 h	PO, IM, IV

  b. Many drug interactions can occur when taken concurrently with the macrolides: carbamazepine (Tegretol), cyclosporine (Sandimmune), warfarin, and theophylline result in increased effects of these drugs

6. Significant food interactions: none reported

7. Significant laboratory studies

  a. Monitor WBC with differential to monitor therapeutic response

  b. Monitor for hepatotoxicity, e.g., ALT, AST, alkaline phosphatase, bilirubin elevations

  c. Monitor for nephrotoxicity, e.g., adverse changes in serum creatinine, BUN, creatinine clearance, urinalysis

8. Side effects

  a. Stimulation of smooth muscle and GI motility results in diarrhea (may be used therapeutically as a GI stimulant to facilitate passage of intestinal tube or to prevent gastroesophageal reflux)

  b. Palpitations and chest pain

  c. Headache, dizziness, vertigo, lethargy, somnolence, confusion, hearing loss usually preceded by tinnitus

  d. Stomatitis, flatulence, epigastric distress, anorexia, nausea, vomiting; abnormal taste (clarithromycin/Biaxin)

  e. Jaundice, rash, pruritis, urticaria

  f. Thrombophlebitis at peripheral intravenous site

9. Adverse effects/toxicity

  a. Hepatotoxicity

  b. Nephrotoxicity

  c. Ototoxicity: erythromycin (Erythrocin)

  d. Superinfections, e.g., pseudomembranous colitis, candidiasis

10. Nursing considerations

  a. Collect data such as age, hypersensitivity to drugs, hepatic and renal function; also check cardiac status if appropriate for drug ordered

  b. Ensure client takes complete course of antibiotic for full beneficial effects, even if clinical manifestations resolved; premature discontinuation can result in regrowth of organisms as well as development of drug resistance

  c. Collect specimen from infection site for C & S before initiating therapy, if possible

  d. Assess GI function and elimination pattern

  e. Observe for bleeding if taking oral anticoagulants

  f. Observe for superinfections

  g. Review OTC and, prescribed client medications for drug-drug interactions

    h. Monitor ALT, AST, bilirubin, and alkaline phosphatase as indicated for hepatic dysfunction prior to and during therapy

    i. Monitor serum creatinine, BUN, creatinine clearance, I & O as appropriate for development of renal dysfunction

    j. Assess baseline hearing and monitor for hearing loss; arrange for discontinuation of drug if occurs

    k. Hydrate with at least 2,000 to 2,400 mL/day if not contraindicated

11. Client education

    a. Know drug name, dose, route, purpose, schedule regimen, and whether to take with or without food

    b. Report signs and symptoms of increasing infection such as fever, pain, redness, drainage, edema, lethargy, or exacerbation of presenting manifestations

    c. Report signs and symptoms of superinfection

    d. Complete full course of treatment to prevent regrowth of bacteria or development of resistant strains

    e. Take as prescribed, including around the clock dosing at regular intervals but not interrupting sleep, to maintain therapeutic level of antibiotic

    f. Include protein in diet since these drugs are highly protein bound and need protein for therapeutic efficacy

    g. Discard any outdated or unused medications to ensure use of drugs with decreased potency or self-administration will not occur (decreases risk for drug resistance developing)

E. Monobactams

    1. Action and use

        a. Bactericidal against gram-negative rods

        b. *E. coli, K. pneumoniae, proteus species, enterobacter species* and *P. aeroginosa, N. Gonorrhoeae, H. influenza*

        c. Have similar activity as beta-lactam antibiotic (penicillins) and cephalosporins

        d. Used for urinary tract, lower respiratory tract, integumentary, intraabdominal, and gynecologic infections and septicemia

        e. Often used in combination with other anti-infectives to provide lower doses of each drug enhancing the therapeutic effect, decreasing degree of side effects, and decreasing risk for developing drug resistance

    2. Common medications (Table 2-5)

    3. Administration considerations: given IM or IV

    4. Contraindications: known hypersensitivity to aztreonam, penicillin, or cephalosporins

    5. Significant drug interactions: no significant interactions

    6. Significant food interactions: none reported

Table 2-5	Generic/Trade Names	Usual Adult Dose	Administration Route
Miscellaneous Antibiotics	Aztreonam (Azactam)	0.5–1 g q 8–12 h	IM, IV
	Imipenem/Cilastatin (Primaxin)	IV 250–500 mg infused over 20–30 min q 6–8 h up to 1 g; IM 500 or 750 mg q 12 h	IM, IV
	Meropenem (Merrem)	1 g q 8 h	IM, IV
	Quinupristin/dalfopristin (Synercid)	7.5 mg/kg q 8–12 h infused over 1 hour	IV
	Vancomycin (Vancocin)	IV 500 mg q 6 h or 1 g q 12 h infuse over 60–90 min; PO 125–500 mg q 6 h	PO, IV

7. Significant laboratory studies

   a. Monitor ALT, AST, bilirubin, and alkaline phosphatase for hepatotoxicity

   b. Monitor creatinine, creatinine clearance, and BUN for nephrotoxicity

   c. Monitor WBC with differential to monitor therapeutic effectiveness

8. Side effects

   a. Headache, dizziness, mental changes, paresthesias, insomnia, diplopia, seizures

   b. Tinnitus, nasal stuffiness, sneezing

   c. Nausea, vomiting, diarrhea

   d. Urticaria, purpura, rash, pruritus, phlebitis

9. Adverse effects/toxicity: hepatotoxicity, nephrotoxicity, eosinophilia, superinfections with gram-positive organisms

10. Nursing considerations

    a. Collect appropriate specimen for C & S, if possible, prior to initiating antibiotic to ensure appropriate drug employed; empiric therapy is usually begun before test results are available because of seriousness of infection

    b. Ensure client takes complete course of drug for full beneficial effects, even if clinical manifestations of infection resolved; premature discontinuation can result in regrowth of organisms as well as development of drug resistance

    c. Monitor laboratory results as noted earlier

    d. Arrange for dose adjustment or discontinuation if nephrotoxicity or hepatotoxicity develops

    e. Maintain nutritional status including positive nitrogen balance and good hydration

    f. Assess for allergies, adverse reactions, and effectiveness of client teaching

11. Client education: same as for penicillins/cephalosporins

F. **Miscellaneous antibiotics (Table 2-5)**

   1. Quinupristin/dalfopristin (Synercid)

      a. Action and use

         1) Two streptogramin antibacterials work synergistically

2) Used to treat bacteremia and life-threatening infections caused by *Enterococcus faecium* (VREF); also complicated skin/skin structure infections caused by *Staphylococcus aureus,* including vancomycin-resistant strains, and *Streptococcus pyogenes*

b. Administration considerations: IV use only, preferably via central line

c. Contraindications: known hypersensitivity to Synercid, pristinamycin or virginiamycin

d. Significant drug interactions: do not mix with other drugs

e. Significant food interactions: none reported

f. Significant laboratory studies

1) Monitor CBC with WBC and differential to monitor therapeutic effectiveness

2) Baseline, and as needed, liver and renal serum tests

g. Side effects: arthralgias, myalgias (possibly severe)

h. Adverse effects/toxicity: with peripheral IV administration, frequently pain, inflammation, edema, and thrombophlebitis

i. Nursing considerations: same as with other antibiotics

j. Client education: same as with other antibiotics

2. Vancomycin (Vancocin)

a. Action and use

1) Bactericidal

2) Mechanism different from other antibiotics

3) Antibiotic of choice for methicillin-resistant *Staphylococcus aureus* (MRSA) and other gram-positive bacteria, yeast, fungi

4) Oral: for antibiotic-induced pseudomembranous colitis caused by *Clostridium difficile* and for staphylococcal enterocolitis

5) IV: for bone and joint infections or septicemia caused by staphylococcal organisms

b. Administration considerations

1) Poorly absorbed from GI tract so oral therapy for treatment of local, surface infected areas of the GI tract

2) IV administration should be through a central venous access device because of drug's high propensity for causing phlebitis; can cause necrosis if it extravasates

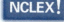

3) Increasing reports of resistance to enterococcus strains; concern about MRSA resistance developing; quinupristin/dalfopristin (Synercid) used in place of vancomycin sometimes to limit evolution of resistance to vancomycin

c. Contraindications

1) Known hypersensitivity

2) Caution in renal dysfunction, prior hearing loss, elderly, in pregnancy and lactation, and in neonates

3) IM administration

d. Significant drug interactions

1) Do not mix intravenously with other drugs

2) Increased risk of ototoxicity and nephrotoxicity when used with other drugs having potential for these toxicities

e. Significant food interactions: none reported

f. Significant laboratory studies

1) Serum creatinine, BUN, creatinine clearance, urinalysis (for casts in urine)

2) Peak and trough drug levels

3) ALT, AST, bilirubin, alkaline phosphatase

4) CBC with WBC and differential

5) Audiometry testing

g. Side effects

1) Nausea, hypotension, flushing

2) "Red neck (or man) syndrome": too rapid IV infusion results in profound hypotension, erythematous rash on face, neck, upper chest, and arms

3) Too rapid infusion can cause increased sense of warmth, nausea, and generalized tingling/paresthesia

4) Pain and thrombophlebitis at injection site

h. Adverse reactions/toxicity

1) Ototoxicity of auditory branch of the 8th cranial nerve; possible irreversible hearing loss; hearing loss may continue after discontinuation of drug

2) Nephrotoxicity with possible uremia

3) Hypersensitivity: anaphylaxis

4) Superinfections

5) Leukopenia/eosinophilia: temporary

i. Nursing considerations

1) Monitor baseline and regular lab results for early detection of toxicities

2) Ensure central venous access available

3) Assess baseline hearing; assess regularly for early detection of hearing loss, and tinnitus and loss of hearing high-pitched tones that may precede deafness

4) Record accurate I & O

5) Assess for improvement in clinical manifestations of infection

6) Monitor for side effects, particularly of too rapid administration

7) Monitor for hypotension and tachycardia during infusion

8) Collect appropriate specimen for C & S, if possible, prior to institution of vancomycin therapy to ensure appropriate drug employed

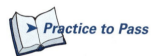

9) Ensure client takes complete course of drug for full beneficial effects

10) Consult with prescriber for dose adjustment or drug discontinuation if toxicities develop

11) Ensure adequate nutrition and hydration

12) Evaluate effectiveness of teaching plan

j. Client education

1) Know drug, dose, route, purpose, schedule regimen

2) Take full course of drug ordered

3) Keep appointments for laboratory testing, drug administrations at home when indicated, and follow-up visits with health care provider

4) If to receive IV therapy in home, ensure appropriate person's knowledge and ability to perform procedures correctly, including monitoring blood pressure (BP) and heart rate

5) Report ringing in ears or change in hearing

6) Report sore throat, watery stools more than 4 to 6 per day or if blood or mucus in stools, severe nausea, vomiting, change in color or consistency of urine, which may indicate superinfection or toxicity

3. Imipenem/cilastatin (Primaxin), meropenem (Merrem), ertapenem (Invanz)

a. Action and use

1) Classified as broad-spectrum carbapenems

2) May be used in serious infections of urinary tract, lower respiratory tract, bones, joints, skin/skin structures, intraabdominal, gynecologic, and mixed infections

3) Used in bacterial septicemia and endocarditis

4) Meropenem (Merrem) used in bacterial meningitis because of its ability to enter the CSF, especially if inflammation present

b. Administration considerations

1) If administering IM, inject deep IM into gluteal muscle

2) Caution: preparations are specific for IM or for IV use; do not interchange

3) Imipenem/cilastatin and ertapenem (Invanz) are not to be given IV push

c. Contraindications

1) In known hypersensitivities to components of drugs or penicillins or cephalosporins; also allergy to amide local anesthetics

2) Use caution in clients with CNS disorders, renal dysfunction, asthma, or in pregnancy and lactation

➤ Practice to Pass

The client states, "I don't know why the doctor wants me to have the vancomycin every 6 hours now instead of every 8 hours as I had been getting it. It seems as though I am so tied down." How do you respond?

        3) Imipenem/cilastatin: stable in dextrose-containing solutions only 4 hours; incompatible in Lactated Ringer's IV solution

   d. Significant drug interactions

        1) Aztreonam (Azactam), cephalosporins, penicillins may interfere with bactericidal action

        2) Synergistic effect with aminoglycosides against some strains of *Pseudomonas aeruginosa*

        3) Probenecid (Benemid) increases possibility of toxicity

   e. Significant food interactions: none reported

   f. Significant laboratory studies

        1) Electrolytes

        2) CBC including WBC with differential

        3) ALT, AST, bilirubin, alkaline phosphatase

        4) Serum creatinine, BUN, creatinine clearance

   g. Side effects

        1) Headache, dizziness, mental changes, somnolence, tremors, paresthesia

        2) Heartburn, nausea, vomiting, diarrhea, glossitis

        3) Rash, pruritis, urticaria, candidiasis, flushing, sweating, facial edema, fever, pain/phlebitis at injection site

        4) Drug fever

        5) Hyperkalemia, hyponatremia, polyuria, oliguria, weakness, arthralgias

   h. Adverse effects/toxicity

        1) CNS effects such as seizures, especially in elderly, with compromised renal function, or when concurrently taking ganciclovir (DHPG)

        2) Transient hearing loss

        3) Hypersensitivity reaction with fever, chills, dyspnea, chest discomfort, hyperventilation, pruritis

   i. Nursing considerations

NCLEX!

NCLEX!

        1) Assess allergies including to penicillin and cephalosporins and the amide local anesthetics

        2) Monitor for neurotoxicity, nephrotoxicity, hepatotoxicity, transient hearing loss; provide safety measures for seizures or other alterations in CNS function if appropriate

        3) Arrange for dose adjustment or discontinuation if adverse effects occur

        4) Observe for signs and symptoms of superinfections

        5) Monitor for clinical manifestations of electrolyte disturbances

        6) Collect appropriate specimen for C & S, if possible, prior to starting the drug to ensure appropriate drug employed

7) Ensure full drug regimen completed to enhance therapeutic effects, decrease risks of reinfection and drug resistance

8) Ensure good nutrition and hydration

9) Evaluate effectiveness of teaching plan

j. Client education

1) Know drug, dose, purpose, route, schedule regimen

2) Take full course of drug ordered

3) Take safety precautions, especially if CNS side effects occur

4) Eat small frequent meals with high quality protein

5) Drink at least 6 to 8 glasses of fluids a day

6) If parenteral therapy will be given at home, ensure proper person is knowledgeable about drug, is able to manage the venous access device maintaining sterile technique, and is able to perform procedure correctly

7) Keep appointments for lab testing and for follow-up with health care provider

G. Penicillins (beta-lactams) and penicillinase-resistants

1. Action and use

a. Beta-lactams are chemical structure of penicillins

b. Derived from fungus or mold evidenced on bread or fruit

c. There is similarity among penicillins, cephalosporins, monobactams, carbapenems, and beta-lactamase inhibitors; they share many of the same actions and uses; cross-sensitivity is possible

d. Penicillin is least toxic of these drugs; usually is the antibiotic of choice because of low toxicity potential in non-allergic client

e. Bactericidal; bacteriostatic effect with adequate dosing/blood levels

f. Increased efficacy during replication of the bacterial cells

g. Only cross blood-brain barrier if meningeal inflammation present

h. Most effective against gram-positive organisms; less effective against gram-negative organisms

i. Used to treat infections caused by meningococci, pneumococci, streptococci, treponema pallidum, staphylococci as in upper respiratory infections, pneumonia, STDs such as syphilis but not gonorrhea, wound infections, and urinary tract infections

j. Used prophylactically against endocarditis for oral, GI, pulmonary procedures when bacteria may enter circulation; usually amoxicillin (Amoxil) or ampicillin (Omnipen) are used

k. Used in beta-hemolytic streptococci Group A infections that can be associated with rheumatic fever or acute glomerulonephritis, such as pharyngitis; penicillin V (V-Cillin); PO route preferred

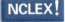

l. Increasing resistance developing, especially in facility-acquired or nosocomial infections

m. Gonorrhea mostly resistant to penicillins

n. *Streptococcus pneumoniae* most frequent microorganism in otitis media and sinusitis; increased resistance to penicillins, tetracyclines, macrolides, and sulfonamides

2. Common medications (Table 2-6)

   a. Penicillins: penicillin G benzathine (Bicillin), penicillin G potassium (Pfizerpen), penicillin G (Pentids), penicillin V (Beepen VK)

   b. Extended spectrum penicillins: ampicillin (Omnipen), amoxicillin (Amoxil), carbenicillin (Geopen), mezlocillin (Mezlin), piperacillin (Pipracil), ticarcillin (Ticar)

   c. Penicillinase-resistant penicillins: bacampicillin (Spectrobid), cloxacillin (Apo-Cloxi), methicillin (Staphcillin), nafcillin (Unipen), oxacillin (Bactocil)

3. Administration considerations

   a. Oral dosing needs to be 3 to 4 times the parenteral dose because of the hepatic first-pass effect and the instability of penicillin in the acid environment of the stomach

   b. For serious systemic infections, parenteral route is recommended

   c. Absorption erratic from IM route; limit due to irritability of tissue; IM injection should be slow and steady over 12 to 15 seconds to minimize discomfort and prevent obstructing the needle, especially with thick preparations

   d. Nafcillin (Unipen): IV extravasation can cause necrosis; avoid IM or, if not possible, inject by Z-tract method

4. Contraindications

   a. Not for use in hypersensitivity reaction and anaphylaxis, serum sickness, exfoliative dermatitis, blood dyscrasias

Table 2-6	Generic/Trade Names	Usual Adult Dose	Administration Route
Penicillins (Beta-lactams) and Penicillinase-Resistants	Amoxicillin (Amoxil)	250–500 mg q 8 h	PO
	Ampicillin (Omnipen)	PO 250–500 mg q 6 h; IM/IV 250 mg–2 g q 6 h	PO, IM, IV
	Bacampicillin (Spectrobid)	400–800 mg q 12 h	PO
	Piperacillin (Pipracil)	8–16 g/d divided q 6–8 h	IM, IV
	Ticarcillin (Ticar)	200 mg/kg/d in 4 divided doses or 1–2 g q 6 h	IM, IV
	Carbenicillin (Geopen)	382–764 mg q 6 h for 10 d	PO
	Mezlocillin (Mezlin)	1.5–2 g q 6 h	IM, IV
	Cloxacillin (Apo-Cloxi)	250–500 mg q 6 h	PO
	Methicillin (Staphcillin)	1–2 g q 4–6 h up to 12 g/d	IM, IV
	Nafcillin (Unipen)	IM/IV 500 mg–2 g q 4–6 h up to 12 g/d; PO 250–1000 mg q 4–6 h	PO, IM, IV
	Oxacillin (Bactocil)	IM/IV 500 mg–2 g q 4–6 h up to 12 g/d; PO 250–1000 mg q 4–6 h	PO, IM, IV
	Penicillin G (Pentids)	PO 1.6–3.2 million U divided q 6 h; IV/IM 1.2–2.4 million U divided q 4 h	PO, IM, IV
	Penicillin V (V-Cillin)	125–500 mg q 6 h	PO

    b. Penicillin G procaine or benzathine not to be given IV: lethal

    c. Most likely drug category to cause allergic reactions

    d. Use caution in anemia, thrombocytopenia, bone marrow depression and concurrently with anticoagulants because some penicillins cause increased bleeding

5. Significant drug interactions

    a. Loop and thiazide diuretics may exacerbate hypokalemia and rash

    b. Potassium-sparing diuretics may contribute to hyperkalemia

    c. Decreased efficacy of oral contraceptives

    d. Probenecid (Benemid) delays excretions and increases serum levels

    e. Avoid co-administration with tetracycline because it may interfere with effectiveness of penicillins

    f. Atenolol (Tenormin) levels may be decreased when given with ampicillin (Omnipen); increased risk for anaphylaxis

    g. Allopurinol (Zyloprim) increases risk for rash

    h. Mezlocillin (Mexlin) and piperacillin (Pipracil) may alter elimination of lithium

    i. Nafcillin (Unipen) may cause lowered levels of cyclosporine (Sandimmune)

    j. Aspirin, phenylbutazone (ibuprofen-like), sulfonamides, furosemide, thiazide diuretics, and indomethacin prolong half-life of penicillin-G (Pentids)

6. Significant food interactions

    a. Take on empty stomach

    b. Amoxicillin not affected by food

7. Significant laboratory studies

    a. CBC with WBC/differential

    b. PT/INR if on oral anticoagulants; APPT if on parenteral anticoagulants

    c. ALT, AST, bilirubin, alkaline phosphatase

    d. Electrolytes, especially potassium and sodium

8. Side effects

    a. Most common allergic responses are skin rash, urticaria, pruritis, angioedema; a maculopapular, pruritic rash that is like measles with ampicillin or amoxocillin is not a true allergic reaction, but develops after 7 to 10 days of therapy and may last few days after discontinuation of PCN; is not a contraindication to give drug in the future

    b. Most common adverse effects are GI, such as nausea, vomiting, diarrhea, epigastric distress, abdominal pain, colitis, elevated liver enzymes; also taste alteration, sore mouth, or dark/discolored/sore tongue

    c. Anemia, bone marrow suppression, granulocytopenia, increased bleeding time

NCLEX!

NCLEX!

NCLEX!

NCLEX!

NCLEX!

NCLEX!

    d. Lethargy, anxiety, depression, hallucinations, twitching, convulsions, coma

    e. Hypokalemia or hyperkalemia, metabolic alkalosis

9. Adverse effects/toxicity

    a. Type I hypersensitivity often fatal immediately if untreated within 2 to 30 minutes

        1) Nausea, vomiting

        2) Urticaria, pruritis

        3) Severe dyspnea, stridor, tachycardia, hypotension

        4) Diaphoresis, vertigo, loss of consciousness/circulatory collapse

    b. Serum sickness–like reaction: skin rash, arthralgia, fever

    c. Exfoliative dermatitis: red, scaly skin

    d. Blood dyscrasias: hemolytic anemia, neutropenia, leukopenia

    e. Superinfections with broader-spectrum penicillins, especially with prolonged therapy; pseudomembranous colitis possible up to several weeks after drug discontinued; treated with anti-infectives such as Flagyl PO or IV or vancomycin PO

10. Nursing considerations

    a. Assess for allergies/hypersensitivity history

    b. Assess all medications taken to avoid drug-drug interaction

    c. Collect appropriate specimen for C & S, if possible, prior to initiating antibiotic therapy to ensure appropriate drug employed; empiric therapy is usually begun before test results available because of seriousness of infection

    d. Ensure client takes complete course of antibiotic for full beneficial effects, even if clinical manifestations of infection resolve; premature discontinuation can result in regrowth of organisms as well as development of drug resistance

    e. Monitor renal studies, liver enzymes, and electrolytes; many of the penicillins contain sodium salts that can result in hypokalemia

    f. Arrange for dose/drug adjustment as indicated by lab results

    g. Monitor for evidence of clinical improvement of infection

    h. Monitor for adverse effects; may not be necessary to discontinue PCN if mild diarrhea develops; give yogurt or buttermilk to restore normal flora; use absorbent anti-diarrheal agents (Kaolin and Pectin/Kao-tin); avoid antiperistaltic agents that delay or prevent elimination of intestinal toxins

    i. Provide good nutrition and hydration

    j. Some penicillins cause false-positive results on urine glucose testing; use Clinistix, or Testape for glucose urine testing or use blood glucose monitoring

    k. Evaluate effectiveness of teaching plan

11. Client education

    a. Know drug, dose, purpose, route, and schedule regimen for improved compliance

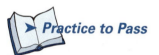

NCLEX!

b. Take full course of drug ordered to avoid regrowth of bacteria or development of drug resistance; take at regular intervals around the clock, as long as sleep not disrupted, in order to maintain therapeutic levels

c. Take oral drug on empty stomach; take 1 hour before meals or 2 hours after meals, except amoxicillin (which is not affected by food)

NCLEX!

NCLEX!

d. Chewable tablets must be crushed or chewed in order for the penicillin to be effectively absorbed

e. Shake suspensions to disperse particles prior to measurement; use a calibrated device to measure liquid since kitchen teaspoons may vary by 2 to 10 mL; most suspensions maintain potency for 14 days if refrigerated

f. Ensure antibiotic drops used for correct route, i.e., oral, eye, ear

NCLEX!

g. Take missed doses as soon as possible; do not take a double dose at the next administration time

h. Report rash, urticaria, pruritis, difficulty breathing

i. Report sore throat, watery stools equal to or greater than 4 to 6 stools/day or stools with blood/mucus, severe nausea, vomiting, unusual bleeding or bruising

j. Discard any outdated or unused medication to ensure drugs with decreased potency will not be used for self-administration, which could adversely affect future treatment and increase risk for developing drug resistance

k. Before taking any OTC drugs, check with health care provider

l. Take small frequent meals with high-quality protein and drink equal to or greater than 6 to 8 glasses of water per day, if not contraindicated by other conditions

H. Sulfonamides

1. Action and use

a. First effective group of antibiotics (1935)

b. Bacteriostatic

c. Used to treat urinary tract infections (especially caused by *Escherichia coli,* the most common cause of cystitis), *Chlamydia trachomatis* causing blindness, pneumonia, brain abscesses, mild to moderate ulcerative colitis, active Crohn's disease, and rheumatoid arthritis; with pyrimethamine as only effective drug treatment for toxoplasmosis; drugs of choice for treatment of nocardiosis

d. Sulfacetamide (silver sulfadiazine) to prevent bacterial growth in burns and wounds

e. Cross-sensitivity possible with penicillins and cephalosporins

2. Common medications (Table 2-7)

3. Administration considerations

NCLEX!

a. Fluid intake should be 3,000 to 4,000 mL/day to promote urinary output at least 1,500 mL/day to prevent crystalluria/stone formation; if not possible,

Practice to Pass

The client taking an antibiotic develops diarrhea. What assessments and interventions would you perform?

Table 2-7	Generic/Trade Names	Usual Adult Dose	Administration Route
Sulfonamides	Sulfisoxazole (Gantrisin)	2–8 g/d in 4–6 divided doses	PO, vaginal
	Sulfadiazine (Microsulfon)	2–4 g/d in 4–6 divided doses	PO
	Sulfamethoxazole–Trimethoprim (Bactrim)	160 mg TMP/800 mg SMZ q 12 h; IV 8–10 mg/kg/d q 6–12 h infused over 60–90 min	PO, IM, IV
	Sulfasalazine (Azulfidine)	1–2 g/d in 4 divided doses up to 8 g/d	PO

may administer antacids or sodium bicarbonate to alkalinize urine; alkaline ash diet may be helpful, which includes fruit (except plums, prunes, and cranberries), vegetables, and milk

   b. Store in light-resistant, tightly closed container at room temperature

4. Contraindications

   a. History of hypersensitity to sulfonamindes, salicylates, penicillins, cephalosporins

   b. In lactation and in children younger than 2 months unless used to treat congenital toxoplasmosis

   c. In porphyria, advanced or severe renal or hepatic dysfunction, or with intestinal and urinary blockage; use with caution in impaired renal or hepatic function, asthma, blood dyscrasias, or G6PD deficiency

5. Significant drug interactions

   a. Increased risk for bleeding with oral anticoagulants

   b. Increased drop in blood glucose with oral hypoglycemic agents

   c. Increased risk for phenytoin toxicity with phenytoin (Dilantin)

   d. Trimethoprim and sulfamethoxazole (Bactrim): combines sulfonamide with folic acid antagonist; increases synergistic effect

   e. Iron and some antibiotics may interfere with absorption of sulfonamide, such as sulfasalazine (Azulfidine)

6. Significant food interactions

   a. Some drugs, such as sulfamethoxazole (Gantanol), may be crushed and taken with liquids of choice

   b. Some, such as sulfasalazine, are best taken after meals to prolong time in intestine

7. Significant laboratory studies

   a. Creatinine, BUN, creatinine clearance, urinalysis to monitor renal function

   b. ALT, AST, bilirubin, alkaline phosphatase to monitor hepatic function

   c. CBC to monitor for blood dyscrasias and response to therapy

8. Side effects

   a. Rash common; most are urticaria and maculopapular

   b. Nausea, vomiting, diarrhea, abdominal pain, jaundice, stomatitis

      c. Headache, insomnia, drowsiness, depression, psychosis

      d. Photosensitivity

      e. Crystalluria

  9. Adverse effects/toxicity

      a. Peripheral neuritis/neuropathy

      b. Tinnitus, hearing loss, vertigo

      c. Ataxia, convulsions

      d. Hepatitis, pancreatitis

      e. Anemia, agranulocytosis, thrombocytopenia, leucopenia, eosinophilia, prothrombinemia

      f. Exfoliative dermatitis, **Stevens-Johnson syndrome** (an adverse reaction of skin that resembles appearance of the 2nd degree burns)

      g. Serum sickness, drug fever

  10. Nursing considerations

      a. Collect appropriate specimen for C & S, if possible, prior to beginning therapy to ensure appropriate drug employed; empiric treatment is usually begun before test results are available because of seriousness of infection

      b. Assess for allergies/history of hypersensitivity

      c. Assess drugs being taken to avoid drug-drug interaction

      d. Assess baseline laboratory findings for liver and renal function and monitor during therapy

      e. Provide hydration to assure daily urinary output of equal or greater than 1,500 mL to prevent stone and crystal formations; alkalinize urine as indicated; keep accurate I & O record

      f. Consult prescriber for dose adjustment or discontinuation of drug if toxicities develop

      g. Provide for safety if neurotoxicities develop, such as ataxia or convulsions

      h. Provide small frequent, nutritious meals with high quality proteins; drugs that may be taken with food may decrease GI upset

      i. Ensure client takes complete course of sulfonamides for full beneficial effects, even if clinical manifestations of infection resolved; premature discontinuation can result in regrowth of organisms as well as development of drug resistance

      j. Assess for clinical improvement, adverse effects, and effectiveness of client education

  11. Client education

      a. Know drug, dose, purpose, route, schedule regimen

      b. Take full course of sulfonamide therapy as ordered

c. Take at evenly spaced intervals around the clock without disrupting sleep to maintain serum levels

d. Take safety precautions if client experiences vertigo, ataxia, seizures

e. Avoid driving or performing hazardous tasks if drowsiness occurs

f. Take with food, if not contraindicated, to minimize GI upset

g. Eat small, frequent meals with at least 2,500 to 3,000 mL fluid intake a day

h. Empty bladder frequently, at least every 2 hours while awake

i. Report flank/suprapubic pain, increased dysuria, disruption of skin integrity to health care provider

j. Discard any outdated or unused medication to deter self-administration of drugs with decreased potency, which could adversely affect future treatment and increase risk for developing drug resistance

I. Urinary tract antiseptics

1. Action and use

   a. Drugs that act against bacteria in the urine but have little or no systemic antibacterial effects

   b. Used for UTIs only

2. Common medications (Table 2-8)

3. Administration considerations: shake suspensions well just prior to measuring with a calibrated device (household teaspoons may vary by 2 to 10 mL)

4. Contraindications

   a. Methenamine hippurate (Hiprex): avoid concurrent use of drugs that could alkalinize the urine and interfere with effectiveness of methenamine hippurate, e.g., antacids, carbonic anhydrase inhibitors, citrates, sodium bicarbonate, thiazide diuretics

   b. Sulfamethizole (Thiosulfil Forte): increased risk for crystalluria

   c. Caution with nitrofurantoin (Furadantin): can increase neurotoxicity in clients with neurological disorders such as peripheral neuropathy and seizures, and can cause pulmonary reaction in clients with pulmonary conditions

   d. Use caution in clients with impaired renal and/or hepatic function

   e. Use caution during lactation and pregnancy

Table 2-8	Generic/Trade Names	Usual Adult Dose	Administration Route
Urinary Tract Antiseptics	Cinoxacin (Cinobac)	1 g/d in 2–4 divided doses	PO
	Methenamine mandelate (Mandelamine)	1 g qid	PO
	Methenamine hippurate (Hiprex)	1 g bid	PO
	Nalidixic acid (NegGram)	Acute therapy 1 g qid; chronic therapy 500 mg qid	PO
	Nitrofurantoin (Furadantin)	50–100 mg qid	PO

5. Significant drug interactions

   a. See contraindications listed above

   b. Probenecid (Benemid): may increase risk for toxicity with sulfinpyrazone; decreased urinary tract effectiveness may occur with nitrofurantoin

6. Significant food interactions

   a. Controversial if pH of urine has any effect on UTI

   b. Alkaline ash diet may interfere with the required acidity of the urine for antiseptic action; alkaline ash foods include fruits (except cranberries, prunes, plums), milk, vegetables

   c. Acid ash foods that may or may not increase urine acidity include meat, cheese, eggs, whole grains as well as cranberries, prunes, and plums

   d. Fluids that may acidify the urine and potentially facilitate the action of the drugs include cranberry or prune juice

7. Significant laboratory studies

   a. Urinalysis and urine C & S: baseline and repeated regularly

   b. CBC with WBC and differential

   c. Baseline ALT, AST, alkaline phosphatase, and bilirubin; repeat as necessary

   d. Baseline creatinine, BUN, creatinine clearance; repeat as needed

   e. Pulmonary tests with nitrofurantoin

8. Side effects: (do not commonly occur)

   a. Nausea, vomiting, anorexia, diarrhea, epigastric distress

   b. Rash, pruritus, photosensitivity, photophobia, tinnitus, insomnia, headache, dizziness, drowsiness

   c. Low back pain, dysuria

   d. Nitrofurantoin: urine may become brown

9. Adverse effects/toxicity: see contraindications and significant drug interactions sections above

10. Nursing considerations

    a. Review client history for allergies, previous renal or liver dysfunction

    b. Assess current drugs being taken to avoid drug interactions

    c. Ensure the client takes the full course of treatment for optimal benefit and to deter risk for development of drug resistance

    d. Discard any unused or outdated drug to ensure drug not taken with decreased potency or self-treatment will not occur in future infections

    e. Monitor for evidence of drug effectiveness

       1) Upper urinary tract infection or pyelonephritis: resolution of pain in lower back, flank, epigastric area, fever, diaphoresis, piloerection, nausea, vomiting, headache, generalized weakness

2) Lower urinary tract infection or cystitis: resolution of urinary urgency, burning, frequency and of suprapubic discomfort; improvement in increasing the amounts of urine on voiding; resolution of incontinence if occurs

3) Resolution of hematuria and pyuria

4) No red or white blood cells, no casts, protein, crystals or bacteria in urine

5) Normalization of CBC with WBC differential

f. Monitor for clinical manifestations of adverse effects

g. Encourage at least 3,000 mL/day fluids, including cranberry juice if not contraindicated by fluid restriction, diabetes mellitus, or other conditions

h. Monitor urine pH at bedside with test strip as indicated

i. Give medication with or after food to limit GI adverse effects

11. Client education

a. Know drug, name, dose, purpose, schedule regimen

b. Take as prescribed around the clock at evenly spaced intervals, without disrupting sleep, in order to maintain therapeutic level

c. Take full course of treatment to optimize benefits of drug and to decrease risk of development of drug resistance

d. Take with or after food to minimize GI distress

e. Drink at least 3 liters of fluid a day including cranberry and prune juice unless contraindicated by other conditions

f. Include acid ash foods in diet, such as cranberries, prunes, plums, cheese, eggs, meat, whole grains; limit or avoid alkaline ash foods, such as citrus fruits and juices, vegetables

g. Do not take other medications unless approved by the prescriber; avoid drugs that may alkalinize the urine, such as antacids, Alka-Seltzer,™ sodium bicarbonate (baking soda)

h. Report to the health care provider if improvement not noted in 2 to 3 days or if severe adverse effects occur

i. Nalidixic acid (NegGram) can cause photophobia, and client should avoid bright sunlight, wear sunglasses, and report any visual disturbances; photosensitivity can also occur several weeks after drug is discontinued so client should avoid direct sunlight or ultraviolet light

j. Nitrofurantoin may cause urine to be brown; may stain

k. Do not drive or perform hazardous tasks if drowsiness or dizziness occurs

l. If diabetic, urine testing for glucose with Clinitest can yield a false-positive result; use TesTape, Clinistix, or Diastix for urine glucose testing or test blood glucose

J. Tetracyclines

1. Action and use

a. Broad spectrum; bacteriostatic; can be bactericidal in high concentrations

    b. Effective against most chlamydia, mycoplasmas, rickettsiae, cholera, and certain protozoa

    c. Suppress *Proprionibacteriium acnes* in treating acne; topical application may be as effective as oral preparation for acne; both forms may be used for severe acne

    d. Used prophylactically for traveler's diarrhea

    e. Used to treat Rocky Mountain Spotted Fever, **amebiasis** (a protozoan infection), brucellosis, shigellosis, cholera, tetanus, chronic bronchitis, Lyme disease

    f. If PCN-allergy, used to treat syphilis and gonorrhea

    g. Used as a sclerosing agent for pleural and pericardial effusion, such as in metastasis of cancer; causes inflammation resulting in fibrosis, leaving scar tissue that does not allow fluid to accumulate

    h. Used in *Helicobacter pylori* peptic ulcer disease, Q fever, Rickettsia pox, typhus, Mycoplasma pneumonia, epididymo-orchitis, pelvic inflammatory disease (PID)

    i. Used with quinine for treatment of malaria

    j. Anti-infective prophylaxis for rape victims

    k. Treat syndrome of inappropriate antidiuretic hormone (SIADH) with demeclocyline (Declomycin) by inhibiting antidiuretic hormone (ADH)

2. Common medications (generic name ends in "-cycline"; Table 2-9)

3. Administration considerations

    a. Avoid administering outdated drug: Fanconi-like syndrome with polyuria, polydipsia, nausea/vomiting, glycosuria, proteinuria, acidosis can occur; renal tubular dysfunction and lupus-erythematosis-like syndrome have occurred and are attributed to preparations used beyond expiration date

    b. Oral: give with full glass of water on empty stomach at least 1 hour before or 2 hours after meals; food, milk, and milk products decrease absorption by one-half

    c. Shake oral suspension well to distribute particles

    d. Use calibrated measuring device (kitchen teaspoon can vary by 2 to 10 mL)

Table 2-9	**Generic/Trade Names**	**Usual Adult Dose**	**Administration Route**
Tetracyclines	Demeclocycline (Declomycin)	150 mg q 6 h or 300 mg q 12 h	PO
	Oxytetracycline (Terramycin)	PO 250–500 mg q 6–12 h; IM 100 mg q 8–12 h; IV 250–500 mg q 12 h	PO, IM, IV
	Tetracycline (Achromycin)	250–500 mg bid–qid; IM 250 mg QD or 300 mg/d in 2–3 divided doses	PO, IM, topical
	Doxycycline (Vibramycin)	100 mg q 12 h on day 1, then 100 mg/d as single dose up to 100 mg q 12 h	PO, IV
	Minocycline (Minocin)	200 mg followed by 100 mg q 12 h	PO, IV

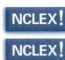

e. IM injection contains procaine so assess for allergies to local anesthetics ending with "-caine"

f. Administer deep IM into large muscle as the gluteus; alternate sites

g. If topical, clean area with soap and water, rinse and dry well prior to application

h. Not to be administered IV

4. Contraindications

   a. Hypersensitivity to tetracyclines

   b. Severe renal or hepatic dysfunction

   c. Tetracyclines bind to calcium, preventing normal bone growth and causing tooth hypoplasia in developing fetus or child younger than 8 years old; contraindicated during last half of pregnancy when tooth development occurs, from birth to 8 years of age, and in lactating women

   d. Use caution with history of renal or liver dysfunction, allergy, asthma, hay fever, urticaria, or in myasthenia gravis

   e. Use caution with concurrent use of oral anticoagulants

   f. Tetracyclines may antagonize other antibiotics, see product literature

5. Significant drug interactions

   a. Antacids and antidiarrheal agents with kaolin and pectin decrease absorption

   b. Oral anticoagulants potentiate hypoprothrombinemia

   c. Decreased effectiveness of oral contraceptives

   d. Increased effect against brain abscess with sulfonamide

   e. Decreased effect of penicillin

   f. Increased or decreased level of digoxin (Lanoxin) depending on specific tetracycline

   g. Can cause fatal nephrotoxicity with methoxyflurane, an anesthetic

6. Significant food interactions

   a. Milk and dairy products and iron supplements interfere with absorption

   b. Take on empty stomach

7. Significant laboratory studies

   a. Obtain C & S of infection site prior to initiation of drug therapy; obtain follow-up culture from gonoccocal infection site 3 to 7 days after end of drug treatment to ensure elimination of infection, or culture from other sites if improvement not observed

   b. Baseline and periodic renal function tests: serum creatinine, BUN, creatinine clearance, urinalysis

   c. Baseline and periodic hepatic function tests: ALT, AST, alkaline phosphatase, bilirubin

    d. CBC including WBC with differential to monitor response to therapy (decreased WBC), to check for thrombocytopenia, and for hemolytic anemia

8. Side effects

    a. Nausea, vomiting, diarrhea, epigastric distress, abdominal discomfort, flatulence, dry mouth, dysphagia, bulky/loose stools, steatorrhea

    b. Headache, photosensitivity, increased intracranial pressure (rare)

    c. Maculopapular rash, urticaria, exfoliative dermatitis, angioedema

    d. Stinging/burning with topical application

    e. Discoloration of developing teeth

    f. Pigmentation of conjunctiva related to drug deposits

    g. Discoloration and loosening of nails

    h. Retrosternal pain

9. Adverse effects/toxicity

    a. Elevated liver function tests and decreased cholesterol level

    b. Drug fever, serum sickness, and anaphylaxis

    c. Hepatotoxicity, pancreatitis, nephrotoxicity

    d. Blood dyscrasias such as thrombocytopenia, hemolytic anemia

    e. Superinfections: increased risk for candidiasis in clients taking oral contraceptives, with diabetes mellitus, leukemia, systemic lupus erythematosis (SLE); stomatitis, glossitis, black hairy tongue (lingua nigra), and pseudomembranous colitis possible

    f. Fatty degeneration of liver results in jaundice, azotemia, increased nitrogen retention, hyperphosphatemia, and metabolic acidosis

    g. Topicycline topical application can cause itching, wheezing, anaphylaxis in client with asthma allergies

10. Nursing considerations

    a. Collect C & S specimen from infection site prior to initiation of drug therapy, if possible; re-check C & S 3 to 7 days after therapy completed for gonococcal infection to assure infection eradicated or culture other infected sites if improvement not observed

    b. Assess for history of renal/liver problems and related laboratory results

    c. Assess history of immunosuppression

    d. Check CBC including WBC with differential, RBC indices, and platelet count

    e. Assess other medications being taken to avoid drug-drug interactions

    f. Collaborate with prescriber regarding dosage or drug change if indicated by adverse effects

    g. Observe for superinfections such as candidiasis and pseudomembranous colitis; consult prescriber for discontinuation of drug if they occur

    h. Monitor I & O

    i. Check IM injection sites every day for induration, redness, edema

11. Client education

a. Know drug name, dose, purpose, and schedule regimen (taken at evenly spaced intervals around the clock, without disrupting sleep, in order to maintain therapeutic serum level)

b. Complete full course of treatment to avoid recurrence or progression of infection and to reduce risk of developing drug resistance

c. Discard any expired or unused drug to avoid using drug with decreased potency or self-treatment of future infections, adversely affecting therapeutic value and increasing risk for drug resistance

d. Unstable with age and light exposure; store in tightly covered container in dry area, protected from light at room temperature

e. Report side effects, particularly severe diarrhea

f. Practice good oral care and hygiene

g. Avoid exposure to direct sunlight or ultraviolet light or tanning beds; wear hat, long sleeves, long-leg pants, and sunglasses outside during and for a few days after treatment; sunscreen or sunblock may not prevent erythema

h. If on long-term treatment, report onset of severe headache or visual disturbances that may indicate increased intracranial pressure (rare); requires discontinuation of tetracycline to prevent irreversible vision loss

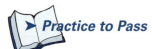

i. Take oral doses with full glass of water on empty stomach (1 hour before or 2 hours after meal or dairy product) to promote absorption and decrease risk of esophagitis; report sudden dysphagia to health care provider

j. Topical form may stain clothing

k. Topical application can cause affected skin to reflect yellow or green fluorescence under an ultraviolet or "black" light

II. Antimycobacterials

A. Antituberculins

1. Action and use

a. Inhibit cell wall synthesis, protein synthesis, RNA synthesis

b. Effects limited primarily to *Mycobacterium tuberculosis* and then certain other mycobacterium strains

c. Prophylaxis or treatment of pulmonary tuberculosis

d. Extrapulmonary tuberculosis in adults and children

e. Often used in combination with other antituberculin agents

f. Used to prevent or delay onset of *Mycobacterium avium* bacteremia in clients with advanced human immunodeficiency virus (HIV); in combination with other antituberculin antibiotic

g. Rifampin eradicates meningococci from nasopharynx of asymptomatic *Neisseria meningitides* carriers when there is increased risk for infection outbreaks among a community

➤ Practice to Pass

Tetracycline capsules have been prescribed for an 18-year-old female client to treat acne. What specific teaching would you include on the client education plan?

NCLEX!

h. Rifampin is used prophylactically with exposure to *Haemophilus influenzae* type B (hib) infection

i. Antituberculins are used in combination to treat leprosy

j. Used to treat endocarditis with methicillin-resistant staphylococci, chronic prostatitis with staphylococcal organisms, and antiinfective-resistant pneumococci

k. Used as combination treatment for mycobacterial infections including tuberculosis

NCLEX!

l. Effective treatment requires compliance and therapy over months to years

2. Common medications (Table 2-10)

3. Administration considerations

a. Effectiveness depends on correct drug, correct combination therapy, adequate dosing, adequate duration of therapy, and compliance

NCLEX!

b. Empiric treatment is initiated with isoniazid, rifampin, pyrazinamide, and ethambutol (Etibi) or streptomycin

NCLEX!

c. Multi-combination drug therapy decreases risk or rate of developing resistance to any single drug

d. Give isoniazid one 1 hour before meals on empty stomach

NCLEX!

e. Give clofazimine (Lamprene) with meals

4. Contraindications

a. Hypersensitivity to drug

b. Hepatic or renal damage

c. Variable by specified drug: caution in pregnancy unless risk is significant

d. Caution in renal or liver dysfunction, history of seizures, ethanol abuse

Table 2-10

Antituberculins

Generic/Trade Names	Usual Adult Dose	Administration Route
Capreomycin (Capostat sulfate)	1 g/d for 60–120 d	IM
Clofazimine (Lamprene)	100 mg/d in combination with 1 or more antileprosy drugs for 3 yrs, then 100 mg/d as monotherapy	PO
Ethambutol HCL (Myambutol)	15 mg/kg q 24 h	PO
Ethionamide (Trecator-SC)	0.5–1 g/d divided q 8–12 h	PO
Isoniazid (INH)	5 mg/kg up to 300 mg/d	PO, IM
Pyrazinamide (Tebrazid)	15–35 mg/kg/d in 3–4 divided doses	PO
Rifampin (Rifadin)	600 mg qd in conjunction with other antituberculosis agents	PO, IV
Streptomycin (also an aminoglycoside)	15 mg/kg up to 1 g/d as single dose	IM
Rifabutin (Mycobutin)	300 mg qd	PO
Cycloserine (Seromycin)	250 mg q 12 h for 2 wk up to 500 mg q 12 h	PO
Kanamycin (Kantrex)	PO 1 g q 1 h for 4 doses then q 6 h for 36–72 h; IM/IV 15 mg/kg/d q 8–12 h	PO, IM, IV

    e. Caution in older clients, children, diabetics, those with gout or blood dyscrasias, and optic neuritis or defects

5. Significant drug interactions

    a. Increased effect of antituberculin agent

        1) Anti-gout agents such as probenecid (Benebid) and sulfinpyrazone (Antazone)

        2) Ketoconazole (Nizoral), an antifungal

        3) Glucocorticosteroids, such as methylprednisolone (Medrol) and prednisolone (Pred-Forte)

        4) Metoclopramide (Reglan), a GI stimulant

        5) Nicardipine, verapamil, and diltiazem (calcium channel blockers)

        6) Nonsteroidal anti-inflammatory drugs (NSAIDS), aminoglycosides, and testosterone agents

    b. Increased toxicity

        1) Salicylates, other antitubercular agents, nephrotoxic and hepatotoxic drugs, alcohol

        2) Increased neurotoxicity: cycloserine (Seromycin), isoniazid (INH), ethionamide (Trecator-C), and phenytoin (Dilantin)

    c. Hyperkalemia with potassium-sparing diuretics and angiotensin converting enzyme (ACE) inhibitors

    d. Crystalluria with ascorbic acid (Vitamin C)

    e. Decreased effect of anti-tubercular drugs and/or other drugs from many drug classifications

    f. Decreased efficacy of oral contraceptives

6. Significant food interactions: decreased rate/extent of absorption of isoniazid (INH) when taken with food (take 1 hour before meals)

7. Significant laboratory studies

    a. Monitor for hepatic dysfunction with ALT, AST, alkaline phosphatase, bilirubin

    b. Purified protein derivative (PPD) tuberculin skin test to check for positive reaction indicating prior exposure to *M. tuberculosis* and T-lymphocyte production; cellular response to tubercle bacillus occurs 3 to 10 weeks after infection and does not diagnose active infection; chest x-rays and sputum tests for tubercle bacillus are done to clarify actual status

    c. Chest x-ray if PPD positive

    d. Sputum smear culture if chest x-ray positive

    e. Drug levels if suspected toxicity, such as with phenytoin

8. Side effects

    a. Fairly well tolerated

    b. Nausea, vomiting, anorexia, constipation, diarrhea, dyspepsia

NCLEX!

NCLEX!

NCLEX!

NCLEX!

NCLEX!

    c. Headache, dizziness, malaise, fever, chills, arthralgia, flu-like symptoms, weakness

    d. Skin rash, dry skin, peripheral paresis, photophobia, photosensitivity, vision changes

    e. Dysrhythmias

    f. Urinary retention (in males)

    g. Change in color to orange-red of excretions/secretions as urine, tears, feces, perspiration (with rifampin and rifabutin)

    h. Electrolyte imbalances

    i. Metallic taste with ethionamide (Trecator-SC)

NCLEX!

    j. Disulfiram-like effect with alcohol ingestion

9. Adverse effects/toxicity

    a. Nephrotoxicity

    b. Hepatotoxicity

    c. Hematologic disorders: agranulocytosis, thrombocytopenia, eosinophilia, anemia

    d. Seizure, depression, confusion, ataxia, paresis, paresthesias, drowsiness

    e. Ototoxicity: tinnitus, hearing loss

10. Nursing considerations

    a. Assess baseline laboratory findings and monitor during therapy the client's liver and renal function, C & S results, CBC with WBC/differential, RBC indices, platelet count

    b. Assess concurrent medications being taken to avoid adverse drug-drug interactions

    c. Assess for pregnancy

    d. Evaluate drug effectiveness by resolution of fever and other signs and symptoms of infection

NCLEX!

    e. Coadminister pyridoxine (vitamin B_6) and/or cyanocobalamin (vitamin B_{12})

    f. Evaluate client compliance

    g. Ensure full course of therapy is completed to lessen risk of re-infection or development of drug resistance

NCLEX!

    h. Encourage food high in B-complex vitamin, (especially pyridoxine) such as meat (chicken, beef, and pork), liver, soybeans, baked potato with skin, raw avocado

    i. Encourage good hydration and good nutrition with high-quality protein

11. Client education

    a. Know drug name, dose, purpose, route, administration schedule, purpose of prolonged/combination therapy

b. Take complete course of therapy to lessen risk of re-infection or development of drug resistance

c. Take isoniazid (INH) 1 hour before meals

d. Report adverse reactions

e. Rifampin (Rifadin): may discolor urine, tears, saliva, and stain contact lens and undergarments

f. Keep follow-up appointments with health care provider and for tests

g. Infection control measures to protect self and others

h. Avoid alcohol because of increased risk for hepatitis or disulfiram-like effect

i. Use alternative contraception during therapy and for at least 1 month after therapy is discontinued if using oral contraceptives

j. For dry skin, use emollients or oils

B. Leprostatics

1. Action and use

a. Treat leprosy and some acquired immunodeficiency syndrome (AIDS)-related opportunistic infections

b. Bacteriostatic against *Mycobacterium leprae, Pneumocystis carinii, Plasmodium, Mycobacterium tuberculosis:* dapsone (DDS)

c. Bacterocidal against *Mycobacterium leprae* and *Mycobacterium avium:* clofazimine (Lamprene)

2. Common medications (Table 2-11)

3. Administration considerations: give clofazimine with food

4. Contraindications

a. Hypersensitivity to DDS and possible sulfonamides

b. Use cautiously in clients with hepatic disease or glucose-6-phosphate dehydrogenase (G6PD) deficiency (an inherited type of hemolytic anemia associated with stress or certain drug interactions)

c. Not established for safe use in pregnant and lactating clients

5. Significant drug interactions

a. Rifampin decreases levels of dapsone by 7- to 10-fold

b. Trimethoprim (Proloprim, Trimpex), a urinary tract anti-infective, and pyrimethamine (Daraprim), an anti-infective/anti-malarial; each increases levels and risk for adverse effects

Table 2-11	Generic/Trade Names	Usual Adult Dose	Administration Route
Leprostatics	Dapsone (DDS)	100 mg/d for minimum of 3 y	PO
	Clofazimine (Lamprene)	100 mg/d in combination with 1 or more antileprosy drugs for 3 y, then 100 mg/d as monotherapy	PO

6. Significant food interactions: none reported

7. Significant laboratory studies: monitor CBC with hemoglobin and hematocrit for hemoglobin decline and reticulocyte count increase

8. Side effects

    a. Skin pigmentation changes, as pink to brownish-black color; may resolve in weeks to months

    b. Dry skin

    c. Nausea, vomiting, diarrhea, abdominal pain

    d. Headache, insomnia, malaise, paresthesias, nervousness, tinnitus, vertigo, vision changes

9. Adverse effects/toxicity

    a. Agranulocytosis

    b. Hepatotoxicity

    c. Dose-related hemolysis (increased in G6PD deficiency)

    d. Methemoglobinemia may occur resulting in rhinitis, fatigue, difficulty breathing, cyanosis

    e. Phototoxicity

    f. Male infertility with DDS

10. Nursing considerations

    a. Ensure client takes complete therapy

    b. Give clofazimine with food

    c. Monitor laboratory test for hemoglobin and reticulocyte count

    d. Assess concurrent medication being taken to avert or minimize drug-drug interactions, such as with rifampin and trimethoprim

    e. Evaluate for drug effectiveness with resolution of infection

11. Client education

    a. Know drug, name, dose, purpose, route, and schedule regimen

    b. Report adverse reactions

    c. Take clofazimine with meals; skin discoloration may be pink to brownish-black; resolves in months to years after drug is discontinued

    d. Keep follow-up appointments with health care provider and for tests

    e. Ensure infection control measures are used

    f. Encourage hydration and good nutrition with complete or complementary proteins for tissue healing

III. Antivirals

A. Medications to treat herpes and cytomegalovirus

1. Action and use

   a. Virustatic; drugs convert to compound that is a counterfeit nucleotide; it is taken into the viral cell where the DNA chain is developing and terminates the chain, resulting in cell death with help from the host's immune system

   b. Drug has little effect on host cells; effective only during acute phase of infection, not during latent phase; virus must be in living cell to survive and replicate

   c. Used to treat broad spectrum of diseases including cold sores, viral encephalitis. shingles, and genital infection

   d. Viruses include **herpes simplex** virus-1 (HSV-1) in oral herpes or herpes labialis, herpes simplex virus-2 (HSV-2) in genital herpes, **herpes zoster** in shingles, **herpes varicella** zoster virus (VZV) in chickenpox, and some Epstein-Barr viruses

   e. Acyclovir (Zovirax) is the drug of choice in herpes simplex encephalitis; genital herpes treatment is its most frequent use; used prophylactically with immunosuppressed seropositive clients before bone marrow transplantation and after other organ transplants; not found to be beneficial in treating those who are not immunosuppressed, although it may help prevent shedding of virus

   f. Ganciclovir (DHPG) is approved to treat only cytomegalic retinitis (caused by **cytomegalovirus** or CMV) in immunosuppressed clients; has good intraocular penetration; foscarnet (Foscavir) is used to treat ganciclovir-resistant CMV retinitis; cidofir (Vistide) is also given by IV administration for CMV-induced retinitis

   g. Famclovir (Famvir) is used to treat acute herpes zoster (shingles)

   h. Trifluridine is a topical treatment for keratoconjunctivitis caused by herpes simplex

   i. Valacyclovir (Valtrex) is the drug of choice for genital herpes; it is an improved oral form of acyclovir

   j. Penciclovir (Denavir) is used to treat herpes infections; topical only; it is negligibly absorbed so is well tolerated and shortens pain/healing by one-half day

   k. Cidofir (Vistide) IV to treat CMV retinitis in client with AIDS

2. Common medications (Table 2-12)

3. Administration considerations

   a. Hydrate client to decrease risk or extent of nephrotoxicity

   b. Administer as soon as possible to improve effectiveness

   c. Wear gloves for topical application to limit exposure to drug or lesions

   d. Preferred central venous access for IV administrations

   e. Foscarnet: precipitates with many drugs when used as IV administration; use with D5%W or NaCl solutions

Table 2-12	Generic/Trade Names	Usual Adult Dose	Administration Route
Antivirals: Medications to Treat Herpes and Cytomegalovirus	Acyclovir (Zovirax)	Genital herpes simplex: PO 200 mg q 4 h 5 times/d, IV 5 mg/kg q 8 h; herpes zoster: PO 800 mg q 4 h 5 times/d	PO, IV
	Cidofovir (Vistide)	5 mg/kg once weekly for 2 wk, also give 2 g probenecid 3 h prior to infusion and 1 g 8 h after infusion	IV
	Ganciclovir (DHPG)	IV 5 mg/kg over 1 h qd; PO 1,000 mg tid	PO, IV
	Famiclovir (Famvir)	500 mg q 8 h for 7 days	PO
	Foscarnet (Foscavir)	40–60 mg/kg q 8 h for 2–3 wk	IV
	Penciclovir (Denavir)	Q 2 h while awake for 4 d	Topical
	Trifluridine (Viroptic)	1 drop 1% ophthalmic solution into affected eye q 2 h until healing	Ophthalmic
	Valacyclovir (Valtrex)	1 g tid for 7 days	PO
	Vidarabine (Ara-A)	15 mg/kg/d infused over 12–24 h	Ophthalmic, IV

4. Contraindications

   a. Hypersensitivity to drug

   b. Use caution in preexisting hepatic or renal dysfunction or concurrent use of nephrotoxic drugs

   c. Use caution in pregnant and lactating women

5. Significant drug interactions

   a. Increased drowsiness with zidovudine (AZT)

   b. Nephrotoxic drugs potentiate renal effects

   c. Probenecid (Benemid) can prolong effects of anti-viral agent

6. Significant food interactions: none reported

7. Significant laboratory studies

   a. CBC including WBC with differential, T-cell count, and platelet count

   b. Serum and urine creatinine, BUN, and creatinine clearance to monitor renal function

   c. ALT, AST, alkaline phosphatase, and bilirubin to monitor liver function

8. Side effects

   a. Anemia, headache, mood changes, seizures

   b. Nausea, vomiting, diarrhea

   c. Local irritation including phlebitis at IV site

   d. Neutropenia; often dose-dependent because of bone marrow suppression

   e. Fever, hypocalcemia, hypomagnesemia, hypokalemia, metabolic acidosis, dysrhythmias

   f. Increased risk for CNS disturbances and fluid overload in clients with impaired hepatic or renal function

   g. Ocular hypotony

9. Adverse effects/toxicity

   a. Additive neutropenia with zidovudine

   b. Carcinogenic, embryotoxic, ant teratogenic in experimental animals

   c. Infertility in males and females; ganciclovir

   d. Nephrotoxicity

   e. Hepatoxicity

   f. Thrombocytopenic purpura

   g. Pancreatitis

10. Nursing considerations

    a. Check allergies, including allergy to anti-viral agents

    b. Assess baseline data to monitor effectiveness of drug and side effects

    c. Assess for neutropenic infection if immunosuppressed

    d. Assess renal function: creatinine, BUN, creatinine clearance, I & O

    e. Check hepatic function: ALT, AST, alkaline phosphatase, bilirubin

    f. Collaborate with prescriber if dosage needs adjustment for hepatic or renal dysfunction

    g. Analyze findings of CBC with differential, CD4 count, platelet count to monitor bone marrow activity and for effectiveness of drug therapy

    h. Preexisting CNS disturbances may be exacerbated; assess orientation and reflexes; implement safety measures if CNS disturbances exist

    i. Assess skin and lesions regularly

    j. Hydrate to decrease risk of nephrotoxicity, e.g., 2,000 to 3,000 mL/fluids per day if not contraindicated by other conditions

    k. Monitor relief of infection and of pain

    l. Monitor platelets and evidence of petechiae or increased risk of bleeding

    m. Monitor electrolytes and fluid balance

    n. Monitor nutritional status, especially if GI side effects occur; ensure adequate protein intake

    o. Provide safety measures if CNS effects occur to protect from injury

11. Client education

    a. Drug, dosage, administration schedule; importance of completing full course of therapy with evenly distributed dosing that does not interrupt sleep (to improve effectiveness and to prevent drug resistance)

    b. Self-administration techniques if indicated

    c. Clinical manifestations to report: severe side effects; evidence of increased bleeding, edema, fatigue; severe rash, especially if accompanied by blisters, fever, and other indications of infection to avert serious complications

    d. Avoid sexual intercourse if genital herpes being treated

NCLEX!

NCLEX!

NCLEX!

NCLEX!

e. Avoid tactile contact of lesions by self and others to avoid spreading infection to new sites

f. Avoid hazardous tasks and driving if drowsiness, dizziness, seizure activity occurs

g. Ensure client follows up with labs and appointments with health care provider

h. Offer frequent, small, high protein meals

NCLEX!

i. Encourage 2,000 to 3,000 mL/day intake

j. Female clients should have annual pap smear since there is increased risk of cervical cancer with genital herpes infection

NCLEX!

k. Anti-viral agents do not cure herpes and CMV infections

l. Notify health care provider if lesions do not heal or recur

B. Medications for HIV and AIDS

1. Antiretroviral protease inhibitors

a. Action and use

1) Most potent of antiviral agents; inhibits cell protein synthesis that interferes with viral replication

NCLEX!

2) Is not curative but slows progression of disease and prolongs life

3) Used prophylactically because viral replication peaks before clinical manifestations of infection emerge and anti-viral efficacy is then more limited; virus relies on using resources within the live host cell and there is increased risk for toxicity to host cell

4) Used in AIDS and AIDS-related complex (ARC) to decrease viral load and opportunistic infections

5) Used in combination to decrease viral load, increase CD-4 counts, and decrease incidence or rate of development of drug resistance

b. Common medications (Table 2-13)

c. Administration considerations

1) Saquinavir (Invirase): take with high fat meals or within 2 hours of full meal

2) Ritonavir (Norvir): unpalatable; take with chocolate milk, nutritional supplement, or food

3) Indinavir (Crixivan) requires an acidic gastric environment for absorption; take 1 hour before or 2 hours after light, low-fat snack; drink greater than 1.5 liters of fluid daily

Table 2-13	Generic/Trade Names	Dose	Administration Route
Antiviral Medications for HIV and AIDS: Antiretroviral Protease Inhibitors	Indinavir (Crixivan)	800 mg q 8 h 1 h before or 2 h after meal	PO
	Ritonavir (Norvir)	600 mg bid 1 h before or 2 h after meal	PO
	Saquinavir (Invirase)	600 mg tid taken 2 h after a full meal	PO

    d. Contraindications

        1) Not recommended for pregnant or lactating women

        2) Not recommended for children

        3) Hypersensitivity

    e. Significant drug interactions

        1) To decrease risk of resistance, drug may be combined with reverse transcriptase agents

        2) Rifampin and rifabutin lower blood levels of protease inhibitors; mycobacterium prophylaxis may be changed to clarithromycin

    f. Significant food interactions (see section on administration considerations)

    g. Significant laboratory studies

        1) Aminotransferase and triglyceride levels may be elevated with ritonavir

        2) ALT, AST, alkaline phosphatase, bilirubin

        3) CBC

        4) Creatinine, blood urea nitrogen, creatinine clearance

    h. Side effects

        1) Headache, fatigue, nausea, vomiting, diarrhea, abdominal discomfort, anemia, taste perversion, asthenia, circumoral paresthesia with ritonavir

        2) Reversible hyperbilirubinemia and nephrolithiasis with indinavir (Crixivan): greater than 1.5 liters fluid daily are needed to prevent nephrolithiasis

    i. Adverse effects/toxicity: hepatotoxicity; reduce dose in liver dysfunction

    j. Nursing considerations

        1) Assess current medications to avoid drug interactions

        2) Assess allergies

NCLEX!

        3) Monitor for hepatotoxicity: ALT, AST, alkaline phosphatase, bilirubin; observe for nausea, vomiting, jaundice, upper right abdominal quadrant enlargement and tenderness

NCLEX!

        4) Monitor for nephrotoxicity: creatinine, BUN, creatinine clearance, urinalysis; keep accurate I & O

        5) Monitor CBC for blood dyscrasias such as neutropenia, thrombocytopenia, or anemia, and for improvement as evidenced by increased T-cell count

NCLEX!

        6) Monitor for side effects; if neutropenic, observe for occult signs of infection, e.g., low back, flank, or suprapubic pain, normal temperature or low-grade fever related to UTI

        7) Collaborate with prescriber if dosage change indicated by analysis of data collected related to adverse effects

8) Saquinavir (Invirase): take with high fat foods or within 2 hours of full meal

9) Ritonavir (Norvir): take with chocolate milk, nutritional supplement or food to counteract unpleasant taste

10) Infivair (Crixivan): take 1 hour before or 2 hours after light, low-fat snack; drink more than 1500 mL/day of fluids

11) Provide neutropenic care as appropriate

k. Client education

1) Know drug, name, purpose, dose, schedule regimen

2) Take full course for duration as prescribed for optimal benefit and to minimize risk of drug resistance

3) Ensure fluid intake of at least 1,500 mL/day

4) Take with food: saquinavir (Invirase) (high fat foods recommended) and ritonavir (unpalatable taste)

5) Take 1 hour before or 2 hours after light, low-fat snack: indinavir

6) Report adverse effects to health care provider

7) Eat small, frequent meals with complete or complementary proteins

8) Report severe side effects to health care provider

9) Keep appointments for follow-up examinations and laboratory testing

10) Use neutropenic precautions

2. Reverse transcriptase inhibitors

a. Action and use

1) Block viral reverse transcriptase; stops replication/growth

2) Are used for all symptomatic, HIV clients with a CD4 count less than $500/mm^3$ and some with higher counts

3) Penetrates blood–brain barrier

4) Possible prophylaxis for known occupational HIV exposure

5) Effectiveness diminishes over time

6) AZT is used to prevent maternal transmission of HIV

7) A major advantage of non-nucleoside reverse transcriptase inhibitors is that they not adversely affect development of blood cells

8) There is no cross-resistance between nucleoside and non-nucleoside reverse transcriptase inhibitors

9) Are used in combination because resistant strains rapidly evolve if used as single agent therapy

b. Common medications (Table 2-14)

1) Nucleoside reverse transcriptase inhibitors: didanosine (Videx), lamivudine (Epivir), stavudine (Zerit), zalcitabine (Hivid), zidovudine (AZT)

Table 2-14	Generic/Trade Names	Usual Adult Dose	Administration Route
Antiviral Medications for HIV and AIDS: Reverse Transcriptase Inhibitors	***Nucleoside Reverse Transcriptase Inhibitors***		
	Didanosine (DDI)	35–49 kg, tablets, 125 mg bid; 50–74 kg, tablets, 200 mg bid; ≥ 75 kg 300 mg bid	PO
	Lamivudine (Epivir)	150 mg bid; 2 mg/kg bid if weight < 50 kg	PO
	Stavudine (Zerit)	≥ 60 kg, 40 mg q 12 h; < 60 kg, 30 mg q 12 h	PO
	Zalcitabine (Hivid)	0.75 mg q 8 h given with zidovudine 200 mg q 8 h	PO
	Zidovudine (AZT, Retrovir)	200 mg q 4 h, after 1 month reduce to 100 mg q 4 h; IV 1–2 mg/kg q 4 h	PO, IV
	Non–Nucleoside Reverse Transcriptase Inhibitors		
	Nevirapine (Viramune)	200 mg qd for first 14 d then increase to 200 mg bid	PO
	Delavirdine (Rescriptor)	400 mg tid	PO
	Efavirenz (Sustiva)	600 mg qd	PO
	Abacavir sulfate	300 mg bid in combination with other antiretroviral agents	PO

2) Non-nucleoside reverse transcriptase inhibitors: nevirapine (Viramune), delavirdine (Rescriptor), efavirenz (Sustiva), acabavir (Ziagen)

c. Administration considerations

1) Crush or chew buffered tablets that are chewable because drug has acid lability

2) Food may slow absorption but does not affect total absorption

3) May administer at bedtime for better tolerance of CNS adverse effects

d. Contraindications

1) Concurrent use of drugs that cause peripheral neuropathy, such as choramphenicol (Chloromycetin), vinca alkaloids (vincristine [Oncovin], vinblastine [Velban], etoposide [VP 16], cisplatin [Platinol]), dapsone (DDS), hydralazine (Apresoline), isoniazid (INH), metronidazole (Flagyl), nitrofurantoin, phenytoin (Dilantin), and ribavirin

2) Avoid or use with caution drugs that can increase toxicity, such as probenecid (Benemid), acetaminophen (Tylenol), lorazepam (Ativan), indomethacin (Indocin), and cimetidine (Tagamet)

3) If neurotoxic signs occur, discontinue drug until signs are resolved

4) Not contraindicated in clients with AIDS dementia

e. Significant drug interactions

1) Many drug class interactions; see contraindications section above

2) May be given with other drugs to enhance antiviral effect: acyclovir, interferon (Intron-A), didanosine (ddl), granulocyte colony-stimulating factor (GCSF) such as epoetin alfa (Procrit)

f. Significant food interactions: none reported

g. Significant laboratory studies

1) Amylase, cholesterol, liver function tests as ALT, AST, alkaline phosphatase, bilirubin

2) CBC including WBC with differential, platelet count, and CD4 count

3) Electrolytes

4) Serum creatinine, BUN, creatinine clearance

h. Side effects

1) Neurological side effects of insomnia, confusion, peripheral neuropathies, and seizures

2) Diarrhea

3) Hypermagnesemia

4) Discolored fingernails, rash

5) Myalgias, numbness and tingling of extremities, altered taste sensations, dizziness, anxiety, tremors

6) Cough

i. Adverse effects/toxicity

1) Pancreatitis

2) Anemia, leukopenia, thrombocytopenia with nucleosides

3) Nevirapine (Viramune): severe hepatotoxicity and dermatologic effects such as Stevens-Johnson syndrome

j. Nursing considerations

1) Assess for hypersensitivity

2) Assess current drug therapies for drug interactions

3) Assess baseline renal and liver tests and monitor at intervals; arrange to decrease dosage as needed

4) Ensure client takes complete course and all drugs included in the regimen to improve effectiveness and retard risk for resistant strains emerging

5) Administer around the clock as needed to maintain therapeutic levels

6) Stop administration if severe rash or other hypersensitivity reaction occurs

NCLEX!

7) Assess client for complications of HIV infection, e.g., opportunistic infections, cancer, neurologic disease

8) Monitor level of consciousness (LOC), strength, appropriateness of activity, short-term memory, ability to follow complex commands, reasoning and calculation abilities, and peripheral sensation

9) Assess for compromised respiratory or cardiovascular status

NCLEX!

10) Provide safety measures to protect from injury if CNS adverse effects occur

11) Assess nutritional intake and tolerance

12) Monitor skin and mucous membranes frequently

13) Monitor renal function with labs, I & O, daily weight

14) Monitor for alleviation of clinical manifestations of AIDS or ARC and for increase in CD4 count

    k. Client education

1) Teach importance of taking full course of therapy and as prescribed to enhance effectiveness and deter drug resistance from developing

2) Caution about risks of dizziness or altered mentation; do not drive or perform hazardous tasks

3) Avoid crowds and persons with infections

4) Drug, dosage, frequency, schedule regimen, take with or without food

5) Proper self-administration techniques if indicated

6) Hair loss possible with zidovudine (AZT)

7) Drug does not cure but helps manage infection; it reduces viral load, decreases risk for complications, and extends survival

8) Practice good hygiene and safe sex practices

C. Medications for influenza and respiratory viruses

    1. Action and use

      a. Virustatic

      b. Most of viral replication has occurred before clinical evidence appears; bacterial replication occurs as clinical manifestations of infection emerge so antibacterial agents more effective against bacterial infections than antiviral agents are against viral infections, since drug therapy relies on viral replication for effectiveness

      c. Ribavirin (Virazole)

1) Aerosolized administration for respiratory syncytial virus (RSV) or severe infections of the respiratory tract secondary to RSV, usually in infants

2) Virustatic

3) May decrease length of disease

4) Efficacy demonstrated in influenza A and B and in hepatitis A

      d. Amantadine (Symmetrel) and rimantadine (Flumadine)

1) Used prophylactically for influenza A; increased efficacy if initiated at time of exposure or at least within 48 hours

2) Adjunctive therapy for temporary immunization of influenza A

3) May limit severity of clinical manifestations of influenza and/or decrease length or duration

    2. Common medications (Table 2-15)

      a. Amantadine (Symmetrel): prophylactically and therapeutically used for respiratory viral infections; also used to treat Parkinson's disease

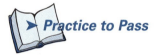

▶ Practice to Pass

The client with HIV states, "I quit taking the acyclovir. I don't have any symptoms. I don't want to take it now and risk becoming resistant to it when I may really need it." How do you respond?

Table 2-15	Generic/Trade Names	Usual Adult Dose	Administration Route
Medications for Influenza and Respiratory Viruses	Amantadine (Symmetrel)	200 mg qd or 100 mg q 12 h	PO
	Ribavirin (Virazole)	Child, 20 mg via SPAG nebulizer over 12–18 h for 3–7 d	Inhalation
	Rimantadine (Flumadine)	100 mg bid for 7 d	PO

    b. Ribavirin (Virazole): treat influenza A, RSV, and herpes infections

    c. Rimantadine (Flumadine): prophylactically against influenza A

  3. Administration considerations

    a. Initiate drug therapy as soon as possible to enhance effectiveness and to deter complications of infection

    b. Administer before flu season for prophylactic purpose

  4. Contraindications

    a. Known hypersensitivity

    b. Ribavirin (Virazole) contraindicated in pregnancy; others use with caution in pregnant or lactating clients or children

    c. Caution in clients with renal or liver dysfunction

    d. Caution in clients with psychotic problems or seizures

  5. Significant drug interactions

    a. Alcohol increases CNS effects

    b. Anticholinergics increase atropine-like effects

    c. Ribavirin with digoxin increases risk for digitalis toxicity

  6. Significant food interactions: none reported

  7. Significant laboratory studies

    a. CBC with WBC differential

    b. Possible C & S of pharynx or of sputum

    c. ALT, AST, alkaline phosphatase, bilirubin to evaluate liver function

    d. Creatinine, BUN, creatinine clearance to evaluate renal function

  8. Side effects

    a. Most are transient and resolve quickly after drug discontinued

    b. Dizziness, light-headedness, headache, palpitations, mood and mental changes, drowsiness, insomnia, irritability, nightmares

    c. Dyspnea, rash, peripheral edema

    d. Orthostatic hypotension, nausea, vomiting, mouth dryness, urinary retention

  9. Adverse effects/toxicity

    a. Slurred speech, ataxia, convulsions

    b. Leukopenia

    c. Possible digitalis toxicity with concurrent digoxin therapy

    d. Possible teratogenic

10. Nursing considerations

    a. Assess for allergies

    b. Assess hepatic and renal dysfunction

    c. Assess baseline neurological status, e.g., orientation, affect, coordination, reflexes

    d. Assess drugs currently taking to avoid drug interactions

    e. Maintain hydration with 2,000 to 3,000 mL fluids/day if not contraindicated by other conditions

    f. Initiate drug therapy as soon as possible after exposure

    g. Ensure complete course of therapy taken to enhance drug effectiveness

    h. Evaluate for resolution of signs/symptoms, such as fever, lethargy, respiratory difficulty

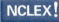

    i. Monitor for adverse effects; monitor for respiratory deterioration in infants

    j. Provide safety precautions if CNS adverse effects develop

    k. Keep accurate I & O; monitor for urinary retention

    l. Avoid commercial mouthwashes that may potentiate dryness of mouth; provide oral care with water or saline rinses

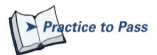

► Practice to Pass

The client taking amantadine (Symmetrel) reports symptoms of xerostomia. What is this complaint? What intervention/teaching would you provide?

11. Client education

    a. Know drug, name, dose, purpose, schedule regimen

    b. Initiate therapy as soon as possible when prescribed

    c. Complete the entire course of therapy for full benefits

    d. Change position slowly to minimize risks of orthostatic hypotension

    e. Report increased respiratory distress or severe adverse effects to health care provider

    f. If drowsiness, dizziness, lightheadedness, confusion, ataxia, or blurred vision occur, do not drive or perform hazardous tasks

    g. If improvement is not noted within 2 to 3 days, notify health care provider

    h. If dryness of mouth develops, rinse mouth as needed with warm water or glass of warm water with one teaspoon of salt; commercial mouthrinses with alcohol content and hydrogen peroxide may increase dryness of mouth; hard sugarless candy may stimulate salivation

    i. Drink at least 6 to 8 glasses of fluids a day

    j. Keep appointments with health care provider and for tests

D. Locally active antiviral agents

    1. Action and use: not absorbed systemically

    2. Common medications (Table 2-16)

        a. Idoxuridine (Herplex): topical ophthalmic agent to treat herpes simplex keratitis

	Generic/Trade Names	Usual Adult Dose	Administration Route
Table 2-16 **Locally Active Antiviral Agents**	Idoxuridine (Herplex)	1 drop instilled in conjunctival sac q 1 h during day and q 2 h at night	Topical
	Imiquimod (Aldara)	5% cream applied 3 times/wk and left on the skin for 6–10 h	Topical
	Penciclovir (Denavir)	q 2 h while awake for 4 d	Topical
	Trifluridine (Viroptic)	1 drop 1% ophthalmic solution into affected eye q 2 h until healing	Ophthalmic
	Vidarabine (Vira–A)	Instill 1 cm in ribbon of ointment into lower conjunctival sac q 3 h 5 times/d	Ophthalmic

    b. Imiquimod (Aldara): genital and perianal warts

    c. Penciclovir (Denavir): herpes simplex 1 or herpes labialis; cold sores on face and lips; do not apply to mucous membranes

    d. Fomivirsen (Vitravene): ophthalmic solution injected into eye to treat CMV retinitis in clients with AIDS

    e. Trifluridine (Viroptic): ophthalmic agent to treat herpes simplex infection of the eye

    f. Vidarabine (Vira-A): ophthalmic agent to treat herpes simplex infection of eye not responsive to idoxuridine (Herplex)

3. Administration considerations

    a. Wash hands well before applying medication

    b. Wear gloves or use cotton-tip applicator to apply to skin lesions being cautious not to contaminate drug or other sites on skin

    c. Ensure proper administration technique

    d. Stop drug if severe local adverse effect or open lesions develop

4. Contraindications: caution if known hypersensitivity, pregnancy, lactation

5. Significant drug interactions: do not apply other topical agents to same lesions

6. Significant food interactions: none reported

7. Significant laboratory studies: none reported

8. Side effects

    a. Local burning, stinging, discomfort may occur at time of application but usually resolve without intervention

    b. Temporary visual impairment possible with optic application

9. Adverse effects/toxicity

    a. Skin eruptions

    b. Hypersensitivity

10. Nursing considerations

    a. See previous Administration Considerations

    b. Assess for allergies

     c. Monitor for therapeutic response

     d. Monitor for adverse effects

     e. Evaluate effectiveness of teaching plan

     f. Monitor for comfort, safety, and compliance

11. Client education

     a. Know drug name, dose, route, purpose, schedule regimen

     b. Ensure proper administration technique

     c. Does not cure but alleviates pain/discomfort and prevents extended damage to uninvolved tissue

     d. Report severe local discomfort/reaction to health care provider

IV. Antifungals

A. Systemic

1. Action and use

     a. Is fungistatic or fungicidal depending on therapeutic serum levels and sensitivity to fungi

     b. Treats candida infections, cryptococcus, blastomycosis, histoplasmosis, and aspergillus fumigates, **tinea** infections (a fungal infection caused by ringworm)

     c. Increased permeability of cell membranes better enables other drugs to enter fungus cell

2. Common medications (Table 2-17)

3. Administration considerations

     a. Administer carefully as ordered, especially intravenous dosages

     b. Combination of antifungal agents may deter or retard drug resistance

     c. Amphotericin B

       1) May premedicate with an antipyretic such as acetaminophen (Tylenol), an antihistamine such as diphenhydramine (Benadryl), an antiemetic, and meperidine (Demerol) to reduce severity of fever/chills response; heparin or hydrocortisone (Cortaid) added to the IV solutions may reduce risk for thrombophlebitis at IV site

       2) Give with heparin or hydrocortisone and over 4 to 6 hours to avert clinical manifestations of hypersensitivity or drug toxicity

       3) Hydrate with IV fluids usually 2 hours before and 2 hours after drug administration to decrease risk for nephrotoxicity

       4) To test for hypersensitivity prior to administration, deliver 1 mg/20 mL D_5W (IV) over 10 to 30 minutes; if test elicits hypersensitivity response, a lipid preparation as amphotericin B liposomal complex (Ambisome) may be given to minimize the severe fever, shaking, and chills; premedicate as above

       5) Mix in D_5W only; precipitates form in any solution containing sodium chloride

Table 2-17	Generic/Trade Names	Usual Adult Dose	Administration Route
Systemic Antifungal Medications	Amphotericin B (Fungizone)	250 mcg/kg/d up to 1.0 mg/kg/d (an IV test dose is recommended to lessen the risk of an anaphylactic reaction)	IV
	Amphotericin B Liposomal Complex (Ambisome)	3–5 mg/kg/d infused over 1–2 h	IV
	Amphotericin B Cholesteryl Sulfate Complex (Amphotec)	3–4 mg/kg/d, infuse at rate of 1 mg/kg/h (an IV test dose is recommended)	IV
	Fluconazole (Diflucan)	Systemic candidiasis: 400 mg day, then 200 mg qd for 4 wks	PO, IV
	Flucytosine (Ancobon)	50–150 mg/kg/d divided q 6 h	PO
	Itraconazole (Sporanox)	Vaginal candidiasis: 200 mg qd for 3 d	PO
	Ketoconazole (Nizoral)	200–400 mg qd; topical apply 1–2 times/d to affected area	PO, topical
	Miconazole (Monistat)	Apply cream bid for 2–3 d	Topical, vaginal suppository and cream, spray, shampoo, IV rarely due to cardiotoxicities
	Nystatin (Mycostatin)	500,000–1,000,000 U tid; 1–4 troches 4–5 times/d; suspension 400,000–600,000 U qid; vaginal 1–2 tablets daily for 2 wk	PO tablet and suspension, troches, vaginal, topical
	Clotrimazole (Mycelex)	PO 1 troche 5 times/d q 3 h for 14 d; topical apply small amount bid	PO, lozenges, topical, vaginal
	Griseofulvin (Grifulvin)	500 mg microsize daily in single dose or divided doses	PO
	Terbinafine (Lamisil)	PO 250 mg qd for 6 wk; topical qd or bid	PO, topical

6) Abelcet (another name for Amphotericin B Liposomal Complex): shake gently to distribute drug particles; use 5-μm filter needle to inject agent into container of D_5W and thoroughly disperse drug throughout solution; redisperse drug in solution every 2 hours if infusion time extends beyond 2 hours; no in-line filter used

4. Contraindications

   a. Hypersensitivity

   b. If IV test dose of amphotericin B elicits hypersensitivity response, the lipid preparations (which are much more expensive) may be given to avoid the severe response of fever, shaking, chills

   c. Avoid H_2 histamine antagonists unless scheduled so not to interfere with absorption of antifungals

   d. Use caution with IV administration of miconazole (Monistat) because of risk of cardiotoxicity

   e. Use caution in pregnant and lactating clients

   f. Use caution with amphotericin B agents in renal impairment/severe bone marrow depression

5. Significant drug interactions

   a. Increased risk for bleeding with concurrent administration of anticoagulants or corticosteroids

b. Dysrhythmias with concurrent administration of astemizole (Hismanol), or cisapride (Propulsid)

c. Increased risk for nephrotoxicity if given concurrently with other nephrotoxic drugs, such as aminoglycosides, cisplatinum (Platinol) and other antineoplastic agents, Furosemide (Lasix), vancomycin (Vancocin), cisapride (Propulsid), fluconazole (Diflucan), and cyclosporine (Sandimmune)

d. Anti-diabetic agents given concurrently with miconazole, fluconazole, and itraconazole may exaggerate hypoglycemia effect

e. Ketoconazole and itraconazole depend on acid environment; give antifungal agent 1 hour before or 2 hours after administration of antacid

f. Ketoconazole and fluconazole prolong effect of cyclosporine (Sandimmune)

g. Ketoconazole: rifampin decreases effect of the antifungal

h. Fluconazole: increases phenytoin (Dilantin) level and decreases serum levels of fluconazole with administration of rifampin (Rifadin)

i. Amphotericin B (Fungizone): synergistic effect with tetracyclines, rifampin or 5-flucytosine (Ancobon)

j. Griseofulvin (Grifulvin V)

   1) Flushing and tachycardia with alcohol

   2) Decreased antifungal effect with barbiturates

   3) Increased risk bleeding with anticoagulants

   4) Decreased efficacy of oral contraceptives and risk for breakthrough bleeding

6. Significant food interactions

  a. Itraconazole (Sporanox): take with food to enhance absorption

  b. Ketoconazole: take with food to decrease nausea and vomiting

7. Significant laboratory studies

  a. Creatinine, BUN, creatinine clearance as baseline and at intervals to evaluate renal function

  b. ALT, AST, alkaline phosphatase, bilirubin as baseline and at intervals to evaluate liver function

  c. PT/INR if taking oral anticoagulants

  d. Electrolytes, especially potassium, magnesium, and sodium

  e. Monitor metabolic acidosis development during amphotericin B therapy

  f. Monitor CBC with hemoglobin and hematocrit, RBC indices, and platelet count

8. Side effects

  a. Thrombophlebitis with administration through peripheral vein

  b. Fever, chills, shaking, headache

  c. Anorexia, nausea, vomiting during or after administration; heartburn, diarrhea, flatulence

    d. Myalgia, arthralgia, weakness, hypotension

    e. Insomnia, vertigo, confusion

    f. Taste acuity diminished or causes unpleasant taste

    g. Photosensitivity

    h. Rash, pruritus, dry skin, urticaria

    i. Hypokalemia, hypomagnesemia: especially with concurrent use of gluco-corticosteroids or diuretics

    j. Furry tongue with griseofulvin (Grifulvin V)

    k. Ketoconazole (Nizoral): sexual impotency, hair loss, and gynecomastia

9. Adverse reactions/toxicity

    a. Bone marrow depression resulting in neutropenia, thrombocytopenia, anemia

NCLEX!

    b. Ototoxicity and nephrotoxicity with amphotericin B preparations

    c. Superinfections

NCLEX!

    d. Drug toxicity or hypersensitivity: fever, chills, shaking, piloerection, headache, anorexia, nausea/vomiting

    e. Stevens-Johnson syndrome

    f. Renal dysfunction with amphotericin B may result in severe hypokalemia

NCLEX!

    g. Cardiovascular collapse with too rapid infusion

    h. Hepatic necrosis: rare

10. Nursing considerations

    a. Assess concurrent medications to avert drug interactions; check for incompatibility of solutions as there are many

    b. Ensure C & S specimen of infection site is collected before starting agent

    c. Assess for pregnancy, lactation, liver or renal dysfunction; monitor liver and renal laboratory studies throughout therapy

    d. Monitor serum levels of antifungal agents

    e. Monitor WBC for improvement and for early detection of developing neutropenia, thrombocytopenia, anemia

    f. Ensure complete course of medication taken for full benefit of therapy and to minimize risk of re-growth of fungus or development of drug resistance

    g. Evaluate for resolution of clinical signs of infection, such as fever

    h. Give potassium supplements if hypokalemia occurs

NCLEX!

    i. Amphotericin B (IV)

        1) Use in-line filter with pores greater than 1.0 micron

        2) Premedicate with Tylenol, Benadryl, an antiemetic, and Demerol as indicated

3) Assess vital signs and for adverse reactions every 15 minutes × 2, then every 30 minutes × 4 hours with initial administration and thereafter as indicated; administer IV over 2 to 6 hours

4) Hydrate with 2,000 to 3,000 mL/day unless contraindicated by other conditions

5) Keep accurate I & O

6) Use strict aseptic technique since there is no preservative in solution and client may be compromised

7) Use in life-threatening infections

8) Protect drug solution from light with foil covering

11. Client education

   a. Know drug name, purpose, dose, route, length of therapy (e.g., Amphotericin B may be given over weeks or months)

   b. Ensure complete regimen given for full benefit

   c. Explain administration procedure

   d. Report adverse effects as burning at IV site, increased bleeding/bruising, evidence of superinfection

   e. Explain febrile reaction may decrease over time

   f. Fluid intake of 2,000 to 3,000 mL/day if not contraindicated by other conditions

   g. Eat small, frequent meals with high quality protein

   h. Take oral agents with food to minimize gastrointestinal distress

B. Topical antifungals

   1. Action and use

      a. Local infections of skin and mucous membranes of oropharnyx, vagina, or intestines caused by Candida species; infections of tinea pedis (athlete's foot), tinea cruris (in scrotal, crural, anal, and genital areas, called "jock itch"), tinea corporis (skin), tinea unguium or onychomycosis (nail fungus), tinea manus, tinea versicolor (infection of skin with yellow or beige-colored brawny patches)

      b. Use vaginal tablets up to 6 weeks prior to delivery to prevent newborn thrush

   2. Common medications (Table 2-18)

   3. Administration considerations

      a. Oral tablets or lozenges/troches not to be chewed or swallowed whole; swallow saliva as lozenge/troche dissolves slowly over 5 to 30 minutes; avoid food or drink during and for 30 minutes after administration

      b. For oral infections in client with dentures, remove dentures at bedtime; with oral suspension, remove dentures before each rinse or before each oral lozenge/troche

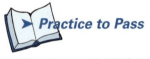

▶ *Practice to Pass*

The client with AIDS is to be given a first dose of Amphotericin B intravenously after a central line is inserted. The client states, "I'm scared to get this stuff. The doctor told me all the bad things that can happen." How would you respond?

Table 2-18	Generic/Trade Names	Usual Adult Dose	Administration Route
Topical Antifungal Medications	Amphotericin B (Fungizone)	250 mcg/kg/d up to 1.0 mg/kg/d (an IV test dose is recommended to lessen the risk of an anaphylactic reaction)	Topical, IV
	Ketoconazole (Nizoral)	200–400 mg QD; topical apply 1–2 times/d to affected area; topical shampoo twice a week for 4 wks	PO, topical, shampoo, vaginal
	Miconazole (Monistat)	Apply cream bid for 2–3 days	Topical, vaginal suppository and cream, spray, shampoo, IV rarely due to cardiotoxicities
	Nystatin (Mycostatin)	500,000–1,000,000 U tid; 1–4 troches 4–5 times/d; suspension 400,000–600,000 U qid; vaginal 1–2 tablets daily for 2 wks	PO tablet and suspension, troches, vaginal, topical
	Clotrimazole (Mycelex)	PO 1 troche 5 times/d q 3 h for 14 d; topical apply small amount bid	PO, lozenges, topical, vaginal
	Butenafine (Mentax)	Apply to affected area qd for 4 wks	Topical
	Edorazole nitrate (Spectazole)		Topical
	Haloprogin (Halotex)	Apply liberally to affected area bid for 2–3 wks	Topical
	Terbinafine cream (Lamisil)	PO 250 mg qd for 6 wks; topical qd or bid	Topical, PO

NCLEX!

  c. For application to skin: wear latex gloves, cleanse area with tepid water (soap if prescribed), dry thoroughly (without application of heat) and apply to infected area sparingly; do not cover with an occlusive dressing or tight clothing; wash hands well after gloves removed

NCLEX!

  d. For treatment of tinea pedis (athlete's foot), apply antifungal powder such as nystatin (Mycostatin) to inside of shoes and stockings

NCLEX!

  e. For vulvovaginal use: insert one applicator full or one vaginal tablet into vagina at bedtime as instructed; continue therapy during menstruation

  f. Avoid contact of antifungal with eyes; with certain agents, avoid contact with mucous membranes

NCLEX!

  g. Do not apply occlusive dressing unless prescribed; client to avoid restrictive clothing in areas of infection

  h. Store creams, vaginal application, and topical preparation at room temperature; if specified for vaginal tablets and troches, refrigerate but do not freeze

  4. Contraindications: hypersensitivity

  5. Significant drug interactions: do not apply other preparations on same surface area

  6. Significant food interactions: none reported

  7. Significant laboratory studies: liver enzymes in hepatic impairment

  8. Side effects

   a. Topical: stinging, burning, erythema, edema, dry skin, vesication, pruritus, urticaria, desquamation, skin fissures

       b. Vaginal: slight burning, lower abdominal discomfort, bloating, erythema, itching, vaginal soreness during intercourse

       c. Oral troches or swish and swallow: nausea and vomiting

  9. Adverse effects/toxicity: possible hepatotoxicity in client with liver impairment

  10. Nursing considerations

       a. Ensure complete course of therapy taken

       b. Observe for clinical signs of improvement

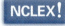

       c. Observe for clinical evidence of liver dysfunction, such as upper right quadrant tenderness, abdominal discomfort/bloating, lethargy, mentation changes, icterus, enlarged liver, elevated liver enzymes (ALT, AST, alkaline phosphatase, bilirubin)

       d. Stop application if severe burning or exacerbation of lesions occur and collaborate with prescriber

  11. Client education

       a. Know drug name, purpose, dose/strength, how to apply/instill, schedule of administration, length of therapy

       b. Observe for resolution of signs/symptoms within first week of therapy; some infections require 2 to 4 weeks of treatment; notify health care provider if condition worsens or no improvement noted in 1 to 2 weeks

       c. Store in tightly covered container at room temperature; if vaginal tablet/suppository, store as recommended, usually in refrigerator or above 59 degrees F; avoid freezing or excess heat of all products

       d. If taken vaginally, refrain from sexual intercourse or have partner wear condom to avoid burning or irritation of penis or urethra

       e. Clothing and linens in contact with infectious sites should be washed after each treatment with soap and water; ointments may be removed from fabric with commercial cleaning products

       f. If severe burning, stinging, or eruptions occur, discontinue use and notify health care provider

       g. See previous administration considerations for specific information regarding types of applications

V. Antiprotozoals

A. Antimalarials

  1. Action and use

       a. Therapeutic use to treat acute episodes or prophylaxis to prevent malarial infection

       b. Chloroquine treatment for **giardiasis** (a protozoan intestinal infection) and amebiasis outside the GI tract

       c. Quinacrine (Atabrine): treat dwarf tapeworm giardiasis and cestodiosis (infestation with tapeworms) ; pleural sclerosing agent to prevent recurrence of pneumothorax

Table 2-19	Generic/Trade Names	Usual Adult Dose	Administration Route
Antiprotozoal Medications	*Antimalarials*		
	Chloroquine HCl (Aralen HCl)	600 mg base/d for 2 d, then 300 mg base/d for 2–3 wks	PO
	Chloroquine phosphate (Aralen Phosphate)	600 mg base followed by 300 mg at 24 and 48 h; IM 200 mg base q 6 h prn	PO, IM
	Hydroxychloroquine sulfate (Plaquenil Sulfate)	Malaria: 620 mg base followed by 310 mg base at 6, 18, and 24 h	PO
	Mefloquine HCl (Lariam)	1250 mg as single oral dose taken with at least 8 oz of water	PO
	Primaquine phosphate	15 mg QD for 14 d concomitantly with chloroquine on first 3 d of acute attack	PO
	Pyrimethamine (Daraprim)	25 mg once/wk	PO
	Quinacrine (Atabrine)	200 mg with 600 mg sodium bicarbonate q 10 min for 4 doses	
	Quinine sulfate (Quinamm)	650 mg q 8 h for 3 d	PO
	Other Antiprotozoal Medications		
	Emetine HCl	1 mg/kg bid for 3–10 d	IM, deep SC
	Paromomycin (Humatin)	25–35 mg/kg divided in 3 doses for 5–10 d	PO
	Pentamidine isoethionate (Pentam 300)	4 mg/kg once/d for 14–21 d, infuse IV over min	IM, IV
	Lindane (Kwell)	Apply to all body area except face, leave lotion on 8–12 h then rinse off	Topical
	Atovaquone (Mepron)	750 mg bid for 21 d	PO
	Iodoquinol (Dioquinol)	630–650 mg tid for 20 days	PO (effective only against intestinal amebic infections)
	Metronidazole (Flagyl)	500–750 mg tid	PO (for other infections, available for PO, IV, vaginal routes)
	Primaquine phosphate	15 mg qd for 14 d concomitantly with chloroquine on first 3 d of acute attack	PO

2. Common medications (Table 2-19)

3. Administration considerations

    a. Separate drug from antacid administration by 4 hours before or after antacids

    b. Take quinine sulfate with food to decrease gastric distress and mask bitter taste; do not crush capsule

    c. Quinacrine HCL (Atabrine): take after food with full glass of water, tea, or juice

    d. Chloroquine HCL (Aralen HCL), hydroxychloroquine sulfate (Plaquenil Sulfate), and pyrimethamine (Daraprim): take with food to minimize gastric distress

    e. For prophylaxis, take as prescribed, such as same day every week when entering high-risk area and for 10 weeks after departing

    f. Mefloquine HCL (Lariam): take with at least 8 ounces water; separate by at least 8 hours from ingestion of quinine or quinidine, an antiarrhythmic

NCLEX!

4. Contraindications

   a. Quinine sulfate: tinnitus, optic neuritis, myasthenia gravis, G6PD deficiency, pregnancy

   b. Quinine sulfate: caution with dysrhythmias and cardiac disorders

   c. Pyrimethamine (Daraprim): caution with antiseizure agents

   d. Mefloquine HCL (Lariam): hypersensitivity; with calcium channel blockers; in dysrhythmias, psychotic or seizure disorders; in pregnancy and in infants

   e. Chloroquine HCL: renal disease; caution in hepatic dysfunction, ethanol abuse, eczema, G6PD deficiency, children, blood dyscrasias, GI and neurological disorders

5. Significant drug interactions

   a. Quinine sulfate: may increase digoxin levels; increased vagolytic effects with anticholinergics; decreased effectiveness if concurrent use of rifampin, antiseizure agents, or barbiturates; increased risk for toxicity with systemic and oral antacids; increased anticoagulant effects with oral anticoagulants; decreased mefloquine HCL levels; increased risk for seizures from possible lowered levels of valproic acid

   b. Disulfiram-like effects with alcohol and some antimalarials

   c. Pyrimethamine: decreased effectiveness against **toxoplasmosis** (protozoan systemic infection transmitted by contact with oocysts in feces of domesticated animals) with concurrent use of folic acid or para-aminobenzoic acid (PABA)

   d. Mefloquine HCL: beta blockers, calcium blockers, and digoxin can prolong cardiac conduction

   e. Decreased absorption with antacids or laxatives containing aluminum or magnesium

   f. May interfere with rabies vaccine

6. Significant food interactions: none reported

7. Significant laboratory studies

   a. ALT, AST, alkaline phosphatase, bilirubin

   b. CBC with differential, reticulocyte count, red blood cell indices, hemoglobin, hematocrit, platelet count

   c. Evaluate electrolytes affected by GI side effects

   d. Prior to therapy, test for G6PD deficiency in African-Americans and clients of Mediterranean descent

8. Side effects

   a. Dizziness, vertigo, headache, visual impairment, angina

   b. Nausea, vomiting, diarrhea, gastric distress, abdominal cramps

   c. Confusion, apprehension, insomnia, nightmares, syncope, delirium

   d. Cutaneous flushing, pruritus, rash, paresthesia, dyspnea, weight loss, fatigue

    e. Quinacrine HCL: may cause reversible yellowing of skin or gray-blue hue to ears, nasal cartilage, and nail beds (not jaundice/cyanosis)

    f. Chloroquine HCL and hydroxychloroquine sulfate: alopecia, bleaching of scalp or hair (including eyebrows and body hair) and freckles; bluish-black hue of skin or mucous membranes, rash, pruritis; photophobia

9. Adverse effects/toxicity

    a. Tinnitus, hearing loss

    b. Cardiotoxicity in clients with atrial fibrillation

    c. Leukopenia, thrombocytopenia, agranulocytosis, hypoprothrombinemia, hemolytic anemia

    d. Hypotension, tachypnea, tachycardia, hypothermia

    e. Convulsions, coma, cardiovascular collapse, blackwater fever (extensive intravascular hemolysis with renal failure), death

    f. Visual halos, blurring, inability to focus

10. Nursing considerations

    a. Ensure complete course of medication is taken for full benefit

    b. Assess drugs being taken to avoid drug interactions

    c. Assess hepatic and cardiac function at intervals

    d. Assess for electrolyte disturbances, blood disorders as anemia, thrombocytopenia

    e. If taking anticonvulsants, monitor drug levels of these agents

    f. Ensure regular ophthalmic exams, electcardiograms, and lab tests as ordered

    g. Assess for G6PD deficiency as indicated

    h. Assess for muscle weakness and depressed deep tendon reflexes periodically

    i. Assess for CNS side effects; collaborate with prescriber regarding discontinuation of agent

11. Client education

    a. Know drug, dose, purpose, and schedule

    b. If weekly, take on same day every week

    c. Do not drive or perform hazardous tasks if drowsiness, dizziness, vertigo, visual disturbances occur

    d. Report fever, sore throat, myalgias, visual disturbances, anxiety, mental changes, hallucinations

    e. Chloroquine HCl: sunglasses may decrease risk of photophobia or ocular changes; urine may become rusty yellow or brown

B. Other antiprotozoals

1. Action and use

   a. Amebic dysentery, hepatic amebiasis or abscess

   b. Some are bacteriocidal as well as amebicidal, especially in GI tract

   c. Paromomycin (Humatin): bactericidal and amebicidal related to tape worms

   d. Destroy intestinal bacteria that forms nitrogen to decrease ammonia in hepatic disease and coma

   e. Pentamidine isethionate (Pentem 300): treat *pneumocystis carinii pneumonia,* an opportunistic infection in client with AIDS

   f. Kills insects-parasites and their ova as in head lice, body lice, and scabies

2. Common medications (Table 2-19)

3. Administration considerations

   a. Pentamidine isoethionate: decreased doses in renal dysfunction

   b. Rotate IM injection sites

   c. Administer atovaquone with high fat meal greater than 23 grams to increase absorption

4. Contraindications

   a. Caution in pregnancy and lactation

   b. Hypersensitivity to drug or to iodine, iodoquinol (Dioquinol), or primaquin

5. Significant drug interactions: none reported

6. Significant food interactions: none reported

7. Significant laboratory studies

   a. Electrolytes including potassium, magnesium, and calcium if GI problems

   b. CBC with WBC and differential: check for infection/blood disorders such as leukopenia, anemia, neutropenia, thrombocytopenia if indicated

   c. Blood glucose for hypoglycemia if pancreatitis develops

8. Side effects

   a. Hypotension, tachycardia, dizziness, headache, syncope

   b. Flushing, pruritis, dyspnea

    c. Abdominal cramps, diarrhea, nausea, vomiting, epigastric distress, unpleasant taste

    d. Myalgia, precordial stiffness

    e. Tremors, restlessness

9. Adverse effects/toxicity

    a. Nephrotoxicity: mild/reversible

    b. Leukopenia, neutropenia, anemia, thrombocytopenia

    c. Dysrhythmias

    d. Hypoglycemia related to pancreatitis

    e. Large doses can cause abscess, cellulitis, or lesion in muscle in the GI tract, heart, liver, and kidneys

    f. Pain at injection site

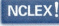

    g. Lindane (Kwell) topical/shampoo can cause CNS problems such as convulsions, or eczematous eruptions

10. Nursing considerations

    a. Ensure complete course of therapy is taken for full benefit

    b. Assess other drugs being taken to avoid drug interactions

    c. Assess skin for scabies, tracking, lesions, nits

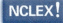

    d. For scabies: warm (not hot) shower and apply topical Kwell, then rinse off after 24 hours

    e. For lice: massage Kwell into head or area infected; leave on for 5 minutes and shampoo out; do not get agent into eyes or on face; do not repeat in less than one week

11. Client education

    a. Know drug, dose, purpose, schedule, proper administration technique

    b. Take full course of therapy for best effect

    c. Report side/adverse effects to health care provider

    d. Wash clothes and linens after treatment to prevent re-infection

    e. Know clinical manifestations of infections to recognize and report

VI. Antihelminthics

A. Action and use

1. *Ascaris lumbricoides* (intestinal worm infestation)

2. *Enterobius vermicularis* (pinworm)

3. *Ancytostoma duodenale* (hookworm)

4. *Necator americanus* (hookworm)

5. *Trichostrongylus* (intestinal worm infestation)

Table 2-20	Generic/Trade Names	Usual Adult Dose	Administration Route
Antihelminthics	Mebendazole (Vermox)	100 mg as single dose	PO
	Piperazine citrate (Antepar)	Roundworms 3.5 g qd for 2 d; pinworms: 65 mg/kg qd for 7–8 d	PO
	Pyrantel pamoate (Antiminth)	11 mg/kg as a single dose	PO
	Thiabendazole (Mintezol)	PO < 70 kg, 25 mg/kg bid for 2 d; ≥ 70 kg, 1.5 g bid for 2 d	PO

B. Common medications (Table 2-20)

C. Administration considerations

   1. Mebendazole: may be chewed, swallowed whole, crushed, mixed with food

   2. Pyrantel pamoate: may take with food

   3. Thiabendazole: take after meals

D. Contraindications

   1. Known hypersensitivity

   2. Paromomycin: in intestinal obstruction

   3. Piperazine citrate: in renal or hepatic impairment, convulsive disorders

   4. Caution with other anthelmintics in clients with hepatic or renal dysfunction

   5. Safety not established in pregnancy and lactation

E. Significant drug interactions

   1. Piperazine citrate: may decrease pyrantel pamoate (Antiminth) levels

   2. Phenothiazines: may increase extrapyramidal effects or risk for convulsions

F. Significant food interactions: none reported

G. Significant laboratory studies

   1. ALT, AST, alkaline phosphatase, bilirubin for liver assessment

   2. Creatinine, BUN, creatinine clearance for renal assessment

   3. Stool for ova and parasites (O & P) for accurate diagnosis of **helminths** (disease-producing parasites)

H. Side effects

1. Nausea, vomiting, diarrhea, abdominal cramps, anorexia

2. Rash, urticaria, erythema multiforme, photosensitivity, purpura, lacrimation, rhinorrhea

3. Dizziness, drowsiness

4. Fever, productive cough, anemia

5. Vision changes

6. Thiabendazole: urinary odor

I. Adverse effects/toxicity

1. Low toxicity; adverse effects usually with large doses

2. Neurotoxicity: headache, vertigo, ataxia, tremors, jerking movements, muscle weakness, paresthesia, depressed reflexes, mental changes abnormal ECG, seizures

3. Dose-related neutropenia; reversed with discontinuation of drug

J. Nursing considerations

1. Assess other drugs being taken to avoid drug interactions

2. Assess laboratory findings for hepatic, renal, or blood disorders and to verify diagnosis

3. Assess allergies

4. Ensure complete regimen taken to optimize therapeutic benefit

5. Collect stool specimen for ova and parasites (O & P) for baseline and follow-up to verify eradication of infectious agents

K. Client education

1. Know drug, dose, purpose, schedule regimen

2. Recognize and report evidence of effectiveness as well as adverse effects that may require discontinuation of drug

3. Agents may be taken with or after food to minimize gastric disturbances

4. Store drug at room temperature protected from light and heat

5. Do not repeat drug therapy for continued infection until one week after initial treatment

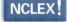

6. Practice personal hygiene to prevent transmission

7. Urine odor may occur with thiabendazole

8. Mebendazole may be chewed, swallowed whole, crushed, or mixed with food

Case Study

A 25-year-old married female client has tested positive for group A streptococcus of the oropharyngeal area. The sensitivity report is not yet available. Amoxicillin (Amoxil) PO is to be initiated as empiric treatment.

❶ What baseline assessment, including laboratory findings, is indicated prior to administering the first dose of amoxicillin?

❷ How would you evaluate drug effectiveness?

❸ If the client developed diarrhea, how would you differentiate the diarrhea from pseudomembranous colitis? What interventions would you implement to manage the diarrhea? For what fluid and electrolyte imbalance would you monitor?

❹ Why is it important to ensure completion of the antibiotic therapy? What two infectious sequela may occur with inadequate therapy against group A streptococcus?

❺ What client education would be appropriate?

For suggested responses, see pages 636–637.

Posttest

1 While teaching the client about taking newly prescribed oral metronidazole (Flagyl), the nurse advises the client about which of the following?

(1) To take with food to minimize the metallic or bitter taste
(2) That visual disturbances are a common side effect
(3) To monitor for urinary retention
(4) That alcohol should be avoided until the last dose is taken

2 The nurse evaluates that the immunocompromised client best understands use of topical acyclovir (Zovirax) for treating genital herpes when the client makes which of the following statements?

(1) "I need to wash my hands for at least 10 seconds with a teaspoon of antibacterial soap before and after application of the drug."
(2) "My sister isn't immunocompromised, but she has genital herpes and should use acyclovir, too."
(3) "I need to use a different finger cot when getting ointment and applying the ointment to each sore to prevent self-inoculation in other areas."
(4) "Acyclovir has been around a long time. I know there have to be newer drugs that are better to treat my genital herpes."

3 The nurse prepares to initiate therapy with acyclovir (Zovirax) to a client with AIDS. What intervention is most appropriate for the nurse to perform?

(1) Assess bilirubin
(2) Assess for hypokalemia
(3) Assess for other nephrotoxic drugs being taken
(4) Assess the number of stools in the past 24 hours and their consistency

4 The nurse anticipates that the client will be premedicated with an antipyretic, an antihistamine, and an antiemetic to decrease infusion-related reaction. Which of the following anti-infectives is most likely prescribed?

(1) Amphotericin B (Fungizone)
(2) Acyclovir (Zovirax)
(3) Cefazolin Sodium (Ancef)
(4) Methicillin (Staphcillin)

5 Knowing that serum protein is needed to bind with anti-infectives in order to maintain therapeutic response rate, the nurse recommends which of the following desserts?

(1) Sherbet
(2) Pudding
(3) Fruit gelatin
(4) Egg custard

6 The nurse assesses the client receiving gentamicin (Garamycin) for what two most specific toxicities?

(1) Hepatotoxicity and neurotoxicity
(2) Nephrotoxicity and ototoxicity
(3) Leukocytosis and thrombocytopenia
(4) Pseudomembranous colitis and crytalluria

7 The nurse assesses for what most significant side effect in a client with tuberculosis taking isoniazid (INH)?

(1) Paresthesias in limbs
(2) Hearing loss
(3) Visual acuity
(4) Crystalluria

8 During administration of vancomycin (Vancocin), the nurse recognizes which of the following clinical manifestations as a specific response to the drug being infused too rapidly?

(1) Hypertension
(2) Projectile vomiting
(3) "Red neck syndrome"
(4) Pseudomembranous colitis

9 Tetracycline has been ordered for a 2-year-old child. What intervention by the nurse is most appropriate?

(1) Teach the child to drink liquid tetracycline to avoid discoloration of the teeth.
(2) Collaborate with the prescriber about appropriateness of the order.
(3) Evaluate renal function prior to initiation of therapy.
(4) Administer with 6 to 8 ounces of water.

10 The nurse teaches a client taking a tetracycline or a sulfonamide to do which of the following?

(1) Have regular evaluation of the prothrombin time (PT) and international rationalized ratio (INR).
(2) Wear long sleeves and long-legged pants, hat, and sunglasses when in the sunlight.
(3) Take with milk or food to minimize gastrointestinal disturbances.
(4) Change position slowly to avoid orthostatic hypotension.

See pages 97–98 for Answers and Rationales.

Answers and Rationales

Pretest

1 Answer: 4 *Rationale:* Administration of vitamin B_6 is recommended during therapy with isoniazid (INH) to reduce the incidence of peripheral neuritis, which may be associated with isoniazid. Monitoring motor reflexes would not be indicated (option 1). Paresthesia is not usually a clinical manifestation of hypercalcemia (option 2). Antacids interfere with absorption of INH when taken within 1 to 2 hours of the INH, but would not cause the symptoms reported by the client (option 3).
Cognitive Level: Application
Nursing Process: Assessment; *Test Plan:* PHYS

2 Answer: 3 Rationale: Rifampin causes an orange-red discoloration of body fluids including urine. The client needs to be aware of this. The drug is being ordered prophylactically to prevent the development of meningitis, not to treat it (option 1). Adverse effects are generally minor with rifampin (option 2). Because the drug is metabolized by the liver, regular liver function tests should be monitored (option 4). Rifampin should be used with caution in the presence of elevated liver enzymes or hepatic dysfunction.
Cognitive Level: Application
Nursing Process: Implementation; *Test Plan:* PHYS

3 Answer: 1 *Rationale:* Amantadine (Symmetrel) can cause anticholinergic effects, one of which is bladder relaxation and detrusor muscle contraction. Urinary retention may become more of a problem for a client with BPH on this medication. Hypermotility of the bowel and increased lacrimation are cholinergic effects, not anticholinergic effects (options 2 and 3). Amantadine is not particularly nephrotoxic (option 4).
Cognitive Level: Application
Nursing Process: Planning; *Test Plan:* PHYS

4 Answer: 4 *Rationale:* Agents for herpes virus as herpes zoster can be nephritic. Important interventions include monitoring renal function and ensuring good hydration to decrease toxic effects. This drug is not reported to be particularly hepatotoxic (option 1). Sexual intercourse is to be avoided if the client was being treated with the acylovir for genital herpes (option 2). Insomnia is not a side effect of acyclovir (option 3).
Cognitive Level: Application
Nursing Process: Implementation; *Test Plan:* PHYS

5 Answer: 1 *Rationale:* A full course of antibiotic therapy must be taken to decrease the risk for resistance to the antibiotic or recurrence of infection. Missed doses should be taken as soon as they are remembered, but the dose should not be doubled by taking two doses at the same time (option 2). Antibiotic doses are to be taken at regular intervals spaced throughout the 24 hours, without interrupting sleep when possible, in order to maintain effective therapeutic blood level of the antibiotic (option 3). Chewable tablets must be crushed or chewed, or the drug may not absorb adequately (option 4).
Cognitive Level: Analysis
Nursing Process: Evaluation; *Test Plan:* PHYS

6 Answer: 4 *Rationale:* More than 4 to 6 watery stools per day and/or stools with blood is a clinical manifestation of pseudomembranous colitis. *C. difficile* is the causative microorganism for this superinfection. The client is at risk for developing metabolic acidosis because of increased loss of bowel contents with loss of base (option 1). Peristaltic agents can promote retention of toxins and should not be given (option 2). Antidiarrheal agents may be given for mild diarrhea but not when toxins need to be eliminated (option 3).
Cognitive Level: Application
Nursing Process: Planning; *Test Plan:* PHYS

7 Answer: 4 *Rationale:* Specific indicators of improvement, such as the resolution of pulmonary infiltrates, improved breath sounds, and normalization of pulse oximetry, are important outcomes to monitor in pneumonia. Systemic signs including fever as well as malaise, and leukocytosis are expected to demonstrate improvement within 48 to 72 hours of antibiotic therapy (option 1). Option 2 does not indicate therapeutic effectiveness, and option 3 is unrelated to the question.
Cognitive Level: Application
Nursing Process: Evaluation; *Test Plan:* PHYS

8 Answer: 1 *Rationale:* The penicillins are structured with a sodium or potassium salt. When a high sodium content penicillin is administered, serum sodium may be elevated, which often results in hypokalemia. This client is demonstrating clinical manifestations of hypokalemia. With the elevated sodium, the accompanying anion would most likely be chloride resulting in hyperchloremia and not hypochloremia (option 2). Options 3 and 4 are not associated with this medication.
Cognitive Level: Analysis
Nursing Process: Assessment; *Test Plan:* PHYS

9 Answer: 4 *Rationale:* A cross-allergenicity with penicillin may exist in this client. Cephalosporins cannot be assumed to be an absolutely safe alternative to penicillin in PCN-allergic clients. If the cephalosporin in this client is administered, the nurse needs to administer cautiously observing for manifestations of hypersensitivity, especially respiratory difficulty. Emergency equipment should be readily accessible. The BUN is within normal limits (option 1). It is expected that the granulocytosis would occur in response to a bacterial infection (option 2). To wait several hours for the results of the C & S may compromise the client's response to the treatment (option 3). If the C & S findings reveal the bacteria is resistant to the prescribed antibiotic, the drug can be changed although the original antibiotic has been continued in some cases if clinical improvement is seen.
Cognitive Level: Application
Nursing Process: Implementation; *Test Plan:* PHYS

10 Answer: 1 *Rationale:* A "shift to the left" refers to an increase in neutrophils, and in immature neutrophils called bands or stab cells. Production of these white blood cells is stimulated by an acute bacterial infection. Lymphocytes, T cells and B cells, are increased primarily in viral infections. Monocytes also fight bacterial infection by phagocytic action. Eosinophils and basophils are elevated in allergic reaction.
Cognitive Level: Analysis
Nursing Process: Analysis; *Test Plan:* PHYS

Posttest

1 **Answer: 1** *Rationale:* Metronidazole (Flagyl) has several gastrointestinal side effects including metallic or bitter taste. It can be taken with food except for Flagyl ER, which should be taken 1 hour before or 2 hours after meals. There is no evidence that Flagyl causes visual disturbances or urinary retention (options 2 and 3). Alcohol taken during drug therapy or within 48 hours after the drug is discontinued may induce a disulfiram-like effect (option 4).
Cognitive Level: Application
Nursing Process: Implementation; *Test Plan:* PHYS

2 **Answer: 3** *Rationale:* A different gloved finger or a different finger cot should be used to apply acyclovir to each lesion not only to prevent spread on client's own body, but also to prevent transmission to others. Caution needs to be taken as well to not contaminate the ointment in the container by obtaining ointment with a contaminated finger cot/glove. Handwashing is important but is not a barrier protection (option 1). Acyclovir is the drug of choice for primary herpes lesions in the immunosuppressed client, but it has not been proven that acyclovir benefits the immunocompetent client, although it may reduce viral shedding (option 2). Option 4 is a false statement.
Cognitive Level: Analysis
Nursing Process: Evaluation; *Test Plan:* PHYS

3 **Answer: 3** *Rationale:* The nurse assesses hydration status, intake and output, creatinine, BUN, creatinine clearance, and other laboratory tests for renal dysfunction. The nurse also assesses for concurrent nephrotoxic agents being taken since these drugs could increase the risk for nephrotoxicity developing with administration of acyclovir (Zovirax). The bilirubin differentiates jaundice caused by liver impairment or by hemolysis (option 1). Bowel pattern and hypokalemia are not particular to acyclovir therapy (options 2 and 4).
Cognitive Level: Application
Nursing Process: Assessment; *Test Plan:* PHYS

4 **Answer: 1** *Rationale:* Almost all clients receiving IV amphotericin B experience adverse reactions involving fever, chills, piloerection, hypotension, tachycardia, malaise, myalgia, arthralgia, anorexia, nausea, vomiting, and headache. The other agents listed do not cause this cluster of severe side effects. Meperidine (Demerol) may also be given to help manage the side effects.
Cognitive Level: Application
Nursing Process: Analysis; *Test Plan:* PHYS

5 **Answer: 4** *Rationale:* Complete proteins are higher quality proteins and contain all nine essential amino acids in sufficient amounts to meet the body's needs. Sources of these proteins are of animal origin, such as eggs, milk, cheese, and meat. Gelatin, an animal product, is an exception since it is an incomplete protein. The pudding contains milk, but the egg custard contains the largest quantity of animal proteins such as eggs and milk.
Cognitive Level: Application
Nursing Process: Implementation; *Test Plan:* PHYS

6 **Answer: 2** *Rationale:* The most significant adverse effects related to the aminoglycosides, of which gentamycin (Garamycin) is a member, are nephrotoxicity and ototoxicity. Risk for ototoxicity is increased in the presence of nephrotoxicity.
Cognitive Level: Application
Nursing Process: Assessment; *Test Plan:* PHYS

7 **Answer: 1** *Rationale:* The most common adverse effect of isoniazid (INH) is peripheral neuritis manifested as paresthesia of the extremities. The items in the other options are not side effects of this therapy.
Cognitive Level: Application
Nursing Process: Assessment; *Test Plan:* PHYS

8 **Answer: 3** *Rationale:* "Red neck syndrome" or "red man syndrome" is flushing of the face, neck, and upper chest associated with too rapid IV administration of vancomycin (Vancocin). Hypotension with shock (not hypertension) also can result from the histamines released with too rapid infusion (option 1). Option 2 does not occur. Pseudomembranous colitis (option 4) is the result of a superinfection.
Cognitive Level: Analysis
Nursing Process: Analysis; *Test Plan:* PHYS

9 **Answer: 2** *Rationale:* Tetracycline should not be given to children under 8 years of age. The drug forms deposits in the bone and primary dentition in growing children that can cause underdevelopment of the child's bones and teeth, temporary stunting of the child's growth, and discoloration of the teeth of the child. Discoloration of the teeth is not caused by direct contact of teeth with the medication, as can happen with iron preparations (option 1). Since the drug should not be administered to a child under 8 years of age, options 3 and 4 are less important and therefore incorrect.
Cognitive Level: Application
Nursing Process: Implementation; *Test Plan:* PHYS

10 **Answer: 2** *Rationale:* Photosensitivity is a side effect of these two classes of antibiotics. The client

avoids sun exposure and tanning beds. Milk or food interferes with effectiveness of the tetracyclines so tetracyclines are taken on an empty stomach (option 3). These drugs are not associated with increased

bleeding or orthostatic hypotension (options 1 and 4).
Cognitive Level: Application
Nursing Process: Implementation; *Test Plan:* PHYS

References

American Society of Health-System Pharmacists (2002). *AHPS drug information 2002.* Bethesda, MD: American Society of Health-System Pharmacists, Inc.

Drug Facts & Comparisons® (Updated Monthly). St. Louis: A. Wolters Kluwer, p. 1242.

Grajeda-Higley, L. (2000). *Understanding pharmacology: A physiologic approach.* Stanford, CT: Appleton and Lange, pp. 3–251.

Ignatavicius, D. D. & Workman, M. L. (2002). *Medical-surgical nursing: Critical thinking for collaborative care* (4th ed.). Philadelphia: W. B. Saunders, p. 1924.

Karch, A. M. (2003). *Focus on nursing pharmacology* (2nd ed.). Philadelphia: Lippincott, Williams, & Wilkins, pp. 34–136.

LeMone, P. & Burke, K. M. (2003). *Medical-surgical nursing: Critical thinking in client care* (3rd ed.). Upper Saddle River, NJ: Prentice Hall, pp. 141–1692.

Lilley, L. L. & Aucker, R. S. (2001). *Pharmacology and the nursing process* (3rd ed.). St. Louis: Mosby, pp. 26–647.

McKenry, L. M. & Salerno, E. (2003). *Pharmacology in nursing* (21st ed. revised reprint). St. Louis: Mosby, pp. 568–1085.

Pagana, K. D. & Pagana, T. J. (2002). *Manual of diagnostic and laboratory tests.* St. Louis: Mosby, pp. 17–520.

Shannon, M. T., Wilson, B. A., & Stang, C. L. (2003). *Health professional's drug guide 2003.* Upper Saddle River, NJ: Prentice Hall.

Williams, S. R. (2001). *Basic nutrition and diet therapy.* (11th ed.). St. Louis: Mosby, pp. 48–415.

Wynne, A. L., Woo, T. M., & Millard, M. (2002). *Pharmacotherapeutics for nurse practitioner prescribers.* Philadelphia: F. A. Davis Company, pp. 60–739.

CHAPTER 3

Antineoplastic Medications

Susan K. Steele, MN, RN, AOCN

CHAPTER OUTLINE

OBJECTIVES

■ Describe the general goals of antineoplastic therapy.

■ Describe the common side effects of antineoplastic medications.

■ Identify the primary toxic effects associated with antineoplastic therapy.

■ Identify the nursing interventions for the client with depressed white blood cell production, bleeding tendencies, or stomatitis.

■ List the significant client education points related to antineoplastic medications.

[Media Link]

Use the CD-ROM enclosed with this text, or log onto the address given to access the free, interactive Companion Website created for this series. The CD-ROM and Companion Website accompanying this book offer additional practice opportunities and information—NCLEX Review, Case Studies, Glossary, In Depth with NCLEX, and more.

www.prenhall.com/hogan

REVIEW AT A GLANCE

acral erythema *red palms*

alopecia *partial or complete hair loss*

anticipatory nausea *conditioned response resulting from repeated association of chemotherapy-induced nausea and vomiting and a stimulus from the environment*

cell cycle specific *chemotherapy agent that exhibits its cytotoxic effect at a certain stage of cell division*

cell cycle nonspecific *chemotherapy agent that exhibits its cytotoxic effect regardless of the stage of cell division*

hemorrhagic cystitis *chemical irritation of the bladder that causes bleeding and hematuria*

irritant *a chemotherapy agent that causes redness and irritation of the skin upon extravasation, but without sloughing*

nadir *the lowest point to which blood counts will drop after chemotherapy administration*

myelosuppression *decrease in blood counts usually related to chemotherapy*

pancytopenia *decrease in all blood cell components; may take 1 month to 2 years to recover*

radiation recall *erythema that develops in a previously irradiated field*

vesicant *medication that causes severe skin and tissue necrosis if it extravasates from the vein*

Pretest

1 Neurological assessment is an important parameter when administering plant (vinca) alkaloids. Which of the following assessed by the nurse indicates an early warning sign of pending impairment?

(1) Confusion
(2) Short-term memory loss
(3) Depression of the Achilles reflex
(4) Decreased hand-grasp strength

2 Which of the following items should be included in the therapeutic management to prevent doxorubicin-related congestive heart failure from cardiotoxicity in a client who has cancer?

(1) Exercise and smoking cessation
(2) Smoking cessation and oxygen administration
(3) Exercise and administration of dexrazoxane (Zinecard)
(4) Oxygen administration and a low-fat diet

3 A client is receiving chemotherapy that has pulmonary toxicity as an adverse effect. Which of the following breathing techniques is important to teach the client to improve the efficiency of breathing?

(1) Exhaling through the nose
(2) Exhaling through pursed lips
(3) Exhaling one half and then inhale
(4) Exhale using accessory muscles

4 The nurse assesses for chemotherapy-induced pulmonary toxicity in a client receiving which of the following antineoplastic agents?

(1) Fluorouracil (5-FU)
(2) Bleomycin (Blenoxane)
(3) Etoposide (Vepesid)
(4) 6-mercaptopurine (Purinethol)

5 A nurse is administering chemotherapy to a group of clients. The nurse implements measures to reduce the risk of mucositis for which of the following most important reasons?

(1) To increase comfort
(2) To decrease infection
(3) To improve self-image
(4) To reduce cancer recurrence

6 Which of the following clients is most likely to experience chemotherapy-induced nausea?

(1) A mother of 2 who experienced severe morning sickness during both of her pregnancies
(2) A navy pilot who experienced motion sickness as a child
(3) A 38-year-old male who has alcoholism
(4) A young woman with no significant history of emesis

7 Which of the following interventions should the nurse plan to use for a client experiencing neutropenia?

(1) Insert an indwelling urinary catheter to maintain accurate intake and output.
(2) Leave all wounds open to the air for better healing.
(3) Encourage daily hygiene, regular oral care, and perianal care after each stool.
(4) Flush all lumens of a long-term catheter with heparinized saline every 8 hours.

8 Which of the following interventions would be recommended for the client with the nursing diagnosis of Risk for altered oral mucous membranes related to side effects of fluorouracil (5-FU)?

(1) Schedule oral hygiene Q 2 hours with a soft toothbrush and nonfluoride toothpaste.
(2) Rinse mouth Q 2 hours during the day and Q 4 hours at night with a baking soda and peroxide rinse.
(3) Schedule oral care Q 2 to 4 hours with a soft toothbrush, fluorinated toothpaste, and a baking soda with isotonic saline rinse.
(4) Continue oral hygiene BID with toothettes and baking soda, and rinse with commercial mouthwash to decrease mouth odor.

9 Which lifestyle changes should the nurse teach the client to decrease the risk of developing constipation after receiving vincristine (Oncovin)?

(1) Decrease physical activity.
(2) Add fiber to the diet.
(3) Increase laxative usage.
(4) Decrease fluid intake.

10 The nurse explains to a client that an important advantage of combination chemotherapy over single-drug regimens is that this will do which of the following?

(1) Reduce the potential for nausea and vomiting.
(2) Reduce the potential for tumor resistance.
(3) Spare the normal cells from severe toxicity.
(4) Decrease the likelihood of drug-induced gonadal sterility.

See pages 139–140 for Answers and Rationales.

I. Alkylating Agents

A. Action and use

1. Interfere with DNA replication through cross-linking of DNA strands, DNA strand breaking, and abnormal base pairing proteins

2. Most agents are **cell cycle nonspecific,** which means that they exhibit a cytotoxic effect regardless of the cell cycle stage (see diagram on companion web site)

3. Major toxicities occur in the hematopoietic, gastrointestinal (GI), and reproductive systems

B. Common medications (Table 3-1)

C. Administration considerations

1. Cyclophosphamide (Cytoxan)

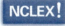

   a. Administer PO on an empty stomach; if nausea and vomiting are severe it may be taken with food; antiemetic agent should be given before the drug is administered

   b. Should be administered by intravenous piggyback (IVPB) over 60 to 90 minutes

2. Busulfan (Myleran)

   a. Should be taken as directed at the same time every day

   b. Taking drug on an empty stomach may minimize nausea and vomiting

   c. Store drug tightly capped in a light-resistant container

Generic (Trade) Name	Route
Altretamine (Hexalen)	PO
Busulfan (Myleran)	PO, IV
Carboplatin (Paraplatin)	IV
Chlorambucil (Leukeran)	PO
Cisplatin (Platinol)	IV
Cyclophosphamide (Cytoxan)	PO, IV
Dacarbazine (DTIC-Dome)	IV
Ifosfamide (Ifex)	IV
Mechlorethamine (Nitrogen mustard)	IV, IT, T
Melphalan (Alkeran)	PO, IV
Procarbazine (Matulane)	PO,
Thiotepa (Thioplex)	PO, IC

Table 3-1

Common Alkylating Agents

PO = oral; IV = intravenous; IT = intrathecal; IC = intracavitary, T = topical

3. Cisplatin (Platinol)

   a. Provide hydration with 1 to 2 liters of IV fluid before and after administration

   b. Administer a parenteral antiemetic agent 30 minutes before cisplatin therapy is instituted and give it on a scheduled basis throughout the day and night as long as necessary

4. Carboplatin (Paraplatin)

   a. Needles or IV sets containing aluminum should not be used

   b. Premedication with an anti-emetic 30 minutes before and on a scheduled basis thereafter is generally recommended

   c. Dosage should not be repeated until the neutrophil count is at least 2,000/mm^3

   d. Store unopened vials at room temperature, protect from light

5. Mechlorethamine (Nitrogen mustard, Mustargen)

   a. Potent **vesicant** (causes severe skin and tissue necrosis if medication extravasates from the vein)

   b. Should be administered through the side-arm portal of a freely running IV to avoid extravasation

   c. If the drug should extravasate, subcutaneous and intradermal injection with isotonic sodium thiosulfate and application of ice compresses may reduce local irritation

   d. Short **nadir** period (6–8 days), which is the lowest point to which the blood counts will drop after chemotherapy administration

D. Contraindications

1. Cyclophosphamide (Cytoxan)

   a. Men and women in childbearing years

   b. Serious infections including chicken pox and herpes zoster

   c. Immunosuppression

    d. Pregnancy (category C) and nursing mothers

  2. Busulfan (Myleran)

    a. Therapy-resistant chronic lymphocytic leukemia

    b. Blast crisis of chronic myelogenous leukemia

    c. Bone marrow depression

    d. Pregnancy (category D) and nursing mothers

  3. Cisplatin (Platinol)

    a. History of sensitivity to cisplatin or other platinum-containing compounds

    b. Impaired renal function and/or hearing

    c. History of gout and urate renal stones

    d. Safe use in pregnancy (category D) and nursing women not established

  4. Carboplatin (Paraplatin)

    a. History of severe reactions to carboplatin or cisplatin

    b. Severe bone marrow depression

    c. Impaired renal function

    d. Cautious use in pregnancy (category D) and with other nephrotoxic drugs

  5. Ifosfamide (Ifex)

    a. Severe bone marrow suppression or known hypersensitivity to ifosfamide

    b. Cautious use in clients with impaired renal function, prior radiation therapy, or prior cytotoxic agents

    c. Cautious use in pregnancy (category D) and nursing mothers

  6. Mechlorethamine (nitrogen mustard, Mustargen)

    a. Myelosuppression: a decrease in blood counts usually related to chemotherapy

    b. Infectious granuloma

    c. Known infectious diseases, including herpes zoster

    d. Pregnancy (category D) and lactation

E. Significant drug interactions

  1. Cyclophosphamide (Cytoxan)

    a. Succinylcholine (Anectine): prolonged neuromuscular blocking activity

    b. Doxorubicin (Adriamycin): may increase cardiotoxicity

  2. Busulfan: probenecid (Probalan), an antigout/uricosuric agent, may increase uric acid levels

  3. Cisplatin (Platinol)

    a. Aminoglycosides, amphotericin-B, vancomycin, and other nephrotoxic drugs increase risk of nephrotoxicity and acute renal failure

        b. Aminoglycosides and furosemide (Lasix) increase risk of ototoxicity

        c. Incompatible with 5 percent dextrose solutions, sodium bicarbonate, and metoclopramide (Reglan)

    4. Carboplatin (Paraplatin)

        a. Aminoglycosides may increase the risk of ototoxicity and nephrotoxicity

        b. May decrease phenytoin (Dilantin) levels

        c. Incompatible with dextrose-containing solutions

    5. Ifosfamide (Ifex)

        a. Barbiturates, phenytoin (Dilantin), and chloral hydrate (Aquachloral) may increase hepatic conversion of ifosfamide to active metabolite

        b. Corticosteroids may inhibit conversion to active metabolite

    6. Mechlorethamine (nitrogen mustard, Mustargen): may reduce effectiveness of antigout agents by raising serum uric acid levels

F. Significant food interactions: Procarbazine

    1. Avoid foods high in tyramine (e.g., beer, wine, cheese, brewer's yeast, chicken livers, and bananas) while taking procarbazine, since it may lead to hypertension and possible intracranial hemorrhage

    2. Disulfiram-like reaction can occur if client consumes alcohol and procarbazine

G. Significant assessment parameters

    1. Cyclophosphamide (Cytoxan)

        a. Determine total differential leukocyte count, platelet count, and hematocrit initially and at least every 2 weeks thereafter

        b. Obtain baseline and periodic determinations of liver and kidney function in addition to serum electrolytes

        c. Microscopic urine examinations are recommended after large doses

    2. Busulfan (Myleran)

        a. Determine total differential leukocyte count, platelet count, and hematocrit initially and at least every 2 weeks thereafter

        b. There may be an abrupt onset of hematotoxicity; recovery from busulfan-induced **pancytopenia** (a decrease in all blood cell components) may take from 1 month to 2 years

        c. Ovarian suppression, amenorrhea, and menopausal symptoms are common

    3. Cisplatin (Platinol)

        a. Pre-treatment electrocardiogram (ECG) is indicated because of possible myocarditis or focal irritation

        b. Monitor urine output and specific gravity for 4 consecutive hours before therapy and for 24 hours after therapy; report an output of less than 100 mL/hr or a specific gravity of greater than 1.030 to physician; a urine output of less than 75 mL/hr necessitates medical intervention

c. Audiometric testing should be performed before the initial dose

d. Anaphylactic reactions may occur within minutes of drug administration

e. BUN, serum uric acid, serum creatinine, and urinary creatinine clearance should be assessed before initiating therapy and every subsequent course

f. Nephrotoxicity usually occurs within 2 weeks after drug administration and becomes more severe and prolonged with repeated courses

g. Suspect ototoxicity if client manifests tinnitus or difficulty hearing in the high-frequency range

h. Assess blood pressure, mental status, pupils, and optic fundi every hour during therapy since hydration increases the danger of elevated intracranial pressure

i. Monitor and report abnormal bowel patterns since constipation may be an early sign of neurotoxicity

4. Carboplatin (Paraplatin)

a. Allergic reaction can occur within first 15 minutes of administration, monitor closely for signs of anaphylaxis during the first 15 minutes of infusion

b. Frequently monitor peripheral blood counts; nadir usually occurs at day 21

c. Periodically monitor kidney function and creatinine clearance, although it has less renal toxicity than cisplatin

d. Monitor for peripheral neuropathy, ototoxicity, and visual disturbances, although they occur less frequently than with cisplatin

e. Monitor clients on diuretic therapy closely since carboplatin may also decrease serum sodium, potassium, calcium, and magnesium levels

5. Ifosfamide (Ifex)

a. Monitor complete blood count (CBC) with differential before each dose; hold ifosfamide if WBC is below 2,000/mm^3 or platelet count is below 50,000/mm^3

b. Monitor urine before and during each dose for microscopic hematuria

c. Hydrate with at least 3,000 cc of fluid daily to reduce risk of **hemorrhagic cystitis** (excessive bleeding from the bladder due to chemical irritation)

H. Side effects/toxicity

1. Cyclophosphamide (Cytoxan)

a. Cardiotoxicity, acute cardiomegaly with high dose; prior radiation therapy and prior anthracycline therapy increases risk

b. Hemorrhagic cystitis (occasionally chronic and severe)

c. Metallic taste on administration

d. Acute myelosuppression

e. **Acral erythema** (palmar redness) and sloughing of the skin on palms of hands and feet

f. Diffuse hyperpigmentation

       g. Gonadal dysfunction

       h. Nausea and vomiting

   2. Busulfan (Myleran)

       a. Myelosuppression

       b. Severe nausea and vomiting

       c. Severe mucositis

       d. Pulmonary fibrosis, sometimes referred to as "busulfan lung"

       e. Hepatic dysfunction leading to veno-occlusive disease

       f. Diffuse hyperpigmentation; development of bullae

       g. Chronic **alopecia:** partial or complete hair loss usually on the scalp

   3. Cisplatin (Platinol)

       a. Renal and hepatic toxicity

       b. Eighth cranial nerve damage because of ototoxicity

       c. Myelosuppression

       d. Peripheral neuropathy; neurotoxicity

       e. Intense nausea and vomiting

       f. Metallic taste on administration

   4. Carboplatin (Paraplatin)

       a. Myelosuppression with pronounced thrombocytopenia

       b. Severe nausea and vomiting

       c. Hepatotoxicity

       d. Auditory toxicity

       e. Mild renal toxicity

   5. Ifosfamide (Ifex)

       a. Hemorrhagic cystitis, occasionally chronic and severe

       b. Neutopenia and thrombocytopenia

       c. Nausea and vomiting

       d. Hepatic dysfunction

       e. Nephrotoxicity

       f. Somnolence, confusion, and hallucinations

I. Client and family education

   1. Cyclophosphamide (Cytoxan)

       a. Because of the mutagenic potential, teach client to employ adequate means of contraception during and for at least 4 months after termination of drug therapy

    b. Instruct client to void frequently and maintain hydration with oral fluids to at least 3,000 mL/24 hours

  2. Cisplatin (Platinol)

    a. Continue maintenance of adequate hydration with oral fluids to at least 3,000 mL/24 hr; report reduced urinary output, anorexia, nausea and vomiting uncontrolled by antiemetics, fluid retention, and weight gain

    b. Keep vestibular stimulation to a minimum to avoid dizziness or falling

    c. Tingling, numbness, tremors of extremities, loss of position sense and taste, and constipation are early warn signs of neurotoxicity

  3. Carboplatin (Paraplatin)

    a. Give special attention to strategies to prevent nausea

    b. Inform client about potential for infection and hemorrhagic complications related to bone marrow suppression

    c. Instruct client to report paresthesias, visual disturbances, or symptoms of ototoxicity (hearing loss/tinnitus)

  4. Ifosfamide (Ifex)

    a. Instruct client to void frequently and to maintain hydration

    b. Advise client that the susceptibility to infection will increase

    c. Teach client to report any unusual bleeding or bruising

II. Antimetabolites

A. Action and use

  1. Inhibit protein synthesis, substitute erroneous metabolites or structural analogues during DNA synthesis, and inhibit DNA synthesis

  2. Most agents are **cell cycle specific;** that is, they exhibit a cytotoxic affect during a specific phase of the cell cycle, such as the S phase (see diagram on companion Web site)

  3. Most toxicity occurs in the hematopoietic and GI systems

  4. Used to treat leukemia, solid tumors, and lymphoma

B. Common medications (Table 3-2)

> **Practice to Pass**
>
> List 3 measures to assist in the prevention of renal toxicity secondary to cisplatin (Platinol) administration.

Table 3-2	Generic (Trade) Name	Route
Common Anti-Metabolites	Cytarabine (Ara-C, Cytosar-U)	IV, SC, IT
	Fludarabine (Fludara)	IV
	Fluorouracil (5-FU, Adrucil)	IV
	Gemcitabine (Gemzar)	IV
	Mercaptopurine (Purinethol)	PO
	Methotrexate (Folex)	PO, IV, IM, IT
	Thioguanine (generic only)	PO, IV

PO = oral; IV = intravenous; IT = intrathecal; IM = intramuscular, SC = subcutaneous

C. Administration considerations

1. Rotate IV sites every 48 hours to decrease hyperpigmentation

2. Determine whether the dosage ordered is standard versus high dose and obtain appropriate rescue therapy before administration (i.e., methotrexate with leucovorin)

3. Dosage of mercaptopurine should be reduced by 75 percent if given concurrently with allopurinol (Zyloprim); however, no dosage reduction is required with thioguanine

4. Fludarabine (Fludara) should be given as a 30-minute infusion

D. Contraindications

1. Myelosuppression

2. Pregnancy (category D) and nursing women

3. Concurrent administration of hepatotoxic drugs and hematopoietic depressants

4. Cautious use in the following situations

   a. Clients with major surgery during the previous month

   b. Previous use of alkylating agents

   c. History of high-dose pelvic irradiation

   d. Preexisting bone marrow impairment

   e. Men and women during childbearing years

   f. Hepatic or renal impairment

E. Significant drug interactions

1. Fluorouracil (5FU): cimetidine (Tagamet) increases pharmacological effects; thiazide diuretics increase risk of myelosuppression; leucovorin (Wellcovorin) increases cytotoxicity

2. Cytarabine (Ara-C): decreases bioavailability of digoxin (Lanoxin)

3. Methotrexate (Folex)

   a. Protein-bound drugs (i.e., aspirin, phenytoin, tetracycline) increase toxicity

   b. Nonsteroidal inflammatory drugs (NSAIDS), sulfamethoxazole/trimethoprim (Bactrim), and pyrimethamine (Daraprim) increase and prolong methotrexate levels

4. Thioguanine (6-Thioguanine): busulfan (Myleran) increases hepatotoxicity

5. 6-mercaptopurine (Purinethol)

   a. Allopurinol (Zyloprim) increases 6-mercaptopurine levels

   b. Warfarin (Coumadin) affects prothrombin time (PT) levels

   c. Non-depolarizing muscle relaxants: decreased neuromuscular blockade

6. Fludarabine (Fludara): fatal pulmonary toxicity can occur if administered concurrently with pentostatin (Nipent), an enzyme-inhibitor type of antineoplastic

F. Significant food interactions: none known

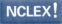

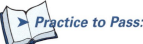
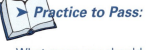

G. Significant assessment parameters

    1. Assess baseline CBC, WBC differential, and platelet count prior to administration

    2. Assess for signs and symptoms of infection or bleeding

H. Side effects/toxicity

    1. General toxicities for this drug group

        a. Myelosuppression

        b. Nausea and vomiting

        c. Mucosal inflammation: stomatitis

        d. Photosensitivity with or without hyperpigmentation

        e. Diarrhea (most commonly associated with antimetabolites)

    2. Fluorouracil (5-FU): specific side effects/toxicity

        a. Cardiotoxicity mimicking an acute myocardial infarction (MI), angina, cardiogenic shock

        b. Photosensitivity and hyperpigmentation

        c. Cerebellar toxicity

    3. Cytarabine (Ara-C): specific side effects/toxicity

        a. Maculopapular rash, with or without fever

        b. Cytarabine syndrome (rash with or without fever, myalgia, bone pain, malaise)

        c. Chemical conjunctivitis

        d. Acute neurotoxicity: cerebellar toxicity; clients > 50 years of age are at highest risk

        e. Hepatotoxicity

        f. Acral erythema

I. Client and family education

    1. Teach importance of self-care measures to avoid infection and bleeding

        a. Avoid large crowds

        b. Avoid proximity to people with infections

        c. Avoid over-the-counter (OTC) aspirin-containing medications

    2. Teach oral assessment and the importance of maintaining scheduled mouth care and to report development of stomatitis to healthcare professional

    3. Teach client to maintain a low residue diet after discharge and to report excessive diarrhea (> 3 loose stools in 24 hours) to healthcare professional

    4. Teach client that darkening of the veins, mucous membranes, and fingernails may occur

    5. Photosensitivity precautions should be followed year-round

        a. Encourage use of sunscreen with a sun protection factor (SPF) of at least 15

        b. Avoid sun exposure between 10 A.M. and 2 P.M.

➤ *Practice to Pass:*

What measures should the nurse take to prevent or decrease the severity of stomatitis secondary to the administration of fluorouracil (5-FU)?

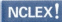

c. Wear long sleeves and a large brimmed hat

III. Anti-tumor Antibiotics

A. Action and use

1. Interfere with nucleic acid synthesis and function, inhibit ribonucleic acid (RNA) synthesis, and inhibit DNA synthesis

2. Most agents are cell cycle nonspecific

3. Major toxicities occur in the hematopoietic, GI, reproductive, and cardiac systems (cumulative doses)

B. Common medications (Table 3-3)

C. Administration considerations

1. Most anti-tumor antibiotics are severe vesicants except for bleomycin (see signs and symptoms of extravasation in Table 3-4 and antidotes for vesicant drugs in Table 3-5)

2. Administer slowly by IV push (IVP) via the side-arm portal of a freely flowing IV

3. Maintain clear visualization of the injection site during administration

4. IV catheter should have an excellent blood return, be recently placed, and not more than 48 hours old before administering vesicant therapy

5. If possible, avoid use of antecubital veins, dorsum of the hand, or wrist, where extravasation could damage underlying tendons and nerves

6. Avoid venous access in an extremity with compromised venous or lymphatic drainage

D. Contraindications

1. Doxorubicin (Adriamycin)

   a. Myelosuppression

   b. Impaired cardiac function

   c. Obstructive jaundice

   d. Crosses placenta and is distributed in breast milk; therefore, safe use in pregnancy is not established

   e. Impaired hepatic or renal function

Table 3-3	Generic (Trade) Name	Route
Anti-Tumor Antibiotics	Bleomycin (Blenoxane)	IV, IM, SC
	Dactinomycin (Cosmegen)	IV
	Daunorubicin (Cerubidine)	IV
	Doxorubicin (Adriamycin)	IV
	Plicamycin (Mithracin)	IV
	Idarubicin (Idamycin)	IV
	Mitomycin (Mutamycin)	IV
	Mitoxantrone (Novantrone)	IV

IV = intravenous; IM = intramuscular, SC = subcutaneous

Table 3-4

Signs and Symptoms of Extravasation

Assessment Parameter	Immediate Manifestations	Delayed Manifestations	Irritation of the Vein	Flare Reaction
Pain	Severe pain or burning that lasts minutes to hours and eventually subsides; usually occurs while drug is being given around needle site	Up to 48 hours	Aching and tightness along the vein	No pain
Redness	Blotchy redness around the needle site; not always present at time of extravasation	Later occurrence	Full length of the vein may be reddened or darkened	Immediate blotches or streaks along the vein, which usually subside within 30 min with or without treatment
Ulceration	Develops insidiously; usually occurs 48 to 96 hours later	Later occurrence	Not usually	Not usually
Swelling	Severe swelling; usually occurs immediately	Up to 48 hours	Not likely	Wheals may appear along the vein line
Blood Return	Inability to obtain a blood return	Good blood return during drug administration	Usually	Usually
Other	Change in quality of infusion	Local tingling and sensory deficits	NA	Urticaria

2. Bleomycin (Blenoxane)

   a. History of hypersensitivity or idiosyncrasy to bleomycin

   b. Pregnancy (category D) and women that are of childbearing age

   c. Cautious use in clients with compromised hepatic, renal or pulmonary function, or previous cytotoxic drug or radiation therapy

Table 3-5

Antidotes for Vesicant Therapy

Chemotherapeutic Drug	Antidote
Nitrogen mustard (Mustargen), Cisplatin (Platinol)	Thiosulfate
Dactinomycin (Cosmegen)	Apply ice and elevate, heat may enhance tissue damage
Doxorubicin (Adriamycin)	Cold pack with circulating ice water first 24 to 48 hrs
Vinblastine (Velban), Vincristine (Oncovin), Vinorelbine (Navelbine)	Hyaluronidase; apply warm pack for first 24 to 48 hrs
Paclitaxel (Taxol)	Hyaluronidase; apply ice for first 24 hours

3. Plicamycin (Mithramycin)

   a. Bleeding and coagulation disorders, myelosuppression

   b. Electrolyte imbalance, especially hypocalcemia

   c. Pregnancy (category C)

   d. Cautious use in clients with prior abdominal or mediastinal radiation

4. Mitoxantrone (Novantrone)

   a. Hypersensitivity to mitoxantrone

   b. Myelosuppression

   c. Pregnancy (category D) and lactation

   d. Cautious use in impaired cardiac, renal, or hepatic function

5. Mitomycin-C (Mitomycin)

   a. Hypersensitivity to Mitomycin-C

   b. Pregnancy (category D) and lactation

   c. Thrombocytopenia and coagulation disorders

E. Significant drug interactions

1. Doxorubicin (Adriamycin)

   a. Barbiturates may decrease pharmacological effects of doxorubicin by increasing hepatic metabolism

   b. Streptozocin (Zanosar, another antitumor antibiotic) may prolong the half-life of doxorubicin

   c. Incompatible with aminophylline, dexamethasone, diazepam, fluorouracil, hydrocortisone, heparin, vinblastine, and furosemide

2. Bleomycin (Blenoxane)

   a. Decreases effects of digoxin (Lanoxin) and phenytoin (Dilantin)

   b. Incompatible with aminophylline, carbenicillin, diazepam, hydrocortisone, methotrexate, mitomycin, nafcillin, penicillin, and terbutaline

3. Plicamycin (Mithramycin): concurrent administration of vitamin D may enhance hypercalcemia

4. Mitoxantrone (Novantrone)

   a. May impair immune response to vaccines

   b. Incompatible with heparin, hydrocortisone, and paclitaxel (Taxol), an antineoplastic agent

5. Mitomycin-C (Mitomycin): incompatible with dextrose-containing solutions

F. Significant food interactions: none known

G. Significant assessment parameters

1. Doxorubicin (Adriamycin)

   a. Assess hepatic, renal, hematopoietic, and cardiac function prior to administration and at regular intervals thereafter

   b. Begin a flowchart to establish baseline data, including temperature, pulse, respiration, blood pressure, body weight, laboratory values, intake and output (I & O) ratio and pattern, and cardiac ejection fraction

   c. Give prompt attention to complaints of stinging or burning sensation at the injection site

   d. Be alert to and report early signs of cardiotoxicity and hepatic dysfunction

   e. Stomatitis is greatest at 2 weeks following therapy, begins with a burning sensation

   f. Nadir usually occurs 10 to 14 days after administration

   g. **Radiation recall,** erythema that develops in previously irradiated field, is common

2. Bleomycin (Blenoxane)

   a. Inject a test dose of 2 units or less deeply into the muscle to assess anaphylactic response before IV administration

   b. Assess vital signs; a febrile reaction is relatively common

   c. Bone marrow toxicity is rare

   d. Pulmonary toxicity occurs in about 10% of clients, most usually in clients > 70 years of age and when the cumulative dose reaches 400 units

   e. Radiation recall is common

3. Plicamycin (Mithramycin)

   a. Assess bowel function to prevent high impaction

   b. Assess liver, hematological, and renal function before and periodically throughout therapy

   c. Thrombocytopenia is common and is frequently evidenced by a single or persistent episode of epistaxis or hematemesis

4. Mitoxantrone (Novantrone)

   a. Assess IV insertion site; transient blue discoloration may occur

   b. Assess cardiac function throughout course of therapy, report signs and symptoms of CHF

   c. Assess uric acid levels and initiate hypo-uricemic therapy before anti-leukemia therapy

5. Mitomycin-C (Mitomycin)

   a. Assess serum creatinine since drug is rarely given if > 1.7 mg/dL

   b. Assess platelet count, PT, and bleeding times

   c. Assess I & O ratio and pattern, dysuria, hematuria, and oliguria; maintain hydration since drug is nephrotoxic

H. Side effects/toxicity

1. Anthracycline(s)

   a. Vesicant: flare reaction is common and may be difficult to distinguish from an extravasation

   NCLEX!

   b. Cardiotoxicity leading to degenerative cardiomyopathy occurs over time

   c. Lifetime dosage is 450 to 550 mg/m^2

   d. Prior radiation therapy to the chest wall may predispose client to enhanced cardiotoxicity

   e. Alopecia

   NCLEX!

   f. Severe mucositis, stomatitis

   NCLEX!

   g. Hyperpigmentation of nail beds and dermal creases

   h. Acute myelosuppression

2. Bleomycin (Blenoxane)

   NCLEX!

   a. Pulmonary toxicity that is dose- and age-related

   NCLEX!

   b. Anaphylactic reaction may occur

   c. Mild febrile reaction commonly occurs

   d. Diffuse alopecia, hyperpigmentation of the skin, vesiculation, acne, thickening of the skin and nail beds

3. Plicamycin (Mithramycin)

   a. Vesicant

   NCLEX!

   b. Depression of platelet count, usually severe; thrombocytopenia may be of rapid onset and occur at anytime during the therapy

   c. Hypocalcemia (because it is often given to treat hypercalcemia)

4. Mitoxantrone (Novantrone)

   a. Is an **irritant:** a drug capable of causing pain and inflammation at the administration site if extravasation occurs

   NCLEX!

   b. Sclera and urine may turn blue to blue-green

   NCLEX!

   c. Potent myelosuppression

   d. Increased cardiotoxicity with cumulative dose > 180 mg/m^2

5. Mitomycin-C (Mitomycin)

   NCLEX!

   a. Vesicant; has the unique ability to produce ulceration at distal sites

   b. Myelosuppression is delayed and cumulative initial nadir is 4 to 6 weeks

   NCLEX!

   c. Nephrotoxic; can cause hemolytic uremia syndrome

I. Client and family education

1. Anthracycline agents

Practice to Pass

    a. Alopecia, which may also involve eyelashes, eyebrows, beard/mustache, and pubic and axillary hair; regrowth of hair usually begins 2 to 3 months after completion of administration

    b. Advise client that urine may turn red

  2. Mitoxantrone (Novantrone)

    a. Advise client that blue-green urine is common for 24 hours after the drug therapy and that sclera may also take on a bluish color

    b. Stomatitis and mucositis may occur within one week of therapy

IV. Plant Alkaloids (Mitotic Inhibitors)

A. Action and use

  1. Arrest or inhibit mitosis

  2. Most agents are cell cycle specific, M-Phase

  3. Major toxicities occur in the hematopoietic, integumentary, neurologic, and reproductive systems; also, hypersensitivity reactions may occur

B. Common medications (Table 3-6)

C. Administration considerations

  1. Etoposide (VP-16): administer by slow IVPB over 60 to 90 minutes to avoid hypotension

  2. Paclitaxel (Taxol)

    a. Do not use equipment or devices containing polyvinyl chloride (PVC)

    b. Tissue necrosis occurs with extravasation

    c. Administer via nitroglycerine tubing with an in-line filter of 0.22 micron or less

    d. Requires strict premedication (preferably with dexamethasone, diphenhydramine, and either cimetidine or ranitidine) per protocol order set before administration to prevent anaphylaxis

  3. Vincristine (Oncovin)

    a. Vesicant: administer into the side arm portal of a freely flowing IV

    b. Hyaluronidase is the antidote should extravasation occur; also apply moderate heat to disperse drug and minimize sloughing

Table 3-6		
Plant Alkaloids (Mitotic Inhibitors)	**Generic (Trade) Name**	**Route**
	Etoposide (VP-16, VePesid)	IV
	Paclitaxel (Taxol)	IV
	Teniposide (VM-26, Vumon)	IV
	Vinblastine (Velban)	IV
	Vincristine (Oncovin)	IV
	Vinorelbine (Navelbine)	IV

IV = intravenous

D. Contraindications

1. Etoposide (VP-16)

   a. Severe bone marrow depression

   b. Severe hepatic or renal impairment

   c. Existing or recent viral infection or bacterial infection

   d. Safe use in pregnancy (category D) and nursing mothers not established

2. Paclitaxel (Taxol)

   a. Hypersensitivity to paclitaxel

   b. Baseline neutropenia of less than 1,500 cells/mm^3

   c. Cautious use in the presence of cardiac arrhythmias and impaired liver function

   d. Pregnancy (category X)

3. Vincristine (Oncovin)

   a. Obstructive jaundice

   b. Demylinating neurological diseases; preexisting neuromuscular disease

   c. Pregnancy (category D)

E. Significant drug interactions

1. Etoposide (VP-16): don't administer concurrently with other medications

2. Paclitaxel (Taxol)

   a. Increased myelosuppression when administered with cisplatin

   b. Avoid using PVC bags and infusion sets due to leaching of DEPH (plasticizer)

3. Vincristine (Oncovin): bronchospasm may occur in clients previously treated with mitomycin; hepatic metabolism of vincristine may be decreased when given with asparaginase (doses need to be separated by 12 to 24 hours)

F. Significant food interactions: none known

G. Significant assessment parameters

1. Etoposide (VP-16)

   a. Assess IV site before and after infusion; extravasation can cause thrombophlebitis and necrosis

   b. Be prepared to treat an anaphylactic reaction

   c. Monitor vital signs during and after infusion; if hypotension occurs, stop infusion

   d. Assess CBC, WBC and differential, and hepatic and renal function before administration and periodically during treatment

2. Paclitaxel (Taxol)

   a. Monitor for sensitivity reaction during the first and second administration of the drug; development of angioedema and generalized urticaria requires immediate discontinuation

b. Monitor VS frequently; bradycardia occurs in 12% of clients who receive the drug

    c. Assess for peripheral neuropathy

3. Vincristine (Oncovin)

    a. Assess for leukopenia, which occurs in a significant number of clients

    b. Assess hand grasps and deep tendon reflexes; depression of the Achilles reflex is the earliest sign of neuropathy

H. Side effects/toxicity

1. Etoposide (VP-16)

    a. Severe mucositis

    b. Acral erythema and sloughing of the skin on palms and soles

    c. Myelosuppression

    d. Severe blood fluctuations

    e. Fever and chills during infusion

2. Paclitaxel (Taxol)

    a. Transient bradycardia

    b. Peripheral neuropathy

    c. Neutropenia, thrombocytopenia

    d. Hypersensitivity reaction including hypotension, bronchospasm, urticaria, and angioedema

    e. Alopecia

3. Vincristine

    a. Neurotoxicity, loss of sensation on the soles of the feet and the finger-tips

    b. Depression of the Achilles reflex is the earliest sign of neuropathy

    c. Paralytic ileus

I. Client and family education

1. Etoposide (VP-16)

    a. Inform about possible adverse effects, such as blood dyscrasias, alopecia, and carcinogenesis

    b. Caution client to make position changes slowly, particularly from a recumbent position

    c. Inspect mouth daily for ulcerations and bleeding and avoid obvious irritants

2. Paclitaxel (Taxol)

    a. Instruct to report dyspnea, chest pain, palpitations, or angioedema

    b. Stress need for periodic labwork

    c. Inform of high probability of developing alopecia

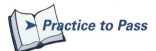

Practice to Pass

Constipation is a primary complication when administering vinca or plant alkaloid medications. What can the nurse do to prevent this treatment side effect?

NCLEX!

3. Vincristine

   a. Maintain a prophylactic regimen against constipation and paralytic ileus

   b. Report a change in bowel habits

   c. Alopecia is the most common side effect and is reversible after the treatment is completed

V. Nitrosoureas

A. Action and use

   1. Interfere with DNA replication and repair

   2. They are not cross-resistant to alkylating agents

   3. Most agents are cell cycle nonspecific

   4. Most agents cross the blood-brain barrier

   5. Major toxicities occur in the hematopoietic and GI systems

B. Common medications (Table 3-7)

C. Administration considerations

   1. Carmustine (BCNU)

   a. Administer over 1 to 2 hours by slow IV infusion with constant monitoring if given peripherally

   b. Vesicant: if possible, avoid starting IV in the dorsum of the hand, wrist, or antecubital veins, since extravasation may cause damage to underlying tissues

   2. Lomustine (CCNU): should be taken on an empty stomach to avoid nausea

   3. Streptozotocin (Zanosar)

   a. Vesicant: administer via the side arm portal of a freely flowing IV

   b. Administer antiemetic routinely prior to dose and Q 4 to 6 hours thereafter for the first 24 hours

D. Contraindications

   1. Carmustine (BCNU)

   a. History of pulmonary function impairment

   b. Decreased platelets, leukocytes, or erythrocytes

   c. Safe use during pregnancy (category D) not established

   2. Lomustine (CCNU)

   a. Decreased platelets, leukocytes, or erythrocytes

   b. Safe use during pregnancy (category D) not established

Table 3-7	Generic (Trade) Name	Route
Nitrosoureas	Carmustine (BCNU)	IV, IT
	Lomustine (CeeNu)	PO
	Streptozotocin (Zanosar)	IV

PO = oral; IV = intravenous; IT = intrathecal

3. Streptozotocin (Zanosar)

   a. Hepatic and renal dysfunction

   b. Safe use during pregnancy (category C) not established

E. Significant drug interactions

  1. Carmustine (BCNU): cimetidine may potentiate neutropenia and thrombocytopenia

  2. Streptozotocin (Zanosar)

   a. Vancomycin, ampotericin B, and cisplatin add to nephrotoxicity

   b. Phenytoin may reduce cytotoxic effect on beta cells

F. Significant food interactions: none known

G. Significant assessment parameters

  1. Carmustine (BCNU)

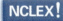

   a. Persistent nausea and vomiting may occur 2 hours after drug administration and persist up to 6 hours; prior administration of an antiemetic will help

   b. Blood counts should be monitored prior to beginning the course of drug therapy and weekly for at least 6 weeks after last dose

   c. Assess results of pulmonary function studies prior to therapy and periodically thereafter

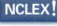

   d. Symptoms of lung toxicity should be reported to the physician: cough, dyspnea, fever

   e. Be alert to hepatic and renal insufficiency

  2. Lomustine (CCNU): blood counts should be monitored prior to therapy and weekly for at least 6 weeks after last dose; liver and kidney function tests should also be performed

  3. Streptozotocin (Zanosar)

   a. Assess for early evidence of renal dysfunction as evidenced by hypophosphatemia, mild proteinuria, and changes in I & O pattern

   b. Monitor CBC prior to therapy and weekly during therapy

   c. Do liver function studies prior to each dose

H. Side effects/toxicity

  1. Carmustine (BCNU)

   a. Severe nausea and vomiting

   b. Ocular infarctions, retinal hemorrhage, suffusion of the conjunctiva

   c. Delayed myelosuppression

   d. Pulmonary infiltration or fibrosis

  2. Lomustine (CCNU)

   a. Delayed myelosuppression

   b. Severe nausea and vomiting

3. Streptozotocin (Zanosar)

    a. Nausea and vomiting

    b. Mild to moderate myelosuppression, can be severe in 10 to 20% of clients

    c. Insulin shock due to effect on the pancreatic beta cells

    d. Nephrotoxicity

I. Client and family education

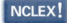

1. Myelosuppression is severe and may be cumulative; teach neutropenic precautions and symptoms of sepsis

2. Teach signs and symptoms of hypoglycemia when administering streptozocin

3. Teach signs and symptoms of pulmonary toxicity when administering carmustine

VI. Hormones and Hormone Modulators

A. Action and use

1. Corticosteroids: lyse lymphoid malignancies and have an indirect effect on malignant cells

2. Estrogens: suppress testosterone production in males and alter the response of breast cancers to prolactin

3. Progestins: promote palliation and tumor cell regression; exact mechanism of action is unknown

4. Anti-estrogens: compete with estrogens for binding with estrogen receptor sites on malignant cells

5. Androgens: hormone therapy that has palliative use in metastatic/advanced carcinoma of the breast; used if surgery and irradiation deemed inappropriate; otherwise, tamoxifen (Nolvadex) is drug of choice for this purpose

6. Anti-androgens: inhibit binding of androgens at androgen receptor sites in target tissues; indicated for use in metastatic/advanced prostate cancer

B. Common medications (Table 3-8)

C. Administration considerations

1. Corticosteroids

    a. Oral forms should be administered with meals and may be crushed

    b. IV form should be given slowly by IVPB to prevent vaginal and anal burning

2. Estrogens

    a. Give orally immediately after solid food

    b. An exception is estramustine (Emcyt), which is a combination estrogen and nitrogen mustard compound; this must be taken with water an hour

Table 3-8	Generic (Trade) Name	Route
Hormones and Hormone Modulators	*Glucocorticoids*	
	Prednisone (Deltasone)	PO
	Dexamethasone (Decadron)	PO, IV
	Hydrocortisone (SoluCortef)	PO
	Methylprednisolone (SoluMedrol)	IV
	Estrogens	
	Chlorotrianisene (TACE)	PO
	Diethylstilbestrol (DES)	PO, IV
	Ethinyl estradiol (Estinyl)	PO
	Polyestradiol (Estradurin)	PO
	Estramustine (Emcyt)	PO
	Anti-estrogens	
	Tamoxifen (Nolvadex)	PO
	Toremifene (Fareston)	PO
	Anastrozole (Arimedex)	PO
	Fulvestrant (Faslodex)	IM
	Progestins	
	Medroxyprogesterone acetate (Depo-Provera)	PO, IM
	Megestrol acetate (Megace)	PO
	Leuprolide (Lupron)—a Gn-RH agonist	IM, SC
	Anti-androgens (androgen receptor blockers)	
	Bicalutamide (Casodex)	PO
	Flutamide (Eulexin)	PO
	Nilutamide (Nilandron)	PO
	Goserelin (Zoladex)—a Gn-RH agonist	SC
	Androgens	
	Testosterone (generic)	PO
	Testolactone (Teslac)	PO
	Fluoxymesterone (Halotestin)	PO

PO = oral; SC = subcutaneous, IM = intramuscular; IV = intravenous

before meals, and requires that no milk, dairy products, or calcium-containing products be used concurrently

3. Progestins: give orally without regard to meals

4. Estrogen antagonists: give orally; dosage may be decreased if side effects are severe

5. Androgens and anti-androgens: give orally

D. Contraindications

1. Corticosteroids

  a. Systemic infections

  b. Ulcerative colitis, diverticulitis, active or latent peptic ulcer disease

    c. Safe use in pregnancy (category C) and nursing mothers has not been established

  2. Estrogens

    a. Known or suspected pregnancy

    b. Estrogen-dependent neoplasms

    c. History of thromboembolic disorders

  3. Progestins

    a. Severe arrhythmias possible if client also takes a calcium-channel blocker

    b. Psychiatric depression

    c. Pregnancy (category C), cautious use in lactation

  4. Anti-estrogens: first trimester of pregnancy (category C)

E. Significant drug interactions

  1. Corticosteroids

    a. Phenytoin (Dilantin) and rifampin (Rifadin) increase steroid metabolism

    b. Increased doses may be required when given with amphotericin-B

    c. Diuretics increase potassium loss

    d. May inhibit antibody response to vaccines and toxoids

  2. Estrogens: phenytoin (Dilantin) and rifampin (Rifadin) decrease estrogen effect by increasing its metabolism

  3. Progestins

    a. Can prolong cardiac conduction in clients taking beta blockers, calcium channel blockers, and possibly digoxin (Lanoxin)

    b. Quinine may decrease plasma levels

    c. Chloroquine may increase risk of seizures

  4. Anti-estrogens may enhance hypoprothombinemic effect of warfarin

F. Significant food interactions: none known

G. Significant assessment parameters

  1. Corticosteroids

    a. Establish baseline and continuing data on blood pressure, I & O, weight, and sleep patterns

    b. Measure 2-hour postprandial blood glucose, serum potassium, and serum calcium prior to therapy and at regular intervals thereafter

    c. Watch for changes in mood, emotional stability, and sleep patterns

  2. Estrogens

    a. Spotting or breakthrough bleeding may occur

    b. Severe hypercalcemia may occur

    3. Progestin

        a. Assess weight periodically

        b. Assess for allergic reactions, rash, urticaria, anaphylaxis, tachypnea

    4. Anti-estrogens: assess CBC, including platelet count, periodically

    5. Androgens: monitor serum calcium levels; hypercalcemia can result, requiring temporary termination of drug therapy and administration of large volumes of IV fluid

    6. Anti-androgens: monitor liver function studies periodically to detect rare complication of hepatitis

H. Side effects/toxicity

    1. Corticosteroids

        a. Euphoria, headache, insomnia, psychosis

        b. Edema

        c. Muscle weakness, delayed wound healing, osteoporosis, spontaneous fractures

        d. Hyperglycemia

    2. Estrogens

        a. Thromboembolic disorders

        b. Nausea

    3. Progestins

        a. Vaginal bleeding and breast tenderness

        b. Abdominal pain, nausea, and vomiting

        c. Increased appetite and weight gain

    4. Anti-estrogens

        a. Thrombosis

        b. About 25% of clients experience nausea and vomiting

        c. Hot flashes, weight gain, changes in menstrual cycle, leaking from breasts

    5. Androgens

        a. Virilization, including clitoral enlargement, increases in facial and body hair, deepened voice, increased libido, and male-pattern baldness

        b. Hypercalcemia

    6. Anti-androgens

        a. Gynecomastia

        b. GI disturbances (nausea, vomiting, constipation, diarrhea)

        c. Hepatitis

I. Client and family teaching: for all drug groups, teach clients about adverse effects and when to report them

VII. Other Antineoplastics

A. Action and use

1. Asparaginase (Elspar) depletes extracellular supply of asparagine, an amino acid essential to DNA synthesis

2. Hydroxyurea (Hydrea) blocks incorporation of thymidine into DNA and may damage already formed DNA molecules

B. Common medications: asparaginase (also referred to as L-asparaginase) and hydroxyurea

C. Administration considerations

1. Asparaginase (Elspar)

   a. Administer intradermal (ID) skin test before initial dose because of the potential for anaphylaxis; a negative skin test does not preclude the possibility of an allergic reaction

   b. Fiber-like particles may develop in vial after reconstitution; use a 5-micron filter to remove particles (will not affect potency)

2. Hydroxyurea: capsule may be opened and mixed with water if client has difficulty swallowing

D. Contraindications

1. Asparaginase (Elspar)

   a. History of or existing pancreatitis

   b. Safe use during pregnancy (category C) and nursing mothers is not established

2. Hydroxyurea: pregnancy (category D)

E. Significant drug interactions

1. Asparaginase (Elspar)

   a. Causes decreased hypoglycemic effects of sulfonylureas and insulin

   b. Antitumor effect is blocked if administered concurrently with vincristine (Oncovin) or methotrexate (Folex)

2. Hydroxyurea (Hydrea): none established

F. Significant food interactions: none known

G. Significant assessment parameters

1. Asparaginase (Elspar)

   a. Prepare for anaphylaxis and have personnel, emergency medications, oxygen, and airway equipment readily available

   b. During administration, monitor vital signs and be alert for hypersensitivity or anaphylactic reaction, which usually occurs 30 to 60 minutes after medication administration

   c. Assess laboratory values prior to treatment and routinely thereafter, including CBC, amylase, serum calcium, coagulation factors, hepatic and renal function studies, and ammonia and uric acid levels

2. Hydroxyurea (Hydrea)

    a. Determine status of kidney, liver, and bone marrow function before and periodically during therapy

    b. Monitor I & O and increase fluid intake, especially in clients with high serum uric acid levels

H. Side effects/toxicity

1. Asparaginase (Elspar)

    a. Severe anaphylaxis is possible; crash cart should be readily available

    b. Severe nausea and vomiting

    c. Potential for bleeding because of reduced clotting factors, decreased circulating platelets, and decreased fibrinogen levels

2. Hydroxyurea (Hydrea)

    a. Bone marrow suppression

    b. Stomatitis

    c. Maculopapular rash

    d. Hyperuricemia

VIII. Safe Handling of Chemotherapeutic Agents

A. Drug preparation and administration

1. All individuals preparing and administering cytotoxic drugs should be specially trained in safety procedures for handling of chemotherapeutic drugs and comply with agency standards, which should be in compliance with government and professional practice standards

2. Chemotherapy doses are generally individualized according to body weight (in kg) or body surface area (in m^2)

3. Most chemotherapy protocol order sets consist of short, intermittent, high-dose courses of medications (often in combination) to maximize cancer cell kill while allowing normal cells time to heal and recover

4. Chemotherapy drugs should be prepared for use in an air-vented space, such as a clean-air workstation or biohazard cabinet; access to this area should be limited

5. Wear a disposable, leak-proof gown, surgical latex gloves, a mask, and eye protection when preparing chemotherapeutic agents

6. Do not prepare or administer IV chemotherapy if pregnant because of possible risk to fetus

B. Safe handling of antineoplastic agents and spill management

1. Use leak-proof, puncture-resistant containers to dispose of antineoplastic drugs and associated vials, needles, syringes, tubing, and other equipment; use double-bagging technique and identify container with a "Biohazard" label

2. Do not separate needle from syringe or break needles to avoid leaking medication from them

3. If drug accidentally touches a nurse or client, wash area well with soap and water; immediately remove any contaminated clothing; copiously flush eyes if involved while keeping eyelids open

4. Double-glove to clean a drug spill, washing hands before and after

5. For powdered medications, wear a mask and eye protection as well

6. Place spilled substance in a plastic bag; wipe remaining area with a damp cloth and place it in the same bag; place this bag into another plastic bag (double-bag) and label it as biohazardous

7. All materials used for drug preparation and administration must be disposed of by incineration

C. Disposal of client's body fluids

1. Handle all body substances cautiously, such as blood, urine, vomitus, stool, and others; carefully follow standard precautions and other procedures as designated by agency policy

2. Wear gloves when in contact with all body substances; carefully dispose of them in toilet; clean containers carefully and thoroughly

IX. Nursing Management of Treatment Side Effects

A. Myelosuppression

1. Neutropenia

   a. Assessment

   1) Neutropenia is defined as an absolute neutrophil count of 1,500/mm^3 or less

   2) The lowest point in the WBC count reached after chemotherapy (the nadir) most commonly occurs 7 to 14 days following chemotherapy administration

   3) Fever of more than 38° C or 100.4° F is the most reliable and often the only sign of infection in clients with neutropenia

   b. Management

   1) Avoid exposure to these substances

      a) Fresh fruits, vegetables, flowers, and live plants

      b) People recently vaccinated with live organisms or viruses

      c) Pet excreta including fish tanks and aquariums

   2) Instruct clients to avoid contact with people who have a contagious illness

   3) Teach people who come in contact with client to wash hands prior to touching client

   4) Encourage client to practice good personal hygiene

   5) Prevent trauma to skin and mucous membranes

   6) Culture urine, peripheral blood, all lumens of central venous catheters (CVCs) and suspected sources of infection; obtain chest x-ray (CXR); administer antibiotics as ordered for empiric therapy

7) Institute neutropenic precautions for hospitalized clients whose absolute neutrophil count drops as described above using previously described measures

8) Administer filgrastim (Neupogen), a granulocyte colony-stimulating factor that increases production of neutrophils, either IV or SC as ordered; client may complain of bone pain 1 to 3 days before blood count increases; this may be controlled with nonopioid analgesics

c. Client and family education

1) Teach client and family to report temperature greater than 38° C or 100.4° F, shaking chills, dysuria, dyspnea, sputum production, or pain

2) Reinforce the need for meticulous hygiene

3) Teach self-administration of granulocyte colony-stimulating factor (G-CSF) for neutropenia or granulocyte/macrophage colony-stimulating factor (GM-CSF) for treatment of blood-forming organ cancers as ordered

2. Thrombocytopenia

a. Bone marrow suppression decreases platelet production

b. Circulating platelets are diminished gradually because the platelet life span is only 10 days

c. Chemotherapy drugs accelerate platelet destruction

d. Assessment

1) Platelet count below 50,000/mm³; risk significantly increases when platelet count falls below 20,000/mm³

2) Petechiae, bruising, and hemorrhage

3) Neurological changes that may indicate intracranial bleeding

4) Hypotension and tachycardia

e. Management

1) Institute bleeding precautions

2) Decrease activity to prevent falls and maintain a safe environment

3) Discourage heavy lifting and Valsalva maneuver, which may increase risk of intracranial bleeding

4) Encourage the client to eat a high-fiber diet and drink adequate liquids

5) Daily care

a) Avoid use of straight-edge razors; use an electric razor instead

b) Avoid using nail clippers; use a nail file instead

c) Avoid using vaginal douches, rectal suppositories, or enemas

d) Use water-soluble lubricant for sexual intercourse

e) Avoid intercourse when platelet count is below 50,000/mm³

f) Instruct menstruating women to monitor pad count and amount of saturation; tampon use should be avoided

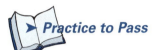

Practice to Pass

What measures should the nurse teach the client to decrease the potential for infection after chemotherapy administration?

NCLEX!

g) Encourage client to blow nose gently

h) Instruct client to avoid dental floss and oral irrigation, and to use a soft toothbrush or sponge-tipped applicator for mouth care

i) Avoid administration of aspirin or aspirin-containing products as well as NSAIDs

j) Apply pressure for 5 to 10 minutes following venipuncture, bone marrow biopsy, or other invasive procedures; platelet transfusion prior to the procedure may be indicated

f. Client and family education

1) Notify MD of symptoms of bleeding

2) Test urine and stool for occult blood

3) Teach other safety recommendations for daily management as above

B. Nausea and vomiting

1. **Anticipatory nausea:** a conditioned response resulting from repeated association of chemotherapy-induced nausea and vomiting and stimulus from environment

2. Acute nausea: occurs 0 to 24 hours after chemotherapy administration

3. Delayed nausea: persistent vomiting lasting 1 to 4 days after chemotherapy administration

4. Assessment parameters

   a. Women have a higher incidence than men

   b. Younger clients experience more nausea than their older counterparts

   c. A history of motion sickness can predispose some to experience chemotherapy-induced nausea

   d. Dehydration may accelerate nausea and vomiting

5. Administer antiemetics to cover the emetogenic period (see Table 3-9); these may include (but are not limited to) ondansetron (Zofran) and metoclopramide (Reglan), a prokinetic GI stimulant

6. Provide additional antiemetics to manage breakthrough nausea

7. Dexamethasone may be the most effective agent in preventing anticipatory nausea/vomiting

8. Client and family education

   a. Eat small frequent meals and avoid fatty, sweet, salty, or spicy foods

   b. Notify healthcare professional if vomiting persists ≥ 24h and client is unable to take oral hydration

   c. Maintain antiemetic schedule for 48 to 72h to avoid delayed nausea

C. Diarrhea

1. Chemotherapy affects rapidly dividing cells of the villae and micro-villae in the GI mucosa

Table 3-9

Emetogenic Potential, Onset, and Duration of Selected Chemotherapeutic Agents

Incidence	Agent	Onset (Hours)	Duration (Hours)
Very High	Cisplatin	1–6	24–72+
	Dacarbazine	1–3	1–12
	Mechlorethamine	0.5–2	8–24
		3–6	6–12
	Melphalan	1–2	4–20
	Dactinomycin		
High	Carmustine	2–4	4–24
	Cyclophosphamide	4–12	12–24
		24–27	Variable
	Procarbazine	4–6	24+
	Etoposide	1–12	24–72
	Methotrexate		
Moderate	Doxorubacin	4–6	6+
	Mitoxantrone	4–6	6+
	Fluorouracil	3–6	24+
	Mitomycin-C	1–4	48–72
	Carboplatin	4–6	12–24
	Ifosfamide	3–6	24–72
	Cytarabine	6–12	3–12
Low	Bleomycin	3–6	–
	Daunorubacin	1–2	–
	6-Mercaptopurine	4–8	–
	Methotrexate	4–12	–
	Vinblastine	4–8	–
	Lomustine	2–6	2–24
Very low	Vincristine	4–8	–
	Paclitaxel	4–8	–

2. Combination chemotherapy and radiation therapy to the pelvis can lead to additional cellular destruction

3. Monitor number of stools, amount, and consistency

4. Replace fluid and electrolytes, including potassium

5. Administer anti-diarrhea medication to reduce peristalsis and the frequency and volume of stools

6. Client and family education

   a. Consume low-residue, high-protein, high-calorie diet to promote bowel rest

   b. Eliminate irritating foods, such as alcohol, coffee, cold liquids, popcorn, and raw fruits and vegetables

   c. Drink 6 to 8 glasses of water per 24-hr period

   d. Implement a liquid diet if diarrhea is severe

   e. Avoid milk products and chocolate

   f. Decrease activity when diarrhea is severe to provide rest and decrease peristalsis

   g. Clean rectal area with mild soap after each bowel movement and apply moisture barrier

   h. Take warm sitz baths

D. Stomatitis

1. Epithelial cells of the oral mucosa are destroyed, causing an inflammatory response and denudation of the oral mucosa

2. Initial presentation: burning sensation with no physical changes in the oral mucosa, sensitivity to heat and cold, and sensitivity to salty and spicy foods

3. Promote a well-balanced intake, including a protein intake of greater than 1 g/kg of body weight

4. Promote consistent, thorough oral hygiene after each meal and at hour of sleep

5. Administer antifungal/antiviral medication for prophylaxis as directed

6. Client and family education

   a. Instruct in consistent oral hygiene

   b. Avoid using lemon/glycerin swabs, hydrogen peroxide, and products containing alcohol, which promote dryness and irritation

E. Constipation

1. Neurotoxic effects of chemotherapy can decrease peristalsis or cause paralytic ileus

2. Assess patterns of elimination including amount and frequency

3. Assess usual fiber and fluid intake

4. Determine laxative and cathartic use, including frequency and amounts taken

5. Initiate a bowel maintenance program for clients receiving neurotoxic chemotherapeutic agents or those at high risk for constipation

6. Recognize complications associated with constipation, such as fecal impaction

7. Client and family education

   a. Drink warm liquids to stimulate bowel movement

   b. Increase fiber intake to increase peristalsis and stool bulk

   c. Drink at least 8 glasses of water per day

   d. Exercise regularly

   e. Develop a regular bowel program, avoiding use of laxatives if possible

F. Alopecia

1. Cells responsible for hair growth have a high mitotic rate and are affected to some degree by most chemotherapeutic agents

2. Hair loss begins approximately 2 weeks after drug administration and will continue until 3 to 5 months after the last chemotherapy treatment is completed

3. Devices to decrease circulation to the scalp are contraindicated since they can also promote micro-metastasis

4. Provide emotional support to client who is experiencing body image change

5. Client and family education

    a. Rationale and expected timeframe of hair loss and regrowth

    b. Provide gentle hair care, avoiding permanent waves, coloring, peroxide, electric rollers, and curling irons until regrowth has been reestablished long enough for two haircuts

    c. Hair prosthesis (wig)

    d. Emotional support strategies to cope with changing body image

G. Cardiotoxicity

1. May occur within 24 hr to up to 4 to 5 weeks after drug administration; is self limiting; warrants immediate drug discontinuation

2. Higher doses over a shorter period of time increase its incidence

3. Baseline ejection fraction should be assessed before administration of cardiotoxic agents

4. Characteristics of cardiotoxicity are outlined in Table 3-10

5. Maintain ongoing documentation of the client's cumulative dose

6. Cardioprotective iron chelating agents (e.g. dexrazoxane) may be administered to prevent cardiotoxicity in clients that have received ¾ of their lifetime dosage

7. Client and family education

    a. Cardiotoxicity is an expected side effect of some chemotherapy medications

    b. It is important to recognize signs and symptoms of CHF and report them to health care professional as directed

    c. Chronic cardiotoxicity is dose-related and possibly irreversible

H. Pulmonary toxicity

1. Lung tissue is sensitive to the toxic effects of chemotherapy, causing direct damage to the alveoli and capillary endothelium

2. Dyspnea is the cardinal symptom

3. Deteriorating creatinine clearance (renal dysfunction) is an important predictor for pulmonary pneumonitis

4. High oxygen concentrations can enhance the pulmonary toxicity of bleomycin

5. The risk of pulmonary toxicity increases significantly after age 70

6. Monitor pulmonary function studies as indicated

7. Client education

    a. Provide education regarding symptoms associated with pulmonary toxicity (e. g., dyspnea, chest pain, shallow breathing, chest wall discomfort)

    b. Teach pursed-lipped breathing and use a small fan to decrease symptoms of dyspnea

	Drug	Characteristics	Comments
Table 3-10 **Cardiotoxicity**	***DNA Intercalators*** Doxorubicin (Adriamycin)	EKG changes, non-specific ST-T wave changes; premature ventricular and atrial contractions; low voltage QRS changes	Chronic effects seen with cumulative dosages greater than recommended
	Daunorubicin (DaunoXome) Dactinomycin (Cosmegen) Mitoxantrone (Novantrone)		
	High-dose Therapy Cylophosphamide (Cytoxan)	Diminished QRS complexes on EKG, cardiomegaly, pulmonary congestion	May result in acute lethal pericarditis and hemorrhagic myocardial necrosis
	Fluorouracil (5-FU)	Angina, palpitations, sweating and syncope	May be treated prophylactically or therapeutically with long-acting nitrates or calcium channel blockers
	Taxanes Paclitaxel (Taxol)	Asymptomatic bradycardia, hypotension, asymptomatic ventricular tachycardia and atypical chest pain	A baseline EKG, client history and cardiac assessment should be performed prior to treatment; routine cardiac monitoring not warranted

c. Encourage the use of opioid analgesia as prescribed to decrease the fear of air hunger

d. Review safety issues related to oxygen administration

e. Explore with the client and significant other their wishes for intubation and resuscitation; breastfeeding should be discontinued

I. Hemorrhagic cystitis

1. Bladder mucosal irritation and inflammation results from contact with acrolein, the metabolic by-product of cyclophosphamide and ifosfamide

2. Prior radiation therapy to the pelvis or bladder increases risk

3. It presents with dysuria, frequency, burning upon urination, and hematuria

4. A chemo-protectant agent (mesna), may be given to bind to acrolein in the bladder, inactivating it and allowing excretion from the bladder

5. Client education

   a. Instruct that hemorrhagic cystitis is a possible side effect of cyclophosphamide (Cytoxan) and ifosfamide (Ifex) therapy

   b. Report signs and symptoms of hemorrhagic cystitis

   c. Encourage client to void frequently and take medication early in the day

   d. Instruct the client to drink a minimum of 6 to 8 glasses of fluid daily and to empty bladder every 4 to 6 hours

J. Hepatotoxicity

1. It is caused by direct toxic effect on the liver when drugs are metabolized; see Table 3-11 for incidence

2. Prior liver infection, tumor involvement in the liver, advanced age, total bilirubin > 2 mg/100 dL, or cirrhosis increase incidence

3. Clinical manifestations include jaundice, ascities, fatigue, anorexia, nausea, hyperpigmentation, upper right quadrant pain, hepatomegaly, and changes in urine and stool

4. Avoid hepatotoxic drugs if liver function tests are abnormal

5. Client and family education

   a. Teach client to avoid alcohol-containing beverages

   b. Instruct client that hepatotoxicity is a possible side effect of some chemotherapeutic medications

   c. Instruct client about signs and symptoms of liver failure

K. Nephrotoxicity

1. It is caused by direct damage to the glomerulus, renal blood vessels, different parts of the nephron, and/or precipitation of metabolites in the acid environment of the urine; leads to obstructive nephropathy

2. Advancing age, pre-existing renal disease, poor nutritional status, and administration of other nephrotoxic agents predispose client to nephrotoxicity

3. It is manifested by increasing serum creatinine, declining creatinine clearance, hypomagnesemia, proteinuria, and hematuria

4. Continuation of nephrotoxic agents should be reviewed if the blood urea nitrogen (BUN) is > 22 mg/dL and or the creatinine is > 2 mg/dL

5. Institute hydration of 3,000 mL/day to prevent or minimize renal damage

6. Induce diuresis with mannitol (Osmitrol) or furosemide (Lasix) when administering cisplatin

Table 3-11	Classification	Incidence	Comments
Hepatotoxicity	***Alkylating agents*** Cyclophosphamide (Cytoxan)	Rare	Exception is > 3 g used in bone marrow transplant (BMT)
	Nitrosoureas Carmustine (BCNU)	26% at low doses	Unusually not clinically significant, however may be associated with veno-occlusive disease when used in BMT
	Lomustine (CeeNu) Streptozocin (Zanosar)	26% 15–67%	
	Antimetabolites Methotrexate (Folex)	24% with oral administration	Cumulative dose is important Seen only when cumulative dosages exceed 2 mg/kg/day
	Fluorouracil (Adrucil) Cytarabine (Cytosar)	Rare Unknown	
	Antitumor Antibiotics Doxorubicin (Adriamycin)	Rare	May be lower than other anthracyclines
	Mitoxantrone (Novantrone) Bleomycin (Blenoxane) Plicamycin (Mithracin)	Rare Rare 16%	
	Plant (Vinca) Alkaloids Vincristine (Oncovin)	Rare	Rarely seen with standard dosages, higher dosages can cause irreversible liver enzyme changes
	Etoposide (VePesid) Paclitaxil (Taxol)	Rare 7–22%	
	Miscellaneous Asparaginase (Elspar)	42–67%	Increases with higher doses

NCLEX!

7. Administer allopurinol (Zyloprim) to decrease uric acid production from high tumor-cell kill (e.g., leukemia, lymphoma, small cell lung cancer)

8. Maintain alkalinization of urine with sodium bicarbonate to a pH level greater than 8 to prevent renal damage when giving high-dose methotrexate (Folex)

9. Avoid administration of aspirin and NSAIDs

10. Client and family education

    a. Instruct that nephrotoxicity is a possible side effect of selected chemotherapeutic agents

b. Reinforce importance of compliance with measures to prevent nephrotoxicity

        1) Accurately obtain 12- or 24-hr urine for creatinine clearance

        2) Increase fluid intake

        3) Comply with instructions to alkalinize urine, complete leucovorin rescue, and/or allopurinol (Zyloprim) therapy

L. Neurotoxicity

    1. Caused by direct toxicity on the nervous system, metabolic encephalopathy, or intracranial hemorrhage related to chemotherapy-induced coagulopathy

    2. Risk factors

      a. Administration of agents that cross the blood-brain barrier

      b. Specified chemotherapeutic agents, especially cumulative doses of vinca alkaloids

      c. Concurrent radiation therapy to the brain

      d. Incidence increases with age

      e. Impaired renal function

    3. Use assessment guidelines to determine fine motor losses, numbness, tingling, gait disturbance, constipation, and change in mentation, which are early warning signs

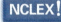

    4. Use measures outlined in Table 3-12 for collaborative management of neurotoxicity

    5. Client and family education

      a. Instruct client that neurotoxicity is a possible side effect of some chemotherapy agents

      b. Instruct client and family about early warning signs and importance of notifying physician

M. Sexual and reproductive dysfunction

    1. Infertility occurs in men primarily through depletion of the germinal epithelium that lines the seminiferous tubules

    2. Women experience reproductive dysfunction primarily as a result of hormonal alterations or direct effects that cause ovarian fibrosis and follicular destruction

    3. Chemotherapy compromises fertility by exerting cytotoxic effects on gametogenesis; the degree is related to the therapeutic agent and the duration of treatment

    4. Approximately 40 to 100% of clients experience some sexual dysfunction following treatment; it is frequently underreported because it often not assessed by healthcare personnel

    5. Males should be encouraged to bank sperm before starting treatment

    6. Although expensive (and not always successful), females should be informed of the opportunities to bank oocytes or cryopreserve embryos

	Area Affected	Chemotherapy Agent	Assessment	Collaborative Management
Table 3-12 **Neurotoxicity**	Cerebrum	Asparaginase Cisplatin Carboplatin Ifosfamide	Assess for confusion, memory loss, and level of consciousness	1. Use positive support and encouragement 2. Maintain a consistent schedule
	Sensory	Cisplatin Carboplatin Cytarabine Etoposide Paclitaxil Vincristine	Assess for decreased deep tendon reflexes, numbness, decreased sensation, jaw pain, paresthesia of hands or feet	1. Avoid extreme temperatures 2. Use assistive devices as required 3. Use opioids, antidepressants, and anticonvulsants for neuropathic pain
	Autonomic	Vincristine	Assess for abdominal pain, constipation, ileus, bladder atony	1. Recommend a high fiber diet 2. Increase fluid intake 3. Administer stool softeners and laxatives as required 4. Initiate a bowel management program ½ hour after meals 5. Monitor for bladder infection with urinary retention
	Auditory	Cisplatin Prednisone	Assess for tinnitis, hearing loss	1. Report auditory changes 2. Reduce or discontinue chemotherapy

7. Water-based lubricants or estrogen supplements may help to decrease vaginal dryness

8. Client education and counseling

    a. Provide an unbiased, sexually neutral environment that promotes open discussion

    b. Identify whether sexual issues pose a problem for the client and/or partner

    c. Explain the implications of treatments on sexuality

    d. Provide information related to contraception

    e. Discourage pregnancy during treatment

    f. Advise the client of possible long-term side effects on reproductive function

    g. Encourage communication between client and significant other

NCLEX!

NCLEX!

NCLEX!

Case Study

A 64-year-old male client is admitted for his first dose of chemotherapy. His wife died 6 months ago of a massive heart attack. He has two daughters who live out of state; one is a lawyer, while the other is a pediatrician. The client is the chief executive officer (CEO) of his own electronic business, is self-insured, and has no oncology supplement.

Chemotherapy orders include:

- Cytoxan 800 mg IVPB
- Methotrexate 160 mg IVPB
- Adriamycin 40 mg in 1000 mL normal saline IV infusion over 24 hr times 2 doses
- Leucovorin 75 mg IVPB Q 6 hrs times 4 doses; begin Leucovorin 24 hr after methotrexate
- 5-FU 80 mg IVPB after second dose of leucovorin

Other medication orders include:

- Zofran 35 mg IVPB prior to starting chemotherapy and prior to the second liter of Adriamycin
- Zofran 15 mg IVPB 4 and 8 hr after each 35 mg loading dose
- Benadryl 12.5 mg, Reglan 5 mg, and Decadron 2 mg IVPB Q 6 hours around the clock

Diagnostic studies include MUGA scan, ultrasound of the liver, CBC, and chemistry profile.

❶ What are the most important nursing diagnoses, and what is your rationale for prioritizing them the way you did?

❷ What important diagnostic/assessment values need to be obtained before initiating the chemotherapy?

❸ Outline a pre-treatment teaching plan for this client.

❹ What orders need further clarification with the physician?

❺ How will you prepare the client for discharge from the hospital?

For suggested responses, see pages 637–638.

Posttest

1 Which of the following interventions represents the best nursing action should an extravasation of a vesicant occur?

(1) The infusion of the drug should be stopped and a new site chosen for administration.
(2) The site should be treated with the appropriate antidote and observed for 3 to 4 weeks.
(3) A plastic surgeon should be consulted immediately.
(4) Emergency medical care, including corticosteroids and epinephrine, should be administered immediately.

2 The nurse is especially careful to assess for hematuria and dysuria when a client is receiving which of the following chemotherapeutic agents?

(1) Cyclophosphamide (Cytoxan)
(2) Doxorubicin (Adriamycin)
(3) Fluorouracil (5-FU)
(4) Cytarabine (Ara-C)

3 After noting altered gait, altered reflexes, and ileus in a client receiving chemotherapy, the nurse would report to the oncologist that which of the following types of organ damage is occurring?

(1) Hepatic
(2) Neurologic
(3) Renal
(4) Gastrointestinal

4 The nurse places highest priority on assessing for which of the following most common and most lethal side effect of chemotherapy?

(1) Increased respiratory rate
(2) Electrolyte imbalance
(3) Myelosuppression
(4) Elevated liver function studies

5 Which of the following is the initial step that the nurse takes in client and family education regarding chemotherapy administration?

(1) Clarify information and dispel misconceptions.
(2) Obtain informed consent.
(3) Choose an appropriate venous access.
(4) Demonstrate safe gloving and gowning.

6 A client asks the nurse to explain the term "cell cycle specific," which was overheard when the health care team made rounds. The nurse replies that chemotherapy drugs that are cell cycle specific act preferentially on cells that:

(1) Are well developed.
(2) Have entered a resting phase and are not growing.
(3) Are actively getting ready to divide or are dividing.
(4) Are no longer alive.

7 When administering vesicant chemotherapy to a client the nurse should do which of the following?

(1) Instruct the client to report any pain or burning experienced during the infusion.
(2) Infuse this type of medication in the large veins of the hands or wrist.
(3) Assess for a blood return after each 5 to 10 mL of chemotherapeutic drug administered.
(4) Apply a warm compress during the infusion to dilate the vein.

8 The nurse assesses for cardiotoxicity most carefully in a client receiving which of the following chemotherapeutic agents?

(1) Vincristine (Oncovin)
(2) Doxorubicin (Adriamycin)
(3) Nitrogen mustard (Mustargen)
(4) Cisplatin (Platinol)

9 When administering chemotherapy, the nurse should be aware of which of the following drug interactions?

(1) Cytotoxic chemotherapy drugs should never be given concurrently with another drug.
(2) Drug interactions can result in additive toxicity, decreased effectiveness, or altered activity of non-chemotherapeutic medications.
(3) Chemotherapy should never be administered in sequence with another drug.
(4) The number of drugs a client is taking does not influence the incidence of drug interactions.

10 The nurse reinforcing health teaching with a client explains that dose limitations of chemotherapy are determined by which of the following client or drug related factors?

See page 140 for Answers and Rationales.

(1) Physical status and medical history
(2) History of previous treatments
(3) Number of cancer cells in the body
(4) The toxicities of a particular drug

Answers and Rationales

Pretest

1 Answer: 3 *Rationale:* A decreased Achilles reflex is the earliest sign of neuropathy. Other assessment findings listed are adverse medication effects that occur later in the trajectory of toxicity.
Cognitive Level: Analysis
Nursing Process: Assessment; ***Test Plan:*** PHYS

2 Answer: 3 *Rationale:* Exercise strengthens cardiac muscle, thus increasing function. Dexrazoxane protects the cardiac muscle against the toxic effects of doxorubicin. The other options do not apply to this situation.
Cognitive Level: Application
Nursing Process: Implementation; ***Test Plan:*** HPM

3 Answer: 2 *Rationale:* With pursed-lip breathing, back pressure is created to keep the airways open. This promotes a more complete exhalation and, in addition, facilitates removal of secretions from the bronchial tree. The methods outlined in the other options do not achieve this effect.
Cognitive Level: Application
Nursing Process: Implementation; ***Test Plan:*** HPM

4 Answer: 2 *Rationale:* Pulmonary toxicity is a known adverse effect of bleomycin. The other responses are incorrect. It is helpful to think of "blue for bleomycin" to recall that it has respiratory adverse effects.
Cognitive Level: Analysis
Nursing Process: Assessment; ***Test Plan:*** PHYS

5 Answer: 2 *Rationale:* Intact skin is the body's first defense against infection. Although altered mucous membranes are uncomfortable and can affect the client's self-image, they are not the most important reasons. Occurrence of mucositis has no relationship to cancer recurrence.
Cognitive Level: Application
Nursing Process: Analysis; ***Test Plan:*** HPM

6 Answer: 1 *Rationale:* A client's prior nausea history is indicative of his or her individual nausea threshold and is predictive of how chemotherapy-induced nau-

sea will be handled. Women are at higher risk for developing chemotherapy-induced nausea than are men.
Cognitive Level: Analysis
Nursing Process: Analysis; ***Test Plan:*** PHYS

7 Answer: 3 *Rationale:* Since most clients become septic from organisms on their skin and in their environment, meticulous hygiene is the best way to prevent infection. An indwelling catheter is a source of infection and should only be used if the client is immobile and has a high risk for skin breakdown. Dressings should cover all open wounds to prevent contamination. Long-term catheters should be flushed after use or every 8 hours to prevent clotting; however this will not decrease the client's risk for infection.
Cognitive Level: Application
Nursing Process: Planning; ***Test Plan:*** HPM

8 Answer: 3 *Rationale:* Once stomatitis develops, meticulous oral hygiene must continue with a soft toothbrush or toothettes, fluoride-containing toothpaste, and rinsing with a dilute baking soda solution. Dilute hydrogen peroxide mouth washes are not recommended since they can dry the mouth and inhibit granulation tissue formation. Commercial mouthwashes are never recommended since they usually contain alcohol, which is drying and can burn irritated tissues.
Cognitive Level: Application
Nursing Process: Planning; ***Test Plan:*** HPM

9 Answer: 2 *Rationale:* Increasing fiber in the diet increases bulk and gastric motility, thereby decreasing constipation. Increasing activity and fluids are also helpful. Stool softeners should be encouraged, but laxative usage should be kept to a minimum to prevent becoming laxative-dependent.
Cognitive Level: Application
Nursing Process: Implementation; ***Test Plan:*** HPM

10 Answer: 2 *Rationale:* In most cancers, single-drug therapy has proven unsuccessful and leads to major tumor drug resistance. Combination chemotherapy has demonstrated long-term remission, more effective

prevention of drug resistance, and tolerable treatment side effects.
Cognitive Level: Application
Nursing Process: Analysis; *Test Plan:* PHYS

Posttest

1 **Answer: 2** *Rationale:* Vesicant therapy will cause tissue irritation with eventual sloughing without the appropriate antidote. Protocols should be in place to administer the antidote immediately after an extravasation is observed to neutralize the vesicant and minimize tissue trauma. The site should be observed for 3 to 4 weeks, but a plastic surgeon need only be consulted if tissue damage occurs (option 3).

   While the infusion must be stopped, the priority is not choosing a new site for administration (option 1). Emergency care is needed for anaphylaxis, not extravasation (option 4).
   Cognitive Level: Application
   Nursing Process: Implementation; *Test Plan:* SECE

2 **Answer: 1** *Rationale:* Cystitis can occur in the bladder as a result of chemotherapy with cyclophosphamide or ifosfamide. Nephrotoxicity can occur higher in the renal tubules as a result of therapy with cisplatin, methotrexate, streptozocin, and more rarely with mitomycin.
   Cognitive Level: Application
   Nursing Process: Assessment; *Test Plan:* PHYS

3 **Answer: 2** *Rationale:* The symptoms exhibited are most descriptive of neurotoxicity. Symptoms can arise as direct or indirect damage to the central nervous system, peripheral nervous system, cranial nerves, or any combination of the three.
   Cognitive Level: Application
   Nursing Process: Assessment; *Test Plan:* PHYS

4 **Answer: 3** *Rationale:* Myelosuppression is the most common and lethal side effect of chemotherapy. Since hematopoietic cells divide rapidly, they are most vulnerable to chemotherapy. Although respiratory failure may be lethal, an increased respiratory rate does not indicate respiratory failure (option 1).

   Electrolyte imbalances and liver function study elevations can occur with greater or lesser severity, and are therefore not the most lethal (options 2 and 4).
   Cognitive Level: Analysis
   Nursing Process: Planning; *Test Plan:* PHYS

5 **Answer: 1** *Rationale:* Clarifying information and dispelling the myths that surround cancer and cancer treatment is the initial step in client and family education. Most institutions do not require a signed informed consent to administer chemotherapy. Choosing the venous access device and the necessary safety

equipment occur after the initial education has been completed.
Cognitive Level: Analysis
Nursing Process: Implementation; *Test Plan:* HPM

6 **Answer: 3** *Rationale:* Drugs that are cell cycle specific act preferentially on cells that are proliferating (dividing). Cells in the G_0 phase or resting phase are dormant and are out of the cell cycle. Cells that are differentiated are also out of the cell cycle.
   Cognitive Level: Application
   Nursing Process: Implementation; *Test Plan:* PHYS

7 **Answer: 1** *Rationale:* The client should be instructed to notify the nurse of any burning or pain during administration so that the treatment can be stopped. Vesicant therapy should be administered in the large veins midway between the wrist and elbow. A blood return should be checked with every 1 to 2 mL of drug administered. Warm compresses should not be applied during administration, since a potential extravasation may be missed.
   Cognitive Level: Application
   Nursing Process: Implementation; *Test Plan:* SECE

8 **Answer: 2** *Rationale:* Vincristine, doxorubicin, and nitrogen mustard are all vesicants. Doxorubicin has a dose-limiting cardiotoxic effect. The major side effect of vincristine is peripheral neuropathy. The major side effects of nitrogen mustard are severe nausea and vomiting and thrombocytopenia. The major side effects of cisplatin are severe nausea and vomiting and nephrotoxicity.
   Cognitive Level: Analysis
   Nursing Process: Analysis; *Test Plan:* PHYS

9 **Answer: 2** *Rationale:* The incidence of drug interactions increases with the number of medications the client takes. Pretreatment and ongoing assessment is essential to detect potential interactions and avert or minimize an adverse outcome. Contrary to options 1 and 3, it is often necessary to administer chemotherapeutic agents concurrently or sequentially with other drugs.
   Cognitive Level: Comprehension
   Nursing Process: Analysis; *Test Plan:* SECE

10 **Answer: 4** *Rationale:* Although a client's physical well-being and response to previous treatments are important to know, toxicities of the drug commonly determine the maximum amount of the drug that can be administered safely. The number of cancer cells in the body has little to do with the dose limitations of the medications.
   Cognitive Level: Analysis
   Nursing Process: Analysis; *Test Plan:* PHYS

References

Bender, C. (1998). Nursing implications of antineoplastic therapy. In J. K. Itano & K. N. Taoka (Eds.), *Core curriculum for oncology nursing.* Philadelphia: W. B. Saunders.

Fishman, M., & Mrozek-Orlowski, M. (Eds.) (1999). *Cancer chemotherapy guidelines and recommendations for practice.* Pittsburgh: Oncology Nursing Press.

Held-Warmkessel, J. (1998). *Chemotherapy complications.* Springhouse, PA: Springhouse Corporation. Retrieved May 10, 2002 from the World Wide Web: http://www.findarticles.com/cf_0/m3231/n4_v28/20512633/print.jhtml.

Hurst, M., & Schulmeister, L. (1999). Oncology nursing update: Symptom management to enhance outcomes (Part III). *American Journal of Nursing, 99* (4). Retrieved April 24, 2002 from the World Wide Web: http://216.251.241.178/ce/test/article.cfm?id=B58F9363-4E49-11D4-83DF-00508B605149.

Lehne, R. (2004). *Pharmacology for nursing care* (5th ed.). Philadelphia: W. B. Saunders.

LeMone, P., & Burke, K. M. (2003). *Medical-surgical nursing: Critical thinking in client care* (3rd ed.). Upper Saddle River, NJ: Prentice-Hall, Inc., pp. 311–370.

McKenry, L. M., & Salerno, G. (2003). *Mosby's pharmacology in nursing* (21st ed). St. Louis: Mosby, Inc., pp. 928–965.

National Cancer Institute (1999). *Chemotherapy and you: A guide to self help during treatment* (Pub # 99-1136). Bethesda,

MD: Author. Retrieved May 10, 2002 from the World Wide Web: http://cancernet.nci.nih.gov/chemotherapy/chemoside.html.

Pace, N. L. (2001). *Treatments for chemotherapy side effects.* Philadelphia: OncoLink/University of Pennsylvania. Retrieved May 10, 2002 from the World Wide Web: http://www.oncolink.upenn.edu/support.html.

Potter, K. L., & Schafer, S. L. (1999). Oncology nursing update: Symptom management to enhance outcomes (Part I). *American Journal of Nursing, 99* (4). Retrieved April 24, 2002 from the World Wide Web: http://216.251.241.178/ce/test/article.cfm?id=B9713302-04C9-11D4-83DE-00508B92C4AE.

Shannon, M. T., Wilson, B. A., & Stang, C. L. (2003). *Health professional's drug guide: 2003.* Upper Saddle River, NJ: Prentice Hall, Inc., pp. 164–165, 383–384, 601–602.

Weis, P. A., & O'Rourke, M. E. (1999). Oncology nursing update: Symptom management to enhance outcomes (Part II). *American Journal of Nursing, 99* (4). Retrieved April 24, 2002 from the World Wide Web: http://216.251.241.178/ce/test/article.cfm?id=B9713335-04C9-11D4-83DE-00508B92C4AE.

Wilkes, G. M., Ingwersen, K., & Barton-Burke, M. (2001). *2001 oncology nursing handbook.* Boston, MA: Jones and Bartlett Publishers.

Wilson, B. A., Shannon, M. T., & Stang, C. L. (2003). *Nursing drug guide: 2003.* Upper Saddle River, NJ: Prentice Hall, Inc., pp. 842, 1464–1466.

CHAPTER 4

Blood Modifying Agents

Daryle Wane, MS, APRN, BC

CHAPTER OUTLINE

OBJECTIVES

- Describe goals of therapy related to the various blood-modifying medications.

- Identify significant nursing interventions for the client receiving an anticoagulant, antiplatelet, or thrombolytic medication.

- Identify antidotes for hemorrhage caused by various anticoagulants.

- Identify common side effects of medications used to lower serum cholesterol.

- Discuss nursing considerations related to administration of iron, vitamin B_{12}, or folic acid.

- Identify dietary sources of iron, vitamin B_{12}, and folic acid.

- Describe action and use of epoetin alfa (Epogen, Procrit).

- List significant client education points related to various blood-modifying medications.

[Media Link]

Use the CD-ROM enclosed with this text, or log onto the address given to access the free, interactive Companion Website created for this series. The CD-ROM and Companion Website accompanying this book offer additional practice opportunities and information—NCLEX Review, Case Studies, Glossary, In Depth with NCLEX, and more.

www.prenhall.com/hogan

REVIEW AT A GLANCE

activated partial thromboplastin time (APTT) *a diagnostic blood test used to determine intrinsic clotting response that is measured in seconds; it is used to monitor and evaluate a client's response when on a heparin protocol*

aggregation *an accumulation of substances such as platelets in the blood that form a group or cluster*

anticoagulants *substances that prevent or delay the coagulation of the blood*

antithrombin III (ATIII) *a specific substance in the clotting cascade that prevents the activation of three clotting factors (thrombin, activated IX, and activated X)*

clotting cascade *a coagulation pathway in which enzymes and specific blood factors interact to effectively maintain normal hemostasis in the body; it includes both the extrinsic and intrinsic pathways and leads to the conversion of prothrombin to thrombin*

extrinsic pathway *the pathway in the clotting cascade that forms fibrin and acts within seconds; the PT and INR measure extrinsic pathway function*

fibrinolysis *the process whereby the dissolution of a clot takes place utilizing specific plasminogen activators in the body in order to prevent excessive clotting which could lead to vascular obstruction*

fibrinolytic system *the fibrinolytic system involves releasing plasmin (through the use of plasminogen activators) to act on the fibrin (blood) clot and cause it to dissolve*

hemostatics *substances, devices, or procedures that stop the flow of blood*

heparin-induced platelet aggregation (HITT) *a potentially fatal complication of heparin therapy, whereby the client develops new clot formation with severe thrombocytopenia; it is also called white clot syndrome; HITT stands for heparin-induced thrombocytopenia and thrombosis*

hypercoagulation *a process whereby blood coagulates faster, leading to potential problems in the coagulation cascade*

International Normalized Ratio (INR) *a standard reference range used to establish consistency in reporting PT levels that takes into account normal variations seen in lab testing; INR levels lead to a better consensus of therapeutic management and assure that test results are being evaluated based on common standards*

intrinsic pathway *the pathway in which fibrin formation occurs and takes several minutes; intrinsic pathway function is measured by the APTT*

low molecular weight heparin (LMWH) *a term that refers to a group of heparin*

products that are comparable in molecular weight and have a higher bioavailability than traditional heparin

pernicious anemia *a specific type of megaloblastic, macrocytic anemia that is related to the lack of intrinsic factor necessary for absorption of vitamin B_{12} in the GI tract*

pica *the ingestion of nonfood substances, such as chalk, dirt, or paint, that can lead to nutritional deficiency states (and sometimes potential toxicity); it can be seen as a type of craving whereby the client seeks out these substances*

protamine sulfate *antidote used for heparin*

prothrombin time (PT) *a diagnostic blood test used to measure extrinsic clotting response that is measured in seconds; a control level is run with the test to determine a standard response; it is used to monitor and evaluate a client's response when on oral anticoagulation therapy*

purple toe syndrome *a complication of oral anticoagulation therapy, whereby vascular emboli are released leading to microemboli formation in the toes and disruption of circulation*

thrombolytics *a group of substances that break down existing clots in the vascular system to restore blood flow and circulation*

Pretest

1 A client has been diagnosed with iron deficiency anemia (IDA) and wants to know what foods would help to maintain adequate iron levels in the body. Which of the following items regarding diet information would be beneficial to include in a teaching plan for achieving the goal of increased iron levels?

(1) Maintain a strict vegetarian diet.
(2) Eat ice cubes that are present in beverages.
(3) Increase tea and cereal in the diet.
(4) Use adequate sources of vitamin C in the diet.

2 A client is taking antiplatelet medication for several weeks and presents with a noticeable bruise on the arm. What information should the nurse assess first in order to determine if this skin manifestation is related to drug therapy?

(1) Whether the bruising is a result of a specific injury, and therefore not caused by drug therapy
(2) Whether the client has taken the medication for the last several days
(3) Whether the client self-monitors for skin manifestations
(4) Whether the client has bruising and discoloration on other areas of the body

3 In order to verify iron stores in the body, which priority laboratory test result would the nurse look for in a client's medical record?

(1) Ferritin level
(2) Transferrin level
(3) Hemoglobin and hematocrit
(4) Complete blood count (CBC)

4 A client is being treated with alteplase (Activase) in the emergency department following a cerebrovascular accident (CVA or stroke). What is the priority nursing intervention related to the care of a client receiving this drug therapy?

(1) Perform vital signs every 15 minutes until the client's blood pressure is stabilized.
(2) Place the client on a cardiac monitor and observe for potential dysrhythmias as this medication can have cardiac effects.
(3) Insert a urinary catheter and maintain accurate hourly output measures.
(4) Monitor the client for hypothermia, as this is a common side effect of this medication.

5 A client is taking epoetin alfa (Epogen) for treatment of anemia related to chronic renal disease. What clinical finding reveals that this medication is working effectively?

(1) The client is not experiencing any related bone pain when the medication is being administered.
(2) The client's hemoglobin and hematocrit levels are rising rapidly based on the latest two daily blood draws.
(3) The client's hematocrit is in the established target range at 33%.
(4) The client is afebrile.

6 A client who has elevated cholesterol levels has been prescribed nicotinic acid (Niacin). What information would you provide to this client?

(1) Niacin treatment is highly individualized and there may be dose adjustments based on lab values.
(2) Expect facial flushing, as this is a common expected effect of this medication.
(3) Dietary sources of niacin are necessary to ensure that the medication works effectively.
(4) Niacin can be taken concurrently with lovastatin (Mevacor) in order to maximize the therapeutic effect.

7 A client with von Willebrand's disease is taking desmopressin (DDAVP) and cryoprecipitate as part of the treatment regimen. The nurse would explain that medication therapy will provide what pharmacologic benefit to this client?

(1) These medications will help to restore and release deficient clotting factors (vW and VIII) that occur in this disease process.
(2) DDAVP is given for its antidiuretic effect to promote fluid management.
(3) Cryoprecipitate and DDAVP must be given concurrently in order to potentiate their therapeutic effect.
(4) These medications will stimulate the client's own production of specific blood factors.

8 The nurse reviewing a client's laboratory test results would conclude that which of the following would affect the client's ability to maintain hemostasis?

(1) Low ferritin level
(2) Elevated triglyceride level
(3) Neutropenia
(4) Thrombocytopenia

9 A client is being discharged on warfarin (Coumadin) following heart valve replacement surgery. What information would the nurse give to the client to provide safe and effective care during the course of therapy?

(1) Follow-up lab testing is required on a weekly basis in order to monitor client response.
(2) Be alert to the possibility of bleeding tendencies caused by this drug therapy and use electric razors and soft toothbrushes.
(3) Take medication upon arising in the morning on an empty stomach to maximize absorption.
(4) Since the therapy is based on achieving a therapeutic blood level, if a dose is missed, double up the next dose.

10 The nurse has just received an order to start intravenous heparin (Liquaemin) therapy on a client admitted for deep vain thrombosis (DVT). What nursing intervention would the nurse employ in order to implement this order?

See pages 185–187 for Answers and Rationales.

(1) Vitamin K should be readily available as long as the client remains on heparin therapy.

(2) The client should remain NPO as long as the medication is infusing.

(3) An infusion pump should be utilized for the administration of heparin.

(4) The client should be weighed twice a day in order to evaluate for potential fluid overload.

I. Anticoagulants

A. Oral medications

1. Action and use

   a. Oral **anticoagulants,** substances that prevent or delay the coagulation of the blood, are a group of medications used both to treat and prevent thromboembolic disorders in clients who are at risk

   b. Oral anticoagulants such as warfarin (Coumadin and its derivatives) exert their effects by preventing conversion of vitamin K, thereby decreasing its production in the liver

   c. Vitamin K plays an active role in the **extrinsic pathway** (a pathway that forms fibrin and acts within seconds) in the **clotting cascade** (a coagulation pathway)

   d. With vitamin K production reduced, several clotting factors (II, VII, IX, and X) are also reduced, thereby affecting the clotting cascade

   e. Coumadin is bound to plasma proteins, most notably albumin; it is metabolized in the liver

   f. Oral anticoagulants are used in the management of clients with actual, potential, and recurrent health problems such as deep vein thrombosis (DVT), pulmonary embolism (PE), acute myocardial infarction (MI), heart valve replacement (bioprosthetic and mechanical), atrial fibrillation, and antiphospholipid syndrome

2. Common medications

   a. Coumarin derivative warfarin sodium (Coumadin) is probably the most frequently used oral therapy utilized in the United States for the management of anticoagulation

   b. Warfarin (Coumadin) is given orally at a usual dose of 1 to 15 mg daily, with dose titrated to keep INR 2 to 3

   c. Bishydroxycoumarin (Dicumarol) is also a coumarin derivative; it is given orally 200–300 mg on day 1, then 25 to 200 mg daily based on PT

3. Administration considerations

   a. The administration of Coumadin requires close monitoring (because of a narrow therapeutic range), frequent dose adjustments (because of individual dose response), and a high potential for the development of interactions (involving food and drug interactions) that can lead to ineffective therapy or toxicity

b. Coumadin's onset of action is slow to materialize, and its full anticoagulant effect is not seen until after approximately 1 week's duration; because of this, this drug may be started while a client is still on heparin therapy and overlap as the heparin drug is tapered once desirable anticoagulation has been reached

c. **Prothrombin time (PT),** a diagnostic blood test used to measure extrinsic clotting response, and the **International Normalized Ratio (INR),** a standard reference range used to establish consistency in reporting PT levels, are both used to monitor the client's response to therapy; the two are used in conjunction because of the variation of the individual dose response

d. Coumadin is usually given in the evening following careful attention to pertinent laboratory test results drawn earlier in the day

NCLEX!

e. Depending on the indication for therapy, the desired range of the PT and INR will vary; PT levels usually are felt to be effective when they are maintained at 1.5 to 2.5 times the control value; INR levels range from a usual 2.0 to 3.0 range to a higher level of 3.0 to 4.5 range if the client has a mechanical cardiac valve replacement

NCLEX!

f. Duration of therapy can range from several months to lifelong depending on the specific client's health problem

g. Refer to specific hospital protocol and physician's order for dose adjustments and monitoring of client's PT and INR levels

NCLEX!

h. Vitamin K is the antidote that reverses the action of Coumadin

4. Contraindications

a. Oral anticoagulants are contraindicated in clients who are pregnant

b. Lactating women can be given bishydroxycoumarin and warfarin as these medications will cross through in the breast milk but there is little effect on an infant's PT; however, if the infant were to require surgery, it would be advisable to obtain the infant's PT as a baseline

c. Oral anticoagulants should not be given to clients who are hemorrhaging or have bleeding tendencies, clients with malignant hypertension, or clients with a past history of allergic reaction to coumarin derivatives

d. Clients with co-morbid conditions such as liver failure and congestive heart failure (CHF) may have problems with metabolism and utilization of the drug

NCLEX!

5. Significant drug interactions

a. Because coumadin competes for binding sites in the liver, there is a high potential for drug interactions relative to enzyme inhibitors and enzyme inducers; these chemical reactions will affect the serum concentration level of coumadin

b. Coumadin is often considered to be one of the primary examples of a medication that has complex interactions with a vast number of medications

Table 4-1	Drugs that Potentiate Action	Drugs that Decrease Action
Partial Listing of Coumadin Drug Interactions	Acetaminophen and acetylsalicylic acid (ASA) Antibiotics H$_2$ histamine antagonists Loop diuretics Nonsteroidal anti-inflammatory drugs (NSAIDS) Sulfonamides Vitamin E	Alcohol Barbiturates Estrogens/oral contraceptives Spironolactone Thiazide diuretics Thyroid drugs Vitamin K

    c. Refer to Table 4-1 for a partial listing of medications that can potentiate and diminish the effect of Coumadin

    d. The use of herbal medications will be discussed under the next subheading because the Food and Drug Administration (FDA) does not currently clearly define the "medicinal" effects of this type of therapy under conventional medical models; they are considered to be dietary supplements

6. Significant food interactions

    a. Increased effects are seen with chondroitin and garlic

    b. There is an increased bleeding risk seen with cayenne, feverfew, garlic, ginger, and Gingko biloba

    c. Decreased effectiveness of the medication is seen with the use of green tea, ginseng, and goldenseal

    d. The action of oral anticoagulants can be dramatically diminished by an increase in dietary sources of vitamin K

    e. Foods high in vitamin K such as liver, cheese, egg yolk, leafy vegetables (broccoli, cabbage, spinach, and kale) and oils (peanut, corn, olive, or soybean) should be avoided or used sparingly during therapy

    f. Dietary supplements of vitamin K should be avoided

    g. The use of alcohol should be restricted (if not avoided) to maintain effective drug therapy

    h. Referral to a dietician is always indicated for clients receiving Coumadin therapy because of the many potential dietary interactions and possibility of prolonged treatment with this type of medication

7. Significant laboratory studies

    a. Discoloration of urine (red-orange) can be seen with the use of coumarin derivatives and may be of concern to the client

    b. A hematologist should evaluate clients who are resistant to anticoagulation treatment with these types of medications for other specific underlying disorders of coagulation that might affect therapy

8. Side effects

    a. Ecchymosis of the skin, or bleeding from any tissue or organ

    b. Gastrointestinal (GI) and dermatologic problems

        c. Hypotension

        d. Thrombocytopenia

  9. Adverse effects/toxicity

        a. Bleeding is the major adverse effect and is usually seen at higher dosage levels

        b. GI: nausea, diarrhea, intestinal obstruction, anorexia, abdominal cramping

        c. Dermatologic manifestations: rash, urticaria, and **purple toe syndrome** (discoloration caused by decreased perfusion from release of microemboli)

        d. Increased serum transaminase levels, hepatitis, jaundice

        e. Burning sensation of feet

        f. Transient hair loss

  10. Nursing considerations

        a. Monitor client's baseline labs with regard to initiation and continuation of therapy (specifically PT and INR)

        b. Review client's medications and dietary history with regard to potential drug and food interactions; be sure to include nutritional and herbal supplements

        c. Notify the physician/practitioner of current PT and INR results, making note of client's current dose

        d. Communicate with the dietician regarding the client's status and anticipate discharge planning needs as the therapy continues

        e. Assess the client's skin for bleeding tendencies and monitor for GI side effects

        f. Client teaching is critically important because of the many potential inter-actions, length of therapy, and close follow-up monitoring required

        g. Vitamin K may be ordered to reverse the action of Coumadin depending on client's pertinent labs (PT and INR); it can be ordered as a single-dose therapy if high PT and INR values persist; additional doses of vitamin K may be given, and the coumadin dose may be withheld

        h. If the client experiences adverse effects or toxicity, stop (withhold) Coumadin therapy; depending on the INR or client manifestations, admin-istration of phytonadione (vitamin K) may be indicated

        i. If there is significant bleeding, the physician may order transfusion of fresh frozen plasma (FFP) or prothrombin concentrate

  11. Client education

        a. Establish individualized teaching goals which will increase client's knowl-edge of the disease process and thereby improve compliance with long-term therapy

        b. Alert client to bleeding problems and how to respond

        c. Frequent follow-up blood tests will be required to make sure safe therapeu-tic therapy is maintained

  d. Point-of-care (POC) testing is available for self-monitoring PT and INR; the physician may establish a home protocol to help manage care and necessary dosage adjustments

  e. The medication is to be taken on a daily basis; medication cannot be stopped unless the physician orders a dose to be held (pending PT and INR results), or the client experiences a bleeding episode

  f. Communication between the client and all members of the health care team is an essential part of therapeutic management

  g. Use a soft toothbrush and electric razor to minimize even mild trauma that could lead to bleeding

  h. Observe for bleeding gums, bruises, nosebleeds, tarry stools, hematuria, hematemesis, and petechiae; report these findings to the prescriber

  i. Teach client to avoid intake of foods high in vitamin K (see previous section)

B. Heparin and related medications

 1. Action and use

  a. Heparin is a heterogeneous group of carbohydrates that exert anticoagulant effects; they have different molecular weights and other chemical properties that influence the vascular system

  b. Heparin plays an active role in the **intrinsic pathway** (the pathway in which fibrin formation occurs and takes several minutes) in the clotting cascade

  c. Heparin combines with a plasma heparin cofactor named **antithrombin III (ATIII),** and this complex causes inactivation of specific clotting factors (II_a, X_a, XII_a, XI_a, and IX_a) in the clotting cascade

  d. The heparin/ATIII complex has a very strong anticoagulant effect that inhibits conversion of fibrinogen to fibrin, prevents formation of a fibrin clot, and inhibits thrombin

  e. The molecular weight of the heparin molecule can range from 3,000 to 30,000 daltons (d), the average weight being around 15,000 d; the standard measurement used is unfractionated heparin (UFH); **low molecular weight heparin (LMWH)** is also available with a molecular weight range of 4,000 to 6,500 d

  f. Because of its immediate effect, heparin is the treatment of choice for clients who have DVT, PE, and embolism as a result of atrial fibrillation

  g. It is also used as a prophylactic measure for clients at risk for developing thrombi as a result of surgical intervention

  h. It is also used in a weak concentration as a flush solution to maintain access and prevent thrombus formation in vascular access devices

 2. Common medications

  a. LMWH is a newer class of the heparin molecule consisting of heparin fragments, with enoxaprin (Lovenox) being the most commonly used

  b. Heparin (Liquaemin) sodium is the most commonly used anticoagulant for treatment, prevention, and recurrent thromboembolic episodes

  c. Refer to Table 4-2 for a listing of heparin anticoagulants

Table 4-2	Generic/Trade Names	Usual Adult Dose	Administration Route
Heparin and Related Medications	Heparin (Liquaemin)	5000 unit bolus dose, then 20,000–40,000 U infused over 24 hour	IV
		10,000–20,000 U followed by 8,000–20,000 U q 8–12 hours	SC
	Ardeparin (Normiflo)	150–500 mg in 1–2 doses	PO, IM, IV, SC
	Dalteparin (Fragmin)	400 mg bid for 3–6 months	PO
	Danaparoid (Orgaran)	400 mg bid for 3–6 months	PO
	Enoxaprin (Lovenox)	Prophylactically: 30 mg bid	SC
		Therapeutic: 1 mg/kg	
	Tinazaparin (Innohep)	175 anti Xa IV q 24 hours	SC

3. Administration considerations

a. Heparin can be administered intravenously (IV) or by subcutaneous (SC) injection

b. Heparin bioavailability is influenced by its mode of administration and its chemical formulation; LMWH have a higher bioavailiability when compared to standard UFH

c. Activated partial thromboplastin time (APTT) is a diagnostic blood test that determines intrinsic clotting response and is measured in seconds; it is used to monitor a client who is receiving heparin therapy; the results are trended over time to determine client response and therapeutic effect

d. Low-dose UFH therapy: used as a prophylactic treatment for DVT; dosage ranges from 5,000 U SC every 8 to 12 hours or 3 doses in the immediate post-operative period dependent on physician protocol; enoxaparin or Lovenox (a LMWH) is used in the clinical setting for this purpose and comes in prefilled syringes ready for individual use

e. High-dose UFH therapy is done to achieve a therapeutic APTT; APTT levels should be stabilized at 1 ½ to 2 times the control value

f. An infusion pump is required for parenteral administration; IV heparin should be infused through a dedicated infusion line because of its incompatibility profile

g. Heparin weight-based therapy protocol is a standard format utilized by physicians in the clinical setting to effectively anticoagulate a client who has need for immediate intervention (refer to Box 4-1 for specific information relevant to protocol management)

h. Be sure to carefully identify strength on product label; several concentrations of IV heparin are available; some are used only as flushes for IV lines

i. Protamine sulfate is the antidote that reverses the action of heparin; the dosage depends on both the amount of heparin that is given and the time period following its administration; however, the nurse should not give more than 50 mg in a 10-minute time period; protamine sulfate is administered IVP

Client weight should be obtained as a baseline for initiation of therapy.
Monitor daily weight and pertinent labs (APTT).
Hemocult all stools to assess for possible adverse effect of bleeding.
Titrate heparin dosage, as needed based on results of APTT.
APTT labs are usually ordered q 6 hours until two consecutive therapeutic levels are obtained. At that time, APTT can be ordered q 24 hours.
Once the client is stabilized, an oral anticoagulant such as Coumadin is usually added if client requires long-term therapy.
Further monitoring of APTT, PT, and INR is required leading to heparin being discontinued and Coumadin being maintained as the method of anticoagulation.

    j. Hypersensitivity or allergic reactions can be seen in clients receiving heparin, so epinephrine 1:1,000 should be readily available if a reaction develops

4. Contraindications

    a. Contraindicated with uncontrolled bleeding, known hypersensitivity, and thrombocytopenia

    b. Should not be given with aspirin (ASA) and nonsteroidal anti-inflammatory drugs (NSAIDS), as this will increase the risk of bleeding

    c. LMWH are contraindicated in clients with active bleeding, thrombocytopenia, and/or heparin or pork allergy

NCLEX!

5. Significant drug interactions: ASA, NSAIDS, and antiplatelet agents can potentiate the anticoagulation effect and increase bleeding

NCLEX!

6. Significant food interactions: allergy to pork products may indicate a potential hypersensitivity to LMWH

7. Significant laboratory studies

    a. Heparin prolongs APPT level that is used to monitor oral anticoagulants

    b. Elevations of serum transaminase levels have been seen

8. Side effects

    a. Hemorrhage, hematuria, epistaxis, bleeding gums

    b. Thrombocytopenia

9. Adverse effects/toxicity

    a. A serious form of thrombocytopenia called **heparin-induced platelet aggregation (HITT),** or white clot syndrome; this can be fatal if not treated aggressively; thrombocytopenia is more pronounced (less than $100,000/mm^3$) and begins between 3 and 12 days following initiation heparin therapy

    b. Clients who are on long-term heparin therapy (longer than 6 months duration) are prone to develop osteoporosis

NCLEX!

10. Nursing considerations

    a. Monitor client's baseline labs with regard to heparin protocol (specifically APTT); trend results and titrate medication according to protocol; with continuous IV heparin infusion, APTT is commonly measured q 6 hours; when level is critically high, infusion may be stopped for 1 or more hours and APTT measured in 2 to 3 hours

b. Obtain daily weight for client on weight-based heparin protocol

c. Monitor client for signs of bleeding, perform a thorough skin assessment, hemocult all stools, and evaluate pertinent labs

d. Verify with pharmacy or another RN the correct dosage of heparin before administering or adjusting the heparin infusion

e. Evaluate dosage for safety and therapeutic range based on normal adult dosage range of 20,000 to 40,000 units/24 hr; heparin is usually infused in units/hr

f. Have antidote available (protamine sulfate)

g. Subcutaneous administration of heparin requires rotation of sites; aspiration and rubbing of the injection site are not done

h. When administering heparin SC, inject into the abdomen using a small (5/8-inch, 25- to 27-gauge) needle at a 90-degree angle

11. Client education

a. Establish specific goals to increase client's knowledge related to heparin administration

b. Inform client that frequent blood work monitoring is required to make sure that effective anticoagulation is achieved

c. Teach client to be alert for bleeding problems and how to respond

d. Instruct client to observe for hematuria, nosebleeds, blood in the stool and petechiae

II. Antiplatelet Agents

A. Action and use

1. Antiplatelet drugs are substances that prevent the formation of the natural clotting mechanism in the body; they are a group of medications used to prevent or disrupt the **aggregation** (an accumulation of substances in the blood that form a group or cluster) of platelets needed to form a clot

2. Act on different aspects of the clotting cascade to prevent formation of a blood clot

3. Used to treat thrombus formation and are often used as adjunctive therapy to other anticoagulant medications such as warfarin (Coumadin)

4. Used as both preventive and treatment measures for clients with history of MI, stroke, and cardiac surgery

5. Inhibit or block certain enzyme pathways to prevent clot formation

B. Common medications

1. Aspirin (or acetylsalicylic acid, ASA) is the most commonly used type of antiplatelet medication

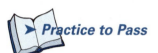

Practice to Pass

What discharge instructions would you provide to a client who has been placed on anticoagulation therapy?

NCLEX!

NCLEX!

2. Ticlopidine (Ticlid) can be used as an antiplatelet medication in those clients who cannot take aspirin therapy

3. In addition to its utility as an antiplatelet agent, dipyridamole (Persantine) is also used in cardiac stress testing

4. ASA has many other therapeutic properties such as analgesic, anti-inflammatory, and antipyretic action

5. Clopidrogrel bisulfate (Plavix) is used as a form of secondary prevention for clients who have had MI, stroke, and peripheral arterial disease

6. Abciximab (ReoPro) is a fab fragment of a specific monoclonal antibody

7. Refer to Table 4-3 for a listing of common antiplatelet medications

C. Administration considerations

1. ASA is administered in dosages ranging from 81 to 325 mg/day (baby ASA to adult strength); it can also be given as an enteric-coated preparation to minimize GI upset

2. Dipyridamole (Persantine) has a better profile when used with clients who have prosthetic mechanical heart valves

3. Ticlopidine (Ticlid) has been used effectively as a preventive measure in clients who are at risk for MI

4. Abciximab (ReoPro) is administered via the parenteral route and the client can receive a bolus dose as well as a constant infusion

D. Contraindications

1. ASA is contraindicated in clients who have a known hypersensitivity to salicylates, have bleeding disorders, asthma, or who have presence of gastrointestinal bleeding; ASA should not be given to pediatric clients because it can be associated with the development of Reye's syndrome

2. Dipyridamole (Persantine) is contraindicated in clients who are pregnant or lactating

3. Abciximab (ReoPro) is contraindicated in clients with evidence of current or recent bleeding, cerebral vascular accident (CVA) within the past 2 years with deficit, and thrombocytopenia

Table 4-3			
Antiplatelet Agents	**Generic/Trade Names**	**Usual Adult Dose**	**Administration Route**
	Abciximab (ReoPro)	0.25 mg/kg	IV
	Aspirin	81–325 mg qd	PO
	Clopidrogrel bisulfate (Plavix)	75 mg qd	PO
	Dipyridamole (Persantine)	75–100 mg qid along with warfarin therapy	PO
	Eptifibatide (Integril)	2 mcg/kg/min	IV
	Ticlopidine (Ticlid)	250 mg bid with food	PO
	Tirofiban (Aggrastat)	0.1 mcg/kg/min	IV

4. Ticlopidine (Ticlid) is contraindicated in clients who are pregnant, those with a known hypersensitivity, liver disease, or evidence of blood dyscrasias

5. Clopidrogrel bisulfate (Plavix) is contraindicated in clients with a known hypersensitivity or who have active bleeding problems as a result of intracranial hemorrhage or peptic ulcer disease

E. Significant drug interactions

1. With ASA: increased effects are seen with the use of ETOH, anticoagulants, methotrexate and sulfonylureas; decreased effects are seen with the use of angiotensin converting enzyme (ACE) inhibitors, beta-blockers, and diuretics

2. Dipyridamole/ASA can lead to additive effects and lead to an increased risk for bleeding

3. Ticlopidine (Ticlid): can increase levels of theophylline and phenytoin; cimetidine can lead to increased levels of Ticlid in the body

4. Clopidrogrel bisulfate (Plavix)/NSAIDS: may increase risk of bleeding episodes

F. Significant food interactions

1. Ticlopidine is best taken on a full stomach to help maximize absorption and not in the presence of antacids

2. ASA is usually taken on a full stomach to minimize gastrointestinal upset

G. Significant laboratory studies

1. ASA can cause false-negative or -positive results for urine glucose and increase uric acid levels

2. Ticlopidine has a potential to cause blood dyscrasias and a rise in serum cholesterol levels

H. Side effects

1. ASA: blood dyscrasias, hemorrhage, GI symptoms, as well as central nervous system (CNS) alterations, increased bleeding tendencies, hemorrhage, nausea and vomiting, dizziness, and confusion

2. Persantine: gastrointestinal complaints, nausea and vomiting, CNS alterations, headache and dizziness

3. Ticlopidine: serious blood dyscrasias such as agranulocytosis and neutropenia; GI symptoms, such as nausea, vomiting, and jaundice

4. Clopidrogrel: flu-like symptoms, chest pain, edema, and hypertension

5. In general: bruising, hematuria, tarry stools

I. Adverse effects/toxicity

1. ASA toxicity: tinnitus and ototoxicity

2. Abciximab: allergic reaction

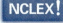

J. Nursing considerations

1. A baseline level of pertinent hematologic labs should be included at the client admission

2. Monitor vital signs

3. Monitor bleeding time

4. Monitor the client for side effects related to bleeding

5. The use of antiplatelet medications should be stopped for at least 7 days prior to a planned surgery

6. Older adult clients may require closer monitoring with antiplatelet therapy to avoid toxicity because it may be harder to assess for tinnitus and ototoxicity if a client's baseline hearing is already diminished

7. Life span concerns: children, pregnant women, and lactating women should not be taking antiplatelet medications

K. Client education

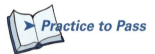

1. Instruct client to carry a Medic-alert bracelet

2. Establish specific individualized goals to increase client's knowledge of treatment therapy and the need for continued compliance

3. Instruct client to monitor for side effects related to bleeding and report them

4. Inform client that communication between the client and health care team members is critical

5. Inform client that adults should not use aspirin for self-medication of pain longer than 5 days without consulting a physician

6. Instruct to maintain adequate fluid intake to prevent salicylate crystalluria

7. Inform female clients that prolonged use of ASA can lead to iron-deficiency anemia

> **Practice to Pass**
>
> A client has been told by his physician to "take an aspirin a day to thin the blood" but is unsure as to the type and dosage. What information would you provide to the client with regard to this dilemma?

III. Thrombolytics

A. Action and use

1. **Thrombolytics:** substances that dissolve or break down a thrombus or blood clot

2. After the thrombus is broken down, blood flow is reestablished to the area (increased perfusion) to maintain vascular integrity and prevent ischemia

3. The use of thrombolytic substances in the body helps activate the **fibrinolytic system** that breaks down the thrombus or blood clot

4. The conversion of plasminogen to plasmin helps break down the clot by digesting fibrin and degrading fibrinogen and other procoagulant proteins into soluble fragments

5. The process of **fibrinolysis** is activated naturally in the body to prevent excessive clotting or vascular compromise

6. Thrombolytic therapy is indicated for clients who are at risk for developing thrombus with resultant ischemia such as acute MI, arterial thrombosis, DVT, pulmonary embolism, and occlusion of catheters or shunts

7. Thrombolytic medications are mostly given in emergency and critical care environments

B. Common medications

1. Streptokinase (Kabikinase, Streptase) is isolated from group-A beta-hemolytic streptococci (bacteria) and is considered to be antigenic; its action is systemic in nature

2. Alteplase (Activase) is a natural substance secreted by vascular endothelial cells in the body and therefore does not cause an antigenic response; its action is specific in nature

3. Urokinase (Abbokinase) was primarily used for the treatment of pulmonary embolism (PE) and catheters that are occluded; however, recent evidence may indicate that it is not the drug of choice for treatment of PE (except in client with a massive PE who has compensated hemodynamically)

4. Refer to Table 4-4 for a listing of common thrombolytics

C. **Administration considerations**

1. Thrombolytic medications are usually given to clients who are acutely ill in emergency and critical care settings where stabilization is the primary goal of intervention

2. Baseline vital signs and pertinent lab results regarding coagulation status are necessary

3. IV administration is carried out through specific protocols and guidelines to maintain safe and therapeutic effects; monitor IV sites for signs and symptoms of infiltration and/or phlebitis

4. If IV site is not patent or if symptoms develop suggesting infiltration or phlebitis, then the site should be changed to the opposite extremity

5. Continuous monitoring of blood pressure (BP), mental status, and response to therapy should be documented; report any signs of chest pain, dizziness, headache or evidence of bleeding to the physician

6. Client should be on a cardiac monitor during the administration of thrombolytics

7. The antidote to streptokinase or urokinase is aminocaproic acid (Amicar)

D. **Contraindications**

1. IM administration of medications is contraindicated when using thrombolytics

2. Contraindicated in clients who are actively bleeding, have a recent history of CVA, severe uncontrolled hypertension, recent trauma and neoplasm

3. Contraindicated during pregnancy

E. **Significant drug interactions:** increased risk of bleeding when taking with anti-coagulant and antiplatelet drugs

Table 4-4

Thrombolytics

Generic/Trade Names	Usual Adult Dose	Administration Route
Alteplase (Activase)	0.75 mg/kg	IV
Anistreplase (Eminase)	30 U push over 2–5 min	IV
Reteplase (Retavase)	10 U over 2 min	IV
Streptokinase (Kabikinase, Streptase)	250,000 IU , then 100,000 IU/h for 48–72 h	IV
Urokinase (Abbokinase Open-Cath)	Initial dose: 4,400 IU/kg	IV

NCLEX!

NCLEX!

NCLEX!

F. Significant food interactions: none reported

G. Significant laboratory studies

1. Reductions in plasminogen and fibrinogen levels are seen with the use of thrombolytic agents

2. Monitoring coagulation profile such as bleeding time, APTT, and PT is required to ensure safe and therapeutic treatment

H. Side effects

1. Hemorrhage

2. Hypersensitivity reactions

3. Nausea, vomiting, and hypotension

4. Cardiac dysrhythmias

I. Adverse effects/toxicity

1. Side effects of the thrombolytic agents are dose-related

2. Dysrhythmias as a consequence of therapy may pose further problems for the client who is already in an acute situation

J. Nursing considerations

1. Monitor pertinent baseline labs and continue to assess client during therapy

2. Monitor client for vital sign changes, as there may be variations in pulse, BP, and temperature caused by thrombolytic administration

3. Maintain adequate IV site for medication administration; observe closely for signs and symptoms of infiltration

4. Limit the nature of invasive procedures when a client is on thrombolytic therapy to reduce the risk of bleeding

5. Assess frequently for signs of bleeding, both obvious and occult

6. If the client is found to be bleeding, the medication should be stopped; fresh frozen plasma (FFP) and packed red blood cells (PRBCs) may be ordered

7. Monitor client closely for development of dysrhythmias

8. Maintain aseptic technique to prevent infection

9. Antidote: aminocaproic acid (Amicar); should be readily available on the clinical unit

10. Provide adequate nutrition and rest in order to support the client during treatment

11. Support the client and family members during the acute-care management period

12. Maintain effective, open, and therapeutic communication among client, family, and all health care team members

K. Client education

1. Instruct client about treatment methods and medication administration

2. Instruct client to use electric razor to reduce risk of bleeding

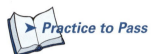

3. Instruct client to brush teeth gently using a soft toothbrush to reduce risk of bleeding

4. Teach client to avoid trauma to skin and other areas of body to reduce risk of bleeding

5. Explain to client that lifestyle changes may be instituted in order to prevent further occurrences of abnormal clotting

6. Inform client that measurable signs of clinical response may not occur for 6 to 8 hours after therapy is started

7. Instruct client to discontinue medication if bleeding occurs and notify physician

IV. Hemostatics

A. Systemic hemostatics

1. Action and use

   a. Systemic **hemostatics** are substances that inhibit bleeding after an injury in order to maintain hematologic balance

   b. Used to stop/or prevent bleeding in clients who are at risk due to injury

   c. Vitamin K is also used as the mandatory treatment to prevent hemorrhagic disease of the newborn

   d. Vitamin K works in the liver to formulate specific clotting factors (II, VII, IX, and X) that are necessary in the coagulation cascade

2. Common medications

   a. Aminocaproic acid (Amicar) and tranexamic acid (Cyklokapron) both impede fibrinolysis

   b. Aminocaproic acid is used to treat hyperfibrinolysis-induced hemorrhage after surgery and for hematologic disorders such as aplastic anemia, hepatic cirrhosis, and some neoplastic disease states; it is also an antidote to thrombolytic drugs

   c. Tranexamic acid is used 1 day prior and 2 to 8 days after dental or other surgery in clients with hemophilia

   d. Phytonadione, vitamin K_1 (Aquamephyton) is the antidote to warfarin and is fat-soluble; it is used to reverse excess effects of oral anticoagulants

   e. Menadiol sodium diphosphate, Vitamin K_4 (Synkayvite) is a water-soluble compound

   f. Refer to Table 4-5 for a listing of common systemic hemostatics

3. Administration considerations

   a. Aminocaproic acid and tranexamic acid are administered via oral or IV route; close continuous monitoring of the client is required

   b. Phytonadione is usually given IM to newborns in the delivery room for treatment and prophylaxis of hemorrhagic disease of the newborn

   c. Vitamin K preparations can be given PO, IM, SC, or IV

Practice to Pass

A client in the emergency department is receiving thrombolytic therapy. What nursing interventions should you employ in order to reduce the likelihood of increased bleeding?

Table 4-5 Systemic Hemostatics		
Generic/Trade Names	**Usual Adult Dose**	**Administration Route**
Aminocaproic acid (Amicar)	1–1.25 q h until bleeding is controlled, max 30 g/24 h	PO/IV
Aprotinin (Trasylol)	500,000 KIU/h	IV
Phytonadione, Vitamin K₁ (AquaMEPHYTON)	2.5–10 mg	PO/SC/IM
Menadiol sodium diphosphate, Vitamin K₄ (Synkayvite)	5–15 mg/d	PO/SC/IM/IV
Tranexamic acid (Cyklokapron)	25 mg/kg 3 to 4 times per day for 2 to 8 days postoperatively	PO
	10 mg/kg 3 to 4 times per day for 2 to 8 days postoperatively	IV

KIU = kallikrein inactivator units

    d. Monitoring of PT levels will provide information relative to dosing and therapeutic management of the client

  4. Contraindications

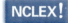

    a. Aminocaproic acid is contraindicated in clients who have disseminated intravascular coagulopathy (DIC), postpartum bleeding, upper urinary tract bleeding, or new burns

    b. Contraindicated in any client with a known hypersensitivity

    c. Vitamin K is contraindicated during the last few weeks of pregnancy and in clients with liver disease

  5. Significant drug interactions

    a. Concurrent use of aminocaproic acid and tranexamic acid with estrogen and oral contraceptives (OCT) can lead to increased coagulation

    b. The use of aminocaproic acid and certain antibiotics can lead to ototoxicity and nephrotoxicity; check individual antibiotic product literature

    c. The use of antibiotic therapy may lead to a decrease in vitamin K synthesis due to destruction of intestinal bacteria, and supplementation may be required

    d. Mineral oil can decrease the absorption of vitamin K

  6. Significant food interactions

    a. Dietary sources of vitamin K are found in green leafy vegetables, milk and meats

    b. Vitamin K is a fat-soluble vitamin and can be synthesized by intestinal flora; deficiency states are usually not identified solely with diet, but are more likely caused by malabsorption problems linked to liver disease or alcohol abuse

      c. The addition of yogurt in the diet helps to provide a medium for bacterial growth that can lead to maintenance of intestinal flora

  7. Significant laboratory studies

      a. PT level must be evaluated as an indicator of response to vitamin K administration

      b. Amicar can cause a decrease in potassium levels when used in clients with decreased renal function

  8. Side effects

      a. GI: nausea, vomiting, diarrhea, and abdominal cramps

      b. Headache, dizziness, and flushing

      c. Localized reaction at the injection site with vitamin K administration

      d. Allergic response with vitamin K products

  9. Adverse effects/toxicity

      a. Most drug effects are mild and are usually dose-related

      b. Overdose with vitamin K can lead to a serious problem if the client is a newborn because of its effect on the coagulation cascade

NCLEX!

  10. Nursing considerations

      a. Monitor client for baseline labs related to renal and liver function

      b. Monitor PT levels and response to therapy for vitamin K administration

      c. Monitor the client's coagulation profile as the administration of antifibrinolytics can cause a **hypercoagulation** or rapid coagulation of blood

      d. Rotate injection sites for the administration of Vitamin K; assess the client for signs of local irritation

      e. Monitor client closely for signs of hypersensitivity and development of allergic reactions

      f. Monitor client closely during the administration of parenteral infusion as there is potential for volume overload and adverse reactions

      g. Use of an infusion pump for IV administration is required

NCLEX!

  11. Client education

      a. Inform client about the dietary sources of vitamin K

      b. Explain to client that periodic PT levels will be drawn to monitor response to therapy

      c. Instruct client to monitor for signs and symptoms of bleeding

      d. Instruct client that use of yogurt and buttermilk products in the diet can help restore normal intestinal flora that will aid in the synthesis of vitamin K; clients who are on antibiotic therapy or who have intestinal problems may benefit from this supportive therapy

      e. Instruct client to report difficulty urinating or reddish-brown urine (caused by myoglobinuria) while taking aminocaproic acid

      f. Instruct client to report chest pain, arm or leg pain, or difficulty breathing

B. Local absorbable hemostatic agents

1. Action and use

   a. Localized hemostatics are utilized to stop or inhibit bleeding at a specific site

   b. The use of topical local hemostatics leads to the absorption of blood in a controlled manner

   c. Thrombin can be used following dental extraction procedures to stop bleeding

2. Common medications

   a. Gelatin products, oxidized cellulose, thrombin, and epinephrine are all examples of topical hemostatic agents

   b. Refer to Box 4-2 for a listing of common local hemostatics

3. Administration considerations

   a. Topical hemostatics are available in pads, powder, sponge, film, and liquid forms

   b. Application involves the adherence of the form to the local bleeding site and then the material is allowed to remain in place to establish hemostasis

   c. Depending on the type of local hemostatic used, removal may be done as early as 24 to 48 hours

   d. Irrigation with normal saline may be necessary to prevent further tissue destruction as the topical is removed

   e. If the product is a sponge or film, it may be completely reabsorbed into the body

4. Contraindications

   a. Contraindicated if client has a previous allergy to animal protein products or gelatin, since they are composed of animal protein

   b. Contraindicated in the presence of infection

Box 4-2

Local Hemostatics

Absorbable gelatin sponge (Gelfoam): a sterile gelatin that absorbs blood when placed in surgical wound and is absorbed within 4 to 6 weeks

Absorbable gelatin film (Gelfilm): a sterile absorbable gelatin film often used in neurosurgery, thoracic surgery, or ocular surgery to absorb blood in tissues, act as dural substitute (neurosurgery) or repair pleural defect (thoracic surgery)

Epinephrine: a medication that reduces bleeding by causing vasoconstriction

Oxidized cellulose (Oxycel): a specially treated form of surgical gauze or cotton that is hemostatic and is absorbable in 2 to 7 days usually; controls bleeding during surgery involving liver, pancreas, spleen, kidney, thyroid, and prostate

Oxidized regenerated cellulose (Surgicel): see oxidized cellulose above

Microfibrillar collagen hemostat (Avitene): an absorbable topical hemostatic substance that attracts platelets and causes platelet aggregation on a bleeding surface

Thrombin (Fibrindex): a sterile powder treated with thromboplastin in the presence of calcium; catalyzes conversion of fibrinogen to fibrin and may cause platelet aggregation; used topically for capillary bleeding or in combination with absorbable gelatins above during surgery

5. Significant drug interactions: none reported

6. Significant food interactions: none reported

7. Significant laboratory studies: none reported

8. Side effects

   a. Hypersensitivity reactions at the site of application

   b. Erythema, pruritus, and localized irritations

9. Adverse effects/toxicity: same as above

10. Nursing considerations

    a. Application of topical hemostatics must be done according to physician protocol and within the guidelines of product information

    b. Assess local site for signs of hypersensitivity and document findings

    c. Remove topical hemostatics as indicated by product guidelines; irrigation of site with normal saline may be required to prevent further tissue destruction; documentation of site should be included in the nursing notes

    d. If client develops an allergic reaction to the product, an antihistamine such as diphenhydramine (Benadryl) may be given; if a potential allergic response is anticipated, the antihistamine may be given prior to product administration as a preventative measure

    e. Switching from one material to another may facilitate a better response

11. Client education

    a. Educate client as to removal of topical hemostatics; it is important not to pull off dry materials as this could cause further skin damage and pain

    b. Inform client that treatment with local hemostatics may occur over a number of days and weeks

    c. Inform client that compliance with the treatment regimen is necessary in order to achieve a good outcome

    d. Instruct client to monitor the site for signs of potential infection

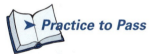

Practice to Pass

A topical hemostatic agent used on the client now has to be removed. What nursing interventions would you employ to perform this action?

C. **Clotting factor replacement therapy**

1. Action and use

   a. Refers to the specific restoration of blood components that are necessary for the body to regain homeostasis so as to maintain hematologic integrity

   b. Congenital deficiencies of specific clotting factors can lead to serious (if not fatal) consequences unless there is adequate replacement therapy

   c. Functional platelet and plasma abnormalities can lead to coagulation problems that include specific syndromes, such as hemophilia and von Willebrand's disease

   d. Used to stop and prevent hemorrhage in clients who have specific identified factor deficiencies

   e. Used to support client with specific factor deficiencies who is undergoing a surgical procedure

2. Common medications or blood products

   a. Cryoprecipitate provides a concentrated form of fibrinogen and is a blood product obtained from fresh frozen plasma (FFP)

   b. Antithrombin III (Atnativ, Thromvate III) works with heparin to provide an anticoagulant effect

   c. Desmopressin acetate (DDAVP) is classified as an antidiuretic hormone, but it has adjunctive effects on increasing factor VIII in the body

   d. Refer to Box 4-3 for a listing of replacement therapy medications

3. Administration considerations

   a. Antihemophilic factor (AHF) medications, such as Hemofil, are administered via parenteral (intravenous) route; dosage is individualized based on client's weight, bleeding status, factor deficiency, presence of factor inhibitor and results of pertinent coagulation lab studies

   b. DDAVP can be administered intranasally; alternate nares when administering the drug and document appropriately on medication record

   c. AHF medications are usually refrigerated

   d. Administration of AHF should be done according to protocol; premedicate with antihistamines if ordered; document vital signs during the first 15 minutes of therapy to determine that they stay within client's baseline

4. Contraindications

   a. Contraindicated in clients with a hypersensitivity to bovine, hamster, or mouse protein

   b. Antithrombin III may cause possible infection and hepatitis in pediatric clients and therefore should be used cautiously

   c. DDAVP is contraindicated in pregnant or lactating clients or clients with known hypersensitivity to the drug

   d. It should be used with caution in pediatric or elderly clients due to its antidiuretic effect and potential to develop hyponatremia

5. Significant drug interactions

   a. Concurrent use of antithrombin III and heparin leads to an increased anticoagulant effect

   b. The effects of DDAVP can be potentiated with the use of chlorpropamide, clofibrate, and carbamazepine

Box 4-3 **Clotting Factor Replacement Therapy**	Antihemophilic factor (Hemofil M, Koate-HP) Cryoprecipitated antihemophilic factor-human Antihemophilic factor-porcine (Hyate: C) Antihemophilic factor-recombinant (Helixate, Kogenate) Antithrombin III (Atnativ, Thrombate III) Desmopressin (DDAVP, Stimate) Factor IX complex, human (Bebulin VH, Konyne-80, Profilnin) Coagulation Factor IX, recombinant (Benefix)

6. Significant food interactions: none reported

7. Significant laboratory studies: sodium levels may need to be monitored with DDAVP therapy because of its effect on this electrolyte

8. Side effects

    a. AHF: hypersensitivity, lethargy, fatigue, nausea, and hypotension

    b. Antithrombin III: none reported

    c. DDAVP: headaches, nausea, nasal congestion, facial flushing, and chills

9. Adverse effects/toxicity

    a. AHF: developing AIDS and hepatitis, as certain AHF products are derived from human plasma

    b. DDAVP overdose: increased symptoms with dyspnea

10. Nursing considerations

    a. Proper reconstitution and administration of the medication is required according to protocol

    b. Monitoring of pertinent baseline hematologic labs is required

    c. Document baseline vital signs during first 15 minutes of therapy and then according to protocol to monitor client's continued response

    d. Observe client closely for signs of hypersensitivity

    e. Infusion may have to be slowed down or discontinued if the client develops increased allergic symptoms

    f. Review client's medication profile for use of concurrent medications that could interfere with clotting

    g. Clients with defined factor deficiencies and their families will need anticipatory support and guidance during a lifetime of therapy

    h. A collaborative health care team approach should be instituted to provide continued care to the client and family

    i. Clients who have hereditary factor antithrombin III deficiency and become pregnant or require surgery are at risk of developing thrombosis; monitor closely during the obstetric and post-surgical time periods

11. Client education

    a. Instruct client regarding medication storage and administration if therapy is to be given at home

    b. Instruct client on disease process and genetic transmission issues; referral to a genetic counselor may be indicated in clients of childbearing age

    c. Refer client to support groups for assistance and strengthening of coping mechanisms

    d. Since client is at risk for bleeding because of factor deficiencies, review concepts of safety as related to lifestyle and job/employment

V. Medications to Treat Anemia

A. Iron salts

1. Action and use

    a. Iron is an essential trace element in the body that participates in oxygen transport, tissue respiration, and enzyme reactions

    b. Iron is stored as ferritin in the body; ferritin levels reflect the visceral stores of iron that are available to the body; transferrin levels reflect how iron is transported in the body

    c. Iron deficiency anemia (IDA) is one of the most common nutritional deficiencies seen in the United States

    d. IDA is classified as a microcytic anemia; iron preparations are indicated for the treatment of this type of anemia

    e. The use of ferrous salts is indicated for the treatment and management of iron deficiency

    f. Iron medications are available through prescription and OTC

2. Common medications

    a. Ferrous iron salts provide the largest amount of elemental iron and are available as oral medications

    b. Ferrous fumarate, ferrous gluconate, and ferrous sulfate are the three oral iron preparations available; all are equally effective but require different doses to provide an equivalent amount of iron

    c. Iron dextran is available as an injection and is given when a client cannot tolerate oral administration or if the oral therapy is ineffective

    d. Refer to Table 4-6 for a listing of common iron preparations

3. Administration considerations

    a. Oral iron is given with meals in order to decrease gastric upset

    b. Z-track administration of iron dextran is required to minimize client discomfort, prevent tissue discoloration, and ensure absorption

    c. There is a potential for anaphylactic reaction to occur following iron dextran administration; therefore, a test dose may be ordered to monitor client response

NCLEX!

Table 4-6 Iron Salts			
	Generic/Trade Names	**Usual Adult Dose**	**Administration Route**
	Ferrous fumarate (Femiron, Fumerin)	200 mg tid or qid	PO
	Ferrous gluconate (Fergon)	325–600 mg/d	PO
	Ferrous sulfate (Feosol)	750–1,500 mg/d	PO
	Iron dextran injection (DexFerrum)	No more than 100 mg within 24 hours	IV/IM

  d. Iron can be found in vitamins and nutritional supplements; monitor client for alternate sources of iron so as to avoid potential overdosing and toxicity

  e. Be aware of potential drug interactions that may limit or increase oral iron medications

  f. Liquid (elixir) iron is administered by straw to avoid discoloration of tooth enamel

 4. Contraindications

  a. Contraindicated in clients with ulcerative colitis, peptic ulcer disease, cirrhosis, and hemolytic anemia

  b. Contraindicated in clients with iron overload syndromes (hemosiderosis and hemochromatosis)

  c. Prior history of reaction could lead to a contraindication for use of iron dextran injection

 5. Significant drug interactions

  a. The use of antacids, antibiotics (quinolones and tetracycline), and thyroid drugs all lead to a decreased absorption of iron; therefore, oral iron medication should not be administered at the same time

  b. Vitamin C can increase the absorption of oral iron medications

 6. Significant food interactions

  a. Iron is composed of both heme (animal) and non-heme (plant) sources in the diet; heme sources have a higher bioavailability and are more beneficial in maintaining iron levels

  b. Clients on a strict vegetarian diet may require supplementation to ensure adequate iron levels

  c. Taking iron with vitamin C can lead to increased absorption

  d. Foods that are high in phytates (grains and cereals) can cause a decreased absorption of dietary iron

  e. Iron should not be taken with milk, as decreased absorption will occur

 7. Significant laboratory studies

  a. Monitor client's reticulocyte count, as this will indicate whether response to treatment has been successful; the reticulocyte count will increase if the bone marrow is responding and RBC production is being increased

  b. If client's hemoglobin and hematocrit levels do not rise following iron therapy, additional testing may be required to determine the exact type of anemia

 8. Side effects

  a. GI: upset stomach, nausea and vomiting, diarrhea, and constipation

  b. Dark and tarry stools

  c. Dermatologic: discoloration of skin and pain upon injection

9. Adverse effects/toxicity

   a. **Pica** (ingestion of nonfood items in the diet) can interfere with iron levels in the body causing individuals to become anemic; pregnant women are the client group most likely to be involved with pica

   b. Iron can accumulate in the body, leading to potentially toxic levels

   c. Symptoms of iron overdose can lead a client to progress to shock, seizures, or coma; serum iron levels evaluated greater than 300 µg/dL is serious and should be treated aggressively

   d. Removal of iron from body during iron overdose is necessary; poison control should be notified if iron overdose is suspected

   e. Chelation therapy should be instituted to remove iron from the body in addition to supportive measures such as airway maintenance, correction of acidosis and administration of IV fluids

NCLEX!

10. Nursing considerations

    a. Monitor client for expected side effects related to iron administration, such as tarry stools

    b. Give oral medication on a full stomach to minimize GI upset

    c. Since anemia is often a symptom of a disease, assess client for the underlying cause; monitor client lab findings to confirm a diagnosis of IDA

    d. If client does not show a clinical response to iron therapy, notify physician

    e. Referral to a dietician may be indicated to support client's food choices in maintaining adequate iron levels

    f. Evaluate client for pica if there is a high index of suspicion

NCLEX!

11. Client education

    a. Teach client the proper administration of oral iron medications

    b. Discuss the importance of adequate food sources in the diet to maintain iron levels; these include foods such as lean meats, liver, egg yolks, dried beans, green vegetables (e.g., spinach)

    c. Inform client about expected changes in the characteristics of stool (black, tarry)

B. Vitamin B_{12} (Cyanocobalamin)

1. Action and use

   a. Vitamin B_{12} is a water-soluble vitamin that is utilized in the body as part of many coenzyme reactions during the process of metabolism of carbohydrate, protein, and fat

   b. Vitamin B_{12} is found primarily in foods of animal origin (liver, meat, shellfish, and dairy food items)

   c. Deficiency of vitamin B_{12} affects neurological, hematological, and GI systems

   d. Vitamin B_{12} is considered to be the extrinsic factor whereas the intrinsic factor is released by the parietal cells in the stomach

e. Clients with GI surgeries that result in partial or complete removal and/or anastomosis of the stomach and end the release of intrinsic factor will require injections of vitamin B_{12} on a lifelong basis

f. **Pernicious anemia** is the classification given to the anemia that is a result of vitamin B_{12} deficiency

g. Vitamin B_{12} deficiency is classified as a megaloblastic macrocytic anemia

h. Atrophic gastritis is associated with vitamin B_{12} deficiency

i. Because B-complex vitamins work together, there is likelihood that there is more than one deficiency existing at the same time

2. Common medications

a. Cyanocobalamin is available as both prescription and OTC

b. Cyanocobalamin is contained in many multivitamin preparations in addition to being sold as a separate vitamin unit

c. Vitamin B_{12} is available in oral and injectable forms

d. Refer to Table 4-7 for a listing of common Vitamin B_{12} preparations

3. Administration considerations

a. Vitamin B_{12} must be administered via the parenteral route in clients who have lost the ability to manufacture intrinsic factor

b. Rotation of sites is indicated with injection of this medication

c. Use the Z-track method to minimize burning and local irritation that is common with this drug

d. Cyanocobalamin injection should be protected from the light, as this will inactivate the medication; it should not be mixed with other medications but given as a separate injection

4. Contraindications: known prior hypersensitivity

5. Significant drug interactions

a. Medications such as anticonvulsants, aminoglycosides, cholestyramine, colchicine, neomycin, and potassium timed-release products will cause decreased absorption of vitamin B_{12}

b. Monitor potassium levels as the use of cyanocobalamin can cause hypokalemia

c. Chloramphenicol antagonizes the hematologic action of this vitamin

Table 4-7			
Vitamin B_{12} Preparations	**Generic/Trade Names**	**Usual Adult Dose**	**Administration Route**
	Vitamin B_{12A} (Hydroxycobalamin, Alphamin)	100–200 mcg/month	IM
	Vitamin B_{12} (Cyanocobalamin, Cobex, Rubramin PC)	100–200 mcg/month	IM/deep SC

6. Significant food interactions

   a. Clients with malabsorption problems may be prone to develop vitamin B_{12} deficiency

   b. Clients with alcoholism are more likely to have malabsorption problems and therefore are likely to have many vitamin deficiencies

   c. A strict vegetarian diet without adequate supplementation may increase a client's risk for developing this vitamin deficiency

7. Significant laboratory studies

   a. Monitor pertinent hematologic labs to confirm diagnosis of pernicious anemia

   b. Monitor client for potential hypokalemia

8. Side effects

   a. Flushing

   b. GI: diarrhea with resultant hypokalemia

   c. Dermatologic: itching and pain at the injection site

9. Adverse effects/toxicity

   a. Vitamin B_{12} is a water-soluble vitamin and as such should not cause toxic levels to be reached in the body

   b. Some clients can have more serious cardiac effects such as development of CHF and pulmonary edema

10. Nursing considerations

   a. Review client's medications, both prescription and OTC, for potential drug interactions

   b. Rotate the injection site and document appropriately on the medication record

   c. Establish baseline pertinent labs and monitor as needed to document response to treatment

   d. Assess client's pulses and vascular status to determine baseline

   e. Clients with pernicious anemia cannot take oral vitamin therapy alone to correct the problem; medication must be administered via the parenteral route

   f. If client's lab values do not indicate a positive response to treatment, notify the physician and further investigate to determine the underlying cause

   g. Refer to dietician for supportive diet management; foods high in vitamin B_{12} (for those who can absorb it) include liver, kidney, fish and milk

11. Client education

   a. Teach clients regarding the lifelong nature of the therapy if they have been diagnosed with pernicious anemia

   b. Discuss food sources of vitamin B_{12} for inclusion in the diet (see previous section)

   c. Discuss the effects of alcohol on the absorption of vitamin B_{12}

      d. Teach client to monitor for signs and symptoms of B_{12} deficiency (numbness and tingling in lower extremities, weakness, fatigue, anorexia, loss of taste, diarrhea, memory loss, and mood changes)

      e. Instruct client that if diarrhea is significant, a change in drug dosage may be required

C. Folic Acid

    1. Action and use

      a. Folic acid (vitamin B_9) is a water-soluble vitamin needed for DNA synthesis and cellular division

      b. Folic acid may be used either to treat deficiency states, or as prophylaxis against a deficiency state, such as in pregnancy

      c. Deficiency states of folic acid have been associated with neural tube defects in the developing fetus and with hematologic manifestations such as megaloblastic macrocytic anemia

      d. Folic acid helps to break down homocysteine (an amino acid) in the body; if there is a folic acid deficiency state, then levels of homocysteine can build up in the body; high homocysteine levels are associated with heart disease

      e. Dietary sources of folic acid are found in fresh green vegetables, yellow fruits and vegetables, liver, yeast and meats

      f. Folic acid supplements in addition to dietary sources are used to treat deficiency states; supplementation is recommended during pregnancy and lactation

    2. Common medications

      a. Folic acid (Folvite) can be obtained as an OTC medication; the therapeutic dose is ≤ 1 mg per day orally and the maintenance dose is ≤ 0.4 mg per day orally

      b. Nutritional supplements and/or multivitamin preparations can contain folic acid

      c. Leucovorin calcium (Wellcovorin) may be given IM or IV at a usual adult dose of not more than 1 mg per day; this form of folic acid is reserved for use as an adjunct to cancer chemotherapy, not folic acid deficiency

    3. Administration considerations

      a. Route of administration can be oral, SC, IM or IV depending on formulation; folic acid can be given IVP or added to an infusion; IV rate should not exceed 5 mcg/minute

      b. Folic acid (0.4 mg) is recommended on a daily basis for all pregnant women in the United States to prevent folate deficiency; it is suggested that therapy should be started 1 month prior to conception and continued throughout the first trimester

      c. Regardless of client's age, the daily dose should not be less than 0.1 mg/day

      d. Folic acid should not be mixed with any other medication and should be given as a separate injection

NCLEX!

e. Clients may experience a rash or hypersensitivity at the site of the injection; rotate injection sites

4. Contraindications

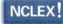

a. Contraindicated for the treatment of other anemias that are not caused by folic acid deficiency

b. Folic acid injections may contain benzyl alcohol and therefore should not be given to neonates; the use of this preservative is contraindicated in neonates

5. Significant drug interactions

a. ASA, phenytoin, and sulfonamides cause decreased folic acid levels

b. There is increased likelihood of seizure activity when used concurrently with phenytoin

c. Oral contraceptives can increase the risk of folic acid deficiency

d. Steroid use increases the need for folic acid in the body

e. Methotrexate, pyrimethamine, triamterene, and trimethoprim act as folic acid antagonists

f. Alcohol use can lead to folic acid deficiency because it increases folic acid requirements

6. Significant food interactions

a. Dietary sources of folic acid should be identified for the client

b. Prolonged cooking of vegetables may destroy the folic acid present

c. Heating can destroy the vitamin, leading to decreased bioavailability

7. Significant laboratory studies

a. If the client has neurological deficits, the use of folic acid will not correct the problem; attention must be directed to other B vitamins, and appropriate therapy must be instituted to correct neurological compromise

b. Continued use of folic acid may interfere with findings associated with vitamin B_{12} deficiency states

8. Side effects

a. Yellow discoloration of urine

b. Nausea

c. Altered sleep and depression

d. Rash

e. Bronchospasm

9. Adverse effects/toxicity

a. No toxic effects are reported with oral folic acid

b. Toxicity can occur if the client is on anticonvulsant therapy concurrently with vitamin B_{12} due to competition for binding sites

c. Hemolytic anemia can occur as a result of increased utilization

10. Nursing considerations

   a. Clients who are pregnant should be taking 0.4 mg of folic acid on a daily basis as neural tube defect prophylaxis

   b. Review client medications for potential drug interactions

   c. Assess and monitor pertinent hematologic labs related to folic acid

   d. Referral to dietician for dietary support and maintenance of folic acid levels

   e. Counsel client as to the effect that alcohol can have on folic acid levels

   f. Monitor client for potential allergic reactions to the medication

   g. Improvement in blood picture and reversal of symptoms of folic acid deficiency (diarrhea, constipation, restless legs, fatigue, diffuse muscular pain, forgetfulness, mental depression) are the therapeutic effects of folic acid therapy

11. Client education

   a. Teach the pregnant client the importance of neural tube prophylaxis

   b. Make client aware of the potential for increased drug interactions with this vitamin

   c. Instruct client that repeated lab tests are necessary in order to monitor response to therapy

   d. Advise client to remain under close medical supervision while taking folic acid

   e. Teach client about food sources high in folic acid, such as green leafy vegetables, yellow fruits and vegetables, yeast, and meats

D. Epoetin Alfa (Epogen, Procrit)

1. Action and use

   a. Epoetin is a recombinant form of erythropoietin that stimulates RBC production; it is chemically identical to erythropoietin that is produced in the kidney and serves the same function, to promote RBC growth

   b. Used to treat clients with anemia with various causes such as renal failure, HIV infection, and nonmyeloid malignancies with associated chemotherapy-induced anemia

   c. Used as a treatment measure to reduce the need for blood transfusions because of its growth potential effect in clients who are undergoing surgery

   d. Ferritin and transferrin saturation levels must be adequate in order to support the activity of RBC formation

2. Common medication dosage of Epogen varies with the client's situation; the dosage is calculated in units/kg; dose may range from 3 to 500 units/kg/dose 3 times/wk and is given SC/IV

3. Administration considerations

   a. Medication is refrigerated; let warm to room temperature before administering to client

   b. Do not use medication that is discolored or contains particulate matter

    c. Do not administer with any other solutions; medication can be administered SC or IV; there is no preservative in the vial, and therefore any unused portion must be discarded

    d. Do not shake the medication as this will lead to inactivation

    e. Administration of Epogen must adhere to physician protocol to avoid overdose

    f. Dosages are individualized depending on clinical condition and whether or not dialysis has been instituted

    g. The hematocrit will serve as the measure of client response; the physician will identify target levels (usually 30 to 36%) and therapy will be titrated to achieve the target level goal; if the hematocrit level rises too quickly or passes the target goal, the client may be at risk for developing hypertension and seizures; if the hematocrit level does not rise in response to therapy, the dose will be increased depending on adequacy of iron stores; initial effects are usually seen in 1 to 2 weeks, while achievement of target goal usually takes 2 to 3 months

    h. Epogen is usually given up to three times a week

4. Contraindications

    a. Contraindicated in clients with uncontrolled hypertension or with known hypersensitivity to human albumin

    b. Contraindicated in clients with complicated anemia from multiple etiologies

    c. Epogen should not be used in pregnant clients unless the benefits outweigh the potential risks

5. Significant drug interactions

    a. The use of myelosuppressive agents can interfere with the ability of Epogen to work because they have an antagonistic effect; Epogen is usually given following chemotherapy to avoid this effect

    b. The use of Epogen is limited in that it cannot correct the underlying problem associated with the specific type of anemia; continued use of Epogen leads to potential long-term ineffectiveness as the body tries to compensate

6. Significant food interactions: the use of iron supplementation is recommended with this medication and can be in the form of dietary sources as well as oral medications

7. Significant laboratory studies

    a. The use of Epogen is expected to have an effect on the RBC lineage and raise the serum level, as well as the hematocrit and hemoglobin concentrations

    b. Adjustment of dosage is related to pertinent lab values such as hematocrit, and adequate iron stores; dose is usually adjusted when the hematocrit is between 30 and 36%

8. Side effects

    a. Hypertension and edema

    b. Diarrhea, constipation, nausea, and vomiting

    c. Fever, joint pain, and pain at the injection site

    d. Thrombocytosis, iron deficiency, sweating, and arthralgias

9. Adverse effects/toxicity

    a. Overcorrecting with Epogen can result in toxic levels leading to the development of polycythemia

NCLEX!

    b. Clients can develop hypertension and seizures with toxic levels or a too rapid therapeutic response

NCLEX!

10. Nursing considerations

    a. Closely monitor client's baseline hematologic labs to provide information relative to treatment response

    b. Monitor BP prior to initiation of therapy and monitor closely during therapy

    c. Rotate injection sites to minimize discomfort

    d. Monitor client for the risk of thrombotic events, such as MI, CVA, and transient ischemic accident (TIA), especially for clients with chronic renal failure (CRF)

    e. Follow administration protocols and monitor ongoing pertinent labs

    f. Clients who are on dialysis may require adjusted dosages caused by stress of the hemodynamic process

    g. Monitor client's iron stores (ferritin) and transferrin levels; use of additional supplementation and or medication may be required to support the effects of Epogen in RBC maturation

    h. Refer to dietician for nutritional support

    i. Monitor client's baseline vital signs and continue to monitor BP following drug administration

NCLEX!

11. Client education

    a. Teach client regarding the need for continued lab follow-up and possible adjustment of dosage

    b. Review the list of possible side effects with the client

    c. Premedicate if necessary with analgesics if bone pain is present or client becomes febrile

    d. Medication can be given in the home setting; client can be taught to self-administer Epogen

    e. Stress importance of keeping follow-up appointments

    f. Instruct client not to drive or be involved in other hazardous activity during the first 90 days of therapy because of possible seizure activity

    g. Reinforce the importance of compliance with dietary and drug therapy

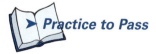

Practice to Pass

A client asks if medication alone can restore adequate blood cell levels to correct anemia. What would be your best response to this client?

VI. Medications to Lower Blood Cholesterol

A. HMG-CoA reductase inhibitors

1. Action and use

   a. They belong to the class of "statins" that work in the liver to affect cholesterol synthesis

   b. They act by competitively inhibiting this rate-limiting enzyme in the liver that leads to a decrease in cholesterol concentration

   c. Use is aimed at lowering LDL cholesterol levels in clients with significant cholesterol elevations and in whom diet therapy has not been effective

   d. Statins also have an effect on HDL cholesterol that is somewhat dose-dependent; lipoprotein levels are not affected by the use of statins

2. Common medications

   a. Lovastatin (Mevacor), simvastatin (Zocor), and pravastatin (Pravachol) are similar in nature and are isolated from fungal cultures

   b. Fluvastatin (Lescol), atorvastatin (Lipitor), and cerivastatin (Baycol) are produced synthetically

   c. Refer to Table 4-8 for a listing and dosage recommendations for common medications

3. Administration considerations

   a. Administration is usually done at night

   b. This dosing schedule increases the effectiveness of the drug, as cholesterol synthesis normally occurs during the evening hours

4. Contraindications

   a. Contraindicated in clients with active liver disease and abnormal serum transaminase levels

   b. Contraindicated in pregnant and nursing mothers

5. Significant drug interactions

   a. Increased risk of myositis when used concurrently with immunosuppressives, antifungal agents, fibric acid derivatives, nicotinic acid and erythromycin

Table 4-8 HMG-CoA Reductase Inhibitors		
Generic/Trade Names	**Usual Adult Dose**	**Administration Route**
Atorvastatin (Lipitor)	10–80 mg QD	PO
Cerivastatin (Baycol)	0.3 mg QD	PO
Fluvastatin (Lescol)	20 mg hs	PO
Lovastatin (Mevacor)	20–40 mg 1–2 times/day	PO
Pravastatin (Pravachol)	10–40 mg QD	PO
Simvastatin (Zocor)	5–40 mg QD	PO

      b. Additive effects are seen when used with cholestyramine (Questran)

      c. Spironolactone and cimetidine can cause decreased levels of HMG-CoA reductase inhibitors

6. Significant food interactions: none reported

7. Significant laboratory studies

      a. Elevation of liver function tests can be seen; baseline measurement is required before starting therapy

      b. Continued monitoring of liver function tests at predetermined intervals (12 weeks and with dose adjustment) is necessary in order to confirm response to treatment and prevent possible adverse/toxic reactions

      c. Monitoring of creatinine phosphokinase (CPK) levels can be done to evaluate the client's potential to develop myositis

      d. Digoxin level should be monitored if taking concurrently

8. Side effects

      a. GI upset, dyspepsia, flatulence

      b. Pain and myalgias

      c. Headache, rash, dizziness

      d. Sinusitis

9. Adverse effects/toxicity: altered liver function tests (elevated serum transaminase levels)

NCLEX!

10. Nursing considerations

      a. Drug selection is dependent on physician preference and client tolerance

      b. They are not recommended for use in clients who are younger than 20 years of age

      c. The client should be instructed to take the medication at the evening meal to coincide with the body's timing of cholesterol production

      d. Measurement of client's baseline liver function is required before initiating therapy; continued monitoring is required at specific intervals

      e. Monitor lipid levels within 2 to 4 weeks after initiation of therapy

      f. May be given without regard to food

NCLEX!

11. Client education

      a. Educate client about proper self-administration in order to promote biochemical activity

      b. Educate client about required lab monitoring to maintain compliance and assess client response

      c. Instruct client to report immediately to the prescriber any unexplained muscle pain, tenderness, yellowing of skin or eyes, or loss of appetite

      d. Advise client that alcohol intake should be minimized or avoided

B. Bile acid sequestrants

1. Action and use

    a. Bile acids are a group of nonabsorbable amine compounds that work in the GI tract to bind with bile acids

    b. The binding of bile acids leads liver cells to respond by sending cholesterol to maintain bile acid synthesis, thereby causing plasma levels of LDL cholesterol to decrease

    c. Indications for use include elevated cholesterol levels with or without high triglyceride levels

    d. Bile acids are also used as an adjunctive therapy to dietary management of cholesterol elevations

2. Common medications

    a. Cholestyramine (Questran) and colestipol (Colestid) are similar in their ability to lower LDL levels

    b. Colestipol is available as a tablet or powder, 15 to 30 grams/day in 2 to 4 doses before meals and at bedtime

    c. Cholestyramine is available as a powder, 4 g bid to qid before meal times and at bed time; a client may need up to 24 grams/day

3. Administration considerations

    a. Colestipol tablets should not be crushed, chewed or cut; they should be taken with adequate fluids

    b. Powdered forms of the drugs should be mixed at the bedside to prevent overthickening and esophageol obstruction; they may be plain or have orange flavoring; cholestyramine powder contains phenylalanine and therefore should not be used in clients who have phenylketonuria (PKU)

    c. Bile acids should be administered alone due to potential for increased binding effects with other concurrent medications; give other drugs 1 to 2 hours before or 4 to 6 hours after bile acid administration

    d. The contents of one packet should be mixed with at least 120 to 180 mL of water or other preferred liquid

    e. The contents of medications should be dissolved before administration as it is irritating to mucous membranes

4. Contraindications

    a. Colestipol is not recommended for use in pediatric clients

    b. Contraindicated in clients with complete biliary obstruction

5. Significant drug interactions

    a. Bile acids can bind to many other medications such as thyroxine, digoxin, diuretics, antibiotics and warfarin; because of this, the medication should not be given concurrently with other medications

    b. Additive effects are seen with the use of bile acids and HMG-CoA reductase inhibitors and nicotinic acid

6. Significant food interactions: powdered forms must be mixed in the appropriate food or fluid to maximize absorption and prevent obstruction

7. Significant laboratory studies

  a. Monitor baseline labs relative to cholesterol and triglyceride levels before starting therapy; continue to trend results to determine client response

  b. Decreased levels of LDL cholesterol should be seen within 1 month of therapy

8. Side effects

  a. Abdominal pain, bloating, reflux, constipation, steatorrhea, and hemorrhoids

  b. Associated vitamin deficiencies (A, D, K)

  c. Rash irritations of skin, tongue, and perianal areas

9. Adverse effects/toxicity

  a. Hypoprothrombinemia

  b. Decreased erythrocyte folate levels

10. Nursing considerations

  a. Proper mixing and administration of medication should be done according to schedule to maximize biochemical activity (see also previous comments on mixing)

  b. Assess and monitor client for side effects of medication

  c. Bile acids are not usually used as a first line therapy in the treatment of elevated cholesterol levels because of poor client tolerance

  d. Vitamin deficiencies may require supplementation, if not discontinuation of bile acids, to restore normal levels

  e. Problems related to hemorrhoids and/or constipation may require intervention to provide client comfort

  f. If the client develops GI complaints, a lower dosage may be necessary in order to maintain client compliance with this drug regimen

  g. Serum cholesterol levels are reduced within 24 to 48 hours after initiation of therapy

  h. Long-term use of cholestyramine can increase bleeding tendency

11. Client education

  a. Teach client proper administration and scheduling of medication to maximize effect

  b. Teach client to be alert for signs and symptoms indicating side effects of these agents

  c. Follow-up blood work will be done to evaluate drug effect on cholesterol levels

  d. Advise client to increase high-bulk diet with adequate fluid intake

  e. Advise client not to omit doses

  f. Instruct client to report constipation immediately

C. Fibric acid derivatives

1. Action and use

   a. They are a group of compounds that affect lipoproteins

   b. They act on very-low lipid-density lipoproteins (VLDL) and chlyomicrons resulting in a reduction of triglyceride levels

   c. HDL cholesterol levels are increased but this is not the primary effect; there is also a variable effect on LDL levels

   d. Fibric acid derivatives are indicated for use in clients with elevated triglyceride levels and whose elevated cholesterol levels have been resistant to dietary management

2. Common medications

   a. Fibric acid derivatives have been shown to decrease triglyceride levels, increase HDL levels, and lower LDL levels

   b. Gemfibrozil (Lopid) is also indicated when there is an increased risk for a client to develop pancreatitis

   c. Refer to Table 4-9 for a listing of fibric acid derivatives

3. Administration considerations

   a. Medication is usually given in divided doses

   b. Medication is usually given 30 minutes prior to morning and evening meals

4. Contraindications

   a. Contraindicated in clients with gallbladder disease, renal problems, liver or biliary cirrhosis

   b. They are not recommended for pregnant or nursing women

5. Significant drug interactions

   a. Drug interactions can be seen with the use of anticoagulants; monitor PT levels

   b. Do not use fibric acid derivatives with statins (HMG-CoA reductase inhibitors) as rhabdomyolysis can occur

   c. Clofibrate increases the hypoglycemic effect of sulfonylureas and should not be used in type 2 diabetes

6. Significant food interactions: fibric acids can cause altered taste perception

Table 4-9		
Fibric Acid Derivatives		
Generic/Trade Names	**Usual Adult Dose**	**Administration Route**
Clofibrate (Abitrate, Atromid-S)	2 g/day in 2–4 divided doses	PO
Fenofibrate (Tricor)	67 mg QD, max 201 mg/day	PO
Gemfibrozil (Lopid)	600 mg BID, max 1,500 mg/day	PO

7. Significant laboratory studies

   a. Baseline lipid levels should be obtained prior to starting therapy; monitor ongoing labs as needed to document response to treatment and evaluate client symptom response

   b. If liver function tests are persistently abnormal after three months, then therapy should be discontinued

   c. Hypokalemia may be seen in response to therapy

   d. Decreased hemoglobin, hematocrit, and white blood cell (WBC) count may be seen with the use of gemfibrozil

8. Side effects

   a. Abdominal or epigastric pain

   b. Jaundice, blurred vision, headache, and depression

   c. Rash, dermatitis, pruritus with gemfibrozil

   d. Back pain, muscle cramps, myalgia, and swollen joints

9. Adverse effects/toxicity

   a. Client may develop gallbladder disease and acute appendicitis

   b. Eosinophilia

   c. Hypokalemia

NCLEX!

10. Nursing considerations

    a. Monitor baseline labs and perform ongoing assessments according to protocol

    b. If there is no response to therapy after 3 months, notify the physician because the medication should be discontinued

    c. Monitor client for potential side effects and adverse effects

    d. Monitor closely for right upper quadrant (RUQ) abdominal pain or vomiting

NCLEX!

11. Client education

    a. Teach client that lab work will be ongoing in nature to determine client response and evaluate for potential side effects

    b. Advise client to report immediately unexplained bleeding

    c. Instruct client to restrict carbohydrate and alcohol intake

    d. Advise client to notify physician immediately if any serious side effects such as acute appendicitis or gallbladder disease should occur

D. **Nicotinic acid (niacin, vitamin B$_3$)**

1. Action and use

   a. It is the active form of vitamin B$_3$ (niacin) in the body and is water-soluble

   b. It works to lower most lipoprotein levels (total cholesterol, LDL, triglyceride and lipoproteins) and to increase HDL levels

   c. Indications for use are high cholesterol levels and as adjunctive therapy for clients where diet management is ineffective; dosage is usually started at 1 g TID in adults

  d. It causes peripheral vasodilation and can be used to treat clients with peripheral vascular disease; dosage is usually 10 to 20 mg/day in adults PO; 25 to 100 mg, 2 to 5 times per day IV/SC/IM

  e. Pellagra (dermatitis, diarrhea and dementia) is the clinical deficiency state associated with niacin deficiency; the required dosage of niacin to treat pellagra is 300 to 500 mg/d orally in divided doses

 2. Common medications

  a. Vitamin B_3 is available both as a prescription and OTC medication

  b. The dosage for lowering cholesterol is higher (greater than 3 g/day) than the normal vitamin dose (500 mg/day in adults)

  c. Nicotinic acid is available in an immediate release form as well as a sustained-release preparation

 3. Administration considerations

  a. Tablets should be taken whole; do not crush or divide the pill

  b. Medication can be taken with meals to prevent GI upset

  c. Flushing is a common side effect of niacin caused by its vasodilator properties

  d. Oral nicotinic acid should be taken with cold water

 4. Contraindications

  a. Contraindicated in clients with liver disease and/or unexplained levels of elevated serum transaminases and with active peptic ulcer disease

  b. Contraindicated in clients with severe hypotension

 5. Significant drug interactions

  a. Nicotinic acid should not be taken concurrently with statins, as there can be an increase in the occurrence of rhabdomyolysis

  b. Nicotinic acid may potentiate the action of other medications, such as antihypertensive and vasoactive drugs

  c. Nicotinic acid should be used cautiously with clients who are on anticoagulant therapy

  d. Diabetic clients may need adjustment of their antidiabetic agents when taking nicotinic acid

  e. Niacin can decrease the uricosuric effect of probenecid and sulfinpyrazone leading to increased uric acid levels

  f. Niacin is often used in conjunction with bile resins to enhance effects

 6. Significant food interactions

  a. Since the medication is available in OTC preparations, there is an increased likelihood of higher dosing

  b. 60 mg of dietary tryptophan (amino acid) is necessary to convert to 1 mg of niacin in the body

  c. Corn in the diet interferes with the conversion of tryptophan to niacin in the body

7. Significant laboratory studies: nicotinic acid leads to increases in blood glucose, uric acid, and serum transaminase levels

8. Side effects

   a. Flushing

   b. Postural hypotension, vasovagal attacks

   c. Pruritus, increased sebaceous gland activity

   d. Dyspepsia, epigastric pain, and nausea

9. Adverse effects/toxicity

   a. Clients who report GI symptoms should be monitored closely for possibility of adverse reactions

   b. Shortness of breath or edema

   c. Megadose therapy has been associated with liver damage, hyperglycemia, hyperuricemia, and cardiac dysrhythmias

10. Nursing considerations

    a. Administer medication as ordered to maximize absorption and minimize potential side effects

    b. Dosing of nicotinic acid is variable depending on whether the medication is being prescribed to reduce cholesterol levels or merely as a vitamin supplement; be aware of specific dosing levels

    c. Expect the side effect of flushing when administering the medication

    d. Evaluate client for food sources that are high in niacin (dairy, meats, tuna, and egg) and assess dietary intake

11. Client education

    a. Review list of medications with the client and determine if there are any possible drug interactions

    b. Instruct client to change position slowly to avoid sudden BP drop

    c. Caution client to avoid direct exposure to sunlight

    d. Instruct client that flushing in face, neck and ears may occur within 2 hours after oral ingestion and immediately after IV administration and may last several hours

    e. Teach client that follow up lab work will be ongoing to determine response to therapy

    f. Inform client that alcohol and niacin cause increased flushing

    g. Instruct client not to self-medicate with additional sources of niacin as this can lead to overdose

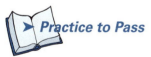

Practice to Pass

Why should cholesterol-lowering medications be taken at bedtime?

E. Estrogens

1. Refer also to Chapter 13

2. The use of estrogen has been found to be an adjunctive therapy in the treatment of elevated cholesterol levels

3. Estrogen has a prior documented cardioprotective effect when found in the body in premenopausal women

4. The continued use of estrogen in the perimenopausal and postmenopausal female is also found to be cardioprotective; it lowers LDL levels and raises HDL levels

Case Study

C. W., 48-year-old-male client, is being admitted for deep vein thrombosis (DVT) of the left lower extremity and is to be placed on a weight-based heparin protocol. You are the nurse that has been assigned to take care of this client.

❶ Why is the weight-based heparin protocol being utilized for this client?

❷ What pertinent lab values and diagnostic tests would help to establish therapeutic care of this client?

❸ C. W. does not understand why blood tests are done so frequently, and he is becoming quite anxious. What measures can you employ to decrease C. W.'s anxiety?

❹ Coumadin is now being added to the treatment regimen and within a few days, C.W. is being discharged. C. W. is concerned about "all the possible risks" associated with Coumadin. What collaborative measures could you include in developing a plan of care with regard to Coumadin therapy?

For suggested responses, see page 638.

Posttest

1 A client is taking lovastatin (Mevacor) for treatment of high cholesterol levels. In conducting medication teaching, the nurse explains that this medication works because of which of the following properties?

(1) Being a bile-acid resin
(2) Being a hormone
(3) Consisting of a fibric acid derivative
(4) Inhibiting cholesterol synthesis

2 A client diagnosed with pernicious anemia is told that vitamin B$_{12}$ injections are required. The client doesn't like "shots" and wants to know why the medication can't be taken orally. How would the nurse respond?

(1) Initially the medication must be given by injection, but it then can be switched over to the oral route once serum levels are maintained.
(2) The medication is only available as an injection, but the length of therapy is only a few months in duration.
(3) The medication cannot be given orally because this type of anemia causes a lack of intrinsic factor that is necessary for the absorption of vitamin B$_{12}$.
(4) The medication can be given once a month by injection and therefore shouldn't be too uncomfortable.

3 A client is receiving intravenous (IV) thrombolytic therapy and complains of pain and redness at the insertion site. Which nursing action is most appropriate?

(1) Continue to monitor the IV site q 15 minutes and check for infiltration or phlebitis.
(2) Restart infusion in the opposite extremity. Further dilute medication per protocol to prevent thrombophlebitis.
(3) Decrease the rate of infusion, monitor IV site q 15 minutes and continue to assess client for complaints of pain.
(4) Reposition client's extremity and continue to monitor IV site.

4 The nurse would monitor the results of which of the following laboratory tests to determine whether a client is responding to ferrous sulfate therapy?

(1) Reticulocyte count
(2) International normalized ratio (INR)
(3) Prothrombin time (PT)
(4) Activated partial thromboplastin time (APTT)

5 A client is taking folic acid (Folvite) for treatment of folic acid anemia. Which one of the following would the nurse recognize as causing a potential drug interaction for this type of therapy?

(1) Vitamin E
(2) Tetracycline
(3) Allopurinol
(4) Oral contraceptives

6 A client being treated with heparin therapy is deemed to have an overdose. The nurse takes which of the following priority actions?

(1) Administer 50 mg of protamine sulfate over a 10-minute period.
(2) Monitor the client's APTT levels prior to and following administration of protamine.
(3) Determine the amount of heparin that was given and the time frame that has elapsed since its administration.
(4) Administer protamine sulfate concurrently with vitamin K to increase its therapeutic effect.

7 A surgical client has suddenly begun to bleed excessively while in the operating room. The nurse anticipates that an order will be given for which of the following medications?

(1) Alteplase (Activase)
(2) Aminocaproic acid (Amicar)
(3) Dipyridamole (Persantine)
(4) Heparin (Liquaemin)

8 A client who has been diagnosed with anemia reports that symptoms have not improved since treatment with folic acid was started. What additional assessments would the nurse want to make to determine the effectiveness of drug therapy?

(1) Obtain current APTT and compare with client's previous APTT to see if the treatment is effective.
(2) Review dietary sources of folic acid with the client to verify if the treatment is effective.
(3) Verify that the client is not taking alcohol to see if the treatment is effective.
(4) Refer the client to the physician for possible deficiencies of other B vitamins, as folic acid and B_{12} deficiencies often occur together.

9 A client taking long-term warfarin (Coumadin) therapy following cardiac valve replacement surgery comes in to the office for a follow-up visit. Upon conducting a diet survey, which one of the following client's dietary patterns would be of concern to the nurse?

(1) The client is drinking a glass of milk at bedtime once a week.
(2) The client is eating yellow wax beans as a vegetable twice a week.
(3) The client has a salad for lunch on weekdays.
(4) The client has a drink of wine once a week with an evening meal.

10 A client is receiving heparin therapy and the activated partial thromboplastin time (APTT) is being monitored. What level does the nurse look for as a therapeutic level?

(1) APTT level of 3 times the control value
(2) APTT level consistent with the control value
(3) APTT level of 3.5 times the control value
(4) APTT level of 1.5 to 2.5 times the control value

See pages 187–188 for Answers and Rationales.

Answers and Rationales

Pretest

1 Answer: 4 *Rationale:* Vitamin C helps to enhance the absorption of iron in the diet and is an easy step in diet management towards improving iron levels in the body. A strict vegetarian diet focuses on non-heme sources of iron that are not as readily absorbable as heme sources (option 1). Eating ice cubes is an example of pica, which is ingestion of a non-food substance (option 2). Nonfood items will not

help to maintain or prevent iron deficiency and in certain cases can actually lead to deficiency states. Tea contains tannic acid and cereals contain phytates and fibers, all of which lead to decreased iron absorption in the diet (option 3).
Cognitive Level: Application
Nursing Process: Planning; *Test Plan:* HPM

2 **Answer: 4** *Rationale:* Inspection of the client's skin is necessary to verify if there are additional areas of bruising or discoloration of which the client may not be aware. It is important to review current findings and compare them with baseline findings as this might provide data to support a potential response to drug therapy. Asking the client if the bruising is related to a particular incident is important (option 1); however, it does not rule out the possibility that drug therapy has made the individual more susceptible to bruising or bleeding tendencies. If the client has not taken the medication as ordered, it would be unlikely that the bruise would be a consequence of drug therapy (option 2). It is important for the client to continue to self-monitor during drug therapy, but that choice by itself does not answer the question (option 3).
Cognitive Level: Application
Nursing Process: Assessment; *Test Plan:* PHYS

3 **Answer: 1** *Rationale:* Ferritin levels reflect the visceral stores of iron in the body. Transferrin levels reflect how iron is transported in the body (option 2). Hemoglobin and hematocrit refer to concentration and proportion measures of red blood cells (RBCs). While they provide information relative to blood count, they are not specific to body iron store values (option 3). A CBC will provide information relative to blood concentration of all three cell lines (red, white and platelets) but again, it is not specific to body iron store values (option 4).
Cognitive Level: Analysis
Nursing Process: Assessment; *Test Plan:* PHYS

4 **Answer: 2** *Rationale:* Activase is used in the emergency setting post stroke and myocardial infarction (MI) in order to dissolve clots and increase perfusion. A client receiving this medication is at risk to develop significant cardiac dysrhythmias and therefore should be placed on a cardiac monitor during treatment. While vital signs (including blood pressure and temperature) are important, they are not the priority intervention (options 1 and 4). The monitoring of urinary output is not a priority unless there are underlying conditions regarding volume management (option 3).
Cognitive Level: Analysis
Nursing Process: Implementation; *Test Plan:* PHYS

5 **Answer: 3** *Rationale:* The target range for hematocrit with epoetin alfa therapy is 30 to 36%. A client who is taking Epogen must be monitored closely so as to prevent adverse side effects that can occur because of either a rapid increase or high-level hematocrit. Rapid or increased hematocrit levels can cause the client to develop seizures and hypertension (option 2). Bone pain and fever are seen in response to administration and are not indicators of effective drug management (options 1 and 4).
Cognitive Level: Analysis
Nursing Process: Evaluation; *Test Plan:* PHYS

6 **Answer: 2** *Rationale:* Facial flushing is an expected side effect of niacin caused by its vasodilator properties. While dosages are often adjusted, it is usually for the purpose of managing side effects related to gastrointestinal complaints and not based on lab values (option 1). Additional dietary sources of niacin are not required to enhance the effect of niacin supplements (option 3). Clients should not take niacin and lovastatin concurrently as this can lead to the development of myopathy (option 4).
Cognitive Level: Application
Nursing Process: Implementation; *Test Plan:* PHYS

7 **Answer: 1** *Rationale:* DDAVP and cryoprecipitate are considered effective treatments for clients with von Willebrand's disease because they contain specific clotting factors (vW and VIII). They are considered a form of replacement therapy but do not stimulate production of blood factors. (option 4). While DDAVP is an antidiuretic, it also has other pharmacological actions in the body; specifically, it stimulates the body to release vW factor (option 2). These medications do not have to be given concurrently in order to potentiate their effects (option 3). Clients can receive them independently based on physician preference.
Cognitive Level: Application
Nursing Process: Implementation; *Test Plan:* PHYS

8 **Answer: 4** *Rationale:* Hemostasis is the ability of the body to prevent bleeding and hemorrhage using platelets in the coagulation process. Thrombocytopenia (a reduced level of platelets in the body) can profoundly affect the body's ability to react to a vascular insult. Neutropenia (a reduced neutrophil count affecting WBCs) can profoundly affect the body's ability to react to an immune response (option 3). Low ferritin levels and elevated triglyceride levels do not directly affect a body's ability to maintain hemostasis (options 1 and 2).
Cognitive Level: Analysis
Nursing Process: Assessment; *Test Plan:* PHYS

9 Answer: 2 *Rationale:* Clients who have valve replacement surgery require life-long anticoagulation therapy. Therefore, they must be instructed as to the possible risks for bleeding and modify their environment and activities of daily living accordingly. Follow-up lab testing is required but is not usually limited to a weekly basis (option 1). Coumadin therapy is usually taken as an evening dose (option 3). Clients are instructed not to double up doses and to take the medication as specifically ordered to assure safe and therapeutic effects (option 4).
Cognitive Level: Application
Nursing Process: Implementation; *Test Plan:* SECE

10 Answer: 3 *Rationale:* Heparin administration requires the use of an infusion pump in order to maintain an accurate level of medication. While vitamin K is important in the coagulation cascade, it is not required to be readily available when heparin is being infused. Protamine sulfate is a heparin antagonist and should be used when reversal is indicated (option 1). The client does not have to be NPO during this type of therapy (option 2). If using weight-based therapy, it is important to weigh the client once a day at the same time with the same scale to verify accuracy (option 4).
Cognitive Level: Application
Nursing Process: Implementation; *Test Plan:* SECE

Posttest

1 Answer: 4 *Rationale:* Mevacor belongs to a group of drugs classified as statins. They work by inhibiting cholesterol synthesis in the liver. Bile-acid resins and fibric acid derivatives also work to decrease cholesterol levels but they work at different sites (options 1 and 3). Bile-acid resins work in the gastrointestinal tract and bind bile salts in the intestine. Fibric acid derivatives work on lipoproteins and triglycerides to reduce cholesterol. Mevacor is not a hormone (option 2).
Cognitive Level: Application
Nursing Process: Implementation; *Test Plan:* PHYS

2 Answer: 3 *Rationale:* It is important for the nurse to understand that both intrinsic and extrinsic factors are necessary for the absorption of vitamin B_{12}. If clients lack intrinsic factor (pernicious anemia), the medication must be administered via the IM or deep SC route. The PO route of administration will not solve the problem if intrinsic factor is absent (option 1). Lifelong administration of vitamin B_{12} is required for clients with this type of therapy (option 2). Injection therapy starts out on a more frequent dosing schedule. Therefore, it is

incorrect to tell the client that injections will be given only once a month (option 4). In addition, this response minimizes the client's concerns, and is therefore not therapeutic.
Cognitive Level: Application
Nursing Process: Implementation; *Test Plan:* HPM

3 Answer: 2 *Rationale:* When administering IV thrombolytic medication, the IV site should be changed to the opposite extremity if the client complains of pain or redness at the infusion site. These symptoms can indicate thrombophlebitis and should be taken seriously and acted on immediately. Continuing to monitor the IV site without appropriate intervention is not considered safe practice (options 1 and 4). Decreasing the rate of solution may be an option based on documented protocol, but the fact that the client complains of pain and redness takes immediate priority (option 3).
Cognitive Level: Analysis
Nursing Process: Implementation; *Test Plan:* SECE

4 Answer: 1 *Rationale:* The reticulocyte count is an indication of the number of immature RBCs found circulating in the body. An increased reticulocyte count will indicate that the bone marrow is functioning and that RBC production has been stimulated. INR, PT, and APTT (options 2, 3, and 4) all refer to coagulation studies that are useful in managing anticoagulation therapy or clients who have coagulation disorders.
Cognitive Level: Application
Nursing Process: Evaluation; *Test Plan:* PHYS

5 Answer: 4 *Rationale:* Oral contraceptives taken concurrently with folic acid will diminish the effectiveness of the folic acid. The nurse should be alert to the potential drug interactions, educate the client, and notify the physician of potential interactions. Vitamin E, tetracycline, and allopurinol (options 1, 2, and 3) all affect the administration of iron.
Cognitive Level: Application
Nursing Process: Analysis; *Test Plan:* HPM

6 Answer: 3 *Rationale:* Because heparin is metabolized quickly in the body, it is important to know both the amount of drug that was given and the elapsed time frame. The dose of protamine sulfate will be calculated based on individual need. While it is true that the maximum dose of protamine is 50 mg over a 10-minute period, that may not be the dosage required since the pertinent information relative to heparin is not stated (option 1). APTT levels would be monitored but are not the priority action at this time (option 2). Vitamin K should not be given with

protamine sulfate, as it is the antagonist to Coumadin (option 4).
Cognitive Level: Analysis
Nursing Process: Implementation; *Test Plan:* SECE

7 **Answer: 2** *Rationale:* Hemostatics such as aminocaproic acid are used to control excessive bleeding. They can be applied topically to stop a local hemorrhage, or they can be administered parenterally to stop a systemic hemorrhage. Thrombolytics are used to dissolve existing clots (option 1). Antiplatelets are used to prevent platelet aggregation and anticoagulants act on the coagulation cascade to prevent clot formation (options 3 and 4). It is important for the nurse to have a basic understanding of each of the drug groupings so that appropriate therapy can be properly monitored.
Cognitive Level: Application
Nursing Process: Analysis; *Test Plan:* PHYS

8 **Answer: 4** *Rationale:* If the client still complains of symptoms of anemia, then it is possible that treatment with folic acid may not be the primary problem. Folic acid and vitamin B_{12} work together to aid the growth of RBCs. Obtaining and comparing APTT results will not demonstrate whether the drug treatment is effective as this test looks at the intrinsic coagulation pathway. While it is true that alcohol has a major effect on folic acid levels and intake, there are many other medications that can affect folic acid levels. This response, while of concern, does not indicate that the drug ther-

apy is effective. A review of dietary sources may be indicated, but if the client were taking drug therapy, then the amount of folic acid in the diet would not indicate whether the drug therapy is effective.
Cognitive Level: Application
Nursing Process: Evaluation; *Test Plan:* PHYS

9 **Answer: 3** *Rationale:* It is very important for the client to be aware of foods that are high in vitamin K while on Coumadin therapy. Green, leafy vegetables are very high in vitamin K and if the client is eating a large amount of these during the week, this might affect the action of Coumadin. While milk is a good source of vitamin K, the amount that the client is taking is not enough to cause concern with regard to Coumadin interaction (option 1). The amount of wine and wax beans is not clinically significant to affect Coumadin interaction (options 2 and 4).
Cognitive Level: Application
Nursing Process: Assessment; *Test Plan:* PHYS

10 **Answer: 4** *Rationale:* The APTT level should be 1.5 to 2.5 times the control value to reach a therapeutic range. A control value is always run with the test to make sure that the results are referenced. Higher APTT levels are not considered to be therapeutic and may require that the medication to be stopped until APTT levels fall back into a safe and therapeutic range.
Cognitive Level: Application
Nursing Process: Evaluation; *Test Plan:* PHYS

References

Bunnell Sellers, J., & Brubaker, M. L. (1999). Cardiovascular disorders. In Youngkin, E. Q., Sawin, K. J., Kissinger, J. F., & Israel, D. S. *Pharmacotherapeutics: A primary care clinical guide.* Stamford, CT: Appleton & Lange, chapter 20, pp. 354–367.

Corbett, J. V. (2000). *Laboratory tests and diagnostic procedures with nursing diagnoses.* Upper Saddle River, NJ: Prentice Hall, pp: 38–337.

Drew-Cates, J., & Gross, R. A. (1999). Neurologic disorders. In Youngkin, E. Q., Sawin, K. J., Kissinger, J. F., & Israel, D. S. *Pharmacotherapeutics: A primary care clinical guide.* Stamford, CT: Appleton & Lange, chapter 29, pp. 635–641.

Eisenhauer, L. A., Nichols, L. W., Spencer, R. T., & Bergan, F. W. (1998). *Clinical pharmacology & nursing management* (5th ed.). Philadelphia: Lippincott, pp. 452–1078.

Estes, M. E. (2002). *Health assessment & physical examination.* New York, Delmar Publishers, pp. 158–235.

Fitzgerald, M. A. (1999). Hematologic disorders. In Youngkin, E. Q., Sawin, K. J., Kissinger, J. F., & Israel, D. S. *Pharmacotherapeutics: A primary care clinical guide.* Stamford, CT: Appleton & Lange, pp. 608–620.

Grajeda-Higley, L. (2000). *Understanding pharmacology. A physiologic approach.* Stamford, CT: Appleton & Lange, pp. 124–271.

Grodner, M. Anderson, S. L., & DeYoung, S. (2000). *Foundations and clinical applications of nutrition. A nursing approach* (2nd ed.). St. Louis, MO: Mosby, pp. 179–199.

Josephson, D. L. (1999). *Intravenous infusion therapy for nurses. Principles & practice.* New York, Delmar Publishers, pp. 81–245.

Kozier, B., Erb, G., Berman, A. J., & Burke, K. (2003). *Fundamentals of nursing: Concepts, process, and practice.* (7th ed.). Upper Saddle River, NJ: Prentice Hall, Inc., pp. 750–1118.

Lemone, P., & Burke, K. (2003). *Medical-surgical nursing: Critical thinking in client care* (3rd ed.). Upper Saddle River, NJ: Prentice Hall, Inc., pp. 206–1301.

Lilley, L. L., & Aucker, R. S. (1999). *Pharmacology and the nursing process* (2nd ed.). St. Louis, MO: Mosby Inc., pp. 349–654.

O'Mara, A. M., & Whedon, M. B. (2000). Hematologic system. In S. M. Lewis, M. McLean Heitkemper, & S. Ruff Dirksen (Eds.), *Medical-surgical nursing: Assessment and management of clinical problems* (5th ed.). St. Louis, MO: Mosby Inc., pp. 719–728.

O'Mara A. M., & Whedon M. B. (2000). Hematologic problems. In S. M. Lewis, M. McLean Heitkemper, & S. Ruff Dirksen (Eds.), *Medical-surgical nursing: Assessment and management of clinical problems* (5th ed.). St. Louis, MO: Mosby Inc., pp. 736–757.

Pickar, G. D. (2002). *Dosage calculations* (7th ed.). New York, Delmar Publishers, pp. 228–231.

Spratto, G. R., & Woods, A. L. (2000). *PDR nurse's drug handbook.* Montvale, NJ: Medical Economics, pp: 20–177.

Weinstein, S. M. (2001). *Plumer's principles & practice of intravenous therapy* (7th ed.). Philadelphia, PA: Lippincott, pp. 452–473.

Weinstein, S. M. (2000). Pharmacology. In A. Corrigan, G. Pelletier, & M. Alexander. *Core curriculum for intravenous nursing* (2nd ed.). Philadelphia: Lippincott, pp. 188–204.

Whitney, E. N., Cataldo, C. B., DeBruyne, L. K., & Rolfes, S. (2001). *Nutrition for health and health care.* New York, Wadsworth Publishing, pp. 176–507.

Whitney, E., & Rolfes, S. (1999). *Understanding nutrition* (8th ed.). New York, Wadsworth Publishing, pp. 143–570.

Wilson, B. A., Shannon, M. T., & Stang, C. L. (2003). *Nurses drug guide 2003.* Upper Saddle River, NJ: Prentice Hall.

CHAPTER 5

Cardiac Medications

Suzanne Kay Marnocha, RN, CCRN, PhD

CHAPTER OUTLINE

Nitrates and Nitrites
Beta-Adrenergic Blockers
Calcium Channel Blockers
Peripheral Vasodilators
Cardiac Glycosides

Antidysrhythmics
Anticoagulants, Antiplatelets,
    Thrombolytics, and Medications to
    Lower Cholesterol

Antihypertensives, Antihypotensives, Diuretics, and Potassium
Supplements

OBJECTIVES

▮ Describe general goals of therapy when administering cardiovascular medications.

▮ Identify specific nursing interventions related to administering digoxin (Lanoxin).

▮ Identify signs and symptoms of digitalis toxicity.

▮ List side effects of the most commonly used antidysrhythmics.

▮ Identify the nursing considerations when administering antidysrhythmics.

▮ Discuss side effects and adverse reactions of beta-adrenergic blockers, calcium channel blockers, and nitrates.

▮ Identify specific client teaching points related to the administration of nitroglycerin.

▮ List significant client education points related to the various cardiovascular medications.

[Media Link]

Use the CD-ROM enclosed with this text, or log onto the address given to access the free, interactive Companion Website created for this series. The CD-ROM and Companion Website accompanying this book offer additional practice opportunities and information—NCLEX Review, Case Studies, Glossary, In Depth with NCLEX, and more.

www.prenhall.com/hogan

REVIEW AT A GLANCE

afterload *resistance to the blood being ejected by the left ventricle; resistance in the aorta and peripheral blood vessels*

automaticity *the heart can initiate impulses on its own without any external stimulation*

cardiac output *the amount of blood ejected in liters/minute by the heart: consists of input from preload, afterload, contractility and heart rate*

chronotropic *affecting the heart rate (HR); positive chronotropic medications increase HR; negative chronotropic medications decrease HR*

conductivity *impulses spread throughout all fibers in the heart despite the absence of specialized conduction tissue*

contractility *amount of force and pressure to pump blood out of the ventricles: amount of or ability of the ventricles to "squeeze"*

dromotropic *affecting the speed with which impulses pass through the conduction system; positive dromotropic medications increase speed of impulses, while negative dromotropic medications decrease speed of impulses*

dysrhythmia *a general term that refers to abnormalities in the electrocardiogram (EKG, ECG) pattern produced by the heart; these refer to electrical activity and not mechanical pumping action (contraction) of the heart*

inotropic *affecting force of contraction; positive inotopic medications increase force of contraction and therefore increase cardiac output (CO), negative inotropic medications decrease force of contraction and therefore decrease CO*

irritability *a state in which heart muscle responds to a variety of external stimuli,*

including hypoxia, ischemia, abnormal electrolyte levels, particular hormones, medications and physical trauma

preload *fiber stretch; or volume just prior to contraction*

refractory period *either relative (able to respond only to a strong stimulus) or absolute refractory period (unable to respond even to a strong stimuli); refers to the recovery period in the cardiac cycle when the heart varies in its depolarization (electrical activity leading to contraction)*

titrate *the act of adjusting medication (usually intravenous medications) according to a predetermined parameter*

Pretest

1 A client is being discharged with a diagnosis of angina. The nurse is teaching the client about the use of nitroglycerine (NTG) tablets at home. What client teaching is needed related to this medication?

(1) "Keep NTG tablets in your pants pocket next to your body to keep them handy at all times. Take two NTG tablets with a glass of water and then go back to your activities."
(2) "Stop your activities and sit down near a telephone if possible, place one NTG under your tongue. Take no more than three tablets, one every 5 minutes. If the pain is unrelieved after a total of three NTG tablets seek help."
(3) "Stop your activities, take two NTG tablets and drive immediately to your doctor's office."
(4) "Continue your activities slowly. Take three NTG tablets every five minutes until your chest pain is gone."

2 The client states, "I always put my nitroglycerin (NTG) patch in the same place so I do not forget to take it off." Your best response would be:

(1) "This is good, but it is very important to take the patch off each night."
(2) "Sometimes the patch should be placed over hairy areas to vary the absorption."
(3) "You should rotate the NTG patch to a different hairless area each day."
(4) "It does not matter if you leave your patch on when you put the next one on. The medication is all gone."

3 A client is hospitalized for heart failure and is receiving digoxin (Lanoxin) IV push. The nurse should withhold the drug and notify physician if the client's:

(1) History reveals depression.
(2) Pulse is 53 beats per minute.
(3) Respiratory rate falls below 18.
(4) Blood pressure is 148/90.

4 A physician orders a nitroglycerine (NTG) drip to be titrated. The nurse carrying out the order would monitor which of the following parameters?

(1) Shortness of breath and level of consciousness
(2) Respirations and urine output
(3) Blood pressure and pulse rate
(4) Headache and blood pressure

5 A client is receiving metoprolol (Lopressor) for hypertension. The nurse should ask the client about a history of which of the following conditions?

(1) Bronchospasm
(2) Seizure
(3) Hypertension
(4) Myasthenia gravis

6 A nurse assesses a client for side effects of verapamil (Calan-SR). Which client manifestation would the nurse anticipate as a side effect of this medication?

(1) Hypertension
(2) Angina
(3) Skin rash
(4) Constipation

7 The client is receiving a lidocaine infusion at a rate of 2 mg per minute via infusion pump. The nurse should discontinue the infusion and notify the physician immediately when the client does which of the following?

(1) Demonstrates slurred speech.
(2) Demonstrates a sinus tachycardia of 102.
(3) States he is concerned about his "heart attack."
(4) Reports leg cramps.

8 The nurse anticipates a positive inotropic effect after administering which of the following medications?

(1) Atropine sulfate
(2) Digoxin (Lanoxin)
(3) Propranolol (Inderal)
(4) Verapamil (Calan)

9 A client asks the nurse to explain why she is receiving lidocaine (Xylocaine) in her IV when her dentist injects it into her gums to numb the teeth before a filling. The best response by the nurse is:

(1) "The medication is more effective intravenously, and you will feel no pain anywhere."
(2) "As an IV medication, it will help you relax and rest so your heart can heal."
(3) "When given IV, this medication reduces the irritability of the cells in your heart and helps reduce dysrhythmias."
(4) "The medication will increase your urine output so that you will be less likely to suffer from heart failure."

10 The nurse provides discharge instructions to a client about the use of amiodarone (Cordarone). Which of the following statements made by the client indicates an understanding of discharge teaching about this medication?

(1) "As soon as the physician says I can stop taking this medication, I will be able to enjoy the sun again."
(2) "The side effects of this medication may not begin to show up for several weeks or even months after I start taking it."
(3) "If my pulse drops below 100 beats per minute, I should call the physician right away."
(4) "If I miss a dose of medication, I should take it as soon as I remember it."

See pages 224–225 for Answers and Rationales.

I. Nitrates and Nitrites

A. Action and use

1. Increase the oxygenated blood flow to the myocardium by dilating the coronary and systemic blood vessels

2. Prophylactic treatment of angina in clients with coronary artery disease (CAD)

3. Dilation of systemic vascular bed leads to pooling of blood in the peripheral vascular system; this reduces the total workload of the left ventricle by reducing both **preload** (volume in the left ventricle just prior to contraction) and **afterload** (resistance to blood being ejected by the left ventricle) and ultimately reducing myocardial oxygen (O_2) demand

Table 5-1	Generic/ Trade Name	Usual Adult Dose	Side Effects	Nursing Implications
Common Nitrates and Nitrites	Isosorbide Denitrate (Dilatrate-SR, Isordil)	PO tablets 10–40 mg BID	Headache Flushing Hypotension Rash	Instruct client to carry NGT tablets at all times as a precaution.
	Isosorbide (Imdur, ISMO, Monoket)	20 mg BID PO given 7 hours apart	Local burning or tingling sensation GI upset with PO use	Tolerance may develop, adjust dosing schedule to allow a "nitrate-free" period.
	Nitroglycerin SL (Nitrostat)	Up to 3 tablets PRN each 5 minutes apart, if not relieved, call MD or Emergency Medical Services	Contact dermatitis with topical use	Do not crush or chew sustained-release or SL tablets.
	Nitroglycerin SR (Nitrong, Nitro-Bid)	2.5–13 mg BID		Do not expose to light or heat.
	Nitroglycerin Topical (Nitrol)	½–1 inch topical every 6 to 8 hours		Wear gloves during application of paste.
	Nitroglycerin Transdermal (Depoint, Transderm-Nitro)	0.2–0.4 mg/hr topical daily		

B. **Common medications (Table 5-1)**

C. **Administration considerations**

1. Instruct client to sit down next to a phone when taking sublingual (SL) nitroglycerine (NTG) tablets in case it becomes necessary to call for help

2. Instruct client to take no more than 3 NTG tablets (one every five minutes); if pain is unrelieved after a total of three tablets, notify physician or call emergency services

3. The client's mucous membranes should be moist when taking sublingual (SL) tablets

4. Instruct client that NTG degrades in heat, light, or moisture, so the medication should be stored in the original container in a cool, dry place

5. Sublingual tablets should be replaced every 3 to 6 months after opening; each tablet should produce a slight stinging or tingling sensation when placed under the tongue

6. Intravenous (IV) NTG must be delivered as a continuous or intermittent infusion (not IV push) and given via an infusion pump

7. Intravenous NTG must be diluted in 5% dextrose or 0.9% normal saline (NS) solution

8. Intravenous NTG should be mixed in glass bottles and only manufacturer-supplied IV tubing should be used; regular IV tubing can absorb 40 to 80% of NTG because of the polyvinyl chloride plastic

9. Nitroglycerine drips are often ordered to control or treat the client's chest pain; the nurse should **titrate** (adjust medication according to a predetermined parameter) the medication accordingly

10. Monitor blood pressure (BP) and heart rate (HR) every 15 minutes when using IV form of NTG and titrating the medication; be prepared to treat hypotension by decreasing or stopping the NTG infusion

11. Wear gloves when applying NTG paste to the client's skin to avoid absorption of the medication into the skin

12. Rotate the location of NTG paste or patch to reduce skin irritation and enhance absorption; place on hairless areas for predictable absorption

13. For a hospitalized client, tablets may be kept at bedside only if policy allows; instruct client to report all attacks; count tablets daily if kept at bedside

14. The dosing regimen should allow for a 6 to 8 hour nitrate-free period to prevent the body's development of tolerance; the NTG patch should be applied in the morning and removed at 10 PM

D. Contraindications

1. Hypersensitivity to nitrates

2. Hypotension and/or hypovolemia

3. Severe bradycardia or severe tachycardia

4. Right ventricular myocardial infarction

5. Use of Viagra within 24 hours

E. Significant drug interactions

1. Do not mix with any other medications in the bottle or IV tubing

2. Use of sildenafil citrate (Viagra) within 24 hours leads to profound hypotension

3. All other antihypertensive and vasodilation medications may interact to cause profound hypotension

4. Intravenous NTG may antagonize heparin anticoagulation

5. Alcohol consumption should be avoided

F. Significant food interactions: none reported

G. Significant laboratory studies

1. Nitroglycerine may increase urinary catecholamines

2. It may cause a false report of decrease in serum cholesterol

3. Prolonged high-dose use of NTG may lead to methemoglobinemia

H. Side effects

1. Headache (50%)

2. Postural hypotension

3. Flushing

I. Adverse reactions/toxicity

1. Blurred vision and dry mouth

2. Central nervous system (CNS): weakness, dizziness, vertigo, and faintness

3. Cardiovascular (CV): severe postural hypotension with resulting tachycardia; when BP falls, the heart rate increases to sustain the **cardiac output** (the amount of blood ejected in liters/minute by the heart)

4. Gastrointestinal (GI): nausea, vomiting, fecal and urinary incontinence, abdominal pain, and dry mouth

J. Nursing considerations

1. Drug forms appropriate for angina prophylaxis include NTG paste, NTG patch, spray, SL tablet and oral sustained-release forms

2. Drug forms appropriate for acute angina include NTG spray, SL tablet, or IV infusion

3. Ensure that client is sitting or lying down when taking NTG to prevent dizziness or fainting

4. Allow the tablet to dissolve naturally under the tongue; if mouth is dry, instruct the client to take a sip of water before placing the tablet under the tongue

5. Give client no more than 3 tablets total, one every 5 minutes; notify the physician or emergency services if the pain is unrelieved after the third dose

6. If using NTG paste or a transdermal patch, do not apply it to areas with extensive body hair or scar tissue; the appropriate areas include chest, upper abdomen, anterior thigh, or upper arm

7. Use gloves or an applicator to spread the ointment evenly and to avoid getting medication on fingers

8. Rotate application sites and check the skin for irritation

9. Remove the paste or patch each day at the designated time before applying additional medication

10. Store ointment in a cool, dry place with the cap attached tightly

11. Intravenous NTG must be diluted in 5% dextrose or 0.9% NaCl solution before administrating; never administer this drug IV push

12. NTG must be prepared in only glass bottles and delivered through tubing manufactured specifically for NTG

13. Nitroglycerine infusions must be delivered via an infusion pump

14. Monitor BP and HR frequently during medication titration (this may be as often as every 5 to 10 minutes)

15. Check the infusion concentration carefully, as many different dilutions are possible

16. Visualize the client's skin and remove any NTG patches that could lead to severe hypotension

K. Client education

1. Instruct client that all forms of NTG might cause dizziness and headache; the client using the SL form of NTG for angina should rest for at least 15 minutes after taking the medication to avoid dizziness

2. Instruct client to report to the health care provider if symptoms become worse or increase in frequency when taking NTG

3. Teach client that if pain persists after three NTG tables (or sprays) at 5-minute intervals, physician should be notified as this could indicate an impending myocardial infarction (MI)

4. Assist client to identify emergency phone numbers and write them down to be placed next to the phone with home address and exact direction

5. Advise client to take a sublingual or spray NTG before an event that might cause angina, such as stair climbing, exercise, or sexual intercourse

6. Instruct client to keep a written record for physician of times, dates, amount of medication required for relief of each attack and possible precipitating factors

7. Advise the elderly to change position slowly to avoid postural hypotension and fall

8. Advise client to shake aerosol spray well prior to use as this affects the metered dose

9. If client is wearing a NTG patch or paste and experiencing an anginal attack, a sublingual NTG tablet may be used following the safety measures outlined above

10. Client may swim or bathe with a NTG patch in place

11. Instruct client that frequent and prolonged use of NTG may reduce efficacy, requiring a medication adjustment

12. Instruct client to avoid over-the-counter (OTC) medications or herbal products without consulting physician

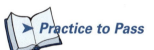

An overweight female client has just told you she is planning to take OTC diet pills to lose 50 pounds. The client is also taking Transderm-Nitro. How would you address this issue? What client teaching is needed related to this medication?

II. Beta-Adrenergic Blockers

A. Action and use

1. In therapeutic doses, they block beta-adrenergic receptors (remember β_1—you have 1 heart) that are found chiefly in cardiac muscle

2. In higher doses, they may cause blocking of the beta-adrenergic receptors in the airways (remember β_2—you have 2 lungs) leading to increased airway resistance especially in clients with asthma or chronic obstructive pulmonary disease (COPD)

3. Blocking beta-adrenergic receptors leads to reduction in renin activity, with resulting suppression of the renin-angiotension-aldosterone system; this results in:

   a. Competition for binding of catecholamines at the beta-adrenergic receptor sites

   b. Reduction in systolic and diastolic BP

   c. A negative **inotropic** (force of contraction) and **chronotropic** (heart rate) effect

4. Beta-blockers are used therapeutically for management of hypertension, angina pectoris, acute myocardial infarction (MI), and supraventricular tachycardia

5. These medications should be administered to all clients with suspected MI and unstable angina in the absence of complications such as congestive heart failure (CHF); help prevent ventricular fibrillation

6. They block cardiac effects of beta-adrenergic stimulation resulting in:

   a. Reductions in HR, myocardial **irritability** (cardiac muscle response to a variety of external stimuli such as hypoxia), and force of contraction

   b. Depression of **automaticity** (the heart's ability to initiate impulses on its own without any external stimulation) of the sinus node

   c. Reduction in AV node and intraventricular **dromotropic** (conduction velocity) effect

7. Also useful in controlling panic attacks and stage fight in some clients

B. Common medications (Table 5-2)

C. Administration considerations

1. Assess client before, during and after the initial dose

   a. Monitor BP, HR, and cardiac rhythm frequently during initial administration; if given orally, assess client 30 minutes before and 60 minutes after the initial dose

   b. Subsequent to the next dose, reassess BP, heart rate, and rhythm

2. Give medication at consistent times with or without meals; it is recommended to take the medication before meals and at bedtime

Table 5-2 **Common Beta-Adrenergic Blocker Medications**	**Generic/ Trade Name**	**Usual Adult Dose**	**Side Effects**	**Nursing Implications**
	Atenolol (Tenormin)	50–200 mg PO daily, with renal insufficiency max. dose: 50 mg daily	Bradycardia Hypotension Worsening CHF Worsening PVD Bronchospasm	Therapy should not be abruptly discontinued. Check apical pulse and BP before administration of drug, especially in client receiving digitalis.
	Sotalol (Betaloc)	10–20 mg PO daily	Impotence GI upset Increased triglyderides	Monitor apical pulse, BP, respirations and peripheral circulation throughout dosage adjustment period. Caution client to make position changes
	Metoprolol (Lopressor, Toprol XL)	50 mg PO BID, max: 400 mg daily	Decreased HDL cholesterol Mask signs of hypoglycemia	slowly. Instruct client to protect extremities from cold and not to smoke. Instruct client to report immediately
	Nadolol (Corgard)	40 mg PO daily, max: 240 mg/day		to physician the onset of ocular symptoms. Client with diabetes mellitus should be
	Propranolol (Inderal)	40 mg PO BID		monitored closely as the mediation may mask some symptoms of hypoglycemia.
	Timolol (Blocadren)	10 mg PO BID, max: 60mg/day		

3. Beta-adrenergic blockers are not the same as calcium channel blockers; simultaneous use of beta-adrenergic blockers and calcium channel blockers may increase the adverse response, including bradycardia and hypotension

4. Tablets may be crushed as needed (PRN) before administration and taken with fluid of choice

5. Intravenous administration: for IV push (IVP) give 1 mg/minute either undiluted or diluted in up to 50mL of 5% dextrose or 0.9%. NaCl and give as an infusion over 15 to 30 minutes

6. Do not discontinue therapy abruptly; dosage is reduced gradually over a period of 1 to 2 weeks, and observe client for paradoxical reactions such as hypertension and tachycardia

D. Contraindications

1. Greater than first-degree heart block (first-degree heart block is a consistent PR interval greater than 0.20 second)

2. CHF

3. Right ventricular failure secondary to pulmonary hypertension

4. Sinus bradycardia

5. Cardiogenic shock

6. Significant aortic or mitral valve disease

7. Hyperactive airway syndrome (asthma or bronchospasm)

8. Severe seasonal allergies (allergic rhinitis during pollen season)

9. Concurrent use of psychotropic drugs that use an adrenergic augmentation or within 2 weeks of an monoamine oxidase (MAO) inhibitor

10. Use cautiously in client with systemic allergies to insect stings and major surgery, renal or hepatic impairment, diabetes mellitus, myasthenia gravis, or Wolff-Parkinson-White (WPW) syndrome

E. Significant drug interactions

1. Phenothiazines have an additive effect, worsening hypotension

2. Beta-adrenergic agonists (e.g., albuterol) antagonize effects (cancel each other)

3. Atropine and tricyclic antidepressants block bradycardia

4. Diuretics and other antihypertensive medications increase hypotension

5. High doses of tubocurarine (a neuromuscular agent used as an adjunct to anesthesia to relax skeletal muscles) may potentiate neuromuscular blockade

6. Cimetidine (Tagamet) decreases clearance and increases effect

7. Antacids may decrease absorption

F. Significant food interactions: none reported

G. Significant laboratory studies

1. They may induce false negative test results in exercise tolerance electrocardiogram (ECG)

2. Elevations in serum potassium, platelet count, uric acid, serum transaminase, alkaline phosphatase, lactate dehydrogenase (LDH), serum creatinine, and blood urea nitrogen (BUN)

3. Increase or decrease in blood glucose levels of diabetic clients

H. Side effects

1. Bradycardia

2. Bronchospasm

3. Hypotension

4. Weight gain

5. Dizziness

6. CHF

I. Adverse reactions/toxicity

1. CNS: sleep disturbances, depression, confusion, agitation, or psychosis

2. CV: hypotension, profound bradycardia, heart block, acute CHF, and peripheral paresthesias resembling Raynaud's phenomenon

3. Laryngospasm or bronchospasm

4. Dry eyes with a gritty sensation, blurred vision, tinnitus, or hearing loss

5. GI: dry mouth, nausea, vomiting, heartburn, diarrhea, constipation, abdominal cramps, and flatulence

6. Agranulocytosis, hypoglycemia, hyperglycemia and hypocalcemia in clients with hyperthyroidism

J. Nursing considerations

1. Take apical pulse and BP before administering drug; evaluate client for fluid volume overload as it may indicate CHF

2. Monitor intake and output (I & O) and daily weight

3. Withhold medication if HR is less than 60 beats per minute (bpm) or if systolic BP is less than 90 mmHg

4. Perform a head to toe physical examination and assess client thoroughly for a history of asthma, allergies, or COPD; beta-blockers may lead to bronchospasm in clients with no history of pulmonary disease

5. Assess HR, BP, and respiratory status carefully during periods of dosage adjustment; maintain effective communication with physician

6. The most common adverse reaction is bradycardia; clients with digitalis toxicity and WPW syndrome are most at risk

7. Client receiving IV beta-blockers should be monitored for ECG rhythm and rate, BP, and occasionally pulmonary capillary wedge pressure (left ventricular end-diastolic pressure or LVEDP) in the intensive care unit (ICU); reduction in sympathetic stimulation may lead to cardiac standstill

8. Adverse reactions are most likely to occur after the IV form of beta-blockers are administered, but may occur in the elderly and clients with impaired renal function after oral doses soon after therapy is initiated

9. Dietary sodium is usually restricted to prevent fluid volume overload; check with physician regarding sodium restriction or concomitant use of a diuretic

10. Fasting longer than 12 hours may induce hypoglycemia which is worsened by the beta-blocker therapy because signs are masked

11. Periodic evaluations of renal, hepatic, cardiac, and hematologic functions should be made in clients receiving prolonged medication therapy

K. Client education

1. Teach client and significant other about checking pulse and BP; discuss the desired range for these values and how to keep a record of daily measurements, as well as when to call physician

NCLEX!

2. Emphasize that abrupt withdrawal of the medication can lead to severe paradoxical or rebound reactions, including sweating, tremulousness, severe headache, malaise, palpitations, hypertension, MI and life-threatening heart rhythm disturbances

3. Emphasize that client should establish a routine for taking the medication and strive to comply with the prescriptive plan to obtain the best results; work with client to write out a daily schedule for medication

NCLEX!

4. Encourage client to change position slowly to avoid postural hypotension

5. Encourage client to notify physician if any dizziness or lightheadedness occurs; instruct client to avoid driving or operating machinery until these symptoms are relieved

NCLEX!

6. Advise client to stop smoking as this might offset the desired outcomes of controlled heart rate, BP, and prevention of angina; smoking also increases hepatic metabolism of beta-blocker medication leading to unpredictable or diminished drug effects

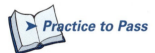

Practice to Pass

Your client is taking a beta-adrenergic blocker medication. Upon auscultation of the lungs, you hear diffuse wheezing throughout the lung fields. What are the appropriate actions to take? What are your rationales for these interventions?

7. Advise client to avoid OTC medications or herbal supplements without consulting physician

8. Teach client taking a beta-blocker medication to notify all healthcare providers regarding the medication

9. Instruct client to notify the ophthalmologist or optometrist while taking this medication as it may lower intraocular pressures

III. Calcium Channel Blockers

A. Action and use

1. Are Class IV antiarrhythmic drugs that inhibit calcium ion influx through slow channels into cells of myocardial and arterial smooth muscle (both cardiac and peripheral blood vessels)

2. Intracellular calcium remains below levels needed to stimulate cell

3. Dilate coronary arteries and arterioles and prevent coronary artery spasm

4. Myocardial O_2 delivery is increased, preventing angina

5. Slow conduction through the sinoatrial (SA) node and atrioventricular (AV) node, resulting in a lower heart rate and decreased strength of the heart muscle contraction (negative inotropic effect)

6. Decrease automaticity and **conductivity** (the amount of force and pressure to pump blood out of the ventricles) by blocking the flow of calcium into the cell

7. Decrease systemic vascular resistance (SVR) and thus afterload by dilating peripheral arteriols

8. Reduce arterial BP (antihypertensive effect) and heart rate

9. They are used for vasospastic angina (Prinzmetal's variant or angina at rest), chronic stable (classic and activity-induced) angina, and essential hypertension; the IV form is useful in treating atrial fibrillation, atrial flutter, and supraventricular tachycardia

B. Common medications (Table 5-3)

C. Administration considerations

1. Administer oral diltiazem before meals and at bedtime and oral verapamil with food to reduce gastric irritation

2. Evaluate BP and ECG before initiation of therapy

3. Monitor for headache; an analgesic may be required

4. Intravenous forms of diltiazem: give undiluted IVP over 2 minutes and repeat in 15 minutes or dilute in D_5W, NS or $D_5W/0.45\%$ NaCl; continuous infusion may be given via infusion pump at a rate of 5 to 15 mg/hr; infusions over 24 h and greater than 15 mg/hr are not recommended

5. Intravenous verapamil may be given IVP when diluted in 5 mL of sterile water for injection at a rate of 10 mg/min

NCLEX!

6. Withhold medication if BP less than 90/60

Table 5-3

Common Calcium Channel Blocker Medications

Generic/ Trade Name	Usual Adult Dose	Side Effects	Nursing Implications
Amlodipine (Norvasc)	2.5–10 mg PO daily	Hypotension Peripheral edema	Monitor pulse and BP for severe hypotension. Withhold medication if BP less than 90/60.
Diltiazem (Cardizem, Dilacor XR, Tiazac)	Regular release PO: 30–120 mg TID or QID Sustained-release: 60–240 mg BID	Tachycardia Flushing Headache GI upset	Monitor heart rhythm for sick sinus syndrome and second or third degree AV blocks. Monitor hepatic and renal labs test results. Assess client for possible headache.
Nifedipine (Adalat, Procardia)	Regular release: 10–20 mg PO TID or QID SR: 30–120 mg daily		Monitor blood glucose levels closely in diabetes. Avoid smoking and alcohol intake.
Verapamil (Calan, Covera HS, Verelan, Isoptin)	Regular release: 40–160 mg PO TID SR: 120–480 mg PO daily		

D. Contraindications

1. Avoid use when there is known hypersensitivity to drug

2. Sick sinus syndrome (unless pacemaker is in place)

3. Second- or third-degree heart blocks

   a. Second-degree Type I or Wenckebach: progressive PR prolongation until a QRS is dropped

   b. Second-degree Type II: P waves are constant until a QRS is dropped

   c. Third-degree heart block: no association between P waves and QRS, usually ventricular HR is between 20 to 40 bpm

4. Severe hypotension, BP less than 90/60

E. Significant drug interactions

1. Beta-blockers and digoxin may have an additive effect on prolongation of the AV node conduction

2. They may increase digoxin or quinidine levels leading to toxicity

3. Cimetidine may increase serum levels of calcium channel blockers

4. Calcium channel blockers may increase serum levels of cyclosporine (an immunosupressant)

5. Furosemide is incompatible in IV solution

F. Significant food interactions: none reported

G. Significant laboratory studies

1. Do not alter total serum calcium levels

2. Monitor baseline and periodic lab tests of hepatic and renal function

3. Monitor diabetics closely; may induce hyperglycemia

4. Cyclosporine levels may become elevated

5. Digoxin and quinidine levels may become elevated

H. Side effects

1. Headache

2. Fatigue

3. Constipation (especially with oral and sustained-release forms)

4. Postural hypotension

I. Adverse effects/toxicity

1. CNS: dizziness, nervousness, insomnia, confusion, tremor, and gait disturbance

2. CV: heart block and profound bradycardia, CHF, profound hypotension with syncope, palpitations, and fluid volume overload

3. GI: nausea, vomiting, and impaired taste

4. Skin rash

J. Nursing considerations

1. Evaluate BP and ECG before the initiation of treatment and monitor them closely during medication adjustment

2. Monitor hepatic and renal lab test results

3. Monitor for headache

4. May induce hyperglycemia; monitor diabetic clients closely

5. Advise client to report gradual weight gain and evidence of edema; may indicate onset of CHF

K. Client education

1. Inform client about the importance of taking radial pulse before each dose (especially verapamil); an irregular pulse or one slower than baseline level should be reported

2. Encourage client to change position slowly to prevent postural hypotension

3. Caution client to avoid driving if dizziness or faintness is noted; these symptoms should be reported immediately

4. Advise client to take medication exactly as prescribed

5. Instruct client not to crush or chew sustained-release tables

6. Stress the importance of follow-up care

7. Inform client to avoid OTC medications and herbal supplements without consulting physician

8. Encourage client to stop smoking

9. Encourage client to avoid alcohol consumption

10. Instruct client to report easy bruising, petechiae, or unexplained bleeding

IV. Peripheral Vasodilators

A. Action and use

1. Potent, non-nitrate hypotensive agents that reduce BP by direct effects on vascular smooth muscles of arteries (some vasodilators such as sodium nitroprusside work equally in all vessel beds)

2. Act directly on vascular smooth muscle to produce peripheral vasodilation, resulting in lowered arterial BP, increased heart rate, and increased cardiac output (CO)

3. Most commonly used to treat hypertension and as an adjunct in treating CHF

4. Certain vasodilators may be ordered to treat peripheral vascular disease (PVD) to increase blood flow to extremities, such as in Raynaud's disease

B. Common medications (Table 5-4)

C. Administration considerations

1. Take oral forms of medications with food to increase bioavailability

2. Intravenous hydralazine may be given undiluted via direct IV push at a rate of 10 mg/min

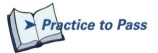

Practice to Pass

Your client is receiving a diltiazem (Cardizem) infusion. The ECG technician notifies you that the PR intervals are becoming progressively longer and occasionally an entire QRS is dropped. What is the most appropriate action for you to take? What is the possible cause of the cardiac rhythm disturbance?

Table 5-4	Generic/ Trade Name	Usual Adult Dose	Side Effects	Nursing Implications
Common Peripheral Vasodilator Medications	Hydralazine HCL (Alazine, Apresoline)	10 mg PO QID up to 300 mg/day in divided doses	Dizziness Hypotension Headache Palpitations Tachycardia Peripheral edema	Monitor BP and HR closely. Do no mix the medication with other IV solutions. Take oral forms of medications with food. Full therapeutic effect of prazosin may not be achieved until 4 to 6 weeks of therapy. Advise not to take OTC medications.
	Nitroprusside (Nipride, Nitropress)	IV 0.5 to 10 µg/ kg/min	Orthostatic hypotension "First dose syncope" with Prazosin	
	Prazosin (Minipress)	1 mg PO BID to TID up to 20 mg/day		

3. Intravenous sodium nitroprusside is diluted by dissolving 50 mg in 2 to 3 mL of D_5W and then diluted in 250 mL D_5W (200 µg/mL); it should be infused cautiously through an IV pump; when mixed, it appears orange and must be covered in a foil pouch to avoid exposure to light during infusion

4. Do not mix with other IV solutions

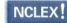

5. All vasodilators should be discontinued slowly to avoid paradoxical hypertensive effects

6. Store medication be in light-resistant container

7. Monitor HR and BP closely during administration to prevent sudden hypotension

D. Contraindications

1. When client has a compensatory hypertension, as in an arteriovenous shunt or coarctation of the aorta

2. Inadequate cerebral perfusion leading to a decreased cerebral perfusion pressure (CPP)

3. Hypovolemia

E. Significant drug interactions

1. All antihypertensive medications, vasodilators (e.g., nitroglycerine), and diuretics may interact to induce profound hypotension

2. Beta-blockers and calcium channel blockers will compound hypotensive effects

3. No additional medication should be infused through the same IV line if given as an infusion

F. Significant food interactions: none reported

G. Significant laboratory studies

1. The various vasodilators have differing laboratory data that is significant; review product literature of individual medications prior to administration

2. When administering hydralazine hydrochloride:

a. Positive direct Coomb's tests can result in hydralazine-induced systemic lupus erythematosus (SLE); this condition mimics SLE and is potentially reversible if identified early

b. Hydralazine interferes with urinary 17-OHCS (modified Glenn-Nelson techniques)

c. Do baseline and periodic LE cell prep and antinuclear antibody (ANA) titer, BUN, creatinine, uric acid, serum potassium, and blood glucose levels

3. During administration of sodium nitroprusside

a. Baseline and periodic BUN, creatinine, uric acid, serum potassium, and blood glucose levels should be done

NCLEX!

b. Monitor serum thiocyanate levels with

1) Prolonged IV infusion

2) Clients who have impaired renal function

c. Monitor plasma cyanogen levels when

1) Prolonged infusion longer than 2 days occurs

2) Clients have impaired hepatic function

d. There are increased or decreased serum cobalamin levels

H. Side effects

1. CNS: headache

2. CV: Palpitations and tachycardia

3. SLE-like syndrome (with hydralazine)

I. Adverse effects/toxicity

1. CNS: dizziness, tremors, apprehension, and muscle twitching

2. CV: angina, tachycardia or bradycardia, flushing, paradoxical pressor response (sudden unexpected elevation in BP), ECG changes, profound hypotension, shock, and dysrhythmias

3. GI: anorexia, nausea, vomiting, constipation or diarrhea, abdominal pain, and paralytic ileus

4. GU: difficulty urinating and glomerulonephritis

NCLEX!

5. Hematologic: decreased hematocrit and hemoglobin, anemia, agranulocytosis (rare)

6. Skin: rash, irritation at IV site, urticaria, pruritus, fever, chills, arthralgia, eosinophilia, and cholangitis

7. SLE-like syndrome, edema

NCLEX!

8. When administering sodium nitroprusside, monitor client for the signs and symptoms of thiocyanate toxicity: profound hypotension, tinnitus, fatigue, pink skin color, metabolic acidosis, and loss of consciousness

J. Nursing considerations

1. Assess carefully baseline vital signs including HR, cardiac rhythm, ECG, and neurological status

2. When administering IV vasodilators:

   a. Establish a large, stable IV site for infusions because they are irritating to tissue; administer the medication with an IV infusion pump

   b. Monitor BP every 5 to 15 minutes with an automatic external BP machine or with an arterial line during the initial infusion and during medication adjustment

   c. Monitor I & O

   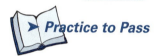

   d. If adverse response is noted (e.g. hypotension), decrease infusion and monitor client closely; if sudden severe hypotension occurs, discontinue medication; maintain airway, breathing and circulation (ABCs); establish IV site; contact physician, and initiate emergency protocols as necessary

3. Obtain baseline vital signs and check BP, heart rate, and cardiac rhythm before each dose when administering orally

Practice to Pass

Your client is receiving a sodium nitroprusside infusion. Upon assessment, you notice a BP of 80/50 and HR of 134 bpm. The client is less responsive. What do you do first? What possible clinical manifestation would you conclude is an adverse effect of this medication?

K. Client education

1. Teach client to monitor pulse and BP

2. Inform client about the possibility of headache and palpitations within 2 to 4 hours after first PO dose

3. Stress the importance of follow-up care

4. Encourage client to write down questions to ask the provider on each follow-up visit

5. Instruct client to avoid all OTC medications and herbal supplements without consulting physician

6. Inform client to stop smoking and avoid alcohol intake as they might negate the positive effects of the medication

7. Instruct client to monitor weight daily and report edema

8. Caution client to change position slowly and avoid hot tubs and hot baths that might induce profound vasodilation and hypotension

V. Cardiac Glycosides

A. Action and use

1. Used primarily in treatment of CHF

2. Used for treatment of atrial **dysrhythmias** (abnormalities in electrical activity of heart)

3. Increase **contractility** (the force of contraction) and efficiency of myocardial contraction

4. Produce a positive inotropic action, which increases the force of myocardial contraction

5. Decrease the conduction velocity through the AV node

Table 5-5	Common Cardiac Glycoside Medications		
Generic/Trade Names	**Usual Adult Dose**	**Side or Toxic Effects**	**Nursing Implications**
Digoxin (Lanoxin, Lanoxicaps)	PO/IV 0.125 to 0.325 mg/QD	Headache Nausea Vomiting Loss of "usual appetite" Anorexia Visual disturbances (blurred, green or yellow vision or halo effect)	Ongoing physical assessment including neurological status, BP, HR, and cardiac rhythm. Before administering the medication, take apical pulse for 1 full minute.
Digitoxin (Crystodigin)	0.05-0.3 mg/QD	Rash Cardiac dysrhythmias	Monitor client closely for digoxin toxicity. Monitor potassium levels and notify prescriber if not within normal range.

B. Common medications (Table 5-5)

C. Administration considerations

1. Cardiac glycosides may be given with or without food

2. Tablet may be crushed and mixed with fluid or food as desired; pediatric elixir is also available

3. Intravenous administration: IVP digoxin may be administered undiluted or diluted in 4 mL of sterile water, 5% dextrose, or NS; administer each direct IV dose over five minutes; the client may receive a loading dose (digitalization) to achieve adequate serum drug levels

4. Never administer digoxin intramuscularly (IM) because it would cause tissue irritation and great variation in bioavailability

5. Infiltration into subcutaneous tissue can cause local irritation and tissue sloughing

D. Contraindications

1. Avoid use in clients with known hypersensitivity to digitalis

2. Full digitalizing dose should not be given if client has received digoxin in the previous week

3. Presence of digoxin toxicity

4. Use cautiously in the following conditions:

   a. Renal insufficiency

   b. Hypokalemia

   c. Advanced heart disease, acute MI, heart block, and cor pulmonale

   d. Hypothyroidism

   e. Lung disease

   f. Pregnant/nursing mothers

   g. Children/premature infants

   h. Elderly

E. Significant drug interactions

1. Antacids, cholestyramine, and colestipol decrease digoxin absorption

2. Diuretics, corticosteroids, amphotericin B, laxatives, and sodium polystyrene sulfonate may cause hypokalemia, increasing the risk of digitalis toxicity

3. Intravenous calcium when given with digoxin may increase the risk of cardiac dysrhythmias

4. Quinidine, verapamil, and amiodarone significantly increase digoxin levels, and digoxin dose should be decreased by 50%

5. Erythromycin and nefazadone may increase digoxin levels

6. Succinylcholine may potentiate dysrhythmias

7. Dobutamine or doxapram should not be injected in the same IV line or mixed in solution with digoxin

F. Significant food interactions: none reported

G. Significant laboratory studies

1. Before initiating digoxin therapy, baseline labs should be drawn

   a. Serum digoxin levels

   b. Potassium

   c. Magnesium

   d. Calcium

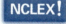

2. Draw serum digoxin level periodically during therapy and if client develops any symptoms of digoxin toxicity; blood sample should be drawn at least 6 hours after the daily dose and preferably just before the next scheduled daily dose

3. Therapeutic range of serum digoxin is 0.8 to 2.0 ng/mL, and the toxic levels are greater than 2.0 ng/mL

H. Side effects

1. Nausea

2. Loss of "usual appetite"

3. Headache

I. Adverse reactions/toxicity

1. CNS: fatigue, muscle weakness, headache, facial neuralgia, depression, paresthesias, hallucinations, confusion, drowsiness, agitation, dizziness, and malaise

2. CV: dysrhythmias, hypotension, AV heart block, and diaphoresis

3. GI: anorexia, nausea, vomiting, diarrhea, and dysphagia

4. Visual disturbances (blurred, green or yellow vision or halo effect)

5. Digoxin toxicity may be unrecognized, since it may present the same manifestations as a "flu"; these include anorexia, nausea, vomiting, diarrhea, or visual disturbances

J. Nursing considerations

1. Obtain baseline data and perform ongoing physical assessments, including neurological status, HR, BP, and cardiac rhythm

2. Check the baseline serum digoxin level prior to initiating digoxin therapy:

   a. The blood level is 0 if no digoxin is being taking before

   b. The therapeutic levels are 0.8 to 2.0 ng/mL

   c. The toxic levels are greater than 2 ng/mL

3. Assess baseline and ongoing laboratory values, including serum electrolytes, creatinine clearance, magnesium, and calcium

4. Monitor closely elderly clients taking digoxin and a diuretic for CHF or atrial fibrillation for digoxin toxicity

5. Take the apical pulse for 1 full minute prior to administering digoxin, noting rate, rhythm and quality; if any changes are noted, withhold medication, and notify the physician; an ECG will likely be ordered

6. Withhold the medication if client has symptoms of digoxin toxicity (anorexia, nausea, vomiting, diarrhea, or visual disturbances)

7. In children, early signs of toxicity include cardiac dysrhythmias; children rarely demonstrate anorexia, nausea, vomiting, diarrhea, or visual disturbances

8. Advise client to eat foods high in potassium such as oranges, bananas, fruit juices, vegetables, and potatoes if taking loop diuretics

9. Monitor I & O and daily weight especially in clients with impaired renal failure; auscultate breath sounds for crackles

10. Antidote: digoxin immune Fab (Digibind) is used in extreme toxicity

11. Assess extremities for edema because it indicates fluid volume overload

12. Concurrent antibiotic-digoxin therapy can precipitate toxicity because of altering of intestinal flora

13. Monitor client closely when being switched from one administration route to another; often a dose adjustment is required (if tablet form is replaced by elixir, potential for toxicity increases)

14. Be cautious to note the differences in dosing between digoxin (0.125 to 0.5 mg) and digitoxin (0.05 to 0.1 mg)

K. Client education

1. Instruct client to check pulse for 1 full minute prior to taking digoxin; advise to contact physician before taking dose if pulse falls below 60 bpm or raises above 110 or if the skipped beats are present

2. Instruct client to suspect toxicity if any of the following occur:

   a. Nausea

   b. Vomiting

   c. Anorexia

   d. Diarrhea

   e. Visual disturbances (halos, green/yellow lights)

3. Teach client to withhold the next dose of medication if digoxin toxicity is suspected and contact the physician immediately

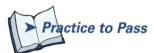

A client is receiving digoxin 0.125 mg PO every morning. Upon arrival to the office, you notice that the HR is 44 bpm. The client reports feeling weak and nauseated. Based on the clinical data, what might cause the low heart rate? What are the priority nursing assessments?

4. Instruct client to weigh self daily with the same clothes and at the same time; report any weight gain greater than 2 lb/day

5. Instruct client to take digoxin as ordered and not to skip or add additional dose if experiencing chest discomfort (a common report from clients admitted with digoxin toxicity is that they take digoxin as a "heart pill" when experiencing a chest pain)

6. Caution client to not take OTC medications or herbal supplements without consulting physician because these medications might have direct adverse effects on the absorption of digoxin

7. Teach client to insist on the original brand of digoxin ordered by the physician to avoid errors in dosing

VI. **Antidysrhythmics**

A. **Class I-A (fast sodium channel blockers)**

1. Action and use

a. Used to treat both atrial and ventricular dysrhythmias; prevent the recurrence of premature ventricular contractions and ventricular tachycardia that are not severe enough to require cardioversion

b. Function by depressing myocardial contractility and excitability and prolonging the **refractory period** (able to respond only to a strong stimulus)

c. Reduce the rate of spontaneous diastolic depolarization in pacemaker cells, thereby suppressing ectopic focal activity

d. Disopyramide shortens sinus node recovery time and increases atrial and ventricular effective refractory period

e. Quinidine is classified as a chemical cardioversion agent useful to convert atrial fibrillation to normal sinus rhythm

2. Common medications (Table 5-6)

3. Administration considerations

a. Give the first dose of disopyramide 6 to 12 hours after the last quinidine dose and 3 to 6 hours after the last procainamide dose

b. Do not administer controlled-release capsules when giving a loading dose, when a rapid control is required, or when the creatinine clearance is less than 40 mL/min

c. Do not crush or open controlled-release capsules as it may deliver a potentially toxic dose of medication

d. Start the controlled-release form of capsule 6 hours after the last dose of the conventional capsule when switching from a conventional capsule to a controlled-release form

4. Contraindications

a. Cardiogenic shock

b. Second or third degree heart block

c. Severe heart failure

Table 5-6	Generic/ Trade Names	Usual Adult Dose	Side Effects	Nursing Implications
Common Antidysrhythmic Medications: Class I–A: Fast Sodium Channel Blockers	Disopyramide (Norpace)	Adult > 50 kg: Total of 400–800 mg/d PO in divided doses Adult < 50 kg: 400 mg/day PO in divided doses	Mild hypotension Blurred vision Dry mouth Urinary hesitancy Constipation GI upset Diarrhea	Check apical pulse before administering the medication. Monitor ECG. Monitor BP, especially during dosage adjustment.
	Moricizine (Ethmozine)	600–900 mg/day PO divided every 8 hr	Drug fever Rash Photosensitivity Pruritis	Monitor I & O. Instruct client to measure daily weight. Instruct client to assess lower extremities for edema daily.
	Procainamide (Pronestyl, Pronestyl SR)	Regular release: 50 mg/kg/ PO q 3 hr PO SR: q 6 hr PO		Advise client to avoid taking OTC medication and consuming alcohol.
	Quinidine (Quinidex)	Regular release: 200-300 mg PO TID to QID SR: 300–600 mg PO q 8-12 hr		

    d. Hypotension

    e. Caution should be used when administering disopyramide in the presence of:

        1) Sick sinus syndrome

        2) Wolff-Parkinson-White (WPW) syndrome

        3) Bundle branch block

        4) Myocarditis or other cardiomyopathy

        5) Hepatic or renal impairment

        6) Urinary tract disease (especially prostatic hypertrophy)

        7) Myasthenia gravis

        8) Angle closure (narrow angle) glaucoma

5. Significant drug interactions

    a. Anticholinergic drugs compound other anticholinergics such as tricyclic antidepressants and antihistamines

    b. Antidysrhythmics compound toxicities

    c. Phenytoin and rifampin may increase metabolism of disopyramide and decrease blood level

    d. Disopyramide may increase warfarin-induced hypoprothrombinemia

6. Significant food interactions: none reported

7. Significant laboratory studies

    a. Baseline and periodic determinations of hepatic and renal function should be made

    b. Assess blood glucose levels and serum potassium levels because hyperkalemia worsens toxic effects; hypokalemia and other electrolyte imbalances should be corrected before therapy is initiated

    c. Electrocardiogram should be followed closely; if the following changes occur, notify physician immediately:

        1) Prolonged QT interval

        2) Worsening of dysrhythmias

        3) Widening of the QRS, greater than 25%

        4) HR less than 60 bpm or greater than 120 bpm

        5) Unusual change in rate, rhythm, or quality of pulse

8. Side effects

    a. Mild hypotension

    b. Blurred vision

    c. Dry mouth

    d. Urinary hesitancy or retention

    e. Constipation

    f. Abdominal cramping, nausea, and vomiting

9. Adverse effects/toxicity

    a. CNS: dizziness, headache, fatigue, muscle weakness, convulsions, paresthesias, nervousness, acute psychosis, and peripheral neuropathy

    b. CV: severe hypotension, chest pain, edema, dyspnea, syncope, bradycardia, tachycardia, increased dysrhythmias, CHF, cardiogenic shock, and heart block

    c. GI: epigastric and abdominal pain, jaundice

    d. GU: profound urinary retention, frequency, urgency, and renal insufficiency

    e. Skin: puritis, urticaria, rash, photosensitivity, and laryngospasm

    f. Drying of nose, throat and bronchial secretions

    g. Uterine contraction during pregnancy, precipitation of myasthenia gravis, agranulocytosis (decreased granulocytes) and thrombocytopenia

10. Nursing considerations

    a. Check apical pulse before administering the medication

    b. Monitor ECG and report any changes to physician immediately

    c. Monitor BP especially during dosage adjustment and if receiving high doses of medication

      d. Monitor I & O especially in elderly and client with impaired renal function, prostatic hypertrophy, and urinary retention/hesitancy

      e. Monitor labs results as appropriate

      f. Assess for peripheral neuritis

  11. Client education

      a. Instruct to measure daily weight and to report weight gain greater than 2 to 4 lb/week

      b. Instruct to assess ankles and tibia daily for edema

      c. Instruct to change position slowly to avoid dizziness and syncope; teach to avoid prolonged periods of standing and to lie down if feeling lightheaded; avoid driving or other hazardous activities if dizzy or lightheaded

      d. Advise to take the medication as prescribed and do not skip doses

      e. Instruct not to stop taking medication abruptly

      f. Advise client not to take OTC medications or drink alcohol without contacting physician

      g. Avoid exposure to sunlight or ultraviolet radiation

      h. Inform client to notify all other healthcare providers of medication and have regular eye exams for glaucoma

  B. Class I-B

    1. Action and use

      a. Decreases the refractory period

      b. Suppresses automaticity in the Bundle of His-Purkinje system

      c. Elevates the electrical stimulation threshold of ventricle during diastole

      d. Treats or prevents ventricular dysrhythmias

    2. Common medications (Table 5-7)

Table 5-7

Common Antiarrhythmic Medications: Class I–B

Generic/ Trade Names	Usual Adult Dose	Side Effects	Nursing Implications
Lidocaine (Anestacon, Xylocaine)	IV:50–100 mg bolus at a rate of 20–50 mg/min, may repeat in 5 min, then start infusion of 20–50 µg/kg/min	Dizziness Vertigo Lightheadedness Hypotension Nausea Drowsiness Worsening CHF Confusion	Assess CNS frequently during infusion (lidocaine). Auscultate breath sounds for crackles. Assess serum blood levels. Instruct client to avoid taking OTC medications.
Mexiletine (Mexitil)	200-400 mg PO q 8 hr up to 1,200 mg/day	Dyspnea Heart block Tinnitus Tremors	
Tocainide (Tonocard)	400-600 mg PO q 8 hr		

3. Administration considerations

   NCLEX!

   a. Bolus dose of lidocaine may be given undiluted via IVP at a rate of 25 to 50 mg/min

   b. Add 1 g lidocaine to 250 to 500 mL of D_5W for infusions; flow rate should not be more than 4 mg/mL

   c. Use microdropper and infusion pump for an infusion

   d. Discontinue IV infusion as soon as the client's basic cardiac rhythm stabilizes

   e. Hypokalemia should be corrected prior to initiating tocainide

4. Contraindications

   a. History of hypersensitivity to amide-type anesthetics

   b. Stokes-Adams syndrome

   c. Untreated sinus bradycardia

   NCLEX!

   d. Severe degrees of SA, AV, and intraventricular heart block

   e. Use cautiously with:

   1) Hepatic or renal disease

   2) CHF

   3) Hypovolemia or shock

   4) Myasthenia gravis

   5) Debilitated clients or elderly

   6) Family history of malignant hyperthermia

5. Significant drug interactions

   a. Barbiturates decrease lidocaine activity

   b. Beta blockers, quinidine, phenytoin, and procainamide increase the effect of lidocaine

   c. Phenytoin and cefazolin are incompatible with lidocaine infusion

6. Significant food interactions: none reported

7. Significant laboratory studies

   a. Lidocaine levels should be assessed

   1) Therapeutic level is 1.5 to 6 μg/mL

   2) Potentially toxic level is greater than 7 μg/mL

   NCLEX!

   b. Assess electrolytes and correct hypokalemia before treating with antidysrhythmics

   c. Check baseline hepatic and renal blood studies

8. Side effects

   a. Drowsiness

   b. Lightheadedness

   c. Mild hypotension

9. Adverse effects/toxicity

   a. CNS: restlessness, confusions, disorientation, irritability, apprehension, euphoria, wild excitement, numbness of lips or tongue and other paresthesias, chest heaviness, and difficulty speaking

   b. Dyspnea and difficulty swallowing, muscular twitching, tremors, psychosis, convulsions and respiratory depression with high doses

   c. CV: hypotension, bradycardia, heart block, cardiovascular collapse, and cardiac arrest

   d. Ear: tinnitus and decreased hearing

   e. Eye: severe blurred vision, double vision, and impaired color perception

   f. GI: anorexia, nausea, vomiting, and excessive perspiration

   g. Skin: urticaria, rash, edema, and anaphylactoid reactions

10. Nursing considerations

   a. Assess ECG for changes including prolonged PR interval, widened QRS, aggravation of dysrhythmias, and heart block

   b. Monitor BP frequently

   c. Assess CNS status at baseline and frequently during infusions

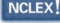

   d. Administer via infusion pump and observe rate carefully

   e. Auscultate breath sounds for crackles and monitor respiratory rate

   f. Assess serum blood levels

11. Client education

   a. Instruct client to notify physician if lightheadedness, dizziness, confusion, numbness or tingling of lips, tongue or fingers, and visual changes or ringing in ears occur

   b. Instruct client to notify physician if unusual CNS changes occur, as well as nausea, vomiting, or yellowish changes in whites of eyes or skin (jaundice) when taking oral forms of medication

   c. Advise client not to take any OTC medications or herbal supplements without consulting physician

   d. Instruct client to take medications as prescribed without skipping doses

C. Class I-C

1. Action and use

   a. Decrease automaticity and conductivity through the AV node and ventricles

   b. Are used to treat life-threatening ventricular dysrhythmias

2. Common medications (Table 5-8)

3. Administration considerations

   a. Medications are available in oral forms

   b. Increasing dosages are not recommended more frequently than every 4 days especially with elderly or clients with previous extensive myocardial damage

	Generic/ Trade Names	Usual Adult Dose	Side Effects	Nursing Implications
Table 5-8 **Common Antiarrhythmic Medications: Class I–C**	Flecainide (Tambocor)	50–100 mg PO q 12 hr up to 300 mg/day	Dizziness Blurred vision Nausea Headache Lightheadedness	Treat hypokalemia before initiating the therapy. Monitor ECG rhythm for any changes. Instruct client to report any visual changes. Advise client to avoid taking OTC medications.
	Propafenone (Rythmol)	150–300 mg PO q 8 hr up to 900 mg/day total dose	Dyspnea Palpitation Fatigue Chest pain Tremors	

c. Dosage reduction should be considered in severe liver dysfunction and with significant widening of the QRS complex

4. Contraindications

 a. Hypersensitivity to flecainide

 b. Severe degrees of heart block

 c. Intraventricular blocks

 d. Cardiogenic shock

 e. Hepatic failure

5. Significant drug interactions

 a. Cimetidine may increase flecainide levels

 b. Flecainide may increase digoxin levels by 25%

 c. Beta-blockers enhance negative inotropic effects

6. Significant food interactions: none reported

7. Significant laboratory studies

 a. Assess baseline electrolytes

 b. Monitor serum levels

  1) Effective trough level is 0.7 to 1 µg/mL

  2) Toxic trough level is greater than 1 µg/mL

 c. Monitor blood levels frequently if client is taking digoxin

8. Side effects

 a. Slight dizziness

 b. Blurred vision

 c. Nausea

9. Adverse effects/toxicity

 a. CNS: headache, prolonged lightheadedness, unsteadiness, paresthesias, fatigue, and fever

    b. CV: worsening dysrhythmias, chest pain, CHF, edema, and dyspnea

    c. Eye: prolonged blurred vision and spots before eyes

    d. GI: prolonged nausea, constipation, and changes in taste perception

10. Nursing considerations

    a. Assess laboratory data and treat hypokalemia/hyperkalemia before initiating therapy

    b. Monitor ECG rhythm for changes, including worsening of dysrhythmias; client may need Holter monitoring for ambulatory assessment

    c. Determine the threshold levels of pacemaker before initiating medication and at regular intervals thereafter

11. Client education

    a. Take medications as prescribed without skipping doses

    b. Instruct to report any visual changes

    c. Do not take any OTC medications or herbal supplements without consulting physician

    d. Stress the importance of follow-up care

D. Class II (Beta-blockers): see previous section II

E. Class III (potassium channel blockers)

    1. Action and use

        a. Prolongs repolarization and refractory period

        b. Decreases intraventricular conduction

        c. Used to treat ventricular tachycardia and ventricular fibrillation

        d. May also be used to treat supraventricular tachycardias

    2. Common medication: amiodarone (Cordarone, Pacerone)

    3. Administration considerations

        a. Gastroenteritis symptoms may occur with high oral dose therapy and loading dose

        b. Intravenous dose for first 24 hours

            1) Prepare loading dose by adding 150 mg amiodarone to 100 mL D_5W; rapidly infuse at 15 mg/mL over 10 minutes via infusion pump

            2) Add 900 mg amiodarone to 500 mL D_5W to yield 1.8 mg/mL; infuse at 1mg/min over 6 hours

            3) Decrease the rate after 6 hours to 0.5 mg/min for the remaining 18 hours

        c. After the first 24 hours:

            1) Use a concentration of 1 to 6 mg/mL and infuse at 0.5 mg/min (720 mg/24h)

2) Use a central line if the rate exceeds 2 mg/mL

3) Infusion rate may be increased to achieve desired effect; must use an infusion pump

4. Contraindications

a. Hypersensitivity to amiodarone

b. Cardiogenic shock

c. Severe sinus bradycardia

d. Severe degrees of heart block

e. Hepatic disease

f. Use cautiously in: Hashimoto's thyroiditis, goiter, hyperthyroidism or hypothyroidism, CHF, electrolyte imbalance, preexisting pulmonary disease, cardiac surgery, and sensitivity to iodine

5. Significant drug interactions

a. Increases digoxin levels

b. Enhances effects and toxicities of disopyramide, procainamide, quinidine, flecainide, lidocaine, cyclosporine

c. Enhances anticoagulant effects

d. Bradycardia effects are greater when used with verapamil, diltiazem, and beta-adrenergic blockers

e. Increases phenytoin blood levels 2- to 3-fold

f. Cimetidine and ritonavir may increase amiodarone levels and toxicity

g. Cholestyramine may decrease amiodarone levels

6. Significant food interactions: none reported

7. Significant laboratory studies

a. Thyroid function test abnormalities (in the absence of thyroid function impairments)

b. Baseline and periodic serum assessments of:

1) Liver enzymes: aspartate aminotransferase (AST) and alanine aminotransferase (ALT)

2) Lung: pulmonary function tests, ABG's

3) Thyroid

8. Side effects

a. Skin and corneal pigmentation (lipofuscinosis) in client receiving drug longer than 2 months; reversible in 7 months after discontinuing drug

    b. Muscle weakness

    c. Hypotension

    d. Mild anorexia, nausea, and constipation

  9. Adverse reactions/toxicity

    a. CNS: peripheral neuropathy, muscle wasting, weakness, fatigue, abnormal gait, dyskinesia, dizziness, paresthesias, and headache

    b. CV: bradycardia, severe hypotension, sinus arrest, cardiogenic shock, CHF, worsening dysrhythmias, and heart block

    c. Eye: corneal microdeposits, blurred vision, optic neuritis, optic neuropathy, permanent blindness, corneal degeneration, macular degeneration, and photosensitivity

    d. Respiratory: alveolitis, pneumonitis, and interstitial pulmonary fibrosis

    e. Skin: slate-blue pigmentation to skin and rash

    f. GI: severe anorexia, nausea, vomiting, and constipation

    g. Angioedema, hyperthyroidism or hypothyroidism, and hepatotoxicity

  10. Nursing considerations

    a. Monitor BP during IV infusion and titrate to prevent hypotension and bradycardia

NCLEX!

    b. Monitor client continually due to unusually long half-life of the medication (10 to 55 days)

    c. Check laboratory and other reports for liver, lung, thyroid, GI and neurological dysfunction

    d. Baseline and regular ophthalmic examinations with a slit-lamp are recommended throughout therapy

NCLEX!

    e. Report adverse reactions promptly

NCLEX!

    f. Be alert to signs of pulmonary toxicity: dyspnea, fatigue, cough, pleuritic pain or fever; auscultate breath sounds for adventitious sounds

    g. Monitor client for CNS changes, which generally develop within a week after amiodarone therapy begins; muscle weakness and tremors are a potential safety risk

    h. Observe client already receiving other antiarrhythmic therapy for adverse effects, especially heart block and worsening dysrhythmias

  11. Client education

NCLEX!

    a. Instruct client to assess pulse daily and report a HR less than 60 bpm

    b. Instruct client to notify all healthcare providers of medication

    c. Advise client to have regular ophthalmic examinations

NCLEX!

    d. Photophobia may be eased by wearing darkened glasses but some clients should avoid daylight entirely

NCLEX!

    e. Alert client to the erythema and pruritus that may develop when exposed to ultraviolet radiation; clients should avoid sunlight, tanning beds and sunlamps

    f. Instruct client to wear protective clothing and a barrier-type sunblock to avoid exposure to the sun (zinc-oxide or titanium-oxide preparations)

    g. Inform client that the blue-gray skin pigmentation (found after 1 year) may slowly disappear after medication is stopped

    h. Instruct client to take the medication as prescribed without skipping doses

    i. Advise client to avoid taking OTC medications or herbal supplements without consulting physician

    j. Stress the importance of follow-up care

F. Class IV (calcium channel blockers): see previous section III

G. Other antiarrhythmics (miscellaneous)

  1. Action and use

    a. Slow conduction through the SA and AV nodes

    b. Interrupt the reentry pathways through the AV node

    c. Depress left ventricular function (very temporary)

    d. Treat supraventricular dysrhythmias

  2. Common medication: adenosine (Adenocard, Adenoscan)

  3. Administration considerations

    a. Rapid IV bolus

      1) Administer directly into vein as proximal to the insertion site as possible; the half-life is only 10 seconds

      2) Administer over 1 to 2 seconds

      3) Follow with a rapid normal saline flush

    b. The solution contains no preservatives so it must be clear; discard any unused portion

    c. Expect sudden slowing of the HR or even asystole for a brief period of time; do not repeat dose if a high grade of AV heart block develops after the first dose

    d. Must be stored at room temperature to avoid crystallization; if crystals appear, dissolve by warming to room temperature

  4. Contraindications

    a. Severe degrees of heart block

    b. Sick sinus syndrome (without a pacemaker)

    c. Atrial fibrillation or atrial flutter

    d. Ventricular tachycardia

    e. Use cautiously with asthma, pregnancy, hepatic failure, and renal failure

  5. Significant drug interactions

    a. Dipyridamole can potentiate the effects of adenosine

    b. Theophylline will block electrophysiologic effects of adenosine

    c. Carbamazepine may increase risk of heart block

  6. Significant food interactions: none reported

  7. Significant laboratory studies: none reported

  8. Side effects

    a. During conversion to sinus rhythm (SR) many dysrhythmias can occur

      1) Sinus bradycardia

      2) Sinus arrest

      3) Sinus tachycardia

      4) Premature ventricular contractions (PVCs)

      5) Premature atrial contractions (PACs)

      6) Various degrees of heart block

    b. Facial flushing

  9. Adverse effects/toxicity

    a. Transient dyspnea

    b. Dysrhythmias

    c. Hypotension

  10. Nursing considerations

    a. Monitor ECG continuously

    b. Evaluate baseline BP, HR, and respiration

    c. Must be administered very quickly over 1 to 2 seconds and followed by a rapid NS flush; if given too slowly, the medication will have no effect

    d. Monitor HR and BP every 15 minutes after administration until stable

    e. Monitor carefully for bronchospasm especially in clients with asthma

  11. Client education

    a. Alert client to various forms of monitoring during the medication administration

    b. Inform client about transient facial flushing

VII. Anticoagulants, Antiplatelets, Thrombolytics, and Medications to Lower Cholesterol: refer to Chapter 4

VIII. Antihypertensives, Antihypotensives, Diuretics, Potassium Supplementation: refer to Chapter 12

Case Study

T. A., a 46-year-old client is being discharged after suffering an acute myocardial infarction (MI). Discharge medications include aspirin (ASA) 600 mg PO daily, Furosemide (Lasix) 20 mg PO every morning, atorvastatin (Lipitor) 10 mg PO daily and propranolol (Inderal LA) 160 mg PO q hs.

❶ What information do you need to know about this client before addressing discharge medications?

❷ What assessments would you make before teaching T. A.? What is the rationale for the selected assessments?

❸ What information would you teach about each medication?

❹ T. A. asks if the medication may be stopped during vacation. How would you respond and what is your rationale?

❺ How would you assess the effectiveness of your teaching?

For suggested responses, see page 638.

Posttest

1 The nurse is caring for a client with chronic angina pectoris. The client is receiving sotalol (Betapace) 80 mg PO daily. Which client manifestation would the nurse conclude is a side effect of this medication?

(1) Difficulty swallowing
(2) Diaphoresis
(3) Dry mouth
(4) Bradycardia

2 The nurse is caring for a client with a history of mild congestive heart failure (CHF) who is receiving diltiazem (Cardizem) for hypertension. The nurse would assess the client for which side effects of this medication?

(1) Tachycardia and rebound hypertension
(2) Wheezing and shortness of breath
(3) Bradycardia and peripheral edema
(4) Chest pain and tachycardia

3 The nurse has just administered a dose of hydralazine (Apresoline) intravenously to a client. After the initial dose, which of the following measurements is the priority assessment?

(1) Cardiac rhythm
(2) Oxygen saturation
(3) Blood pressure
(4) Respiratory rate

4 The nurse has begun a continuous infusion of nitroglycerin (Nitrostat) intravenously. Which of the following indicates to the nurse that the client is experiencing an adverse reaction?

(1) Pulmonary capillary wedge pressure (PCWP) falling from 13 to 11 mm Hg
(2) Central venous pressure (CVP) falling from 10 to 7 mm Hg
(3) Heart rate (HR) falling from 96 to 78
(4) Blood pressure (BP) falling from 130/80 to 90/64

5 The nurse is caring for a client with chronic stable angina receiving amlodipine (Norvasc). In developing a medication teaching plan, the nurse should include which of the following findings as an adverse reaction to this medication?

(1) Hypertension
(2) Hypotension
(3) Constipation
(4) Diarrhea

6 A female client tells the nurse, "since I have been taking that medicine I feel so tired." She is being treated with atenolol (Tenormin) for hypertension. The client's statement is reflective of which nursing diagnosis?

(1) Activity intolerance
(2) Ineffective cerebral tissue perfusion
(3) Ineffective health maintenance
(4) Self-care deficit

7 The nurse is scheduled to administer a dose of digoxin (Lanoxin) to an adult client with atrial fibrillation. The client has a potassium level of 4.6 mEq/L. The nurse interprets that the:

(1) Dose should be omitted only for that day.
(2) Client needs a dose of potassium before receiving the digoxin.
(3) Dose should be withheld and the physician notified.
(4) Dose should be administered as ordered.

8 The nurse is planning to care for a client with congestive heart failure being treated with digoxin (Lanoxin) and furosemide (Lasix). Which of the following dinners would be the best choice from the daily menu?

(1) Beef vegetable soup, macaroni and cheese, and a dinner roll
(2) Beef ravioli, spinach soufflé, and Italian bread
(3) Baked white fish, mashed potatoes, and carrot-raisin salad
(4) Roasted chicken breast, brown rice, and stewed tomatoes

9 The physician has prescribed propranolol (Inderal) for a client with frequent premature ventricular contractions (PVCs). The nurse collects material to conduct an education session with the client. Which of the following should the nurse plan to include in the teaching session?

(1) A description of other effective medications
(2) Information about side effects and adverse reactions
(3) Material about the cellular effect of the medication
(4) Data regarding various dysrhythmias

10 Chemical cardioversion is prescribed for a client in atrial fibrillation. The nurse prepares which of the following medications specifically for chemical cardioversion?

(1) Quinidine (Quinidex)
(2) Verapamil (Calan)
(3) Nifedipine (Procardia)
(4) Lidocaine (Xylocaine)

See pages 225–226 for Answers and Rationales.

Answers and Rationales

Pretest

1 Answer 2 *Rationale:* Teach client that the activity in which he or she engaged may be causing the chest pain. Instruct the client in the exact method of taking NTG to avoid dizziness. The teaching about the frequency of the medication must be accurate and specific to prevent overdose as could happen in option 4. Option 1 is incorrect because NTG becomes unstable when exposed to heat, light, and moisture. Option 3 is incorrect because the client shouldn't drive for safety reasons.
Cognitive Level: Application
Nursing Process: Implementation; *Test Plan:* PHYS

2 Answer: 3 *Rationale:* Nitroglycerine patches and ointments must be rotated daily to a hairless area to reduce skin irritation. Options 2 and 4 are incorrect statements, while option 1 is only partially correct.
Cognitive Level: Application
Nursing Process: Implementation; *Test Plan:* PHYS

3 Answer: 2 *Rationale:* It is important to monitor the apical-radial pulse for a full minute before the administration of digoxin. Record and report significant changes from the client's own baseline data. Without solid data regarding client's baseline, it is prudent to report a heart rate less than 60, since bradycardia could indicate drug toxicity. Depression,

respiratory rate, and blood pressure are unrelated to this medication.
Cognitive Level: Application
Nursing Process: Implementation; *Test Plan:* PHYS

4 **Answer: 3** *Rationale:* The blood pressure and heart rate must be monitored closely during titration to prevent hypotension and tachycardia. Shortness of breath is important but not directly related to NTG infusion. Respirations, urine output, and headache do not determine the titration rate. Headache frequently occurs and is treated commonly with acetaminophen or another mild analgesic.
Cognitive Level: Application
Nursing Process: Assessment; *Test Plan:* PHYS

5 **Answer: 1** *Rationale:* Metoprolol is a beta-blocking agent which blocks the effects of both β_1 and β_2 receptors, leading to a reduction in systemic vascular resistance. This effect also may lead to bronchospasm (from broncho constriction secondary to β_2 blockade), and therefore metoprolol would be contraindicated in clients with bronchospastic illness. The drug has no effect on seizure activity or on myasthenia gravis, a neuromuscular disorder.
Cognitive Level: Application
Nursing Process: Analysis; *Test Plan:* SECE

6 **Answer: 4** *Rationale:* Verapamil is a calcium channel blocker used to treat angina. Constipation is a frequent complaint of clients taking the sustained-release form of verapamil. Many elderly clients have difficulty with this, and the nurse must anticipate the need for teaching about increasing fiber and fluid intake. Hypotension is an adverse reaction to verapamil. Skin rash is unrelated to the medication.
Cognitive Level: Application
Nursing Process: Assessment; *Test Plan:* PHYS

7 **Answer: 1** *Rationale:* Early indications of toxicity to lidocaine include various central nervous system (CNS) complications. These may include slurred speech, dizziness, confusion, and paresthesias. If they are ignored, the client can develop seizures that are often difficult to stop and death may ensue. Sinus tachycardia is unfortunate but unrelated to lidocaine. Concerns about the myocardial infarction are normal and should be addressed. Leg cramps are unrelated to lidocaine use.
Cognitive Level: Analysis
Nursing Process: Analysis; *Test Plan:* PHYS

8 **Answer: 2** *Rationale:* Digoxin is classified as a positive inotropic drug. It increases contractility (inotropy) of heart, whereas propranolol (a beta-blocker)

and verapamil (a calcium channel blocker) are negative inotropic medications. Atropine has a neutral effect on contractility.
Cognitive Level: Comprehension
Nursing Process: Analysis; *Test Plan:* PHYS

9 **Answer: 3** *Rationale:* Lidocaine IV is used to treat ventricular dysrhythmias (premature ventricular contractions, ventricular tachycardia, and ventricular fibrillation), particularly in clients with a myocardial infarction. It is a class 1-A antiarrhythmic. The drug causes no anesthetic effect unless the client receives an overdose that is evidenced by a central nervous system deficit (paresthesias, confusion, and slurred speech). Lidocaine may cause drowsiness but is not used for relaxation (option 2). It is not a diuretic (option 4).
Cognitive Level: Analysis
Nursing Process: Implementation; *Test Plan:* SECE

10 **Answer: 2** *Rationale:* The side effects of amiodarone take several weeks or longer to manifest themselves. Sometimes they persist for up to 4 months, and because photosensitivity is a continuing concern, the client should avoid tanning. The pulse should be monitored and if it remains above 100 the physician should be notified. If a dose is missed, the client should call the physician before taking any more medication.
Cognitive Level: Analysis
Nursing Process: Evaluation; *Test Plan:* SECE

Posttest

1 **Answer: 4** *Rationale:* Sotalol is a beta-adrenergic blocking agent. Side effects include bradycardia, difficulty breathing, wheezing, bronchospasm, GI disturbances, anxiety, nervousness, weakness, mood changes, depression and loss of libido. Options 1, 2, and 3 do not occur.
Cognitive Level: Analysis
Nursing Process: Assessment; *Test Plan:* PHYS

2 **Answer: 3** *Rationale:* Calcium channel blocker agents, such as diltiazem (Cardizem) are used cautiously in clients with aortic stenosis, bradycardia, CHF, acute myocardial infarction, and hypotension. The nurse would assess for signs that indicate worsening of these underlying conditions. Bradycardia and peripheral edema are adverse effects of this class of information, and require follow-up if they occur.
Cognitive Level: Application
Nursing Process: Assessment; *Test Plan:* PHYS

3 **Answer: 3** *Rationale:* Hydralazine (Apresoline) is a powerful vasodilator that exerts its action on the

smooth muscle walls of arterioles. After a parenteral dose, blood pressure is checked every 15 minutes until stable and then every 1 hour. Although options 1, 2 and 4 are components of assessment, they are not directly related to the action of the medication.
Cognitive Level: Application
Nursing Process: Assessment; *Test Plan:* PHYS

4 Answer: 4 *Rationale:* Nitroglycerin is an antianginal of the nitrate type that causes vasodilation of coronary and other arteries. It would be expected to cause a decrease in PCWP and CVP. The heart rate could also decrease with overall improvement in cardiac output. A decrease in BP from 130/80 to 90/64 is excessive and warrants further assessment by the nurse to determine whether perfusion to major organs is adequate.
Cognitive Level: Application
Nursing Process: Analysis; *Test Plan:* PHYS

5 Answer: 2 *Rationale:* Amlodipine (Norvasc) is a calcium channel blocker. Adverse or toxic reactions from overdosage may produce excessive peripheral vasodilation and marked hypotension with reflex tachycardia. Frequent side effects include peripheral edema, headache, and flushing. Some sustained-release forms of calcium channel blockers (such as Calan SR) may lead to constipation, a milder side effect than the others.
Cognitive Level: Application
Nursing Process: Assessment; *Test Plan:* PHYS

6 Answer: 1 *Rationale:* Atenolol is a beta adrenergic blocker that causes a decreased heart rate, blood pressure, and cardiac output. Fatigue is the most common side effect. If fatigue becomes severe enough, it could interfere with the client's activity level. Activity intolerance is the state in which an individual had insufficient energy to complete activities of daily living. There is no evidence that the client has Ineffective cerebral tissue perfusion, Ineffective health maintenance, or Self-care deficit.
Cognitive Level: Analysis
Nursing Process: Analysis; *Test Plan:* PHYS

7 Answer: 4 *Rationale:* The normal reference range for potassium for an adult is 3.5 to 5.1 mEq/L. Hy-

pokalemia can make the client more susceptible to digitalis toxicity. The nurse monitors the results of electrolytes for the potassium level. If the potassium level is low, the dose is withheld, and the physician is notified. This client's result is in the normal range, so the dose should be administered.
Cognitive Level: Analysis
Nursing Process: Analysis; *Test Plan:* PHYS

8 Answer: 3 *Rationale:* Lasix depletes potassium stores, and a client taking digoxin and furosemide needs to maintain normal potassium levels and moderate salt intake. Hypokalemia makes the client more susceptible to digitalis toxicity. Option 3 is the best choice because all three foods are high in potassium and low in sodium.
Cognitive Level: Application
Nursing Process: Planning; *Test Plan:* PHYS

9 Answer: 2 *Rationale:* The medication has side effects that could be disturbing to the client. These include hypotension, insomnia, lethargy, bronchospasm, mood changes, and decreased libido. The client should be alert to these so that they can notify the physician or other healthcare provider. It is not the nurse's role to describe alternatives to the currently ordered medication (option 1). It is unnecessary to teach about effects at the cellular level (option 3) unless the client has interest in this. It is also unnecessary to teach the client about various dysrhythmias (option 4) because this is not pertinent.
Cognitive Level: Application
Nursing Process: Planning; *Test Plan:* HPM

10 Answer: 1 *Rationale:* Quinidine (Quinidex) is a Class I-A antiarrhythmic that is very effective as a chemical cardioversion agent. Verapamil is a calcium channel blocker generally used to control heart rate. Nifedipine is a calcium channel blocker used as a vasodilator. Lidocaine is generally used for control of ventricular dysrhythmias.
Cognitive Level: Application
Nursing Process: Implementation; *Test Plan:* PHYS

References

American Heart Association (2000). *Handbook of emergency cardiovascular care for healthcare providers.* Dallas, TX: American Heart Association.

Black, J., Hawks, J. & Keene, A. (2000). *Medical-surgical nursing: Clinical management for continuity of care* (6th ed.). Philadelphia: W. B. Saunders, p. 1302.

Clark, J., Queener, S., & Karb, V. (2003). *Pharmacologic basis of nursing practice* (7th ed.). St. Louis: Mosby-Year Book, pp. 232–249.

Deglin, J., & Vallerand, A. (2003). *Davis's drug guide for nurses* (8th ed.). Philadelphia, PA: F. A. Davis.

Hartshorn, J., Sole, M., & Lamborn, H. (2000). *Introduction to critical care nursing* (3rd ed.). Philadelphia: W. B. Saunders.

Ignatavicius, D. D., & Workman, M. L. (2003). *Medical-surgical nursing: Critical thinking for collaborative care* (4th ed.). Philadelphia: W. B. Saunders, p. 992.

Kidd, P. S., & Wagner, K. D. (2001). *High acuity nursing* (3rd ed.). Upper Saddle River, NJ: Prentice Hall.

Lemone, P., & Burke, K. M. (2003). *Medical surgical nursing: Critical thinking in client care* (3rd ed.). Upper Saddle River, NJ: Prentice Hall.

McKenry, L., & Salerno, E. (2003). *Mosby's pharmacology in nursing* (21st ed.). St. Louis: Mosby, p. 612.

Shannon, M., Wilson, B., & Stang, C. (2003). *Health professional drug guide 2003.* Upper Saddle River NJ: Prentice Hall.

CHAPTER 6

Endocrine System Medications

Bethany Hawes Sykes, EdD, RN, CEN

CHAPTER OUTLINE

Medications Affecting the Pituitary Gland

Medications Affecting the Adrenal Glands

Medications Affecting the Thyroid Glands

Medications Affecting the Parathyroid Glands

Medications Used to Treat Diabetes Mellitus

OBJECTIVES

▌ Describe the general goals of therapy when administering endocrine system medications.

▌ Describe the action, use, and nursing considerations related to the administration of medications used to treat diabetes insipidus.

▌ Identify the nursing considerations related to the administration of thyroid replacement medications.

▌ Discuss the medications used to treat hyperthyroidism.

▌ List the client teaching points related to the administration of calcium and vitamin D supplements.

▌ Identify the characteristics of various types of insulin.

▌ Identify the side effects and complications associated with the use of glucocorticoids.

▌ Discuss the nursing considerations related to the administration of insulin.

▌ Describe the significant client teaching points related to the administration of medications used to treat diabetes mellitus.

▌ List the significant client education points related to various endocrine system medications.

[Media Link]

Use the CD-ROM enclosed with this text, or log onto the address given to access the free, interactive Companion Website created for this series. The CD-ROM and Companion Website accompanying this book offer additional practice opportunities and information—NCLEX Review, Case Studies, Glossary, In Depth with NCLEX, and more.

www.prenhall.com/hogan

REVIEW AT A GLANCE

Addison's disease *life-threatening disease caused by partial or complete failure of adrenocortical function*

adrenal crisis *an acute, life-threatening state of profound adrenocortical insufficiency requiring immediate therapy*

adrenal insufficiency *a condition in which the adrenal gland is unable to produce adequate amounts of adrenocortical hormones*

catecholamine *any one of a group of sympathomimetic compounds composed of a catechol molecule and the aliphatic portion of an amine; some are produced naturally by the body and function as key neurologic chemicals*

cushingoid state *having the habitus and facies characteristic of Cushing's disease, including fat pads on the upper back and face, ruddy complexion, striae on trunk, thin legs, and excess facial hair*

glucocorticoid *an adrenocortical steroid hormone that increases glycogenesis, exerts an anti-inflammatory effect, and influences many body functions*

glycosylated hemoglobin *concentration representative of the average blood glucose level over the previous several weeks*

Graves' disease *a disorder characterized by pronounced hyperthyroidism usually associated with an enlarged thyroid gland and exophthalmos; also called thyrotoxicosis*

hypercalciuria *the presence of abnormally great amounts of calcium in the urine resulting from conditions characterized by augmented bone resorption*

hyperglycemia *a greater than normal amount of glucose in the blood most frequently associated with diabetes mellitus, post-administration of glucocorticoids, and with excessive infusion of glucose-containing intravenous solutions*

hyperthyroidism *a condition characterized by hyperactivity of the thyroid gland; the gland is usually enlarged, secreting greater than normal amounts of thyroid hormones, and the metabolic processes of the body are accelerated*

hypoglycemia *a less than normal amount of glucose in the blood, usually caused by administration of too much insulin, excessive secretion of insulin by the islet cells of the pancreas, or dietary deficiency*

hypoparathyroidism *a condition of insufficient secretion of parathyroid glands caused by primary parathyroid dysfunction or by elevated serum calcium level*

hypothyroidism *a condition characterized by decreased activity of the thyroid gland caused by surgical removal of all or part of the thyroid gland, over dosage with antithyroid medication, decreased effect of thyroid releasing hormone secreted by the hypothalamus, decreased secretion of thyroid stimulating hormone by the pi-*

tuitary gland, or atrophy of the thyroid gland itself

lipodystrophy *any abnormality in the metabolism or deposition of fats*

mineralocorticoid *a steroid hormone that acts on the kidney to promote retention of sodium and water and excretion of potassium and hydrogen*

myxedema *the most severe from of hypothyroidism characterized by swelling of the hands, face, feet, and periorbital tissues and may lead to coma and death*

osteomalacia *an abnormal condition of the lamellar bone, characterized by a loss of calcification of the matrix resulting in softening of the bone and accompanied by weakness, fracture, pain, anorexia, and weight loss*

osteoporosis *a disorder characterized by abnormal loss of bone density most frequently seen in postmenopausal women, sedentary or immobilized individuals, and clients receiving long-term steroid therapy*

Paget's disease *a common nonmetabolic disease of bone of unknown cause, usually affecting middle-aged and elderly people, characterized by excessive bone destruction and unorganized bone repair*

Pretest

1 A mother comes to the clinic with her 5-year-old son. She is concerned that he is not growing fast enough and asks the nurse if he can receive growth hormone (GH). Which of the following would be the best response by the nurse?

(1) "Growth hormone will only affect your child's short bones."
(2) "Can your son swallow pills easily?"
(3) "Growth hormone is only given to children if there is a documented lack of growth hormone."
(4) "How tall do you want him to be?"

2 A client has been receiving high doses of glucocorticoids for several weeks. The client asks the nurse when he can stop taking the medication. The nurse's response incorporates which of the following information?

(1) Even at high doses, adverse reactions are unlikely if the medication is abruptly withdrawn.
(2) If steroid medication is withdrawn suddenly, a client could die of acute adrenal insuffficiency.
(3) The client may experience severe psychological symptoms when the medication is withdrawn.
(4) Tapering of the medication requires daily assessment of serum chemistries.

3 A client recently diagnosed with diabetes insipidus is to receive desmopressin (DDAVP). The client expresses concern about possible inability to properly self-administer the medication. In responding to the client, the nurse conveys that this medication is not given by which of the following routes?

(1) Intramuscular
(2) Intravenous
(3) Intranasal
(4) Subcutaneous

4 A client with Addison's disease is taking fludrocortisone (Florinef) for replacement therapy. In evaluating the effects of drug therapy, the nurse anticipates that which of the following may occur when high doses of this drug are given?

(1) Excess sodium and water are retained and potassium is depleted.
(2) Sodium and water are depleted, and potassium is retained.
(3) Hypotension and hypokalemia may develop.
(4) It may lead to toxic effects when given with any glucocorticoid.

5 A client newly diagnosed with hypothyroidism is placed on levothyroxine sodium (Synthroid). The client asks when his lack of energy will improve. The nurse's response includes which of the following?

(1) Lack of energy is probably caused by depression and not hypothyroidism.
(2) Dramatic improvement in energy levels can be experienced usually in 1 to 2 days.
(3) The drug works best when taken after a full meal.
(4) Optimum effectiveness of the drug may not occur for several weeks.

6 A client with hypothyroidism is prescribed liotrix (Thyrolar). The nurse teaches the client which of the following signs and symptoms of thyrotoxicosis prior to discharge?

(1) Bradycardia and hypothermia
(2) Tachycardia and hyperthermia
(3) Unusual lethargy and inability to keep awake
(4) Complaints of chills and dry skin

7 A client with Graves' disease who has been taking propylthiouracil (PTU) for 6 weeks complains of a sore throat and fever. The nurse concludes that this complaint may be an early sign of which of the following?

(1) Hyperthyroidism
(2) Hyperpituitarism
(3) Agranulocytosis
(4) Hemophilus influenzae

8 A client with Paget's disease is prescribed calcitonin (Calcimar). The nurse tells the client that the purpose of this drug is to do which of the following?

(1) Decrease mobilization of calcium from the bone
(2) Increase intestinal absorption of calcium
(3) Promote urinary retention of calcium
(4) Provide gradual lowering of blood calcium levels

9 A nurse is caring for a client who is receiving insulin. For which of the following signs of hypoglycemic reaction should the nurse observe the client?

(1) Fruity breath
(2) Flushing of the face
(3) Hunger
(4) Dry, flaky skin

10 The nurse is evaluating the client's knowledge of treatment if an insulin reaction occurs. Which of the following actions is most appropriate for the client to understand?

(1) Notify the doctor
(2) Inject a dose of regular insulin
(3) Lie down and wait for the reaction to disappear
(4) Take an oral form of glucose

See pages 262–263 for Answers and Rationales.

I. Medications Affecting the Pituitary Gland

A. Growth hormone (GH)

1. Action and use

    a. Action: determines adult physical size by regulating growth of organs and tissues, specifically length of long bones

    b. Use: approved only for use in children to treat growth hormone deficiency or inadequate growth hormone secretion related to documented lack of growth hormone

2. Common medications (Table 6-1)

3. Administration considerations

    a. Is only given parenterally (IM or SC); oral route is inactivated by digestive enzymes

    b. Is packaged in powder form and is reconstituted for administration with 1 to 5 mL of approved diluent; mixture must be clear and not cloudy or contain any undissolved particles; label date of reconstitution and discard refrigerated drug according to manufacturer's directions

    c. Rotate IM sites and use appropriate needle length to inject into muscle layer

4. Contraindications

    a. To stimulate growth in children who are short unrelated to growth hormone deficiency; during or after closure of epiphyseal plates in long bones; or with secondary intracranial tumors

    b. Use cautiously if there is diabetes or family history of same, hypothyroidism, or concurrent or previous use of thyroid or hormones in males before puberty

    c. Known sensitivity to benzyl alcohol (a preservative in bacteriostatic water that may also be harmful to newborns); preferred diluent is sterile water, especially for newborns

5. Significant drug interactions

    a. Adrenocorticotropic hormone (ACTH) or corticosteroids may slow the action of growth hormone

Table 6-1 **Growth Hormone Drugs**	Generic Name	Trade Name	Administration/Dosage	Notes
	Bromocriptine	Parlodel	**ORAL:** for acromegaly: 5–30 mg/day in divided doses.	Suppresses growth hormone levels.
	Ocreotide	Sandostatin	**SC:** *Adults*—for acromegaly: 0.1 mg 3×/day. *Children*—0.001 to 0.01 mg/kg/day.	Suppresses intestinal peptide hormones, insulin, glucagons, and growth hormone.
	Sermorelin	Geref	**IV:** *Adults*—for diagnosis of pituitary function: 1 mg/kg.	Stimulates release of growth hormone from intact pituitaries.
	Somatrem	Protropin	**IM, SC:** *Children*—for growth failure: 0.025–0.05 mg/kg qod.	Used as replacement therapy.
	Somatropin	Humatrope Nutropin	**IM,SC:** *Children*—For growth failure: 0.025–0.05 mg/kg qod.	Used as replacement therapy.

   b. Thyroid hormone, anabolic steroids, androgens, or estrogens may hasten closure of epiphyseal plates of long bones

6. Significant food interactions: none

7. Significant laboratory studies

   a. Plasma GH levels to confirm deficiency (< 5 to 7 ng/mL)

   b. Regular measurement of thyroid levels to detect undiagnosed hypothyroidism

   c. Blood or urine glucose levels to detect glucose intolerance in diabetic clients or those with significant family history of diabetes

8. Side effects

   a. Metabolic: glucose intolerance, ACTH deficiency, or hypothyroidism

   b. Renal: **hypercalciuria** (excess calcium excretion in the urine) during first 2 to 3 months of treatment; risk of renal calculi with complaints of flank pain, colic, GI upset, urinary frequency, chills, fever, and hematuria

   c. Other: recurrent intracranial tumor growth or presence of GH antibodies

9. Adverse effects/toxicity

   a. Local allergic reaction: pain and edema at injection site

   b. Systemic allergic reaction: peripheral edema, headache, myalgia, and weakness

   c. Excess dosage: diabetes mellitus, atherosclerosis, enlarged organs, hypertension, and features related to acromegaly

10. Nursing considerations

   a. Make sure there is documentation of growth rate for at least 6 to 12 months prior to initiating treatment

   b. Assess client for any adverse effects or toxicities related to drug administration

   c. Make sure annual bone age assessments are performed, especially for clients undergoing thyroid, androgen or estrogen replacement therapy

11. Client education

   a. Advise parents or caregivers to have regular bone age assessments done at specific times

   b. Tell parents or caregivers that a 3- to 5-inch growth rate is expected in the 1st year and less in the 2nd year, with normal growth rate subsequent years; SC fat is diminished during treatment, but will return later

   c. Teach parents or caregivers how to accurately document monthly height and weight measurements and to report any less-than-expected growth to the physician

   d. Teach parents or caregivers signs and symptoms of slipped femoral epiphysis (hip or knee pain and limp) and to notify physician of same

   e. Advise parents or caregivers that treatment is discontinued when adequate adult height reached, when epiphyseal plates are fused, or when client fails to respond to growth hormone

B. Antidiuretic hormone (ADH)

1. Action and use

   a. Action: on renal tubules to promote reabsorption of water; vasopressor effect due to constriction of smooth muscle; increases aggregation of platelets

   b. Use: is a pituitary hormone for replacement therapy for clients with diabetes insipidus; also for use in Hemophilia A, von Willebrand's disease type 1

2. Common medications (Table 6-2)

3. Administration considerations

   a. Give intranasally, intravenously (IV), subcutaneously (SC), intramuscularly (IM), or intra-arterially according to order and preparation

   b. Infusion pump is needed for intravenous or intra-arterial routes

4. Contraindications: clients with coronary artery or vascular disease; blood pressure elevation is caused by vasoconstriction

5. Significant drug interactions

   a. Demecycline and lithium carbonate may inhibit action and promote continuation of diuresis

   b. Carbamazepine, chlorpropamide, and clofibrate may also extend action of antiduretics

6. Significant food interactions: none known

7. Significant laboratory studies

   a. Serum osmolality and plasma osmolality with diabetes insipidus

   b. Factor VIII coagulation level for hemostasis

8. Side effects

   a. CNS: drowsiness, headache, lethargy

   b. EENT: nasal congestion and irritation; rhinitis

   c. GI: abdominal cramps, nausea, and heartburn

   d. GU: pain in vulva

   e. CV: elevated BP

Table 6-2	Generic Name	Trade Name	Administration/Dosage	Notes
Drugs to Treat Diabetes Insipidus	Desmopressin	DDAVP Stimate	**INTRANASAL:** *Adults*—10 µg HS; up to 40 µg maintenence. *Children*—(3 mo–12 yr)−5 µg at bedtime and up to 4 µg/kg maintenance **IV, SC:** *Adults*—1–2 µg 2×/d.	Used as replacement therapy.
	Lypressin	Diapid	**INTRANASAL:** *Adults*—1–2 sprays ea. nostril 4×/d.	Used as replacement therapy.
	Vasopressin	Pitressin	**IM, IV, SC, IA:** *Adults:*—5–10 U 2–3 ×/d prn. IV or IA by infusion pump. *Children:*—2.5–10 U 3–4 ×/d.	Used as replacement therapy or diagnostic aid.

9. Adverse effects/toxicity

    a. IV route may cause anaphylaxis

    b. Overdose may produce symptoms of water intoxication

10. Nursing considerations

    a. Initial dose is given in the evening and amount is increased until uninterrupted sleep is noted

    b. Check vital signs (BP and pulse) before giving by the IV and SC routes

    c. Assess client for mental status changes such as disorientation, lethargy, and behavioral changes related to fluid overload

    d. Measure daily I & O to monitor water retention and sodium depletion; assess edema in extremities

    e. Weigh daily to monitor water retention

    f. For nasal spray, make sure nasal mucosa is intact by inspecting nares prior to dose

    g. IV dose may be given undiluted over one minute

    h. Store nasal spray at room temperature; all other solutions need refrigeration

11. Client education

    a. Instruct in proper technique for nasal instillation (tube inserted into nostril to instill)

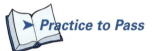

▶ Practice to Pass

A female client who is taking antidiuretic hormone (ADH) intranasally calls to tell you that she has a cold and flu-like symptoms. What will you advise her to do?

    b. Avoid over-the-counter (OTC) meds containing epinephrine that can decrease drug's action

    c. Avoid alcohol use when taking drug

    d. Wear Medic Alert identification

    e. Do not double dose if dose missed; may take skipped dose up to one hour before next dose

    f. Report any nasal congestion or upper respiratory tract infection

II. Medications Affecting the Adrenal Glands

A. Mineralocorticoids

1. Action and use

    a. A **mineralocorticoid** is a steroid hormone that acts on kidneys to retain sodium and water and release potassium

    b. Synthesis is regulated by the renin-angiotensin system

    c. Replacement hormone therapy is required with missing mineralocorticoid action, which occurs in adrenal gland failure or hypofunction

2. Common medications (Table 6-3)

3. Administration considerations

    a. Fludrocortisone acetate is drug of choice

    b. Is given orally from 0.1 mg 3 times/week to 0.2 mg/day

Table 6-3	Generic Name	Trade Name	Administration/Dosage	Notes
Drugs for Adrenal Replacement Therapy (Mineralocorticoids)	Cortisone	Cortone	**ORAL:** *Adults*—25 mg/day or more PRN. *Children*—0.35 mg/kg/day.	Has both mineralocorticoid and glucocorticoid action.
	Fludrocortisone	Florinef	**ORAL:** *Adults*—0.1 mg/day. *Children*—0.05–0.1 mg/day.	Has strong mineralocorticoid action; used with glucocorticoid for replacement therapy.
	Hydrocortisone	Cortef	**ORAL:** *Adults*—20 mg/day or more PRN. *Children*—0.56 mg/kg/day.	Has both mineralocorticoid and glucocorticoid action.

4. Contraindications: hypersensitivity to glucocorticoids; idiopathic thrombocytopenic purpura (ITP); acute glomerulonephritis; viral/bacterial skin infections or infections not being treated with antibiotics; amebiasis; Cushing's syndrome; vaccinations/immunologic procedures

5. Drug interactions

   a. Hypokalemic effect may potentiate action of other drugs

   b. Hypernatremia may result if given with high sodium drugs

   c. Higher dosage may be needed if given with hepatic metabolic enzymes (such as rifampin and phenytoin)

6. Food interactions: high-sodium foods

7. Significant laboratory studies: monitor serum electrolyte levels

8. Side effects: sodium and fluid retention, nausea, acne, and impaired wound healing

9. Adverse effects/toxicity

   a. Adverse reactions occur rarely, but use cautiously in clients with heart disease, congestive heart failure (CHF), or hypertension

   b. Thromboembolism

   c. Aggravation or masking of infection

   d. Anaphyloid reactions rare but may occur in clients hypersensitive to glucocorticoids

10. Nursing considerations

   a. Is used with glucocorticoids for replacement therapy

   b. Monitor serum electrolyte levels

   c. Monitor weight and I & O and report weight gain of five lb/week

   d. Monitor/record BP daily and more frequently during periods of dosage adjustment

   e. Check for signs of overdosage related to hypercorticism (psychosis, excess weight gain, edema, CHF, increased appetite, severe insomnia, and elevated BP)

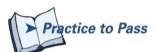

▶ Practice to Pass

A client taking mineralocorticoid therapy tells you that she has gained 5 ½ pounds in the last 2 days. What action will you take?

    f. Check for signs of underdosage: weight loss, poor appetite, nausea, vomiting, diarrhea, muscular weakness, increased fatigue, and low BP

  11. Client education

    a. Instruct to report signs of low potassium associated with high sodium (muscle weakness, paresthesias, circumoral numbness, fatigue, anorexia, nausea, depression, delirium, diminished reflexes, polyuria, irregular heart rate, CHF, ileus)

    b. May advise to eat foods high in potassium

    c. Instruct that salt intake regulates drug's effect and to report signs of edema

    d. Advise to weigh daily and report consistent weight gain

    e. Instruct to report any infections, trauma or unexpected stress

    f. Advise to wear/carry medical identification alert including drug use and MD's name

B. Glucocorticoids

  1. Action and use

    a. A **glucocorticoid** is a steroid hormone that has metabolic effects on carbohydrate, protein and fat metabolism and has anti-inflammatory and immunosuppressive activity; its synthesis is regulated by the pituitary gland via negative feedback effect; may regulate metabolism of skeletal and connective tissues

    b. Is used in acute **adrenal insufficiency** (inability of adrenal glands to produce sufficient adrenocortical hormones) caused by trauma or thrombosis; chronic primary adrenal insufficiency (also known as **Addison's disease**); and secondary adrenal insufficiency (diseased or destroyed adenohypophysis with inadequate production of ACTH)

    c. In allergic conditions (asthma, angioedema, transfusion reactions, and serum sickness)

    d. In dermatological conditions, such as dermatitis and pemphigus

    e. In inflammatory GI disorders, such as Crohn's disease and ulcerative proctitis

    f. In hematologic disorders, such as autoimmune hemolytic anemia and thrombocytopenia

    g. In joint inflammation, bursitis

    h. With antineoplastic agents in leukemias and lymphomas

    i. In ophthalmic diseases, such as allergic conjunctivitis, chorioretinitis, iritis, iridocyclitis, and keratitis

    j. Rheumatic disease (acute inflammatory states of arthritis and systemic lupus erythematosus)

  2. Common medications (Table 6-4)

  3. Administration considerations

    a. Routes of administration for systemic use to treat inflammatory conditions include IV, IM and PO

Table 6-4	Generic Name	Trade Name	Administration/Dosage	Notes
Drugs for Adrenal Replacement Therapy (Glucocorticoids)	Betamethasone	Celestone	**ORAL:** *Adults*—600 µg/day or more PRN. *Children*—5.83 µg/kg 3X/day.	Has little or no mineralocorticoid action.
	Cortisone	Cortone	**ORAL:** *Adults*—25 mg/day or more PRN. *Children*—0.35 mg/kg/day.	Has both mineralocorticoid and glucocorticoid action.
	Hydrocortisone	Cortef	**ORAL:** *Adults*—20 mg/day or more PRN. *Children*—0.56 mg/kg/day.	Has both mineralocorticoid and glucocorticoid action.
	Triamcinolone	Aristacort Kenacort	**ORAL:** *Adults*—4–12 mg/day (single or divided doses). *Children*—0.117 mg/kg (single or divided doses).	Must be used with mineralocorticoid; has little or no mineralocorticoid action.

    b. Routes of administration for nonsystemic use include inhalation, nasal, ophthalmic, otic, and topical

  4. Contraindications: systemic fungal infections and known hypersensitivity

  5. Significant drug interactions

    a. Antibiotics, cyclosporine, estrogen and ketoconazole slow metabolism/clearance

    b. Aminoglutethimide, carbamazepine, cholestyramine, phenobarbital, phenytoin, and rifampin increase metabolism

    c. Antianxiety agents, antipsychotics, anticholinesterases, anticoagulants, antihypertensives, hypoglycemics, vaccines, pancuronium, salicyclates, and sympathomimetics also affect metabolism/clearance

  6. Significant food interactions: none identified

  7. Significant laboratory studies

    a. CBC and differential, serum electrolytes, and blood glucose

    b. With long-term therapy monitor hypothalamic-pituitary-adrenal axis function to check adrenal function

  8. Side effects: few if high doses given for only a few days

  9. Adverse effects/toxicity

    a. Higher doses and prolonged therapy may alter metabolism of tissues and organs leading to muscle wasting, and increased fat tissue deposits in the central portion of the body and face; changes in behavior and personality may also occur

    b. Prolonged therapy may cause growth suppression in children and osteoporosis in adults; impaired glucose tolerance and frank diabetes mellitus may also result

    c. Prolonged therapy can suppress the hypothalamic-pituitary-adrenal axis; **adrenal crisis** (an acute, life-threatening state of profound adrenocortical insufficiency) may result if drug is abruptly withdrawn

d. Toxicity may include anaphylactoid reactions, hypertriglyceridemia, peptic ulcers, acute pancreatitis, aseptic necrosis of bone, cataracts, glaucoma, hypertension, and opportunistic infections

10. Nursing considerations

a. Check vital signs, BP, lung sounds, weight (including any history of gain or loss), nausea and vomiting, and signs of dependent edema

b. Conduct mental status exam and assess for signs of depression, withdrawal, insomnia, and anorexia

c. Check skin for striae, thinning, bruising, change in color, change in hair growth, and acne

d. In children on prolonged therapy, monitor height and growth pattern

e. Advise regular ophthalmic examinations with long-term therapy

f. Check stool for occult blood periodically

g. With prolonged therapy, move and reposition immobilized clients carefully and limit use of adhesive tape on skin

11. Client education

a. Discuss benefits and possible side effects with long-term use and advise to report any new side effects

b. Instruct to take oral doses with meals and avoid alcohol

c. If ordered every other day, take any missed dose as soon as remembered if on same day; if remembered the next day, then take dose and readjust schedule to be every other day; do not double up missed doses

d. Suggest weight reduction diets, limiting sodium intake, and increasing potassium intake if excessive weight gain occurs

e. If client has diabetes, advise to carefully monitor blood glucose levels

f. Instruct to report any blood in stool or black tarry stools, mood changes or insomnia, vision changes or headache, weight gain of more than 5 pounds per week, irregular menses or pregnancy, irregular heart rate, excessive fatigue, severe abdominal pain, serious injury, or infection

g. Avoid strenuous activities if skin is fragile and bruises easily

h. With long-term therapy, tell client to take prescribed doses every day and not discontinue medication without notifying physician; warn client not to increase or decrease dose on own; tapering of dose is necessary

i. Instruct to avoid immunizations during therapy and for 3 months after; avoid contact with anyone with measles or chicken pox or anyone receiving oral polio vaccine

j. Advise to avoid skin testing during therapy

k. Instruct to wear specific medical identification during therapy

l. With long-term therapy, advise to report any fever, cough, sore throat, malaise, and unhealed injuries; avoid contact with anyone with active infection

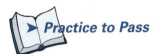

Practice to Pass

A client taking glucocorticoid therapy asks the nurse about wearing some sort of Medic-Alert identification. How should the nurse respond?

  m. Review drug and teach specific administration and that client should not share drug with others

C. Adrenocorticotropic hormone (ACTH)

 1. Action and use

  a. Directly stimulates adrenal cortex to synthesize adrenal steroids

  b. Used in diagnosing adrenal disorders such as Addison's disease and secondary adrenal insufficiency caused by pituitary dysfunction

  c. Used in treatment of adrenocorticoid-responsive diseases, such as multiple sclerosis

  d. Limited use in treatment of adrenal insufficiency

 2. Common medications (Table 6-5)

 3. Administration considerations

  a. Agents may be given IV, IM, SC, or PO

  b. Administer drug according to manufacturer's instructions

  c. Incompatible if mixed with aminophyline or sodium bicarbonate

 4. Contraindications

  a. Ocular herpes simplex; recent surgery

  b. Disorders such as CHF, scleroderma, osteoporosis, systemic fungoid infections, hypertension

  c. Sensitivity to porcine proteins

  d. Conditions related to adrenocortical insufficiency or hyperfunction

 5. Significant drug interactions: aspirin, nonsteroidal anti-inflammatory drugs (NSAIDS), barbiturates, phenytoin, rifampin, estrogens, amphotericin B, and diuretics

 6. Significant food interactions: none

 7. Significant laboratory studies

  a. Baseline electrolyte levels

  b. Baseline plasma cortisol level

Table 6-5	Generic Name	Trade Name	Administration/Dosage	Notes
Drugs Used in Diagnosing Adrenal Gland Disorders	Corticotropin	Acthar	**IV:** *Adults*—to diagnose adrenal/pituitary disorder: 10–25 U in 500 mL D₅W, given over 8 hr. **IV, SC:** *Children*—1.6 U/kg in 3–4 divided doses.	Natural ACTH, protein from pituitary.
	Cosyntropin	Cortrosyn	**IV, IM, SC:** *Adults*—0.25 mg as single injection or IV over 2 min.–6 hr.	Synthetic ACTH.
	Metyrapone	Metopirone	**ORAL:** *Adults*—to check for secondary adrenal insufficiency: 750 mg q 4 hr × 6 doses. *Children*—15 mg/kg q 4 hr × 6 doses.	Blocks cortisol synthesis in adrenals; may cause acute adrenal insufficiency.

8. Side effects: nausea and vomiting, dizziness, drowsiness, or light-headedness

9. Adverse effects/toxicity

   a. Hypersensitivity including urticaria, pruritus, dizziness, vomiting, and anaphylactic shock

   b. Cataracts, or glaucoma; peptic ulcer with perforation; hirsutism and amenorrhea

   c. Sodium and water retention, potassium and calcium loss, and hyperglycemia

   d. Acne, impaired wound healing, fragile skin, petechiae, ecchymosis

   e. **Osteoporosis** (abnormal loss of bone density), decreased muscle mass, **cushingoid state** (having the appearance and facies characteristic of Cushing's disease), activation of latent tuberculosis or diabetes mellitus, vertebral compression fractures

10. Nursing considerations

    a. Individualized dosage and gradual dosage changes should be made only after apparent full effect from drug is seen

    b. Shake bottle well before injecting into deep gluteal muscle; after administration observe closely for 15 minutes for any hypersensitivity reactions; prolonged treatment may increase risk of hypersensitivity reactions

    c. Monitor vital signs and BP and assess for dizziness, fever, flushing, rash and urticaria

    d. Monitor plasma or urinary cortisol levels and serum electrolytes

    e. Be aware that agents may suppress signs and symptoms of chronic disease; new infections may appear during treatment

    f. At high dosage levels, drug must be gradually tapered

    g. Carefully monitor growth and development in children

11. Client education

    a. Advise not to discontinue drug before notifying physician

    b. If ordered, discuss need for low-salt or potassium-rich diet

    c. Take oral doses with food, milk, or meals

    d. If dizziness, drowsiness or light-headedness occur, advise to avoid driving or operating hazardous equipment

III. Medications Affecting the Thyroid Glands

A. Thyroid hormones

1. Action and use

   a. As replacement therapy for **hypothyroidism** (decreased activity of the thyroid gland with a variety of specific causes); have same action as naturally produced thyroid hormones in body

   b. Used to diagnose and treat thyroid deficiency and **myxedema** (most severe form of hypothyroidism characterized by swelling of face, feet, and

	Generic Name	Trade Name	Administration/Dosage	Notes
Table 6-6 **Drugs for Diagnosing Thyroid Disorders or Replacement Therapy**	Levothyroxine	Levothroid Levoxyl Synthroid	**ORAL:** *Adults*—initially 12.5–50 µg/day; gradually increase to maintenance dose (75–125 µg/day). *Children*— 2–6 µg/kg/day in single dose. **IV:** *Adults*—Up to 500 µg/day.	Chemically pure form of T_4 and preferred therapy for hypothythroidism. Given IV for myxedema coma.
	Liothyronine	Cytomel	**ORAL:** *Adults*—Initially 2.5–25 µg/day; gradually increase to maintenance dose (25–50 µg/day).	Chemically pure form of T_3; for adult hypothyroidism; not used for cretinism since T_3 does not cross blood–brain barrier as well as T_4 does.
	Liotrix	Thyrolar, Euthroid	**ORAL:** *Adults & children*— Initially 12.5 µg of T_4 with 3.1 µg of T_3/day; increase slowly to maintenance dose (usually 50–100 mg T_4 with 12.5–25 µg T_3).	Chemically pure T_4 and T_3 in 4:1 ratio; used for hypothyroidism.
	Thyroid	Thyrar	**ORAL:** *Adults & children*— Initially 7.5–15 mg/day; increase slowly to maintenance dose (60–120 mg/day).	Crude thyroid gland preparation containing variable amounts of T_3 and T_4. Dosage difficult to adjust and maintain.
	Protirelin	Relefact TRH	**IV:** *Adults*—0.5 mg. *Children*—7 mg/kg.	Identical to natural hypothalamic hormone. Used in diagnosis.
	Thyrotropin	Thytropar	**IM, SC:** *Adults & children*— 10 IU/day for 1–7 days.	Natural TSH extracted from animals. Used to differentiate primary hypothyroidism from secondary.

periorbital tissues; may lead to coma and death), and to control goiter or thyroid carcinoma

2. Common medications (Table 6-6)

3. Administration considerations

   a. May be given IV, IM, SC, or PO

   b. Administer drug according to manufacturer's instructions

4. Contraindications

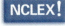

   a. Thyrotoxicosis, acute MI and cardiovascular disease, morphologic hypogonadism, nephrosis, and uncorrected hypoadrenalism

   b. Cautious use with angina pectoris; hypertension; elderly with cardiac disease; renal insufficiency; pregnancy; concurrent use of **catecholamines** (drugs that mimic effects of the sympathetic nervous system); diabetes mellitus; **hyperthyroidism** (hyperactivity of the thyroid gland), and malabsorption states

5. Significant drug interactions: thyroid hormones given with oral anticoagulants, insulin and sulfonylureas, epinephrine, and cholestyramine

6. Significant food interactions: none noted

7. Significant laboratory studies: serum T_4, free thyroxine, T_3 uptake, serum T_3, serum thyroid stimulating hormone (TSH), protirelin test, thyroid uptake of radioiodine, TSH test, and thyroid suppression test

8. Side effects: weight gain, vomiting, and tachycardia

9. Adverse effects/toxicity

   a. Angina pectoris, coronary occlusion, or stroke in elderly or predisposed clients

   b. Relative adrenal insufficiency in clients with inadequate pituitary function related to secondary hypothyroidism and secondary adrenal insufficiency; adrenal crisis

   c. Overdosage causing signs of hyperthyroidism related to thyroid storm with shock and coma; thyrotoxicosis with CHF, angina, cardiac dysrhythmias, and shock

   d. Reactions to thioamides include fever, itching, and skin rash; blood dyscrasias and peripheral neuropathy; pain and swelling of joints or lupus-like syndrome; dizziness; or alterations in taste

   e. Overdosage of thioamides causes hypothyroidism

10. Nursing considerations

   a. Assess vital signs, BP, weight and history of weight change, normal diet, energy level, mood, subjective feeling, and response to temperature

   b. In children, check height

   c. Monitor thyroid function test results and blood glucose levels

   d. Start older adults on lower doses of thyroid hormones and increase dose by small increments; assess for symptoms of stress that could lead to angina or stroke

11. Client education

   a. Teach client how to monitor pulse, weight, and height

   b. With hormone replacement, instruct to adhere to dosage schedule and intervals; emphasize that therapy is life-long; do not to change brand of thyroid medication without discussing with physician because of differences in bioavailability

   c. Immediately report any chest pain or other signs of aggravated cardiovascular disease

   d. With juvenile hypothyroidism therapy, explain dramatic weight loss and catch-up growth

   e. Explain side effects and related treatment if changes in insulin or anticoagulants are needed

   f. Caution client not to discontinue drug and to wear medical alert identification

   g. With radioactive iodine, explain that most clients become hypothyroid and require replacement therapy with thyroid hormones; urge periodic thyroid evaluation

NCLEX!

NCLEX!

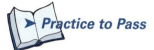

▶ Practice to Pass

A client taking thyroid hormone is also receiving sodium warfarin (Coumadin). What laboratory test should the nurse monitor?

NCLEX!

NCLEX!

NCLEX!

NCLEX!

NCLEX!

B. Antithyroid medications

1. Action and use: used to treat hyperthyroidism and **Graves' disease** (pronounced hyperthyroidism often associated with enlarged thyroid gland and exophthalmos; also called thyrotoxicosis)

2. Common medications (Table 6-7)

3. Administration considerations

   a. Is given PO

   b. Administer drug according to manufacturer's instructions

4. Contraindications

   a. Previous allergic or other severe reactions to thioamides

   b. Impaired hepatic function may require reduced doses

5. Significant drug interactions

   a. Thioamides given with any iodine preparations including amiodarone, iodine solution, potassium iodide, and some contrast imaging dyes or radioactive iodine uptake

   b. Coumarins and other anticoagulants; digitalis

Table 6-7	Generic Name	Trade Name	Administration/Dosage	Notes
Drugs Used to Treat Hyperthyroidism and Graves' Disease	*Thioamides* Methimazole	Tapazole	**ORAL:** *Adults*—Initially 15–60 mg/day in 1–2 doses; maintenance dose 5–30 mg/day in 1–2 doses. *Children*—initially 0.4 mg/kg in 1–2 doses; maintenance dose 0.2 mg/kg/day.	Inhibits thyroid hormone synthesis but not release.
	Propylthiouracil	(Generic)	**ORAL:** *Adults*— Initially 300–900 mg/day. Maintenance dose 50–600 mg/day. *Children* 6–10 yr 50–150 mg/day. *Children* >10 yr 50–300 mg/day.	Inhibits thyroid hormone synthesis but not release; in peripheral tissues inhibits conversion of T_4 to T_3.
	Beta-Adrenergic Blockers Propranolol	Inderal	**ORAL:** *Adults*—10–40 mg 3–4×/day.	Does not lower T_4 and T_3 release from thyroid.
	Iodine Potassium Iodide	Pima	**ORAL:** *Adults*—250 mg tid as preoperative medication.	Has direct action on thyroid and used for short-term inhibition of thyroid hormone synthesis.
	^{131}I as NaI	Iodotope	**ORAL:** *Adults*—4–10 mCi (148–370 megabequerels) as single dose for Graves' disease. For cancer of thyroid: single dose of up to 150 mCi (5.5 gigabecquerels) used. For diagnosis use smaller doses.	Radionuclide concentrated in thyroid. Releases radiation and destroys tissue.

6. Significant food interactions: none noted

7. Significant laboratory studies: serum T_4, serum T_3, free T_4, free T_3, T_3 resin uptake, serum thyroid uptake of radioiodine, and thyroid suppression test

8. Side effects: fever, itching, and skin rash

9. Adverse effects/toxicity

    a. Blood dyscrasias and peripheral neuropathy

    b. Pain and swelling of joints or lupus-like syndrome

    c. Dizziness and alteration in taste

    d. Overdosage results in hypothyroidism

    e. Rare instances of agranulocytosis

10. Nursing considerations

    a. Assess for tingling of fingers and toes

    b. Monitor weight and check for hair loss and skin changes

    c. Check CBC, differential count and thyroid and liver function tests

    d. Dilute oral iodine solutions well in milk, juice, or other beverage

    e. Assess for metallic taste in mouth, sneezing, edematous thyroid, vomiting, and bloody diarrhea

11. Client education

    a. Explain need to wear medical identification tag/bracelet

    b. Explain goals and side effects of medications (side effects may not appear for days or weeks after treatment begun)

    c. Advise to report any fever, chills, sore throat, and unusual bleeding/bruising

    d. Instruct to take med at same time of day and with meals or snack; space additional daily doses throughout the day

IV. Medications Affecting the Parathyroid Glands

A. Medications to treat hypocalcemia

1. Action and use

    a. Consist of calcium supplements

    b. Replaces calcium to supply body's metabolic needs

    c. Helps maintain bone strength and prevent calcium loss from bones

    d. Use to treat mild hypocalcemia and supplementation of dietary calcium

    e. Additional use as antacid

2. Common medications (Table 6-8)

3. Administration considerations

    a. Oral route

    b. Dosage differs among the different oral calcium salts

	Generic Name	Trade Name	Administration/Dosage	Calcium Content
Table 6-8	Calcium acetate	Phos-Ex, PhosLo	ORAL: *Adults*—2.0 gms provides 500 mg of calcium	25%
Drugs Used to Treat Mild Calcium Deficiency	Calcium carbonate	Various names	ORAL: *Adults*—1.3 gms provides 500 mg of calcium	40%
	Calcium citrate	Citracal	ORAL: *Adults*—2.4 gms provides 500 mg of calcium	21%
	Calcium glubionate	Neo-Calglucon	ORAL: *Adults*—7.6 gms provides 500 mg of calcium	6.6%
	Tricalcium phosphate	Posture	ORAL: *Adults*—1.3 gms provides 500 mg of calcium	39%

c. Must be taken with large glass of water and with or after meals

d. When used as antacid, should be taken 1 hour after meals and at bedtime

4. Contraindications: hypercalcemia, renal calculi, and hypophosphatemia

5. Significant drug interactions

a. Glucocorticoids reduce calcium absorption

b. Absorption of tetracyclines and quinolones is reduced if given with calcium

c. Thiazide diuretics decrease renal excretion of calcium

d. May enhance inotropic and toxic effects of digoxin

6. Significant food interactions: spinach, Swiss chard, beets, bran and whole grain cereals can reduce calcium absorption

7. Significant laboratory studies: serum calcium level

8. Side effects: constipation and flatulence

9. Adverse effects/toxicity

a. Hypercalcemia may occur if frequent or high doses

b. May also occur in clients being treated with calcium as part of renal dysfunction therapy

▶ Practice to Pass

A client taking long-term calcium supplements also takes digoxin. What type of drug interaction should the client be prepared to monitor for?

10. Nursing considerations

a. Take 1 to 1½ hours after meals

b. Space additional daily doses throughout the day

c. Note number and consistency of stools, if constipation a problem, then a laxative or stool softener may be ordered

d. With prolonged therapy, monitor weekly serum and urine calcium levels

e. Observe for signs of hypercalcemia if receiving frequent or high doses

f. Monitor for acid rebound if used as an antacid on repeated basis for more than 1 to 2 weeks

11. Client education

a. Explain signs of hypercalcemia and to report any nausea, vomiting, constipation, frequent urination, lethargy, or depression

NCLEX!

    b. Advise not to take with cereals or other foods high in oxalates that form insoluble, nonabsorbable compounds with calcium

    c. If used as antacid explain potential dangers of repeated use for more than 2 weeks

B. Vitamin D

  1. Action and use

NCLEX!

    a. Vitamin D is needed for proper absorption of calcium, is a fat-soluble vitamin that can accumulate in the body

    b. Used to control hypocalcemia or vitamin D deficiency

    c. Used in treatment of rickets, **osteomalacia** (abnormal loss of calcification of the matrix in lamellar bone, resulting in bone softening and fracture), and **hypoparathyroidism** (insufficient secretion of parathyroid glands caused by primary parathyroid dysfunction or elevated serum calcium level)

  2. Common medications (Table 6-9)

  3. Administration considerations

    a. Given orally or intramuscularly

    b. Adequate calcium is needed for optimal response to treatment

  4. Contraindications: clients with hypercalcemia or vitamin D toxicity and malabsorption syndrome

  5. Significant drug interactions

    a. Antacids or other preparations containing magnesium may cause high magnesium blood levels

    b. Digitalis glycosides

  6. Significant food interactions: none noted

  7. Significant laboratory studies

    a. Serum calcium and phosphorus levels

    b. BUN, serum creatinine levels, serum alkaline phosphatase

    c. Urinary calcium and urinalysis

Table 6-9

Drugs Used to Treat Vitamin D Deficiency

Generic Name	Trade Name	Administration/Dosage	Notes
Calcifediol	Claderol	**ORAL:** *Adults*—0.05–0.01 mg/day. *Children*—0.02–0.05 mg/day.	Used for vitamin-D deficiency or rickets.
Calcitrol	Calcijex Rocaltrol	**ORAL:** *Adults*—0.25 µg and increase slowly to maximum of 3 µg/day. *Children*—0.25 µg/day & slowly increase to 0.08 µg/kg. **IV:** *Adults*—0.01 µg/kg rapid IV 3 × week and increase up to 0.05 mg/kg.	Used for hypoparathyroidism or chronic renal failure.
Ergocalciferol	Calciferol Drisdol	**ORAL:** *Adults and Children*—400 units/day for replacement & up to 500,000 units/day for rickets.	Used for hypoparathyroidism and to treat and prevent vitamin-D deficiency.

8. Side effects

   a. Hypercalcemia related to overdosage

   b. These symptoms include ataxia, fatigue, irritability, seizures, somnolence, tinnitus, hypertension, GI tract distress or constipation, and hypotonia in infants

9. Adverse effects/toxicity

   a. Vitamin-D hypercalcemia may lead to dysrhythmias in clients taking digoxin

   b. Hypervitaminosis D caused by large therapeutic doses may lead to hypercalcemia, hypercalciuria, bone decalcification, and calcium deposits in soft tissues

10. Nursing considerations

    a. Assess for any CNS problems

    b. Monitor BP, pulse, and I & O

    c. Monitor BUN, serum creatinine levels, serum calcium and phosphorus levels, serum alkaline phosphatase and urinalysis

    d. If vitamin D toxicity occurs, make sure client stops drug immediately, forces fluid, and eats a low-calcium diet

11. Client education

    a. Make sure oral dose is swallowed intact without crushing or chewing tablet

    b. Instruct client not to increase or decrease dosage before notifying MD

    c. Advise client to check with MD before taking any OTC meds containing calcium, phosphorus, or vitamin D, and any excessive amounts of any substances containing vitamin D

    d. Warn not to drive or use heavy equipment if client develops fatigue, somnolence, vertigo, or weakness

    e. Advise to avoid magnesium-containing antacids

C. Medications to treat hypercalcemia

1. Action and use

   a. Promote urinary excretion of calcium

   b. Decrease mobilization of calcium from bone

   c. Decrease intestinal absorption of calcium

   d. Form complexes with free calcium in blood

   e. Achieve rapid lowering of blood calcium levels

   f. Used in emergency treatment of hypercalcemia, and to control hypercalcemia resulting from malignancies of the bone

2. Common medications (Table 6-10)

3. Administration considerations

   a. May be given SC, IM, IV or PO

   b. Give IM doses at bedtime to minimize effects of flushing following injection

Table 6-10	Generic Name	Trade Name	Administration/Dosage	Notes
Drugs Used to Treat Hypercalcemia	Ededate disodium	Disotate Endrate	**IV:** *Adults*—for hypercalcemia: 50 mg/kg over 24 hr for no more than 4 days and up to 3 g/day. *Children*—40 mg/kg/24 hrs.	Strong chelating agent; used on short-term basis to remove excess calcium.
	Gallium nitrate	Ganite	**IV:** *Adults*—100–200 mg/m² infused over 24 hr × 5 day.	Used for hypercalcemia caused by cancer.
	Pamidronate	Aredia	**IV:** *Adults*—For hypercalcemia: 60 mg over 4–24 hr	Acts directly on bone by slowing bone reabsorption and lowering release of calcium. Also used for Paget's disease.

    c. In emergency situations, dilute IV dose before administration to prevent extravasation; infuse over prescribed period of time

4. Contraindications

    a. Don't give to clients with known hypersensitivity

    b. Avoid in clients with impaired renal function

5. Significant drug interactions

    a. Antacids, mineral supplements, calcium salts, and vitamin D

    b. Decreased effects of digitalis when serum calcium is reduced

    c. Nephrotoxic medications

6. Significant food interactions: calcium-rich dairy products

7. Significant laboratory studies

    a. CBC with differential count

    b. Serum electrolytes, alkaline phosphatase, and creatinine

    c. Liver function tests

    d. Urinalysis

8. Side effects

    a. Nausea, vomiting, diarrhea, and dyspepsia with oral route

    b. Facial flushing, and occasional inflammatory reaction at injection site

    c. Transient influenza-like symptoms with IV route

    d. Nasal dryness and irritation with intranasal spray

9. Adverse effects/toxicity

    a. Allergic reactions with calcitonin salmon

    b. IV administration may cause venous irritation, thrombophlebitis, and nephrotoxicity

    c. Varying effects of hypocalcemia

d. Toxicity with higher doses causes more severe GI distress, such as esophagitis, severe nephrotoxicity, and severe hypocalcemia

10. Nursing considerations

a. Assess for hypercalcemia and hypocalcemia

b. Monitor weight and I & O if vomiting and diarrhea occur

c. Monitor serum electrolytes, serum alkaline phosphatase, serum creatinine, BUN, and liver function tests

d. Monitor vital signs and assess for dysrhythmias with IV infusion

11. Client education

a. Instruct client and receive return demonstration on subcutaneous self-injection

b. Advise not to discontinue therapy without notifying MD

c. Provide emotional support as needed

d. Inform client that taking doses in evening may lessen flushing

e. Instruct client to take PO doses on empty stomach

f. Wear medical alert identification if on long-term therapy

g. Review low-calcium and low-vitamin-D diet (decrease in dairy products, for example)

h. Encourage sufficient fluid intake (at least 6-8 glasses of water per day and possibly more if not contraindicated by other health problems)

D. Medications to treat osteoporosis and Paget's disease

1. Action and use

a. Reduce calcium release from bone

b. Slow bone resorption and remodeling

c. Prevent high serum calcium concentrations

d. Used long-term for **Paget's disease** (a non-metabolic disease of bone) and post-menopausal osteoporosis (abnormal loss of bone density)

e. Also used to treat heterotropic ossification after spinal cord injury and hip replacement

2. Common medications (Table 6-11)

3. Administration considerations

a. Is given SC, IM, PO, IV, and intranasal

b. Nasal spray is given once daily in alternate nostrils

4. Contraindications: do not give to clients with known hypersensitivity or to those with esophageal disorders

5. Significant drug interactions: antacids, mineral supplements, calcium salts, and vitamin D

6. Significant food interactions: calcium-rich dairy products

Generic Name	Trade Name	Administration/Dosage	Notes
Table 6-11 **Drugs to Treat Osteoporosis and Paget's disease**			
Calcitonin human	Cibacalcin	**SC:** *Adults*—Initially 0.5 mg/day; Maintenance 0.25 mg/day.	Used long-term for Paget's disease.
Calcitonin salmon	Calcimar Miacalcin	**IM, SC:** *Adults*—For Paget's disease: Initially 100 IU/day then 50 IU/day or qod. For postmenopausal osteoporosis: 100 IU/day or qod. For hypercalcemia: 4 IU/kg q 12 hr & increase up to 8 mg/kg q 6 hr.	Most active form of calcitonin. Response limited over time by creation of antibodies.
Etidronate	Didronel	**ORAL:** *Adults*—For Paget's disease: 5 mg/kg/day for up to 6 mo. For hypercalcemia: 20 mg/kg/day for up to 90 days.	Slows bone reabsorption and lowers calcium release.

7. Significant laboratory studies

   a. Serum electrolytes, serum alkaline phosphatase, calcium and phosphorus and 24-hour urinary hydroxyproline

   b. Baseline values of bone mineral density (BMD) in hip, vertebrae and forearm

8. Side effects

   a. Nausea, vomiting, diarrhea, and dyspepsia with oral route

   b. Facial flushing, and occasional inflammatory reaction at injection site

   c. Transient influenza-like symptoms with IV route

   d. Muscle spasms; leukopenia with chills, fever, or sore throat

   e. Nasal dryness and irritation with intranasal spray

9. Adverse effects/toxicity

   a. Allergic reactions with calcitonin salmon

   b. IV administration may cause venous irritation, thrombophlebitis and nephrotoxicity

   c. Varying effects of hypocalcemia

   d. Toxicity with higher doses causes more severe hypocalcemia, GI distress such as severe esophagitis with ulceration, and severe nephrotoxicity

10. Nursing considerations

    a. Assess for hypercalcemia and hypocalcemia

    b. Monitor weight and I & O if vomiting and diarrhea occur

    c. Monitor serum electrolytes, serum alkaline phosphatase, calcium and phosphorus and 24-hour urinary hydroxyproline

    d. Monitor bone mineral density (BMD) values

    e. Monitor bone pain in clients with Paget's disease

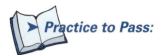

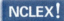

11. Client education

   a. Instruct and receive return demonstration on how to self-administer SC injection and to rotate sites

   b. Advise not to discontinue therapy without notifying MD

   c. Provide emotional support as needed

   d. Inform that taking doses in evening may lessen flushing

   e. Instruct to take PO doses on empty stomach and to remain upright for 30 minutes after taking

   f. Instruct about signs of esophagitis and to discontinue drug and notify MD if difficulty swallowing or worsening heartburn occur

   g. Wear Medic-alert identification if on long-term therapy

   h. Review low-calcium and low vitamin D diet

   i. Encourage sufficient fluid intake

   j. Instruct about how to activate and administer metered dose pump for nasal spray use

V. Medications Used to Treat Diabetes Mellitus

A. Insulin

   1. Action and use

      a. Restores ability of cells to use glucose as an energy source

      b. Corrects the state of **hyperglycemia** (greater than normal amount of glucose circulating in the blood)

      c. Corrects many associated metabolic derangements

      d. Is used to treat both type 1 (formerly insulin dependent or IDDM) and type 2 (formerly non-insulin dependent or NIDDM) diabetes mellitus and diabetic ketoacidosis

      e. Also lowers plasma potassium levels and is used as emergency treatment of hyperkalemia

   2. Types of insulin (Table 6-12)

   3. Administration considerations

      a. Is given only by injection; is inactivated by digestive system enzymes if given orally

      b. May be given SC, IM, or IV; only regular insulin may be given IV

      c. All insulins (except lispro and regular) are mixed in suspension so particles must be dispersed before insulin is drawn up into syringe

      d. Injection sites include: upper arms, thighs, and abdomen, and back in-scapular area

      e. One general location is used at one time to maintain consistent absorption rates although sites within each general location are used only once each month

Table 6-12

Types of Insulin Preparations

Insulin Type	Trade Name	Action	Notes
Lispro	Humalog	**ONSET:** 5 min **PEAK:** 0.5–1 hr **DURATION:** 2–4 hr	Short-acting; modified human type
Regular	Regular Iletin I Regular Iletin II Regular Purified Pork Insulin Humulin R Novolin R Velosulin BR	**ONSET:** 0.5–1 hr **PEAK:** 2–4 hr **DURATION:** 5–7 hr	Short-acting; may be beef/pork, pork or human insulin type.
NPH (Isophane) Insulin	NPH Iletin I Pork NPH Iletin II NPH purified (N) Humulin N Novolin N	**ONSET:** 1–2 hr **PEAK:** 6–12 hr **DURATION:** 18–24 hr	Intermediate-acting; may be beef/pork, pork or human insulin type.
Lente Insulin	Lente Iletin I Lente Iletin II (pork) Lente (L) Purified Pork Humulin L Novolin L	**ONSET:** 1–2 hr **PEAK:** 6–12 hr **DURATION:** 18–24 hr	Intermediate-acting; may be beef/pork, pork or human insulin type.
Ultralente Insulin	Humulin U Ultralente Novolin L	**ONSET:** 4–6 hr **PEAK:** 16–18 hr **DURATION:** 20–36 hr	Long-acting; human insulin type.
NPH/Regular Mixture (70–30%)	Humulin 70/30 Novolin 70/30	**ONSET:** 0.5–1 hr **PEAK:** 5–10 hr **DURATION:** 6–8 hr	Combination Isophane Insulin Suspension and Regular Insulin

NCLEX!

NCLEX!

f. Only mix insulins that are compatible with one another and use according to manufacturer's guidelines

g. Store unopened vials in refrigerator; opened vials can remain at room temperature for up to one month; label vial with date and time opened and/or due to expire according to agency policy

h. Alternate methods of delivery include: jet injectors, pen injectors, portable insulin pumps, implantable pumps, and intranasal insulin

i. Dosage must be monitored and linked with insulin needs

j. Dosing schedules include the following:

    1) Conventional therapy: short-acting and intermediate-acting insulin is given twice a day on a fixed regimen

    2) Intensified therapy: long-acting insulin taken in the evening and a fast-acting insulin given before meals according to blood glucose levels

    3) Continuous SC insulin infusion: a portable infusion pump is connected to a catheter and infuses regular insulin at a steady rate

4. Contraindications: previous allergic response to local or systemic use of drug

5. Significant drug interactions

    a. Hypoglycemic agents that lower blood glucose levels, such as sulfonylureas; acute use of alcohol; and beta-adrenergic blocking agents

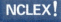

b. Hyperglycemic agents that increase blood glucose levels, such as thiazide diuretic agents, glucocorticoids, and sympathomimetics

    c. Beta-adrenergic blocking agents that delay response of insulin-related hypoglycemia and mask signs of sympathetic nervous system stimulation (tachycardia and palpitations)

6. Significant food interactions: moderate to high alcohol consumption without food enhances hypoglycemic action

7. Significant laboratory studies: random blood glucose, fasting blood glucose, glucose tolerance test, **glycosylated hemoglobin** A_{1c}, (a blood test representative of the average blood glucose level over the past several weeks), urinary glucose and ketones, and serum electrolytes

8. Side effects

    a. Hypoglycemic reactions when blood glucose levels drop below 50 mg/dL

    b. Signs of hypoglycemic reaction include headache, confusion, drowsiness, and fatigue

9. Adverse effects/toxicity

    a. Coma related to inadequate dosage caused by uncontrolled diabetic derangements with high blood glucose levels and ketoacidosis or hyperosmolar coma

    b. Coma related to insulin overdosage caused by inadequate food intake, excessive exercise, or excessive insulin administration

10. Complications

    a. Presence of insulin antibodies that can lead to insulin resistance

    b. **Lipodystrophy** (abnormal deposition of subcutaneous fat at injection sites)

    c. Local allergic reaction related to a contaminant in the insulin preparation

    d. Systemic allergic reaction related to insulin itself and not to any contaminant

11. Nursing considerations

    a. Assess vital signs, weight, condition of skin and nails, serum and urine glucose levels, glycosylated hemoglobin (and electrolyte and arterial blood gas levels) when appropriate

    b. Assess for long-term complications related to acceleration of atherosclerosis (hypertension, heart disease, stroke); retinopathy leading to possible blindness, nephropathy leading to possible renal failure; neuropathy leading to lower limb ulcerations and amputation, impotence, and gastroparesis

    c. Consult with physician regarding insulin management when there is insufficient food intake or when client is NPO for surgery

    d. Adhere to agency policy regarding insulin administration

12. Client education

    a. Develop individual teaching plan about insulin management

    b. Teach all aspects of insulin administration including syringe use, mixing of insulins, stability of mixture, injection technique and sites

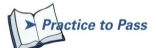

► Practice to Pass

A male client newly diagnosed with type 1 diabetes mellitus is going camping for 6 weeks and asks the nurse how he can store his insulin. What advice should the nurse give?

NCLEX!

NCLEX!

NCLEX!

NCLEX!

NCLEX!

NCLEX!

   c. Instruct not to switch type or source of insulin or brand of syringe and avoid taking any new drug before notifying MD

   d. Teach client and family about signs and symptoms of hyperglycemia and hypoglycemia

   e. Teach how to test blood glucose levels

   f. Teach dietary restrictions and weight control and refer to dietician

   g. Encourage regular exercise

   h. Explain foot care and related aspects of personal hygiene

   i. Teach sick-day management of diabetes and insulin administration (continue to eat and take liquids as able, check blood glucose, maintain insulin schedule, and call prescriber if blood glucose is > 250 mg/dL)

   j. Advise client to obtain and wear a Medic-Alert tag or bracelet

   k. Advise to avoid smoking or drinking alcoholic beverages

   l. Caution female clients to consult with MD before conceiving

   m. Refer to local home care agency and to American Diabetic Association for additional follow-up and access to community-based resources

B. Oral antidiabetic (hypoglycemic) agents—sulfonylureas

  1. Action and use

   a. Stimulate release of insulin from pancreatic islets

   b. Are used as an adjunct to nondrug therapy to reduce blood glucose levels in type 2 diabetes mellitus

  2. Common medications (Table 6-13)

  3. Administration considerations

   a. Dose is given orally 1 to 3 times a day

   b. Different agents possess different durations of action

   c. May be used alone or in combination with insulin

  4. Contraindications

   a. During pregnancy related to teratogenicity in animals

   b. In women who are nursing/lactating

   c. In clients with allergy to sulfa or urea

  5. Significant drug interactions

   a. Nonsteroidal anti-inflammatory drugs (NSAIDS), sulfonamide antibiotics, acute use of ethanol, salicylates, phenothiazines, thiazides, ranitidine, and cimetidine

   b. Beta-adrenergic blocking agents can suppress insulin release and delay response to hypoglycemia

  6. Significant food interactions: none noted

Table 6-13	Generic	Trade Name	Dose & Duration of Action	Notes
Oral Antidiabetics/ Hypoglycemics (Sulfonylureas)	Tolbutamide	Orinase	12–2 g/day in 1–3 doses & up to 2–3 g/day in 1–3 doses **DURATION:** 6–12 hr	First-generation agent
	Acetohexamide	Dymelor	0.25–0.5 g/day in 1–2 doses & up to 1.5 g/day in 1–2 doses **DURATION:** 12–24 hr	First-generation agent
	Tolazamide	Tolinase	100–200 mg/day at breakfast & up to 0.75–1 g in 2 divided doses **DURATION:** 12–24 hr	First-generation agent
	Chlorpropamide	Diabinase	25 mg/day up to 750 mg/day **DURATION:** 24–72 hr	First-generation agent
	Glipizide Standard	Glucotrol	5 mg/day at breakfast & up to 40 mg/day in 2 divided doses **DURATION:** 12–24 hr	Second-generation agent
	Glipizide Sustained release	Glucotrol XL	5 mg/day at breakfast & up to 20 mg/day at breakfast **DURATION:** 24 hr	Second-generation agent
	Glyburide Nonmicronized	Diabeta, Micronase	2.5–5 mg/day at breakfast & up to 20 mg/day in 1–2 divided doses **DURATION:** 12–24 hr	Second-generation agent
	Glyburide Micronized	Glynase PresTab	1.5–3 mg/day at breakfast & up to 12 mg/day in 1–2 doses **DURATION:** 24 hr	Second-generation agent
	Glimepride	Amaryl	1–2 mg/day at breakfast & up to 8 mg/day at breakfast **DURATION:** 24 hr	Second-generation agent

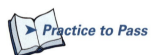

> **➤ Practice to Pass**
>
> A client with type 2 diabetes mellitus has been sick at home for several days with a fever and flu-like symptoms. What instructions should the nurse give to the client regarding sick day diabetes management?

7. Significant laboratory studies

    a. CBC with differential, platelet count

    b. Liver function tests

    c. Blood glucose

8. Side effects

    a. GI tract distress

    b. Neurologic symptoms such as dizziness, drowsiness, or headache

9. Adverse effects/toxicity

    a. Alcohol may cause a disulfiram-like reaction causing flushing, palpitations, and nausea

    b. Allergy related to skin reaction

    c. Hypoglycemia related to drug overdosage, drug interactions, altered drug metabolism, or inadequate food intake

      d. Hypoglycemic reactions are most likely to occur in presence of renal or hepatic dysfunction

  10. Nursing considerations

      a. Assess vital signs, weight, condition of skin and nails, serum and urine glucose levels, glycosylated hemoglobin and electrolyte and arterial blood gas levels when appropriate

      b. Assess for long-term complications of diabetes as noted in previous section regarding nursing considerations with insulin

      c. Consult with physician regarding management when client has insufficient food intake or is NPO for surgery

  11. Client education

      a. Develop individualized teaching plan based on client's previous knowledge, educational level, motivation to learn, and cultural considerations

      b. Teach all aspects of drug therapy and advise to take with food if GI upset

      c. Advise to take medication even if not feeling well

      d. Take dose with first daily meal and take any missed dose as soon as remembered unless time for next dose; do not double-up doses

      e. Teach client and family about signs and symptoms of hypoglycemia and to notify MD if occur

      f. Teach how to test blood glucose levels

      g. Teach dietary restrictions and weight control, and refer to dietician (very helpful for developing effective meal and weight management plans)

      h. Encourage regular exercise that is aerobic and of amount suited to client's health and abilities

      i. Explain foot care and related aspects of personal hygiene

      j. Teach sick day management of diabetes and PRN insulin administration

      k. Advise client to obtain and wear Medic-Alert tag or bracelet

      l. Advise to avoid smoking or drinking alcoholic beverages

      m. Caution female clients to consult with physician before conceiving and to discontinue drug during pregnancy and lactation

      n. Refer to local home care agency and to American Diabetic Association for additional follow-up and access to community-based resources

C. Oral antidiabetics (hypoglycemic) agents—nonsulfonylureas

  1. Action and use

      a. Biguanides lower blood glucose by decreasing production of glucose by the liver

      b. Alpha-glucosidase inhibitors delay absorption of dietary carbohydrates and reduce blood glucose

Table 6-14

Oral Antidiabetics/ Hypoglycemics (Nonsulfonylureas)

Generic	Trade Name	Dose & Duration of Action	Notes
Metformin	Glucophage	500 mg 2×/day & up to 850 mg 2×/day; maximum dose 850 mg 3×/day	Classification: biguanide
Repaglinide	Prandin	0.5 to 2 mg; up to 16 mg/day	Classification: nonsulfonylurea
Acarbose	Precose	25 mg 3×/day & up to 50 mg 3×/day (pts < 60 kg) & 100 mg 3×/day (pts > 60 kg)	Classification: alpha-glucosidase inhibitor
Migitol	Glyset	Individualized, but usually 50 mg 3×/day up to 100 mg 3×/day	Classification: alpha-glucosidase inhibitor
Pioglitazone	Actos	15 to 30 mg once daily up to 45 mg/day	Classification: thiazolidinedione
Rosiglitazone	Advandia	4 mg daily to a maximum of 8 mg	Classification: thiazolidinedione
Nateglinide	Starlit	Usually 60 to 120 mg 3×/day before meals; maximum dose not defined	Classification: D-phenylalanine derivative

    c. Both are used to decrease blood glucose levels after meals in clients with type 2 diabetes mellitus not controlled by diet modification and exercise

2. Common medications (Table 6-14)

3. Administration considerations

    a. Orally 1 to 3 times a day

    b. Biguanides are used alone or in combination with a sulfonylurea

    c. Alpha-glucose inhibitors are used alone or in combination with insulin or a sulfonylurea

4. Contraindications: renal insufficiency and kidney disease

5. Significant drug interactions

    a. Both forms should not be taken together because of the incidence of significant GI distress

    b. Amiloride, cimetidine, digoxin, morphine, procainamide, quinidine, quinine, ranitidine, triamterene, trimethoprin, and vancomycin may decrease renal secretion of antidiabetic agent

6. Significant food interactions: alcohol may increase risk of hypoglycemia or lactic acidosis

7. Significant laboratory studies

    a. CBC with differential, platelet count

    b. Liver function tests

    c. Blood glucose

8. Side effects

    a. Biguanides may cause decreased appetite, nausea, and diarrhea that usually subside over time; also increased absorption of vitamin B_{12} and folic acid may occur

    b. Alpha-glucosidase inhibitors cause flatulence, cramps, abdominal distension, borborygmus, and diarrhea; also may decrease absorption of iron, leading to anemia

9. Adverse effects/toxicity

NCLEX!

    a. Biguanides with hypoglycemia and lactic acidosis result in a mortality rate of 50%

    b. Alpha-glucosidase inhibitors may lead to hypoglycemia if given with insulin or a sulfonylurea

10. Nursing considerations

    a. Assess vital signs, weight, condition of skin and nails, serum and urine glucose levels, glycosylated hemoglobin, and electrolyte and arterial blood gas levels when appropriate

    b. Assess renal function and evidence of renal insufficiency

    c. Assess for early sign of lactic acidosis

    d. Assess for long-term complications of diabetes mellitus

    e. Consult with physician regarding management when client has insufficient food intake or is NPO for surgery

11. Client education

    a. Teach client all aspects of diabetic management as outlined in previous client education section for sulfonylureas.

NCLEX!

    b. Inform about early signs of hypoglycemia and lactic acidosis (hyperventilation, myalgia, malaise, unusual somnolence) and notify physician immediately if occur

D. Glucose-elevating medications—glucagon

1. Action and use

    a. Promotes breakdown of glycogen, reduces glycogen synthesis, and stimulates synthesis of glucose

NCLEX!

    b. Emergency treatment of severe **hypoglycemia** (lower than normal circulating glucose level) in unconscious clients or those unable to swallow and in clients receiving insulin shock therapy

2. Common medication (Table 6-15): glucagon (GlucaGen)

3. Administration considerations

    a. Reconstitute according to manufacturer's directions

    b. Given SC, IM, or direct IVP; flush IV line with 5% dextrose instead of NaCl solution

    c. Incompatible in syringe with any other medication

Table 6-15	Generic	Trade Name	Dose & Duration of Action	Notes
Glucose-Elevating Medication	Glucagon	GlucaGen	**IM, IV, SC:** *Adults*—0.5–1 mg & repeat q 5–20 min if no response for 1–2 doses. *Children*—0.025 mg/kg (max 1 mg/dose & repeat q 5–20 min in no response for 1–2 more doses. *Neonate*—0.3 mg/kg (max 1 mg).	Used in emergency treatment of severe hypoglycemia reactions in unconscious diabetic pts. or pts. unable to swallow.

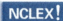

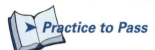

4. Contraindications

   a. Hypersensitivity to glucagon or protein compounds

   b. Cautious use in insulinoma and pheochromocytoma

5. Significant drug interactions: incompatible with sodium chloride solutions or additives

6. Significant food interactions: none noted

7. Significant laboratory studies: blood glucose levels

8. Side effects: nausea and vomiting

9. Adverse effects/toxicity

   a. Hypersensitivity reactions

   b. Hyperglycemia and hypokalemia

10. Nursing considerations

   a. Client usually responds/awakens within 5 to 20 minutes after administration

   b. Give IV glucose if no response to glucagon

   c. After client awakens and is able to swallow give PO carbohydrate

   d. After recovery assess for persistent headache, nausea, and weakness

11. Client education

   a. Teach how to test blood glucose levels

   b. Teach responsible family member how to administer SC or IM in the presence of frequent hypoglycemic reactions

   c. Notify MD immediately after reaction to discover cause

Practice to Pass

A client who has been experiencing frequent hypoglycemic (insulin) reactions at home calls and says that he cannot afford to buy any more blood glucose testing equipment. What should the nurse do?

| **Case Study** | A 52-year-old male client has just been diagnosed with type 2 (formerly non insulin dependent) diabetes mellitus. You are the nurse working in the diabetes management clinic and have been present when the physician told the client about his diagnosis.

❶ What type of initial reaction would you expect the client to exhibit?

❷ What additional assessment data do you need to obtain before you begin client teaching?

❸ What key teaching points should you emphasize during the first teaching session?

❹ What type of follow-up resources would you give this client?

❺ How frequently should you instruct the client to seek follow-up care?

For suggested responses, see pages 638–639.

Posttest

1 A child is about to begin taking growth hormone. Which of the following teaching points should the nurse stress to the parent?

(1) "Your child's expected growth rate is 3 to 5 inches during the first year of treatment."
(2) "You need to measure your child's height and weight daily."
(3) "Growth hormone therapy, once started, must be taken until the child reaches the age of 21."
(4) "The amount of subcutaneous fat your child has will increase during the treatment period."

2 The nurse is instructing the client about insulin administration. Which of the following pieces of client information alerts the nurse that special instruction regarding insulin is necessary?

(1) Client lives in an apartment with spouse.
(2) Client wishes to teach spouse how to administer insulin.
(3) Client jogs 3 to 4 miles every other day.
(4) Client takes a nap in the afternoon.

3 A client with a history of alcoholism has just been diagnosed with type 2 diabetes mellitus and is placed on tolbutamide (Orinase). The nurse explains that which one of the following reactions may occur if the client drinks alcohol while taking this medication?

(1) Decreased diuresis
(2) Disulfiram-like reaction
(3) Anaphylaxis
(4) Increased tolerance to the medication

4 A child is placed on somatrem (Protropin). The parents ask the nurse if the child will keep on growing after the drug has been discontinued. The nurse utilizes which of the following points about this medication in a response?

(1) The drug is not effective until the client has reached teenage years.
(2) The client must take the drug for a lifetime.
(3) The client can expect to grow well into his 4th or 5th decade.
(4) Efficacy of therapy declines as the client grows older.

5 A client is taking metyrapone (Metopirone) and experiences an adrenal crisis. Which of the following most likely predisposed the client to this occurrence?

(1) Cortisol synthesis has increased.
(2) The client has adrenal insufficiency.
(3) The client has type 1 diabetes mellitus.
(4) The client has no adrenal insufficiency.

6 A client is scheduled to have a bilateral adrenalectomy. Which one of the following drugs does the nurse expect to administer in the postoperative period?

(1) Hydrocortisone succinate
(2) Dexamethasone
(3) Adrenocorticotropic hormone (ACTH)
(4) Ketoconazole

7 A client who was recently started on drug therapy with desmopressin (DDAVP) complains of a headache, lethargy, and drowsiness. The nurse concludes that which of the following may be responsible for this reaction?

(1) Streptococcal infection
(2) Excessive ingestion of calcium
(3) Dehydration
(4) Fluid overload

8 A client with hyperthyroidism is being prepared for surgery and propranolol (Inderal) is prescribed. The nurse explains to the client that this drug is being given to control which symptom?

(1) Tachycardia
(2) Hypotension
(3) Dyspnea
(4) Drowsiness

9 A client who is taking digoxin (Lanoxin) is to receive a dose of intravenous calcium. Which of the following drug interactions must the nurse be prepared for?

(1) Severe tachycardia
(2) Severe bradycardia
(3) Severe hypotension
(4) Severe hypertension

10 A client with hypocalcemia needs to increase his calcium absorption. The nurse explains to the client that which of the following vitamins will be most beneficial to the client?

(1) Vitamin A
(2) Vitamin C
(3) Vitamin B$_{12}$
(4) Vitamin D

See pages 263–264 for Answers and Rationales.

Answers and Rationales

Pretest

1 **Answer: 3** *Rationale:* Growth hormone is only approved for use in children to treat a documented lack of growth hormone. It is available as a parenteral medication only, to be given IM or SC (option 2). Only long bones are affected (option 3). Option 4 is incorrect because this response implies that this treatment is appropriate despite the lack of additional diagnostic evidence needed for this therapy.
Cognitive Level: Analysis
Nursing Process: Implementation; *Test Plan:* PHYS

2 **Answer: 2** *Rationale:* Abrupt cessation of long-term steroid therapy can cause acute adrenal insufficiency, which could lead to death. Options 1 and 4 are incorrect statements. Central nervous system symptoms such as confusion and psychosis are adverse effects of steroids such as prednisone (option 3).
Cognitive Level: Application
Nursing Process: Analysis; *Test Plan:* PHYS

3 **Answer: 1** *Rationale:* Desmopressin is not given by the intramuscular route. This medication may be given by the intravenous, subcutaneous, or intranasal routes (options 2, 3, and 4) in the treatment of diabetes insipidus.
Cognitive Level: Application
Nursing Process: Implementation; *Test Plan:* PHYS

4 **Answer: 1** *Rationale:* Fludrocortisone is a mineralocorticoid used to treat Addison's disease. High doses of fludrocortisone may result in excess retention of salt and water and depletion of potassium. Options 2 and 3 contain incorrect statements. In the treatment of Addison's disease, fludrocortisone is commonly used in combination with a glucocorticoid (option 4).
Cognitive Level: Application
Nursing Process: Evaluation; *Test Plan:* PHYS

5 **Answer: 4** *Rationale:* After the start of therapy, peak levels of the drug may not be expected for many weeks to months. Thus, increased energy levels cannot be expected within a few days (option 2). The drug works best when taken before breakfast on an empty stomach (option 3). Lack of energy is a common symptom with hypothyroidism (option 1).
Cognitive Level: Analysis
Nursing Process: Implementation; *Test Plan:* PHYS

6   Answer: 2 *Rationale:* Symptoms of adverse effects and thyrotoxicosis of liotrix (Thyrolar) include tachycardia, angina, tremor, nervousness, insomnia, hyperthermia, heat tolerance, and sweating. Options 1, 3, and 4 represent manifestations that are opposite those of thyrotoxicosis, which are also manifestations of hypothyroidism.
Cognitive Level: Application
Nursing Process: Implementation; *Test Plan:* PHYS

7   Answer: 3 *Rationale:* Agranulocytosis is the most serious toxic effect of this drug, and it can make the client predisposed to a variety of infections. Although rare, this adverse effect may occur within the first few months of treatment. Options 1 and 2 are incorrect conclusions; although option 4 is possible, the manifestations reported are general signs of infection that may or may not be consistent with influenza.
Cognitive Level: Analysis
Nursing Process: Analysis; *Test Plan:* PHYS

8   Answer: 1 *Rationale:* Calcitonin rapidly lowers blood calcium levels by reducing mobilization of calcium from bone, decreasing intestinal resorption, and promoting urinary excretion of calcium. Options 2 and 3 are effects that are opposite to the ones caused by calcitonin, while option 4 is incorrect because of the word "gradual."
Cognitive Level: Application
Nursing Process: Implementation; *Test Plan:* PHYS

9   Answer: 3 *Rationale:* Hunger, nausea, pale, cool skin, and sweating are signs of a hypoglycemic reaction. Fruity breath (option 1) may accompany ketoacidosis. Flushing of the face (option 2) may accompany hyperglycemia. Dry flaky skin (option 4) is unrelated to hypoglycemia.
Cognitive Level: Application
Nursing Process: Assessment; *Test Plan:* PHYS

10   Answer: 4 *Rationale:* The initial action by the client is to take some form of oral glucose in order to raise the blood glucose level. Option 1 would delay appropriate self-treatment. Options 2 and 3 would cause further harm to the client.
Cognitive Level: Analysis
Nursing Process: Planning; *Test Plan:* PHYS

Posttest

1   Answer: 1 *Rationale:* The expected growth rate with growth hormone therapy is 3 to 5 inches in the first year. Height and weight is measured monthly (option 2). Growth hormone is discontinued when optimum adult height is attained, fusion of epiphyseal plates has oc-

curred, or when there is no response to growth hormone (option 3). Growth hormone is related to growth of long bones, not fat deposition (option 4).
Cognitive Level: Application
Nursing Process: Implementation; *Test Plan:* PHYS

2   Answer: 3 *Rationale:* Jogging increases insulin requirements and absorption can be increased if the drug is injected into the thigh. This lifestyle factor of the client requires special instruction. Options 1 and 4 are unrelated to teaching about insulin administration. Option 2 guides the nurse to include the spouse in teaching, but it does not indicate the need for special instruction regarding insulin.
Cognitive Level: Analysis
Nursing Process: Planning; *Test Plan:* PHYS

3   Answer: 2 *Rationale:* Tolbutamide interacting with alcohol can lead to a disulfiram-like reaction causing complaints of headache and flushing of the skin. This is an important teaching point for the client who has a history of alcoholism, even if currently not drinking. The reactions listed in the remaining options do not occur as a result of co-ingestion with alcohol.
Cognitive Level: Application
Nursing Process: Implementation; *Test Plan:* PHYS

4   Answer: 4 *Rationale:* Resistance to growth hormone eventually develops, and the rate of growth begins to slow down with increasing age. Efficacy of the drug is usually lost by the age of 20 to 24 years (options 2 and 3). The medication is quite effective in children (option 1) as long as there is a demonstrated deficiency in growth hormone.
Cognitive Level: Application
Nursing Process: Analysis; *Test Plan:* PHYS

5   Answer: 2 *Rationale:* In the presence of adrenal insufficiency, metyrapone may cause an adrenal crisis by stopping the synthesis of cortisol. Options 1 and 4 are the opposite of what is occurring with the client. Option 3 is an unrelated finding.
Cognitive Level: Analysis
Nursing Process: Analysis; *Test Plan:* PHYS

6   Answer: 1 *Rationale:* Hydrocortisone succinate may be given IV or IM and is the preferred drug for replacement therapy in all forms of adrenocortical insufficiency. ACTH is mostly used for diagnostic testing (option 3). Dexamethasone is used for nonendocrine disorders (option 2) and ketoconazole (option 4) is used to suppress the synthesis of adrenal steroids.
Cognitive Level: Analysis
Nursing Process: Planning; *Test Plan:* PHYS

7 **Answer: 4** *Rationale:* Desmopressin is a drug used to treat diabetes insipidus. The manifestations listed are all signs of water intoxication, which could occur as an excessive effect of the medication. Options 1 and 2 are unrelated to this medication, while option 3 is associated with diabetes insipidus, the underlying condition for which this drug would be ordered.
Cognitive Level: Analysis
Nursing Process: Evaluation; *Test Plan:* PHYS

8 **Answer: 1** *Rationale:* Propranolol is a beta-adrenergic blocker and is used to treat sympathetic nervous system symptoms related to hyperthyroidism such as tachycardia, cardiac dysrhythmias and mental agitation. The manifestations identified in the other options would not be adequately treated with this medication.
Cognitive Level: Application
Nursing Process: Implementation; *Test Plan:* PHYS

9 **Answer: 2** *Rationale:* Parenteral calcium can cause severe bradycardia in clients taking digoxin. Option 1 is the opposite effect of what could occur. Hypertension is not an expected effect (option 4) and hypotension could occur as a result of severe bradycardia, but this is a secondary effect (option 3).
Cognitive Level: Analysis
Nursing Process: Planning; *Test Plan:* PHYS

10 **Answer: 4** *Rationale:* Vitamin D regulates calcium and phosphorus metabolism and increases blood levels of both elements. The vitamins in the other options do not have this beneficial effect.
Cognitive Level: Application
Nursing Process: Planning; *Test Plan:* PHYS

References

Anderson, K., Anderson, L., & Glanze, W. (Eds.). (2001). *Mosby's medical, nursing, & allied health dictionary* (6th ed.). St. Louis: Mosby, Inc.

Clark, J., Queener, S., and Karb, V. (2003). *Pharmacologic basis of nursing practice* (7th ed.). St. Louis: Mosby, Inc.

Kee, J., & Hayes, E. (2003). *Pharmacology: A nursing process approach* (4th ed.). Philadelphia: Elsevier Science, pp. 710–748.

Kozier, B., Erb, G., Berman, A., & Burke, K. (2004). *Fundamentals of nursing: Concepts, process, and practice* (7th ed.). Upper Saddle River, NJ: Pearson Education, Inc.

Lehne, R. (2004). *Pharmacology for nursing care* (5th ed.) Philadelphia: W.B. Saunders Co., pp. 611–676, 803–821.

LeMone, P., & Burke, K. (2003). *Medical-surgical nursing: Critical thinking in client care* (3rd ed.) Upper Saddle River, NJ: Prentice Hall Health.

Skidmore-Roth, L. (2002). *Mosby's 2002 nursing drug reference.* St. Louis: Mosby, Inc., pp. 47, 336, 463, 607, 908–909.

Wilkinson, J. (2000). *Nursing diagnosis handbook* (7th ed.). Upper Saddle River, NJ: Prentice Hall, p. 184.

Wilson, B., Shannon, M., and Stang, C. (2003). *Nursing drug guide 2003.* Upper Saddle River, NJ: Prentice Hall, pp. 414, 1286–1287.

Winningham, M. & Preusser, B. (2001). *Critical thinking in medical-surgical settings* (2nd ed.). St. Louis: Mosby, Inc.

Youngkin, E., Sawin, K., Kissinger, J., and Israel, D. (1999). *Pharmacotherapeutics: A primary care clinical guide.* Stamford, CT: Appleton & Lange.

CHAPTER 7

Gastrointestinal System Medications

Julie Adkins, RN, MSN, APRN-BC

CHAPTER OUTLINE

Gastrointestinal Stimulants
Medications to Decrease GI Tone and Motility (Anticholinergics and Antispasmodics)
Antidiarrheals
Laxatives

Emetics
Antiemetics
Histamine H_2 Antagonists
Proton Pump Inhibitors
Mucosal Protective Agents
Antacids

Antimicrobials for Helicobacter pylori Organisms
Medications Used to Dissolve Gallstones
Pancreatic Enzyme Replacement

OBJECTIVES

▪ Describe general goals of therapy when administering gastrointestinal system medications.

▪ Describe the use and side effects of antacids.

▪ Identify the actions of various forms of laxatives.

▪ Discuss the effects of H_2 receptor antagonists, proton pump inhibitors, and mucosal protectants on the gastrointestinal tract.

▪ Describe nursing considerations related to administration of antiemetics.

▪ Identify specific food and drug interactions associated with various gastrointestinal system medications.

▪ Describe nursing considerations related to administration of pancreatic enzyme replacements.

▪ List significant client education points related to gastrointestinal system medications.

[Media Link]

Use the CD-ROM enclosed with this text, or log onto the address given to access the free, interactive Companion Website created for this series. The CD-ROM and Companion Website accompanying this book offer additional practice opportunities and information—NCLEX Review, Case Studies, Glossary, In Depth with NCLEX, and more.

www.prenhall.com/hogan

REVIEW AT A GLANCE

antacid *agent that reduces or neutralizes acidity*

anticholinergic *antagonist to parasympathetic action or other cholinergic receptors*

antispasmodic *agent that prevents or relieves spasms*

cathartic *agent with purgative action*

emetic *agent that causes vomiting*

H₂ antagonist *antagonist agent against histamine that decreases gastrin secretion*

Helicobacter pylori *bacteria found in gastric mucosa that produces urease and is associated commonly with gastric and duodenal ulcers*

laxative *agent used to cause a bowel movement or loosening of the bowels*

proton pump inhibitor *a class of drugs that inhibit secretion of gastric acid*

surfactant *a surface-active agent also known as a wetting agent, tension depressant, detergent and emulsifier*

Pretest

1 A mother rushes her 2-year-old child to the urgent care clinic. She has given the child two doses of ipecac syrup following ingestion of a bottle of children's aspirin. It has been over 40 minutes and the child has still not vomited. What should the nurse do first?

(1) Call the poison control center.
(2) Give activated charcoal.
(3) Offer milk or carbonated soda.
(4) Wait for physician to assess the client.

2 The nurse is caring for a client with gastroesophageal reflux disease (GERD) who is taking metoclopramide (Reglan). The nurse determines that the client understands the purpose of the medication when the client verbalizes that the medication has which of the following actions?

(1) Increases GI motility
(2) Decreases GI motility
(3) Combats diarrhea
(4) Kills *H. pylori* organisms

3 A client is taking dicyclomine (Antispas) for irritable bowel disorder. The nurse explains to the client that which of the following represents the optimal dosing for dicyclomine?

(1) Take after meals.
(2) Take with meals.
(3) Take only as needed.
(4) Take 30 to 60 minutes before meals and bedtime.

4 A male client has been diagnosed with acute diarrhea. He is allergic to aspirin (ASA) and takes no medications. Which antidiarrheal medication should not be given to this client?

(1) Kaopectate
(2) Pepto-Bismol
(3) Lomotil
(4) Imodium

5 An ambulatory care nurse is working with a client who has come to the clinic because of diarrhea. The nurse determines that the client needs instruction about management of this health problem when the client states to do which of the following?

(1) Avoid dairy products.
(2) Take Kaopectate as directed.
(3) Contact healthcare provider if symptoms not resolved in 2 days.
(4) Use a bulk-forming agent such as Metamucil.

6 The nurse is teaching a client who has a fluid restriction about medications for constipation. During this discussion, the nurse should include which of the following explanations about why a bulk-forming laxative would not be the best choice for this client?

(1) Clients who are on a fluid restriction are already at decreased risk of constipation.
(2) Bulk-forming laxatives should only be used after other types have been tried and found to be unsuccessful.
(3) Bulk-forming laxatives work best for clients with conditions in which they should not bear down or strain at stool.
(4) Bulk-forming laxatives rely on increased water to swell and increase the mass of the intestinal contents.

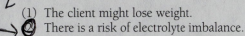

7 The client informs you that he has been taking a laxative for constipation for over a month. What information should you include in the teaching plan regarding prolonged laxative use?

2

(1) The client might lose weight.
(2) There is a risk of electrolyte imbalance.
(3) The client will likely experience decreased appetite.
(4) There is heightened risk of abdominal pain.

8 The client is receiving loperamide (Imodium) prn. The nurse should plan to administer this medication when client has which of the following gastrointestinal conditions?

4

(1) Constipation
(2) Vomiting
(3) Abdominal pain
(4) Diarrhea

9 The client who has just been told that she has a gastric ulcer is asking for information about commonly used therapeutic medications. Which of the following medications should the nurse expect to include in the teaching plan about medication use?

2

(1) Ranitidine (Zantac)
(2) Misoprostol (Cytotec)
(3) Magnesium hydroxide (Milk of Magnesia)
(4) Bethanechol chloride (Davoid)

10 Which of the following symptoms reported by the client would the nurse not attribute to an adverse effect of misoprostol (Cytotec)?

2

(1) Dysmenorrhea
(2) Urinary incontinence
(3) Headache
(4) Diarrhea

See pages 298–299 for Answers and Rationales.

I. Gastrointestinal Stimulants

A. Action and use

1. Decrease reflux by increasing sphincter tone and enhancing acid clearance and decreasing gastric emptying

2. Used for prevention and reduction of nausea and vomiting due to chemotherapy, and for facilitation of small bowel intubations

3. Used for delayed gastric emptying caused by diabetic gastroparesis, gastroesophageal reflux, postoperative nausea, and vomiting

B. Common medications

1. Metoclopramide (Reglan) is currently the only approved prokinetic agent available

2. Metoclopramide dose is 10 mg PO or 1 to 2 mg/kg IV

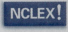

3. Cisapride (Propulsid) was taken off the market in July 2000 due to significant risk of severe cardiac dysrhythmics (QT prolongation)

C. Administration considerations

1. Metoclopramide PO should be taken 30 minutes before meals and bedtime

2. Metoclopramide IV should be given 30 minutes prior to chemotherapy for antiemetic effect

D. Contraindications

1. Concurrent use of macrolides and antifungal agents may cause serious cardiac dysrhythmias (cisapride)

2. Contraindicated in clients where overstimulation may be dangerous, such as with hemorrhage, obstruction, or perforation

3. Use with caution in clients with a history of depression, seizure disorder, hypertension or Parkinson's disease

4. Lactation: excreted in breast milk, so caution should be used in nursing mothers

E. Significant drug interactions

1. Cisapride and metoclopramide are metabolized by P450 liver enzyme system and should not be taken with inhibitors of this enzyme such as macrolides, antifungals, and some protease inhibitors; may decrease absorption of digoxin

2. Concomitant use of metoclopramide, hycosamine, and tricyclic antidepressants may antagonize effects of metoclopramide

3. Levodopa has the opposite effect and may antagonize metoclopramide effect

4. Metoclopramide may increase hypertensive effects of monoamine oxidase (MAO) inhibitors

F. Significant food interactions: none reported

G. Significant laboratory studies: serum electrolyte levels

H. Side effects

1. Drowsiness, diarrhea, restlessness, fatigue

2. Parkinson-like symptoms

I. Adverse effects/toxicity

1. Seizures

2. Agranulocytosis

3. Depression with suicide ideations

J. Nursing considerations

1. Monitor for possible hypernatremia and hypokalemia, particularly if client has congestive heart failure (CHF) or cirrhosis of the liver

2. Extrapyramidal symptoms may occur in young adults and the elderly and with high-dose treatment of metoclopramide

K. Client education

1. Instruct client to report signs and symptoms of side effects

2. Instruct client to report signs of acute dystonia immediately

3. Advise client not to drive for a few hours after taking metoclopramide

II. Medications to Decrease GI Tone and Motility (Anticholinergics and Antispasmodics)

A. Action and use

1. **Anticholinergics** antagonize the action of acetylcholine at the cholinergic receptor sites

2. **Antispasmodics** are similar and they are believed to relax smooth muscle

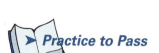

Practice to Pass

What GI drug has been withdrawn by the Food and Drug Administration because of adverse effects of QT prolongation?

Generic/Trade Names	Usual Adult Dosage Range	Route
Dicyclomine hydrochloride (Bentyl)	20 mg qid	PO
Hyoscyamine sulfate (Levsin)	1–2 tablets every 4 hr	PO
Chlordiazepoxide hydrochloride (Librax)	1–2 capsules tid before meals and HS	PO
Glycopyrrolate (Robinul)	1–2 mg 2–3 times a day	PO

Table 7-1

Medications to Decrease GI Tone and Motility- Anticholinergics/ Antispasmodics

3. Used for treatment of spasms of the gastrointestinal (GI) tract such as pylorospasm, ileitis, and irritable bowel syndrome

B. Common medications (Table 7-1)

C. Administration considerations: give medication 30 to 60 minutes before meals and at bedtime for therapeutic effect

D. Contraindications

1. Contraindicated in narrow-angle glaucoma, obstructive GI disease, paralytic ileus, obstructive uropathy

2. Excreted in breast milk, may cause infant toxicity and decreased milk production

3. Use with caution with renal dysfunction

E. Significant drug interactions

1. When taken with any other anticholinergic drug may result in increased anticholinergic side effects

2. Atropine may increase the effect of phenothiazines

3. The effects of atenolol may be increased with anticholinergic drugs

F. Significant food interactions: none reported

G. Significant laboratory studies: serum electrolyte levels

H. Side effects

1. Hypersensitivity

2. Urticaria, rash, dry mouth, nausea, vomiting, constipation, urinary hesitance and retention

3. Impotence, blurred vision, worsening of glaucoma

4. Palpitations, headache, flushing, drowsiness, dizziness, confusion

I. Adverse effects/toxicity

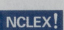

1. May cause dilated, nonreactive pupils, visual changes

2. Tachycardia

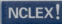

3. Dysphagia, decreased or absent bowel sounds

4. Hyperthermia, hypertension, increased respiratory rate

J. Nursing considerations

1. An understanding of the factors contributing to the diarrhea is essential in effective treatment

2. Clients who lose significant potassium with diarrhea are at risk for the development of paralytic ileus and cardiac dysrhythmias

3. They should also be monitored for metabolic acidosis because of the loss of bicarbonate and impaired renal excretion of acids

4. Document indications and present medications

5. Monitor vital signs, urine output, and visual changes

6. Monitor intake and output (I & O)

K. Client education

1. Instruct client to avoid exposure to high temperatures because of risk of hyperthermia

2. Advise client to report side effects to health care provider

3. Instruct client on dietary/fluid interventions to decrease constipation

4. Instruct client to report any additional medications prescribed

5. Instruct client to monitor I & O

III. Antidiarrheals

A. Action and use

1. Slow and/or inhibit GI motility by acting on nerve endings of the intestinal wall, thereby reducing the volume of stools, increasing viscosity and decreasing fluid and electrolyte loss

2. Used for symptomatic relief of acute nonspecific diarrhea and diarrhea of inflammatory disease

B. Common medications (Table 7-2)

C. Administration considerations

1. Shake suspensions well; chew tablets thoroughly

2. Stool may appear gray-black (may mask GI bleeding)

3. Do not give concurrently with other medications

4. Seek medical care if diarrhea persists for more than 2 days in the adult

5. Do not use to treat diarrhea in children; seek medical attention

Table 7-2	Generic/Trade Names	Usual Adult Dosage Range	Route
Antidiarrheals	Attapulgite (Donnagel)	30 ml after each loose BM	PO
	Loperamide (Imodium)	4 mg initially then 2 mg after each loose BM	PO
	Diphenoxylate HCl (Lomotil)	2 tablets up to 4 times a day	PO
	Difenoxin HCl (Motofen)	2 tablets then 1 tablet after each loose BM	PO
	Bismuth subsalicylate (Pepto-Bismol)	30 ml or 2 tablets every ½ to 1 hour	PO

D. Contraindications

1. Presence of bloody diarrhea, diarrhea associated with pathogens such as *E. coli,* salmonella, shigella or pseudomembranous colitis or other bacterial toxins

2. Avoid use if obstructive bowel disease is suspected

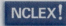

3. Avoid bismuth subsalicylate if allergic to aspirin

4. Difenoxine/atropine sulfate may cause serious side effects in nursing infants; therefore, should not be used for children under 2 years of age

E. Significant drug interactions

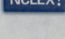

1. Allergies to aspirin or other salicylates since bismuth subsalicylate contains salicylate

2. Avoid aspirin use as concomitant use with bismuth subsalicylate, which may cause aspirin toxicity

3. Bismuth may also decrease tetracycline absorption in the GI tract

4. Diphenosylate/atropine sulfate and difenoxin/atropine sulfate may increase the sedative effects of barbiturates, narcotics, and alcohol

5. Concomitant use with MAO inhibitors may increase the risk of hypertensive crisis

F. Significant food interactions: none reported

G. Significant laboratory studies: diphenoxylate may increase serum amylase levels

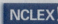

H. Side effects

1. Nausea and vomiting

2. Dry mouth, dizziness, drowsiness, constipation

3. Temporary darkening of stools and tongue may occur with bismuth salicylate

I. Adverse effects/toxicity

1. Clinical signs and symptoms of overdose include drowsiness, decreased blood pressure (BP), seizures, apnea, blurred vision, dry mouth, and psychosis

2. Risk of aspirin toxicity with concurrent use of aspirin, bismuth subsalicylate

3. Other adverse effects include central nervous system (CNS) depression, respiratory depression, hypotonic reflexes, angioedema, anaphylaxis, and paralytic ileus

J. Nursing considerations

1. Note allergies

2. Document onset, duration, and frequency of symptoms

3. Document previous therapies used

4. Note current medications

5. Identify any causative factors; perform stool analysis if necessary and ordered

6. Assess for evidence of dehydration or electrolyte imbalance

7. Monitor vital signs and I & O

8. Note presence of co-morbid conditions

9. Check abdomen for tenderness, distention, bowel sounds, or masses

10. Administer bismuth and tetracycline one hour apart

K. Client education

1. Instruct client to drink fluids to avoid dehydration and alleviate dry mouth

2. Instruct client to follow the BRAT diet: Bananas, Rice, Applesauce, Tea/Toast to avoid dehydration if recommended by healthcare provider

3. Advise client not to exceed prescribed dose

4. Instruct client to consult health care provider if diarrhea persists over 2 days

5. Advise client to use cautious in activities requiring alertness if dizziness/drowsiness is present (possible side effects)

6. Instruct client to report occurrence of fever, nausea and vomiting, abdominal pain or distention

7. Advise client to avoid dairy products

8. Teach good personal hygiene to avoid skin irritation or breakdown because of diarrhea

9. Instruct client to avoid alcohol ingestion while taking medication

10. Instruct client to notify healthcare provider if pregnant or breastfeeding

IV. Laxatives

A. Bulk-forming laxatives

1. Action and use

   a. Include non-absorbable polysaccharide and cellulose derivatives

   b. **Laxatives** swell in water, forming an emollient gel that increases bulk in the intestines

   c. Peristalsis is stimulated by the increased fecal mass, which decreases the transit time

   d. They generally produce a laxative effect within 12 to 14 hours but may require 2 to 3 days for full effect

2. Common medications (Table 7-3)

3. Administration considerations

   a. Since these agents rely on water to increase their bulk, it is essential that adequate fluids be given for bowel absorption

   b. These agents may also cause intestinal and esophageal obstruction when insufficient liquid is administered with the dose

   c. Each dose should be given with a full glass of liquid (240 mL)

   d. Use sugar-free preparations in clients with phenylketonuria

4. Contraindications

   a. Not recommended for clients with intestinal stenosis, ulceration, or adhesions

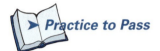

Practice to Pass

How long should a client take an over-the-counter (OTC) antidiarrheal medication before consulting the healthcare provider?

Table 7-3	Generic/Trade Names	Usual Adult Dosage Range	Route
Laxatives	*Bulk forming laxatives*		
	Methylcellulose (Citrucel)	1 tsp (19g) in 8 oz of water 1–3 times a day	PO
	Calcium polycarbophil (Fibercon)	2 tablets 1–4 times a day	PO
	Psyllium (Metamucil)	3–4 g in 8 oz of liquid 1–3 times a day	PO
	Stimulant laxatives		
	Casanthranol (Pericolace)	1–2 capsules at HS	PO
	Senna (Senokot)	2 tablets at HS	PO
	Bisacodyl (Dulcolax)	10–15 mg at HS	PO
		1 suppository	PR
	Castor oil (Neoloid, Purgo)	15 to 60 mL	PO
	Hyperosmotic laxatives		
	Lactulose (Kristalose)	10–20 g in 4 oz water	PO
	Polyethylene glycol (Miralax)	17 g in 8 oz water daily	PO
	Glycerin (Glycerol)	3-g suppository	Rectal
	Stool softeners (surfactants)		
	Docusate sodium (Colace)	50–300 mg daily	PO
	Docusate potassium (Dialose)	100–300 mg daily	
	Docusate calcium (Doxidan)	240 mg daily	PO
	Saline Laxatives		
	Magnesium hydroxide (Milk of Magnesia)	30–60 ml at HS	PO
	Sodium phosphate (Fleets)	1.25 oz enema	Rectal
		2–3 tablets daily	PO
		1 supp. daily	Rectal

    b. Use cautiously in clients with swallowing difficulties to ensure aspiration does not occur

    c. Do not use if fecal impaction is present

5. Significant drug interactions: decreased GI absorption may occur with digitalis, anticoagulants, nitrofurantoin, and salicylates

6. Significant food interactions

    a. Dietary management of constipation can be aided by encouraging the intake of fluid and fiber

    b. Fiber increases stool bulk and water retention in the bowel

    c. A dietary bulk-forming nutrient such as bran is an appropriate adjunctive therapy for constipation

    d. Bran is only partially fermented by bacteria, resulting in increased stool bulk, accelerated transit time, and promotion of normal defecation

    e. Rapid increases in dietary roughage may cause abdominal bloating and flatulence

    f. Adequate fluid intake is also necessary in order to prevent fecal impaction

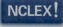

    g. Generally 240 to 360 mL of fluid with each tablespoon of bran is sufficient

7. Significant laboratory studies: none reported

8. Side effects

   a. Abdominal discomfort and/or bloating, flatulence

   b. Nausea and vomiting, diarrhea

9. Adverse effects/toxicity

   a. Rare reports of allergic reactions to karaya such as urticaria, rhinitis, dermatitis, bronchospasm

   b. Esophageal obstruction, swelling, or blockage may occur when insufficient fluid is used in mixing a bulk-forming laxative

10. Nursing considerations

   a. Assess swallowing ability, adequately mix agents in liquid and encourage additional fluid intake

   b. Monitor for aspiration

   c. If administered via feeding tube, it must be a large bore tube, and medication must be adequately dissolved in liquid and given rapidly with adequate flushing

   d. Add at least 8 oz (240mL) of water or juice to drug

   e. Separate psyllium administration from digoxin, salicylates, and anticoagulants by 2 hours

   f. Use sugar-free preparations in diabetic clients

11. Client education

   a. Instruct client that these agents require adequate hydration to be effective

   b. Encourage additional fluids and exercise

   c. Instruct client to mix powder preparation with at least 8 oz fluid and drink immediately and follow with another 8 oz of fluid

   d. Inform client that bulk-forming laxatives may decrease appetite if taken before meals

   e. Instruct client to take them 2 hours after meals and any oral medications

   f. Instruct client in sodium and sugar-free preparations as appropriate to individual diet restrictions

   g. Instruct client that full effect of medication may not occur for 2 to 3 days

B. **Stimulant cathartics**

1. Action and use

   a. Called stimulants because they stimulate peristalsis via mucosal irritation or intramural nerve plexus activity, which results in increased motility

   b. **Cathartics** are agents with purgative actions

   c. It is proposed that stimulant laxatives modify the permeability of the colonic mucosal cells, which results in intraluminal fluid and electrolyte secretion

   d. Defecation occurs between 6 to 12 hours after oral administration of these agents

Table 7-4	Generic/Trade Names	Usual Adult Dosage Range	Route
Antiemetics	Meclizine (Antivert)	25–50 mg 1 hr before activity	PO
	Diphenhydramine (Benadryl)	10–50 mg	IV, IM
	Prochlorperazine (Compazine)	5–10 mg tid–qid	PO
		5–10 mg	IM
		2 ½–10 mg	IV
	Dimenhydrinate (Dramamine)	50–100 mg every 4–6 hours	PO
	Dolesetron mesylate (Anzemet)	100 mg 1 hr before chemo	PO
		100 mg	IV
	Granisetron (Kytril)	10 mcg 1/2 hr before chemo	IV
		2 mg 1 hr before chemo	
	Dronabinol (Marinol)	5 mg/m^2 1 hr before chemo then every 24 hrs prn	PO
	Promethazine HCl (Phenergan)	25 mg every 4–6 hr prn	PO
	Metoclopramide (Reglan)	10 mg ac and hs	PO
	Chlorpromazine (Thorazine)	10–25 mg every 4–6 hr	PO
		50–100 mg every 6–8 hr	PR
	Trimethobenzamide (Tigan)	250 mg 3–4 times a day	PO
		200 mg 3–4 times daily	PR
		200 mg/mL 3–4 times daily	IM
	Scopalamine (Transderm Scope)	1.5 mg patch	Topical
	Phenothiazine (Trilafon)	8–16 mg divided doses	PO
		5 mg	IM
	Ondansetron (Zofran)	24 mg 30 minutes before chemo	IM
		32 mg/50 mL	IV
		2 mg/mL	IV, IM

    e. Rectal administration of bisacodyl and senna produces catharsis within 15 minutes to 2 hours

2. Common medications (Table 7-3, p. 273)

3. Administration considerations

    a. Bedtime administration of dose promotes a morning bowel movement

    b. Swallow tablet whole; do not crush

    c. Do not take within 1 hour of antacids or milk

    d. Mix castor oil with 8 oz of water or juice; this drug is usually limited to use for rapid bowel evacuation, such as before radiological procedures

4. Contraindications

    a. Contraindicated with abdominal pain, nausea and vomiting, symptoms of appendicitis, rectal bleeding, gastroenteritis, intestinal obstruction, fecal impaction

    b. Castor oil may induce premature labor

    c. Use senna cautiously with nursing mothers as senna is excreted in breast milk

5. Significant drug interactions: antacids and drugs that increase gastric pH may result in GI irritation or cramping

6. Significant food interactions: do not take within 1 hour of milk

7. Significant laboratory studies: none reported

8. Side effects

   a. Nausea and vomiting, abdominal cramps, diarrhea, laxative dependence

   b. Muscle weakness, fluid/electrolyte imbalance

   c. Rectal burning or irritation with suppository use

9. Adverse effects/toxicity

   a. Hypokalemia, hypocalcemia

   b. Metabolic acidosis or alkalosis

10. Nursing considerations

    a. Evaluate for nausea and vomiting, abdominal pain or diarrhea

    b. Evaluate for medication effectiveness

    c. Monitor for fluid/electrolyte imbalances

    d. Administer medication 1 hour before or after ingestion of milk or an antacid

    e. Encourage increased fluids and diet alterations to include increased amounts of high-fiber foods

    f. Evaluate for laxative dependence and offer counseling

11. Client education

    a. Discourage client from chronic use of laxatives; use beyond 1 week should be avoided

    b. Instruct client that these agents may produce a cathartic colon if used for several years; the colon develops abnormal motor function, and roentgenography resembles ulcerative colitis; usually discontinuation of laxative use restores normal bowel function

    c. Instruct client to increase fluid intake and diet high in fiber

    d. Advise client to report signs and symptoms of side effects immediately

    e. Instruct to take medications 1 hour before or after ingestion of milk or an antacid

C. **Hyperosmotic cathartics**

   1. Action and use

      a. They increase osmotic pressure within the intestinal lumen, which results in luminal retention of water, softening the stool

      b. Lactulose is an unabsorbed disaccharide metabolized by colonic bacteria primarily to lactic acid, formic and acetic acids

      c. It has been proposed that these organic acids may contribute to the osmotic effect

      d. Used for treatment of occasional constipation

      e. Used to reduce ammonia levels (Lactulose)

   2. Common medications (Table 7-3, p. 273)

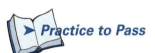

Practice to Pass

What substance can be given to counteract the effects of ipecac syrup?

3. Administration considerations

   a. Glycerin is available only for rectal administration (suppository or enema) for treatment of acute constipation; its laxative effect occurs within 15 to 30 minutes

   b. Lactulose may require 24 to 48 hours for effect; it is also more costly and should be reserved for acute constipation

   c. Dissolve 17 g Miralax in 8 oz of water and drink once daily for up to 2 weeks; it may take 2 to 4 days for results to occur

4. Contraindications

   a. Contraindicated in bowel obstruction

   b. Use lactulose cautiously in clients with diabetes mellitus

5. Significant drug interactions: antibiotics may decrease laxative effect by elimination of bacteria needed to digest active form

6. Significant food interactions: none reported

7. Significant laboratory studies: serum electrolyte levels

8. Side effects

   a. Glycerin: rectal irritation and burning, hyperemia of the rectal mucosa

   b. Lactulose and Miralax: flatulence, abdominal cramps/bloating, diarrhea

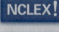

9. Adverse effects/toxicity: fluid and electrolyte imbalances

10. Nursing considerations

    a. Miralax should always be dissolved in 8 oz of water

    b. Dilute lactulose in water or juice to decrease sweet taste

    c. Monitor frequency and consistency of stools

    d. Monitor for electrolyte imbalances especially in the elderly

11. Client education

    a. Instruct client that Miralax should be dissolved in 8 oz water

    b. Instruct client that the medication may take 2 to 4 days for effect

    c. Advise client to contact physician if unusual bloating, cramping or diarrhea occurs

    d. Instruct client that prolonged use may result in electrolyte imbalance and laxative dependence

    e. Instruct client to take medication with juice to improve taste

D. Stool softeners (surfactants)

1. Action and use

   a. Used on a scheduled basis for clients who are likely to become constipated, such as with hospitalization, bedrest, post-surgical status, and for those receiving opioid analgesic medications

   b. Stool softeners are often referred to as emollient laxatives

     c. They are anionic **surfactants** that lower the fecal surface tension in vitro by allowing water and lipid penetration

     d. Softening of the feces generally occurs after 1 to 3 days

     e. Some preparations combine a stool softener such as docusate sodium with a stimulant, such as casanthrol to make a single combination product (e.g., Pericolace)

     f. Used for constipation associated with dry, hard stools and to decrease strain of defecation

NCLEX!

2. Common medications (Table 7-3, p. 273)

3. Administration considerations

     a. Do not give with mineral oil

     b. Offer fluids after each PO dose

4. Contraindications

     a. Contraindicated with any hypersensitivity to the drug

NCLEX!

     b. Contraindicated with intestinal obstruction, undiagnosed abdominal pain, vomiting or other signs of appendicitis, fecal impaction, or acute abdomen

     c. Docusate sodium should not be used by clients with congestive heart failure (CHF) because of sodium content

5. Significant drug interactions: may increase absorption of mineral oil

6. Significant food interactions: none reported

7. Significant laboratory studies: none reported

8. Side effects

     a. Mild abdominal cramping, diarrhea

     b. Dependence with long-term use or excessive use

     c. Bitter taste

9. Adverse effects/toxicity (all rare)

     a. Throat irritation has occurred with docusate sodium solution

     b. Docusate has been associated with hepatotoxicity when used in combination with oxyphenisatin or dantrol

NCLEX!

10. Nursing considerations

     a. Monitor frequency and consistency of stools

     b. Monitor for electrolyte imbalances especially in the elderly

11. Client education

     a. Instruct client to take medication with milk or juice to decrease bitter taste

     b. Encourage client to increase fluid intake

     c. Inform client that it may require 1 to 3 days to soften fecal matter

d. Instruct client to counsel dietitian regarding dietary changes to increase fiber foods

e. Discourage prolonged use

E. Lubricants

1. Action and use

   a. Provide lubrication of feces and hinder water reabsorption into the colon

   b. Used to treat constipation and prepare client for bowel studies or surgery

2. Common medication

   a. Mineral oil

   b. Usual adult dose is 12.5 to 45 mL at HS PO or 120 mL at HS rectal

3. Administration considerations

   a. Mineral oil is indigestible, and its absorption is limited considerably in the nonemulsified formulation

   b. Onset of action when taken orally is 6 to 8 hours

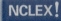

4. Contraindications

   a. Contraindicated with abdominal pain, nausea, and vomiting

   b. Contraindicated with signs and symptoms of appendicitis or acute abdomen, and fecal impaction or bowel obstruction

5. Significant drug interactions

   a. Stool softeners increase mineral oil absorption

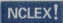

   b. May impair absorption of fat-soluble vitamins (A, D, E, K), anticoagulants, birth control pills, cardiac glycosides, and sulfonamides

6. Significant food interactions: do not give with food as it may delay gastric emptying, separate by 2 hours

7. Significant laboratory studies: none reported

8. Side effects

   a. Nausea and vomiting, diarrhea, abdominal cramps

   b. Decreased absorption of nutrients

   c. Laxative dependence may occur with excessive/long-term use

   d. Anal pruritis, irritation, and hemorrhoids

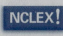

9. Adverse effects/toxicity: aspiration of the product may cause lipoid pneumonia

10. Nursing considerations

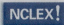

   a. Because of possible aspiration and diminished vitamin absorption, do not administer to young children (younger than 6 years of age), pregnant women, the elderly, and debilitated clients

   b. Do not administer the medication at bedtime

c. Avoid administration of drug to clients lying flat in bed because of risk of aspiration

d. Do not give within 2 hours of food because of possible decrease in gastric emptying

e. Cautionary use in elderly because of increased risk of aspiration

f. Monitor medications and alter administration times to avoid decreased absorption caused by mineral oil

11. Client education

a. Instruct client to avoid chronic use and make aware of impairment of fat-soluble vitamin absorption

b. Instruct client not to take mineral oil with stool softeners because of risk of toxic levels

c. Warn client that mineral oil may leak through the anal sphincter; the side effects should be reported to healthcare provider

d. Instruct client not to take medication when lying flat

e. Advise client not to take medication at bedtime

F. Saline laxatives

1. Action and use

a. Magnesium, sulfate, phosphate, and citrate salts are used when rapid bowel evacuation is required, as in bowel evacuation in preparation for procedures or surgery

b. The mechanism of action of these poorly absorbed ions is unclear, but it is believed that they produce an osmotic effect that increases intraluminal volume and stimulates peristalsis

c. Magnesium may cause cholecystokinin release from the duodenal mucosa promoting increased fluid secretion and motility of the small intestine and colon

d. Orally administered magnesium and sodium phosphate salts are effective within 30 minutes to 6 hours

e. Phosphate-containing rectal enemas evacuate the bowel within 2 to 15 minutes

2. Common medications (Table 7-3)

3. Administration considerations

a. Use magnesium salts cautiously for clients with renal impairment because absorption of magnesium salts may cause hypermagnesemia

b. Use sodium phosphate salts cautiously for clients with CHF when sodium restriction is necessary

4. Contraindications

a. Saline agents are not recommended for children under 2 years of age because of the potential for hypocalcemia in this population

   b. Contraindicated in the presence of abdominal pain, nausea and vomiting, or other signs and symptoms of appendicitis or acute abdomen

   c. Contraindicated with intestinal obstruction, edema, CHF, megacolon or impaired renal function

5. Significant drug interactions: concomitant use with antacids may inactivate both

6. Significant food interactions: none reported

7. Significant laboratory studies: none reported

8. Side effects: cramping and urgency to defecate

9. Adverse effects/toxicity

   a. Safe when administered for short-term management

   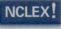

   b. They may cause significant fluid and electrolyte imbalances when used for prolonged periods or in certain clients

10. Nursing considerations

   a. Dehydration and electrolyte imbalances may occur from repeated administration without appropriate fluid replacement

   b. Encourage increased fluid intake

   c. Monitor drug effectiveness

11. Client education

   a. Instruct client on drug dosing

   b. Instruct client to avoid frequent or prolonged use due to laxative dependence

   c. Instruct client to report side effects to health care provider

   d. Advise client to report to health care provider if ineffective

   e. Encourage client to increase fluid intake

V. Emetics

A. Action and use

1. Directly irritate the GI mucosa and stimulate chemoreceptor trigger zone

2. **Emetics** are used to induce vomiting after oral poisoning or drug overdose

B. Common medication

1. Ipecac syrup

2. Dose is 15 to 30 mL orally

C. Administration considerations

1. Onset of action usually occurs in 20 minutes

   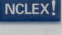

2. Follow dose with 240 cc water for adults and children older than 12, ½ to 1 glass of water for infants up to 1 year, and 1 to 2 glasses of water for children younger than 12 years of age

D. Contraindications

NCLEX!

1. Do not use with corrosive or petrolatum distillates (gasoline, kerosene, volatile oils, or caustic substances)

NCLEX!

2. Do not give to semicomatose or unconscious clients, during intoxication, seizures, shock, or any loss of gag reflex

3. Do not give to infants less than 6 months of age

NCLEX!

E. Significant drug interactions: activated charcoal may inactivate ipecac syrup

F. Significant food interactions

1. Vegetable oil may delay absorption

2. Milk may decrease therapeutic effect

3. Carbonated beverages may cause abdominal distention

G. Significant laboratory studies: none reported

H. Side effects

1. Drowsiness

2. Arrhythmias

3. Diarrhea

4. Mild CNS depression

NCLEX!

I. Adverse effects/toxicity: may be cardiotoxic if not vomited and allowed to absorb, leading to heart conduction disturbances, atrial fibrillation, or fatal myocarditis (treat with activated charcoal to absorb ipecac syrup or gastric lavage)

J. Nursing considerations

1. Evaluate origin of agent ingested

2. There is risk of aspiration of vomitus in children less than 12 months, the elderly, and in anyone with altered level of consciousness or gag reflex

NCLEX!

3. Drug may be abused by clients with eating disorders

4. Monitor medication effect

5. Administer with at least 200 to 300 cc of water

6. Assess respiratory status and level of consciousness

7. Review abuse potential

NCLEX!

K. Client education

1. Instruct client to contact poison control before administering ipecac syrup

2. Advise client to seek immediate medical attention when poisoning is suspected

3. Instruct client to keep all medications out of reach of children

4. Advise client to check the expiration date periodically as drug is available over the counter

5. Avoid drinking milk or carbonated beverages that may alter effectiveness

6. Instruct client that if vomiting does not occur, go immediately to health care provider/emergency room to decrease toxic absorption of drug

VI. Antiemetics

A. Action and use

1. Emesis is a complex reflex brought about by activation of the vomiting center (a nucleus of neurons located in the medulla oblongata)

2. Certain stimuli activate the vomiting center directly (e.g., gastrointestinal irritation) while other stimuli (e.g., drugs, toxins, radiation) act within the medulla to stimulate the chemoreceptor trigger zone (CTZ); presumably, it is by altering the function of these neuroreceptors that emetogenic compounds and antiemetic drugs produce their effects

3. Receptors involved are influenced by acetylcholine, histamine, serotonin, dopamine, benzodiazepines, and cannabinoids

4. Phenothiazines: suppress emesis by blockade of dopamine receptors in the CTZ

5. Butyrophenones: suppress emesis by blocking dopamine receptors in the CTZ

6. Metoclopramide: inhibits dopamine receptors in CTZ

7. Cannabinoids are approved to treat nausea and vomiting associated with cancer chemotherapy; mechanism of action is unknown

8. Dronabinol is also approved as an appetite stimulant for clients with acquired immunodeficiency syndrome (AIDS)

9. Benzodiazepines: primary effect is suppression of anxiety; most effective for management of cancer chemotherapy–associated nausea and vomiting when combined with metoclopramide and dexamethasone

10. Glucocorticoids: mechanism for suppression of emesis is unknown; they are effective alone and in combination with other antiemetics in the treatment of emesis associated with cancer chemotherapy

11. Antihistamines: anticholinergic effect reducing motion sickness and vomiting

12. Ondansetron: blocks serotonin receptors to reduce nausea

B. Common medications (Table 7-4, p. 275)

C. Administration considerations

1. Frequently, antiemetic combinations are more beneficial than single-drug treatment, particularly for cancer chemotherapy management of emesis; this may suggest that there is more than one mechanism triggering the emesis

2. As a rule, prophylactic drugs are generally given by mouth; however, management of active emesis is usually through parenteral or rectal administration of medications

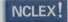

3. Anticipatory nausea and vomiting should be treated 1 hour before meals or treatment

4. Parenteral preparations should be given deep IM to avoid leakage of the drug into the subcutaneous tissues

D. Contraindications

1. Contraindicated with CNS depression and coma

2. Use cautiously in clients with glaucoma, seizures, intestinal obstruction, prostatic hyperplasia, asthma, cardiac, pulmonary, or hepatic disease

E. Significant drug interactions

1. Epinephrine including ephedrine, may increase hypotension

2. Avoid use with MAO inhibitors

3. Antihistamines and CNS depressants may increase CNS depression

4. Levodopa results in decreased levodopa action

5. Phenytoin may increase toxicity

6. Meclizine may mask signs of ototoxicity with such medications as aminoglycosides, salicylates, and loop diuretics

7. Glucocorticoids cause hyperglycemia

F. Significant food interactions: none reported

G. Significant laboratory studies

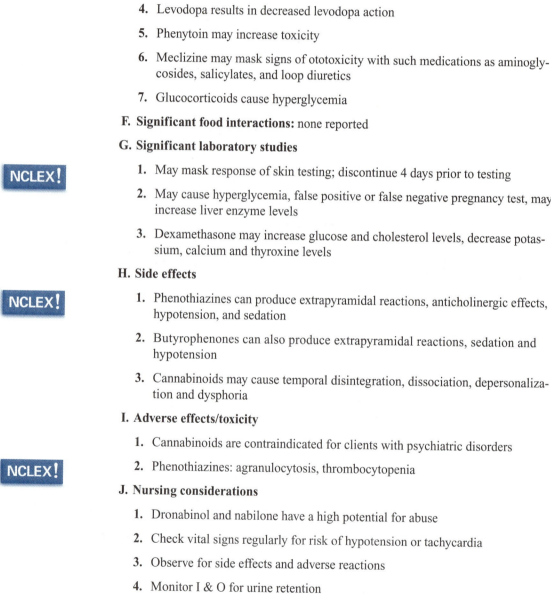

1. May mask response of skin testing; discontinue 4 days prior to testing

2. May cause hyperglycemia, false positive or false negative pregnancy test, may increase liver enzyme levels

3. Dexamethasone may increase glucose and cholesterol levels, decrease potassium, calcium and thyroxine levels

H. Side effects

1. Phenothiazines can produce extrapyramidal reactions, anticholinergic effects, hypotension, and sedation

2. Butyrophenones can also produce extrapyramidal reactions, sedation and hypotension

3. Cannabinoids may cause temporal disintegration, dissociation, depersonalization and dysphoria

I. Adverse effects/toxicity

1. Cannabinoids are contraindicated for clients with psychiatric disorders

2. Phenothiazines: agranulocytosis, thrombocytopenia

J. Nursing considerations

1. Dronabinol and nabilone have a high potential for abuse

2. Check vital signs regularly for risk of hypotension or tachycardia

3. Observe for side effects and adverse reactions

4. Monitor I & O for urine retention

5. Observe for mood changes or involuntary movements

6. Monitor lab values: liver function tests, electrolytes and renal function (blood urea nitrogen and creatinine)

7. Ensure client safety

8. Monitor for anticholinergic effects: dry mouth, constipation, or visual changes

K. Client education

1. Avoid activities that require alertness

2. Teach signs and symptoms to report to health care provider

3. Instruct client to avoid alcohol and CNS depressant drugs

4. Instruct diabetic clients to monitor blood glucose

5. Teach client to take medications as prescribed

6. Instruct client to avoid excessive sunlight/ultraviolet light because of potential photosensitivity

7. Teach client to use sugarless hard candy or ice chips to avoid dry mouth

8. Advise client to increase fluids and dietary fiber to decrease risk of constipation

9. To be more effective, instruct client to take medication 30 to 60 minutes before any activity that causes nausea

VII. Histamine H₂ Antagonists

A. Action and use

1. Reduce gastric acid secretion by blocking histamine 2 in the gastric parietal cells

2. Histamine **H₂ antagonists** (agents against histamine decreasing gastric secretion) are used to treat duodenal ulcer, gastric ulcer, hypersecretory conditions such as Zollinger-Ellison syndrome, reflux esophagitis

3. Used for prevention of stress ulcers in critically ill clients, combination therapy to treat *Helicobacter pylori* (bacteria found in gastric mucosa) infection

B. Common medications (Table 7-5)

C. Administration considerations

1. Intravenous (IV) administered drugs should not be mixed with other medications

2. Avoid antacid use within 1 hour of administration

3. May be given as single dose, twice daily, or with meals and at bedtime

D. Contraindications

1. Hypersensitivity to drug

2. Use caution in clients with impaired renal or hepatic function

Table 7-5	Generic/Trade Names	Usual Adult Dosage Range	Route
Histamine 2 (H₂) Antagonists	Nizatidine (Axid)	150 mg bid or 300 mg HS	PO
	Famotidine (Pepcid)	20 mg bid or 40 mg HS	PO
		20 mg/50 mL	IV
	Cimetidine (Tagamet)	300–400 mg QID	PO
		300 mg/2 mL	IM, IV
	Ranitidine (Zantac)	150 mg bid or 300 mg HS	PO
		25 mg/mL	IM, IV

E. Significant drug interactions

1. Decreased ketaconazole absorption with famotidine

2. Cimetidine: decreased metabolism of beta adrenergic blockers, phenytoin, lidocaine, procainamide, quinidine, benzodiazepines, metronidazole, tricyclic antidepressants, oral contraceptives, and warfarin causing increase risk of toxicity

3. Cimetidine alters absorption of ketoconzole, ferrous salts, indocin and tetracyclines and may decrease concentration of digoxin

4. Nizatidine may increase salicylate levels with high doses of aspirin

5. Ranitidine may increase diazepam absorption, increase hypolycemic effects of glipizide, increase procainamide levels and increase warfarin effect

F. Significant food interactions: none reported

G. Significant laboratory studies

1. Ranitidine: false positive urine prolactin

2. Cimetidine: false negative allergen skin test, increase prolactin, alkaline phosphatase and creatinine levels and may alter gastrocult testing caused by blue dye used in tablets

3. Famotidine may cause false negative allergen results and may increase liver enzyme levels

4. Nizatidine may cause false positive urobilinogen

H. Side effects

1. Somnolence, diaphoresis, rash, headache

2. Taste disorder, diarrhea, constipation, dry mouth

3. Arrhythmia

I. Adverse effects/toxicity

1. Rare but may include agranulocytosis, neutropenia, thrombocytopenia, aplastic anemia, pancytopenia

2. Anaphylaxis

J. Nursing considerations

1. Reduced dosages usually required for clients with hepatic or renal impairment

2. Assess medications for possible interactions

3. Evaluate nutritional status and dietary interventions

4. Evaluate need for smoking cessation and alcoholic abuse programs

K. Client education

1. Instruct client to avoid smoking, which causes gastric stimulation

2. Advise client to avoid **antacid** (agent reducing acidity) use within 1 hour of dose

3. Instruct client to take medications only as directed

4. Inform client that once-a-day dosage should be taken at bedtime; if prescribed more than daily, take before meals

5. Instruct client to avoid gastric irritants such as alcohol, aspirin, or nonsteroidal anti-inflammatory drugs (NSAIDS)

6. Instruct client to report any side effects to health care provider

VIII. Proton Pump Inhibitors

A. Action and use

1. Block acid production by inhibiting the H+−K+ ATPase at the secretory surface of the gastric parietal cells, thereby blocking the formation of gastric acid

2. Used for treatment of erosive or ulcerative gastroesophageal reflux disease (GERD) or duodenal ulcers, active benign gastric ulcers, and nonsteroidal anti-inflammatory drug (NSAID)-associated gastric ulcers (short term)

3. Used for healing and reduction in relapse rates of heartburn symptoms in erosive or ulcerative GERD (maintenance)

4. Used for treatment of pathological hypersecretory conditions such as Zollinger Ellison syndrome (long-term)

B. Common medications (Table 7-6)

C. Administration considerations

1. May give with antacids

2. If unable to swallow capsules, lansoprazole and esomeprazole capsules may be opened and sprinkled on applesauce before taking

3. To give per nasogastric (NG) tube, dilute capsule contents in 40-cc juice

4. Omeprazole, pantoprazole, and rabeprazole must be swallowed whole

5. Pantoprazole IV: should be administered over a period of 15 minutes at a rate not greater than 3 mg/min (7 mL/min)

6. Pantoprazole IV should be administered using the in-line filter provider

D. Contraindications: not recommended in children or nursing mothers

E. Significant drug interactions

1. Rabeprazole and pantoprazole may alter absorption of gastric pH dependent drugs such as ketoconazole, digoxin, iron preparations, and ampicillin

2. Esomeprazole may affect drugs metabolized by CYP2C19

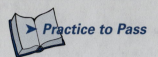

Practice to Pass

What information would you share with a pregnant female client with peptic ulcer disease who asks you about taking misoprostol (Cytotec)?

NCLEX!

Table 7-6			
Proton Pump Inhibitors	**Generic/Trade Names**	**Usual Adult Dosage Range**	**Route**
	Rabeprazole sodium (Aciphex)	20 mg daily	PO
	Lansoprazole (Prevacid)	15–30 mg daily	PO
	Omeprazole (Prilosec)	20–40 mg daily	PO
	Pantoprazole (Protonix)	40 mg daily	PO, IV
	Esomeprazole (Nexium)	20–40 mg daily	PO

3. Lansoprazole may alter theophylline levels; give at least 30 minutes before sucralfate

4. Omeprazole may potentiate diazepam, phenytoin, and warfarin

5. Omeprazole should be taken 30 minutes before sucralfate; it may alter absorption of pH dependent medications

F. Significant food interactions: none reported

G. Significant laboratory studies

1. May increase liver enzymes

2. Monitor theophylline levels with lansoprazole (Prevacid)

3. May need to monitor diazepam and, phenytoin levels and prothrombin times more frequently with omeprazole (Prilosec)

H. Side effects

1. Headache, diarrhea, constipation, abdominal pain, nausea, flatulence

2. Rash, hyperglycemia, dizziness, pruritis, dry mouth

3. Injection site reaction with pantoprazole

I. Adverse effects/toxicity

1. Pancreatitis, liver necrosis, hepatic failure, toxic epidermal necrolysis

2. Stevens Johnson syndrome

3. Agranulocytosis, myocardial infarction (MI), shock, cerebral vascular accident (CVA)

4. GI hemorrhage

J. Nursing considerations

1. Dosage should be reduced in severe liver disease

2. Document reason for therapy, duration of symptoms and drug efficacy

3. Monitor for side effects

4. Monitor laboratory test results including liver function test, CBC, and renal function (BUN, creatinine)

5. Review any diagnostic findings

6. Assess for pregnancy or lactation

K. Client education

1. Review side effects with clients, instruct to report diarrhea

2. Instruct client to take medications as prescribed; do not increase dose

3. Advise client to follow prescribed diet and activities to decrease symptoms

4. Inform client that medication is generally for short-term therapy; instruct client to keep health care appointments for continued signs and symptoms

5. Instruct client that esomeprazole and omeprazole should be taken before meals

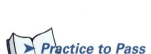

▶ Practice to Pass

A proton pump inhibitor has been ordered for a client with recent cerebral vascular accident (CVA). What nursing assessment should be performed?

6. Advise client to notify health care provider of any difficulty swallowing since omeprazole, pantoprazole, and rabeprazole must be swallowed whole

7. Instruct client that lansoprazole and esomeprazole capsules may be opened and sprinkled

IX. Mucosal Protective Agents

A. Action and use

1. Misoprostol (Cytotec) inhibits gastric secretion, protects gastric mucosa by increasing bicarbonate and mucus production and decreases pepsin levels

2. Sucralfate (Carafate) protects the site of ulcer from gastric acid by forming an adherent coating with albumin and fibrinogen; it absorbs pepsin decreasing its activity

3. Misoprostol (Cytotec) is used for the prevention of gastric ulcers; investigational use with duodenal ulcers

4. Sucralfate (Carafate) is used for short-term treatment of duodenal ulcers with continued maintenance treatment at lower doses; investigational use for gastric ulcers

B. Common medications (Table 7-7)

C. Administration considerations

1. Sucralfate should be taken 1 hour before meals and bedtime or 2 hours after meals

2. Surcalfate should be taken 2 hours after medications and not within 2 hours of antacids

3. Misoprostol should be taken with food

D. Contraindications

1. Misoprostol is contraindicated in clients who are allergic to prostaglandins, or who are pregnant or lactating

2. Use cautiously with clients with renal impairment and clients older than 64 years old

3. Safety has not been established for children under 18 years old

4. Misoprostol may cause miscarriage with serious bleeding

5. No known contraindications with sucralfate but safety in children and during lactation is not fully established

E. Significant drug interactions

1. Sucralfate: decreased absorption of digoxin, fluoroquinolones, ketaconazole, phenytoin, quinidine, ranitidine, tetracycline, and theophylline; dosing medications 2 hours before sucralafate eliminates the interactions

Table 7-7	Generic/Trade Names	Usual Adult Dosage Range	Route
Mucosal Protective Agents	Sucralfate (Carafate)	1 g qid	PO
	Misoprostol (Cytotec)	200 mg qid with meals and HS	PO

2. Antacids may decrease binding of sucralfate

3. Misoprostol decreases the availability of aspirin

F. Significant food interactions: none reported

G. Significant laboratory studies

1. Misoprostal may decrease basal pepsin secretion

2. No laboratory interactions with sucralfate

H. Side effects

1. Dizziness, headache, constipation, diarrhea, nausea, vomiting, flatulence, dry mouth, and rash

2. Misoprostol may cause spotting, cramping, dysmenorrhea, menstrual disorders, and postmenopausal bleeding

I. Adverse effects/toxicity

1. Angioedema

2. Respiratory difficulty, laryngospasm

3. Seizures

J. Nursing considerations

1. Assess GI symptoms

2. Assess for pregnancy

3. Monitor concomitant medications

4. Give medications according to prescription

5. Monitor for side effects

6. Assess respiratory status, swallowing or change in gag reflex

K. Client education

1. Instruct client to avoid gastric irritants such as caffeine, alcohol, smoking, and spicy foods

2. Instruct client to take medication as prescribed and do not share with others

3. Advise client to report side effects to healthcare provider for possible dosage change

4. Instruct client in contraceptive practices while on misoprostol

5. Instruct female clients to report any abnormal vaginal bleeding

6. Instruct client not to take misoprostol if pregnant; if the client becomes pregnant while taking misoprostol, she should stop taking it

7. Inform client to avoid pregnancy at least 1 month or 1 menstrual cycle after stopping medication

8. Instruct client to increase fluids and fiber to decrease constipation

9. Instruct on antacid use to decrease interaction

10. Advise client to report immediately any difficulty swallowing or breathing

X. Antacids

A. Action and use

1. Gastric acid neutralizing agent

2. Used for symptomatic relief of hyperacidity associated with GI disorders

3. Used as an antiflatulent to alleviate symptoms of gas and bloating

B. Common medications (Table 7-8)

NCLEX!

C. Administration considerations: antacids should be taken at least 2 hours apart from other drugs where a drug interaction may occur

D. Contraindications

1. Safety has not been established for use of antacids by lactating women

2. Magnesium hydroxide is contraindicated in the presence of abdominal pain, nausea, vomiting, diarrhea, severe renal dysfunction, fecal impaction, rectal bleeding, colostomy, ileostomy

3. Aluminum carbonate antacids: prolonged use of high doses in presence of low serum phosphate

4. Calcium carbonate antacids: hypercalcemia and hypercalciuria, severe renal disease, renal calculi, GI hemorrhage or obstruction, dehydration

5. Dihydroxyaluminum sodium carbonate: aluminum sensitivity, severe renal disease, dehydration, clients on sodium-restricted diets

E. Significant drug interactions

1. Antacids increase the gastric pH, which may decrease the absorption of other drugs, such as digoxin, ciprofloxacin, ofloxacin, norfloxacin, phenytoin, iron supplements, isoniazid, ethambutol, and ketoconazole

2. Antacids may bind with other drugs, therefore decreasing the drug's absorption and effectiveness, such as tetracycline

F. Significant food interactions: none reported

Table 7-8

Antacids

Generic/Trade Names	Usual Adult Dosage Range	Route
Aluminum carbonate (Basaljel)	10–30 mL or 2 tabs/caps q2h; extra strength 5–15 mL	PO
Aluminum hydroxide (Amphojel)	10 ml 5–6 times daily or 600 mg tablets 5–6 times daily	PO
Magnesium trisilicate (Gaviscon)	1–2 tabs prn	PO
Calcium carbonate (Tums, Dicarbisol)	2 tabs or 10 mL q2h; maximum of 12 doses/day	PO
Magnesium hydroxide and aluminum hydroxide (Maalox)	2–4 tabs prn; maximum 16 tabs/day 10–30 mL 1 to 3 hrs pc and hs	PO
Magnesium hydroxide, aluminum hydroxide, and simethicone (Mylanta, others)	10–20 mL prn; maximum 120 mL/day 2–4 tabs prn; maximum 24 tabs	PO
Dihydroxyaluminum sodium carbonate (Rolaids)	1–2 tabs prn (chew)	PO

G. Significant laboratory studies: prolonged use of antacids may alter aluminum, calcium, sodium, and phosphate levels

H. Side Effects

1. Belching, constipation, flatulence, diarrhea

2. Gastric distention

I. Adverse effects/toxicity

1. Hypophosphatemia (anorexia, malaise, tremors, muscle weakness)

2. Aluminum toxicity (dementia) may occur with repeated dosing

3. Hypercalcemia and metabolic alkalosis may occur with antacids containing calcium carbonate

4. May worsen hypertension and heart failure from increased sodium intake with use of those antacids containing sodium carbonate

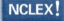

J. Nursing considerations

1. Shake suspension well

2. Flush NG tube with water after administration

3. Observe for signs and symptoms of altered phosphate levels: anorexia, muscle weakness, and malaise

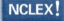

K. Client education

1. Instruct client on methods to avoid constipation

2. Instruct client to take as directed; do not exceed maximum dose

3. Instruct client to keep out of reach of children

4. Advise client to drink plenty of fluids

5. Explain antacids may interact with certain medications; notify health care provider of any prescribed medications

6. Warn client not to use if diagnosed with kidney disease

XI. Antimicrobials for *Helicobacter pylori* Organisms

A. Action and use

1. Antisecretory and antimicrobial action against most strains of *Helicobacter pylori*

2. Used for eradication of *Helicobacter pylori* infection and reduce the risk of duodenal ulcer recurrence

B. Common medications (Table 7-9)

C. Administration considerations

1. Swallow all pills whole except bismuth which should be chewed and not swallowed whole

2. If dose is missed, continue with normal dosage regimen, do not double dose

Table 7-9	Generic/Trade Names	Usual Adult Dosage Range	Route
Antimicrobials for *Helicobacter pylori*	Lansoprazole, amoxicillin, clarithromycin (Prevpak)	bid for 10–14 days	PO
	Bismuth subsalicylate, metronidazole, tetracycline (Helidac)	qid for 14 days	PO
	Omeprazole, clarithromycin (Prilosec/Biaxin)	Omeprazole 40 mg daily and Clarithromycin 500 mg tid for 2 weeks then omeprazole 20 mg daily for 2 weeks	PO
	Ranitidine bismuth citrate, clarithromycin (Titrec/Biaxin)	Ranitidine bismuth citrate 400 mg bid and clarithromycin 500 mg tid for 2 weeks then ranitidine bismuth citrate 400 mg bid for 2 weeks	PO
	Lansoprazole, amoxicillin (Prevacid/Amoxil)	Lansoprazole 30 mg tid and Amoxil 1 g tid for 14 days	PO

D. Contraindications

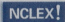

1. Allergy to any component of therapy

2. Avoid coadministration with pimozide or terfenadine because of risk of cardiac dysrhythmias

3. Pregnant women should not take regimens containing clarithromycin

E. Significant drug interactions

1. May alter absorption of drugs dependent on gastric pH: ketoconazole, ampicillin, iron, or digoxin

2. Safety in children is not established

F. Significant food interactions: none reported

G. Significant laboratory studies

1. Abnormal liver function tests

2. May increase theophylline levels

3. May interfere with prothrombin times

4. May alter serum levels of drugs metabolized by P450 enzyme system

H. Side effects

1. Rash, nausea, vomiting, diarrhea, abnormal taste, abdominal pain, dyspepsia

2. Headache, photosensitivity

3. Transient CNS reactions such as anxiety, behavior changes, tinnitus and vertigo

I. Adverse effects/toxicity: ventricular dysrhythmias

J. Nursing considerations

1. Note signs and symptoms, onset, and duration of symptoms

2. Document allergy status

3. Determine pregnancy status

    4. Document previous therapies used

    5. Document confirmation of infection

K. Client education

    1. Educate client regarding importance of compliance

    2. Instruct client to avoid gastric irritants such as smoking, alcohol and caffeine

    3. Educate on stress reduction techniques

    4. Instruct client to report side effects to healthcare provider

    5. Advise client to report continued symptoms to healthcare provider

    6. Inform client that bismuth-containing preparations may cause darkening of tongue and stool

    7. Instruct client to review drug packaging as some preparations are prepackaged

    8. Instruct client to not double dose if dose is missed

    9. Advise client to use additional contraceptive measures as antibiotics can decrease birth control pill effectiveness

    10. Instruct client to avoid prolonged exposure to sun

XII. Medications Used to Dissolve Gallstones

A. Action and use

    1. Urosodiol is used to dissolve gallbladder stones smaller than 20 mm

    2. Absorbed in the small bowel, secreted into hepatic bile ducts and expelled into the duodenum in response to eating

    3. Natural occurring bile acid that inhibits hepatic synthesis and secretion of cholesterol

B. Common medication

    1. Urosodiol (Actigall)

    2. Usual adult dose is 8 to 10 mg/kg/day PO in divided doses or 300 mg bid for prevention

C. Administration considerations: use beyond 24 months has not been established

D. Contraindications

    1. Do not use for clients with calcified cholesterol stones, radiopaque stones, or radiolucent bile pigment stones

    2. Excretion in breast milk is not known, use with caution

    3. Avoid in clients with acute cholecystitis, biliary obstruction, pancreatitis, allergy to bile acids, and chronic liver disease

E. Significant drug interactions: antacids and bile acid sequestrants (cholestyramine, colestipol) may interfere with the action of ursodiol by decreasing its absorption

F. Significant food interactions: none reported

G. Significant laboratory studies: none reported

H. Side effects

1. Nausea, vomiting, abdominal pain, constipation, diarrhea, rash

2. Headache, fatigue, anxiety, sweating

3. Thinning of hair, arthralgia

I. Adverse effects/toxicity: diarrhea

J. Nursing considerations

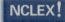

1. If no dissolution of partial stone is observed in 12 months, drug will probably not be effective

2. Gallbladder ultrasound should be done every 6 months the first year of therapy

3. Document indications and length of therapy

4. Determine pregnancy status

K. Client education

1. Instruct client to avoid antacid use with drug unless prescribed

2. Instruct client that therapy may take up to 24 months

3. Inform client that stones may recur

4. Advise client to report any side effects to health care provider

5. Discuss contraceptive methods because birth control pills may decrease drug effect

6. Stress importance of follow up visits and diagnostic tests

XIII. Pancreatic Enzyme Replacement

A. Action and use: enzyme (lipase, amylase and protease) replacement therapy in clients with cystic fibrosis, chronic pancreatitis, ductal obstructions, or pancreatic insufficiency

B. Common medications (Table 7-10)

C. Administration considerations

1. Swallow tablets/capsules whole, do not crush or chew

2. If swallowing is difficult, open capsules and give contents in applesauce or pudding to swallow without chewing

3. Take medications with meals

Table 7-10	Generic/Trade Names	Usual Adult Dosage Range	Route
Pancreatic Enzyme Replacement (Lipase, Amylase, Protease)	Pancrelipase (Creon 5)	2–4 capsules with meals and snacks	PO
	Pancrelipase (Ku-Zyme)	1–2 capsules with meals and snacks	PO
	Pancrelipase (Pancrease)	400 lipase units/kg per meal	PO
	Pancrelipase (Viokase)	1–4 tablets with meals	PO

Note: Dosage is adjusted on an individual basis according to extent of enzyme deficiency, dietary fat content, and enzyme activity of individual drug formulation.

D. Contraindications

1. Hypersensitivity to pork protein or enzymes

2. Contraindicated in acute pancreatitis

E. Significant drug interactions

1. If given with antacids the change in gastric pH may cause the enteric coated capsules to dissolve in the stomach and inactivate the product

2. Pancreatic lipase is inactivated at pH less than 4

3. If antacids allow the enteric coating to dissolve too soon, the drug will be inactivated by the gastric acid

4. This drug needs to travel into the less acidic duodenum before breaking down for therapeutic effect; if given with oral iron supplements the enzymes may decrease the effect of the iron

F. Significant food interactions: none reported

G. Significant laboratory studies: elevated serum uric acid

H. Side effects

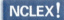

1. Nausea

2. Diarrhea

3. Abdominal cramps

I. Adverse effects/toxicity: hyperuricemia

J. Nursing considerations

1. Monitor for side effects and monitor steatorrhea, as it should diminish with appropriate dose of medication

2. Assess and monitor to maintain good nutritional status

3. Document indications for therapy

4. Document allergies

5. Assess swallowing ability or difficulty

K. Client education

1. Review dietary interventions with clients; consult with dietician for counseling and meal planning

2. Instruct client to take before or with meals with plenty of water

3. Instruct client to report any side effects to health care provider

Case Study

Mr. B is a 74-year-old male who complains of diarrhea for 1 month. He denies abdominal pain, nausea, or vomiting. He states his stools are loose and of soft consistency. Frequency of bowel movements is usually 5 to 10 times in 2 to 3 hours and worse in the morning. He denies blood in the stool or recent weight loss. His only medication is lisinopril (Zestril) 10 mg daily for his blood pressure. Vital signs are: temperature 96.4°F, pulse 84, BP 130/80 mmHg, respirations 18. The client's height is 6 ft and weight is 290 lb.

❶ What other pertinent subjective history should the nurse obtain?

❷ What specific physical assessment should be performed?

❸ What laboratory data would be helpful?

❹ What dietary instructions can the nurse offer?

❺ What are the differential diagnoses?

For suggested responses, see page 639.

Posttest

1 The nurse is teaching a client about the side effects of anticholinergic medications. Which of the following symptoms and signs should be included in this instruction?

(1) Dry mouth, urine retention, constipation, dilated pupils
(2) Polyuria, diarrhea, bradycardia, flushing
(3) Sweating, hypothermia, heartburn, anxiety
(4) Increased salivation, dysphagia, confusion, restlessness

2 A pregnant woman is asking the nurse about laxatives that are safe for use during pregnancy. Which of the following laxatives should the nurse expect to be absolutely avoided during pregnancy?

(1) Bisacodyl (Dulcolax)
(2) Mineral oil (generic)
(3) Castor oil (Neoloid)
(4) Sodium biphosphonate (Fleets Phospho-Soda)

3 A client is receiving a hyperosmotic treatment for occasional constipation. Which of the following medications should the nurse not expect to be used for this condition?

(1) Lactulose (Cephulac)
(2) Polyethylene glycol (Miralax)
(3) Glycerin (Glycerol)
(4) Bisacodyl (Dulcolax)

4 Which of the following would not be one of the actions completed immediately while evaluating the client with poisoning?

(1) Identify the substance
(2) Assess the vital signs
(3) Call poison control
(4) Give ipecac syrup

5 The client is receiving oral mineral oil, a lubricant agent, for constipation. The nurse determines that there is no contraindication for this order if the client has which of the following concurrent conditions?

(1) Dysphagia following a cerebral vascular accident (CVA)
(2) Questionable appendicitis
(3) Fecal impaction
(4) Occasional heartburn

6 The nurse is teaching a group of people in the community about ipecac syrup and its usage. In the discussion, the nurse should include that which of the following population groups has the potential to abuse ipecac syrup?

(1) Elderly clients with congestive heart failure (CHF)
(2) Clients with small children
(3) Clients with eating disorders
(4) Male clients working in food service settings

7 An emetic, ipecac syrup, is being prescribed to a pediatric client. The nurse taking care of the client determines that this medication is contraindicated in which of the following populations?

(1) Toddlers
(2) Schoolage children
(3) Teenagers
(4) Infants younger than 6 months

8 A client has cholelithiasis, but is a poor surgical candidate because of co-morbid disabilities. What medication may help this client?

(1) Urosodiol (Actigall)
(2) Omeprazole (Prilosec)
(3) Cimetidine (Tagamet)
(4) Ibuprofen (Motrin)

9 A client being diagnosed with a gastric ulcer is prescribed an H_2 antagonist medication. Currently, she is taking phenytoin (Dilantin) for seizure activity. The nurse questions a new medication order for which of the following H_2 antagonists that should not be prescribed for this client?

(1) Famotidine (Pepcid)
(2) Cimetidine (Tagamet)
(3) Nizaditine (Axid)
(4) Ranitidine (Zantac)

10 A client has been advised by the health care provider to take bisacodyl (Dulcolax). The nurse should include in the teaching plan that in order to achieving a rapid medication effect, the client should take the medication under which of the following conditions?

(1) On an empty stomach
(2) With plenty of fluids
(3) With meals
(4) At bedtime

See pages 299–300 for Answers and Rationales.

Answers and Rationales

Pretest

1 Answer: 2 *Rationale:* Activated charcoal absorbs ipecac syrup, thus decreasing its effect by inhibiting absorption from the GI tract into the general circulation. While calling the poison control center is important, it is not the highest priority action to ensure the safety of the client. Option 3 is incorrect, and option 4 could result in harm to the client.
Cognitive Level: Analysis
Nursing Process: Implementation; *Test Plan:* SECE

2 Answer: 1 *Rationale:* Metoclopramide is a GI stimulant, increasing motility of the GI tract and shortening gastric emptying time. The other options do not represent correct actions of this medication.
Cognitive Level: Application
Nursing Process: Evaluation; *Test Plan:* PHYS

3 Answer: 4 *Rationale:* Dicyclomine is a cholinergic-blocking agent that decreases hypermotility and spasms of the GI tract. The dose should be taken before a meal to be effective when needed.
Cognitive Level: Application
Nursing Process: Implementation; *Test Plan:* PHYS

4 Answer: 2 *Rationale:* Pepto Bismol (bismuth sub-salicylate) is contraindicated in clients who are allergic to aspirin or salicylates. The other medications can be given to the client safely.
Cognitive Level: Application
Nursing Process: Planning; *Test Plan:* PHYS

5 Answer: 4 *Rationale:* Metamucil is a bulk-forming laxative that could aggravate diarrhea. Kaopectate (option 2) is an antidiarrheal agent that is commonly used to manage this health problem, which is usually self-limiting. The client should contact the health care provider again if diarrhea persists (option 3), because diarrhea lasting more than 2 days requires attention. Dairy products are a food source that may aggravate diarrhea (option 1).
Cognitive Level: Analysis
Nursing Process: Evaluation; *Test Plan:* PHYS

6 Answer: 4 *Rationale:* Bulk-forming laxatives rely on water forming an emollient gel and increasing the bulk of stool in the intestines, stimulating peristalsis. Forcing fluids would be necessary when using this type of laxative. Clients on fluid restrictions are at increased risk of constipation (option 1). Bulk-forming

laxatives are commonly used (option 2), and stool softeners are often used initially for those clients who should not use the Valsalva maneuver (option 3).
Cognitive Level: Application
Nursing Process: Implementation; *Test Plan:* PHYS

7 Answer: 2 *Rationale:* Laxatives can precipitate electrolyte imbalances and dehydration. The underlying cause of constipation should be determined to rule out pathological conditions. Losing weight, decreased appetite and abdominal pain are not directly related to prolonged use of laxative.
Cognitive Level: Application
Nursing Process: Implementation; *Test Plan:* PHYS

8 Answer: 4 *Rationale:* Imodium is an antidiarrheal agent. It is prescribed for acute and chronic diarrhea and to reduce the volume of drainage from an ileostomy. This medication would worsen constipation (option 1) and is not effective in treating vomiting (option 2). It would only be useful in abdominal pain (option 3) if the discomfort was caused by the diarrhea, but there is insufficient information in the question to determine this.
Cognitive Level: Application
Nursing Process: Planning; *Test Plan:* PHYS

9 Answer: 2 *Rationale:* Misoprostol (Cytotec) inhibits gastric secretion and increases bicarbonate and mucus production thereby protecting the gastric mucosa. Ranitidine is used to treat an active duodenal ulcer. Magnesium hydroxide is used to treat constipation. Bethanechol is a direct-acting cholinergic agent that strengthens both peristalsis and micturition.
Cognitive Level: Application
Nursing Process: Planning; *Test Plan:* PHYS

10 Answer: 2 *Rationale:* Misoprostol (Cytotec) is not responsible for urinary incontinence, which represents a pathological condition. It may cause dysmenorrhea (option 1), headache (option 2), and diarrhea (option 3).
Cognitive Level: Analysis
Nursing Process: Evaluation; *Test Plan:* PHYS

Posttest

1 Answer: 1 *Rationale:* Anticholinergic effects include dry mouth, urine retention, constipation, and dilated pupils. Other side effects may include tachycardia, decreased sweating, increased risk of hyperthermia and decreased salivation.
Cognitive Level: Application
Nursing Process: Implementation; *Test Plan:* PHYS

2 Answer: 3 *Rationale:* Castor oil is a pregnancy category X preparation. It may induce premature labor and should not by used by pregnant women. Bisacodyl is pregnancy category C, while mineral oil and sodium biphosphonate are listed as unknown.
Cognitive Level: Application
Nursing Process: Analysis; *Test Plan:* PHYS

3 Answer: 4 *Rationale:* Bisacodyl is a stimulant cathartic producing results in 15 minutes to 2 hours. Hyperosmotic treatment of constipation may not be effective for 2 to 4 days. The other options are hyperosmotic laxatives.
Cognitive Level: Application
Nursing Process: Analysis; *Test Plan:* PHYS

4 Answer: 4 *Rationale:* Ipecac syrup is contraindicated with corrosive or petrolatum-based substances. Assessing stability, identifying the source of poison, and contacting poison control are all first-line interventions.
Cognitive Level: Application
Nursing Process: Implementation; *Test Plan:* PHYS

5 Answer: 4 *Rationale:* There is no contraindication to giving this medication to a client with occasional heartburn, since this is likely caused by food intolerance. Mineral oil should not be given to anyone with swallowing problems because of increased risk of aspiration leading to lipoid pneumonia (option 1). Mineral oil should also not be given unless disease processes are ruled out (option 2). The client with fecal impaction needs to be disimpacted and may require enemas (option 3).
Cognitive Level: Analysis
Nursing Process: Assessment; Test plan: PHYS

6 Answer: 3 *Rationale:* Ipecac syrup is an emetic that causes vomiting. It may be abused by clients with eating disorders. The other groups listed pose no additional risk of abuse. Nursing assessment must include abuse potentials and possible interventions and referrals.
Cognitive Level: Application
Nursing Process: Assessment; *Test Plan:* HPM

7 Answer: 4 *Rationale:* Infants under 6 months of age should not take ipecac syrup because of increased risk of aspiration. Instead, gastric lavage should be performed. There is no evidence that using emetics is contraindicated in the other age populations.
Cognitive Level: Application
Nursing Process: Planning; *Test Plan:* SECE

8 **Answer: 1** *Rationale:* Urosodiol is a naturally oc-
curing bile acid used to dissolve gallstones. Omeprazole is a proton pump inhibitor, cimetidine is a H_2
antagonist, and ibuprofen is a NSAID. None of these
three are indicated for cholelithiasis.
Cognitive Level: Comprehension
Nursing Process: Planning; *Test Plan:* PHYS

9 **Answer: 2** *Rationale:* Cimetidine interacts with the
metabolism of beta-adrenergic blockers, phenytoin,
lidocaine, procainamide, quinidine, benzodiazepines,
metronidozole, tricyclic antidepressants, oral contraceptives, and warfarin. Therefore, it should not be

giving concurrently with phenytoin. The other hista-
mine 2 receptor antagonists are acceptable for use.
Cognitive Level: Analysis
Nursing Process: Implementation; *Test Plan:* PHYS

10 **Answer: 1** *Rationale:* Taking Dulcolax on an empty
stomach will enhance a rapid effect. If taking at bedtime, the client will have a bowel movement in the
morning. Taking the medication with a meal will delay
the absorption. Drinking plenty of fluids is a good
general measure to reduce the risk of constipation.
Cognitive Level: Application
Nursing Process: Planning; *Test Plan:* PHYS

References

Abrams, A. (2004). *Clinical drug therapy: Rationales for nursing practice* (7th ed.). Philadelphia: Lippincott, Williams, & Wilkins, pp. 867–910.

Aschenbrenner, D., Cleveland, L., & Venable, S. (2002). *Drug therapy in nursing.* Philadelphia: Lippincott, Williams, & Wilkins, pp. 671–719.

Burns, C., Brady, M., Dunn, A., & Starr, N. (2000). *Pediatric primary care: A handbook for nurse practitioners.* (2nd ed.). Philadelphia: Saunders, p.741.

Cash, J., & Glass, C. (2000). *Family practice guidelines.* Philadelphia: Lippincott Williams & Wilkins, pp. 278–336.

Karch, A. (2003). *Focus on pharmacology* (2nd ed.). Philadelphia: Lippincott, Williams, & Wilkins, pp. 772–810.

Lehne, R. (2004). *Pharmacology for nursing care* (5th ed.). St. Louis, MO: Mosby, Inc., pp. 847–880.

Lemone, P., & Burke, K. (2003). *Medical-surgical nursing: Critical thinking in client care.* Upper Saddle River, NJ: Prentice Hall, pp. 415–544.

McCance, K., & Huether, S. (2002). *Pathophysiology: The biological basis for disease in adults and children.* (4th ed.). St. Louis, MO: Mosby, p. 1323.

McKenry, L., & Salerno, G. (2003). *Mosby's pharmacology in nursing* (21st ed.). St. Louis, MO: Mosby, Inc., pp. 752–785.

Munden, J. (Ed.). (2002). *Disease management for nurse practitioners.* Springhouse, PA: Springhouse, pp. 381–445.

Spratto, G., & Woods, A. (2000). *PDR: Nurse's drug handbook.* Montvale, NJ: Delmar Publishing & Medical Economics, pp. 105–1341.

Younkin, E., Swain, K., Kissinger, J. & Israel, D.(1999). *Pharmacotherapeutics: A primary care clinical guide.* Stamford, CT: Appleton & Lange, pp. 497–1311.

CHAPTER 8

Immune System Medications

Geralyn M. Valleroy-Frandsen, EdD, MSN, RN

CHAPTER OUTLINE

OBJECTIVES

- Describe the general goals of therapy when administering immune system medications.

- Discuss the primary uses, interactions, major side effects, and adverse/toxic effects of the most commonly prescribed immunosuppressant medications.

- Discuss the primary uses, interactions, major side effects and adverse/toxic effects of the most commonly prescribed immunostimulant medications.

- Describe the recommended childhood immunization schedule.

- Identify side effects and adverse effects associated with the administration of immunizations.

- List contraindications associated with the administration of vaccines.

- Discuss the nursing considerations related to the administration of medications commonly used to treat multiple sclerosis, myasthenia gravis, rheumatoid arthritis, and systemic lupus erythematosus.

- List the significant client education points related to immune system medications.

[Media Link]

Use the CD-ROM enclosed with this text, or log onto the address given to access the free, interactive Companion Website created for this series. The CD-ROM and Companion Website accompanying this book offer additional practice opportunities and information—NCLEX Review, Case Studies, Glossary, In Depth with NCLEX, and more.

www.prenhall.com/hogan

REVIEW AT A GLANCE

active immunity *immunity acquired by having a disease or by injection of the infectious organisms*

antigen *a substance that produces the formation of antibodies*

cellular immunity *immunity of the host that has been enhanced with increases in white blood cells and both helper and suppressor T cell function*

colony-stimulating factors *factors that stimulate glycoproteins to produce blood*

cells, thus stimulating immunity and bone marrow development

glycoprotein *the compounds of carbohydrates and proteins that, when produced, increase blood cell production*

immunosuppression *the ability to suppress the body's response to an antigen*

immune sera *an injection that provides passive immunity following an exposure to certain communicable diseases*

myelosuppression *the suppression of bone marrow function in the manufacture of blood cells*

neutropenia *abnormally low neutrophil count*

thrombocytopenia *abnormally low platelet count*

vaccine *injections of living attenuated organisms or dead organisms that assist the human host to develop protection from a communicable disease*

Pretest

1 Prior to the administration of filgrastim (Neupogen) the client reports a history of hypersensitivity to *E. coli* products. The nurse should take which of the following actions?

(1) Reduce the dosage of filgrastim by 5 micrograms.
(2) Assess the client for leukopenia and fever.
(3) Administer diphenhydramine (Benadryl) prior to administering filgrastim.
(4) Withhold the administration of filgrastim and notify the physician.

2 A client is taking sargramostim (Leukine). The nurse is especially careful to conduct a pulmonary assessment to detect which of the following risks associated with this drug?

(1) Congestive heart failure (CHF)
(2) Respiratory alkalosis
(3) Adult respiratory distress syndrome (ARDS)
(4) Pulmonary embolism

3 A client with rheumatoid arthritis has developed a fever. The nurse suspects that this may be related to which of the following?

(1) The effect of prescribed medications on the immune response
(2) A stable effect unrelated to medication
(3) A known, expected reaction to medication that is not harmful
(4) The client's ability to adapt to the medication regime

4 Following the administration of immune serum globulin the nurse should instruct the client to do which of the following?

(1) Avoid exposure to children
(2) Call the physician with signs of bleeding
(3) Apply heat to the injection site
(4) Repeat the dose within one week

5 A client with a known seizure disorder is taking cyclosporine (Sandimmune) following a kidney transplant. Based on this information, the nurse is aware that which of the following medication dosages will need to be altered?

(1) The standard cyclosporine dose will need to be increased.
(2) The client's anticonvulsant dose will need to be increased.
(3) The standard cyclosporine dose will need to be decreased.
(4) The client's anticonvulsant dose will need to be decreased.

6 A male client calls the physician's office complaining of shortness of breath and edema. He is currently taking hydrochlorothiazide (HCTZ) and digoxin (Lanoxin). Two days ago, he received chemotherapy followed by oprelvekin (Neumega). Based on this information, the nurse should take which of the following actions?

(1) Schedule him an appointment to be seen by the nurse practitioner.
(2) Instruct him to lie down with his head elevated 45 degrees.
(3) Instruct him to call 911 and be transported to the emergency room.
(4) Call the client's family to assess his heart rate.

7 A renal transplant recipient enjoys a grapefruit for breakfast. He is taking cyclosporine (Sandimmune). The nurse should instruct him that ingestion of grapefruit would have which of the following effects?

(1) Cause an increase in edema and renal insufficiency
(2) Increase the serum level of cyclosporine
(3) Assist in relieving his constipation
(4) Increase renal metabolism of cyclosporine

8 It is reported in the news that a restaurant worker at a local burger establishment has been diagnosed with hepatitis A. A patron of this establishment calls the health department for advice. The nurse should provide which of the following instructions to the patron?

(1) Call the physician for guidance.
(2) Assess self for future development of jaundice.
(3) Come to the health department and have a hepatitis blood test.
(4) Come to the health department to receive immune serum globulin.

9 A young mother asks the obstetrics nurse why her baby needs to receive immunizations. Which of the following would be the best response by the nurse?

(1) "Immunizations are required by law."
(2) "Immunizations prevent illnesses that are associated with a high death rate."
(3) "Immunizations are safe without side effects."
(4) "Immunizations are inexpensive and can be provided free from the health department."

10 A client with myasthenia gravis presents in the emergency room with severe ataxia and tremors. The nurse should be ready to administer which of the following medications?

(1) Edrophonium (Tensilon)
(2) Ambenonium (Mytelase)
(3) Neostigmine (Prostigmine)
(4) Atropine (generic)

See pages 325–326 for Answers and Rationales.

I. Immunomodulators

A. Description

1. These are medications used to alter the body's immune system actions

2. These medications can either suppress or enhance the client's immune response

3. Depending on the intended immune response desired the client is either administered an immune stimulant or an **immunosuppressant,** which has the ability to suppress the body's response to an **antigen** (a substance which produces the formation of antibodies)

B. Immunostimulants

1. **Colony-stimulating factors**

   a. Action and use

   1) Colony-stimulating factors are **glycoproteins** that increase the production of blood cells that enhance the individual's **cellular immunity** (immunity of the host that has been enhanced with increases in white blood cells and both helper and suppressor T cell functions) by increasing the number of lymphocytes and inhibiting tumor growth

   2) They can be used to prevent severe **thrombocytopenia** (abnormally low platelet count) from platelet destruction

3) They increase the development of bone marrow, which is adversely affected with the administration of chemotherapy agents used after bone marrow transplantation or to treat cancer

4) These medications reduce **neutropenia** (abnormally low neutrophil count) and decrease the incidence of infection; they assist in the mobilization of stem cells allowing for stem cell collection

b. Common medications (Table 8-1)

c. Administration considerations

1) Sargramostim (Leukine) (GM-CSF): reconstitute with sterile water; during reconstitution avoid shaking vial

2) Epoetin alfa (Erythropoetin): administration in clients with human immunodeficiency virus (HIV) should be for 8 weeks; the goal of therapy is to maintain the hematocrit (HCT) at 30 to 33% (maximum 36%)

3) Filgrastim (Neupogen): with each further chemotherapy administration increase Neupogen 5 mcg/kg; administration of Neupogen with bone marrow transplantation or collection of stem cells 10 mcg/kg/d; administration of Neupogen with severe chronic neutropenia 5 to 6 mcg/kg, 1 to 2 times per day

d. Contraindications

1) Sargramostim: pregnancy, hypersensitivity to yeast products, or *E. coli* products, leukemic myeloblasts in the bone marrow; use cautiously with hepatic or renal insufficiency and lactation

2) Epoetin alfa: uncontrolled hypertension, pregnancy, and hypersensitivity to albumin

3) Filgrastim: pregnancy, hypersensitivity to *E. coli* products

e. Significant drug interactions: lithium increases the effectiveness of sargramostim

f. Significant food interactions: none reported

g. Significant lab studies

1) Obtain a complete blood cell count (CBC) with differential and platelet count prior to beginning treatment with colony-stimulating factors and

Table 8-1 Common Immunostimulant Medications	Generic/Trade Names	Usual Adult Dose	Actions
	Sargramostim (CSF-GM) (Leukine)	250 mcg/m²/day, administer 2 to 4 hours after bone marrow transplantation then continue for 21 days; IV or SC	Increases the production of granulocytes and macrophages before and after bone marrow transplantation
	Epoetin alfa (Erythropoetin)	Chronic renal failure: 50–100 units/kg 3 times/week IV or SC Cancer and HIV:100–150 units/kg/week IV or SC	Increases the RBC count in clients with chronic renal failure, cancer, or human immunodeficiency virus
	Filgrastim (Neupogen)	5 mcg/kg/day IV or SC; dilute dextrose 5%	Increases neutrophil production in cancer clients to prevent infection

twice 2 weekly during drug administration until blood cell levels reach target range

2) Report neutrophil count of 20,000/mm^3 to the physician

3) Assess creatinine, blood urea nitrogen (BUN), liver enzymes before and after administration

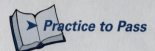
NCLEX!

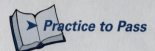
► Practice to Pass

What three assessments for hypersensitivity reaction are necessary for a client with hypersensitivity to *E. coli* products?

h. Side effects

1) Nausea, vomiting, anorexia, constipation, diarrhea

2) Headache, stomatitis, edema, rash, mucositis, generalized pain, bone pain

3) Supraventricular dysrhythmia, tachycardia

4) Renal or hepatic dysfunction, dyspnea, seizures, and porphyria

i. Adverse effects/toxicity

1) Report neutrophil count of 20,000/mm^3 cubed to physician

2) Adult respiratory distress syndrome (ARDS), pleural effusion

3) Myocardial infarction (MI), gastrointestinal (GI) hemorrhage, thrombus formation

j. Nursing considerations

1) Sargramostim (Leukine)

NCLEX!

a) Assess CBC and platelet count before administration and 2 times per week during medication administration

b) Assess renal and hepatic function

c) Assess for excessive myeloid blasts in bone marrow

d) Do not administer during pregnancy

e) Use cautiously with lactation

f) Administer less than 24 hours after cytotoxic chemotherapy

g) Administer less than 24 hours after bone marrow transplant

h) Dilute with normal saline and store in the refrigerator; administer only one dose per vial

2) Epoetin alfa (Erythropoetin)

NCLEX!

a) Assess blood pressure (BP) prior to administration and regularly during therapy; hypertension may occur if hematocrit level rises rapidly

b) Epoetin alfa should be used cautiously during lactation

NCLEX!

c) The client should be on a high-iron diet to increase effectiveness of therapy on red blood cell formation

NCLEX!

d) Assess Homan's sign periodically to detect the development of a thrombus with increased red cell counts

e) Administer cautiously with lactation

f) Do not shake solution after it has been reconstituted

      g) Assess HCT to determine if it has risen 4 points in 2 weeks; an elevation of 4 points may lead to hypertension and seizures

  3) Filgrastim (Neupogen)

      a) Assess results of CBC, differential, and platelet count before administration and 2 times per week during therapy

      b) Do not administer 24 hours before or after chemotherapy

      c) Assess for hypersensitivity to *E. coli* products

      d) Filgrastim is pregnancy category C; use cautiously with lactation

      e) Administer only one dose per vial, and discard after 24 hours; store medication in the refrigerator

      f) Reconstitute in dextrose 5%, and avoid shaking the bottle to prevent damage to the protein

      g) Avoid exposure to infection because client's lowered white cell count indicates increased risk of infection

 k. Client education

  1) Sargramostim (Leukine)

      a) Instruct client to avoid exposure to infection and teach signs and symptoms of infection

      b) Report difficulty breathing and fever

      c) Address body image with client due to alopecia

      d) Instruct client that CBC and platelet counts to be done periodically

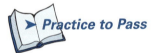
Practice to Pass

  2) Epoetin alfa (Erythropoetin)

      a) Instruct client regarding administration of medication at home with home dialysis

What assessment related to laboratory values should the nurse make when administering colony-stimulating factors?

      b) Instruct client regarding the signs and symptoms of clot formation

      c) Instruct client about action, side effects, and nursing implications associated with epoetin alfa administration

      d) Instruct client to self-evaluate BP

      e) Instruct client to consume a diet high in iron

  3) Filgrastim (Neupogen)

      a) Report pain in the joints and bones

      b) Instruct client to maintain good hygiene and avoid exposure to crowds because of to the susceptibility of infection

 2. Cell-stimulating medications

  a. Action and use

    1) Interleukins are also biologic response modifiers that prevent thrombocytopenia and stimulate platelet production

2) In the helper T cells, cellular immunity is increased along with the number of lymphocytes

3) The interleukins are a group of proteins produced by lymphocytes that have antitumor activity by causing cells to change to a non-proliferative type

4) Aldesleukin (Proleukin) is used for the treatment of renal carcinoma and prevents severe thrombocytopenia

5) Levamisole (Ergamisol) increases the immune response by increasing the activity of B cells and increasing T cells to increase antibody formation and monocyte and macrophage action; it is used in combination with fluorouracil to treat Duke's Stage C colon cancer

6) Oprelvekin (Neumega) is used following **myelosuppressive** (suppresses bone marrow function in manufacture of blood cells) chemotherapy; it increases the thrombocyte and megakaryocyte production to prevent and treat thrombocytopenia in clients receiving chemotherapy

b. Common medications (Table 8-2)

c. Administration considerations

1) Aldesleukin (Proleukin): infuse for 5 minutes 3 times per day for 5 days for a total of 14 doses; following the 7th day hold the medication for 9 days, begin administration again 3 times per day for 14 doses; because of seriousness of side effects, this medication is given in a hospital that has an intensive care unit with medical specialists available

2) Levamisole (Ergamisol): drug therapy should begin 7 to 30 days after bowel resection surgery; maintenance dose is 50 mg every 8 hours for 3 days with fluorouracil

3) Oprelvekin (Neumega): administration can be continued for 21 days or until platelet count is greater than 100,000 cells/mcL

d. Contraindications

1) Aldesleukin

a) Pregnancy and lactation

b) Organ transplant recipient

Table 8-2	Generic/Trade Names	Usual Adult Dose	Actions
Common Cell-Stimulating Medications	Aldesleukin (Proleukin)	600,000 units/kg every 8 hr IV	Increases lymphocytes, platelets and tumor necrosis factor
	Levamisole (Ergamisol)	Administer with fluorouracil 50 mg PO every 8 hr for 3 days	Increases B cell activity and antibody formation by increasing monocyte and macrophage action
	Oprelvekin (Neumega)	25 to 75 mcg/kg/day SC after chemotherapy	Increases thrombocyte and megakaryocyte production, thus preventing thrombocytopenia

        c) Cardiovascular disease

        d) Cardiopulmonary disease

    2) Levamisole: pregnancy and lactation

    3) Oprelvekin: pregnancy and lactation

e. Significant drug interactions: levamisole administered with phenytoin will increase serum phenytoin levels

f. Significant food interactions: none reported

g. Significant laboratory studies

    1) Aldesleukin: platelet count

    2) Levamisole: CBC with differential

    3) Oprelvekin: platelet count

h. Side effects

    1) Aldesleukin: cardiac dyshythmias, fluid retention, lethargy, and myalgia

    2) Levamisole: flu-like symptoms, bone marrow depression, GI upset

    3) Oprelvekin: cardiac arrhythmias, fluid retention

i. Adverse effects/toxicity: aldesleukin and oprelvekin cause cardiopulmonary insufficiency

j. Nursing considerations

    1) Assess CBC, differential, and platelet count

    2) Assess heart rate, BP, respirations, and lung sounds

    3) Maintain fluid and electrolyte balance particularly during flu-like symptoms

    4) Provide good hygiene practices

    5) Reconstitute oprelvekin in an isotonic solution, do not agitate and administer within 3 hours of reconstitution

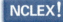

k. Client education

    1) Instruct client and family regarding home medication administration

    2) Instruct client and family about assessment of fluid retention and irregular heart rate

    3) Instruct on measures to assist in preventing infection

    4) Instruct family about care and management of flu-like symptoms

C. Immunosuppressants

  1. Action and use

    a. Immunosuppressants are medications used to inhibit the inflammatory response and block the immune response to an antigen

    b. These medications inhibit T cells

    c. They also block the production of antibodies by the B cells

    d. They are used to prevent rejection of organs that have been transplanted

Table 8-3	Generic/Trade Names	Usual Adult Dose	Actions
Common Immunosuppressant Medications	Azathioprine (Imuran)	Dosage is determined by WBC count, PO	Prevention of rejection in renal transplants; administered for life after the transplant
	Basiliximab (Simulect)	IV; consists of 2 20–mg doses; the first is given within 2 hrs prior to transplant surgery; the second is 4 days postop	Prevent acute renal transplant rejection; must be given in combination with cyclosporine and a glucocorticoid
	Daclizumab (Zenapax)	IV; 1 mg/kg for 5 doses total; given within 24 hrs preop and at 2, 4, 6, and 8 weeks postop	Prevent renal transplant rejection
	Cyclosporine (Sandimmune)	PO or IV; dosage is complex and is based on organ transplanted and other immunosuppressants given	Prevent rejection in solid organ transplant
	Muromonab CD3 (Orthoclone OKT3)	IV; 5 mg/day for 10 to 14 days	Suppresses T cells to prevent renal transplant rejection
	Mycophenolate (Cell Cept)	PO or IV; dosage depends on organ transplanted	Prevent rejection in renal, liver, and cardiac transplants
	Tacrolimus (Protopic, Prograf)	PO; 0.15 to 0.30 mg/kg every day; IV 0.05 to 0.1 mg/kg every day	Prevents rejection in solid organ transplant, primarily liver transplant

2. Common medications (Table 8-3)

3. Administration considerations

   a. Azathioprine (Imuran): it reaches the peak blood concentration in 1 to 2 hours and duration of action is 10 hours

   b. Cyclosporine (Sandimmune): it reaches its peak level in 4 to 5 hours after administration and duration of action is 20 to 54 hours

   c. Basiliximab (Simulect): is administered IV 24 hours after transplant then 4 days after transplant

   d. Declizumab (Zenapax): is administered IV 24 hours after transplant for total of 5 doses

   e. Muromonab CD3 (Orthoclone OKT 3): therapy should begin as soon as rejection is identified

   f. Mycophenolate (Cell Cept): renal transplant clients receive 1 gram 2 times per day; therapy should begin 72 hours after transplant

   g. Tacrolimus (Prograf): is administered 6 hours after transplant

4. Contraindications

   a. Allergy to drug

   b. Lactation

   c. Pregnancy

   d. Use cautiously with renal or hepatic impairment

5. Significant drug interaction

   a. Increased risk of hepatic or renal toxicity in clients taking other renal or hepatotoxic medications

   b. Cyclosporine: anticonvulsant medications decrease cyclosporine levels; oral contraceptives increase cyclosporine levels

6. Significant food interactions: increased serum levels are associated with administration of cyclosporine and grapefruit juice or grapefruit

7. Significant laboratory studies

   a. Aspartate aminotransferase (AST) and alanine aminotransferase (ALT)

   b. BUN and creatinine

   c. CBC and platelet count

8. Side effects

   a. Increased risk for infection

   b. Hepatotoxicity and/or renal toxicity

   c. Hypertension

   d. Flu-like symptoms and/or headache

   e. Acne

   f. Diarrhea, nausea, and/or vomiting

9. Adverse effects/toxicity: renal toxicity and hepatotoxicity are noted with the immunomodulators

10. Nursing considerations

    a. Assess for signs and symptoms of infection

    b. Provide supportive care for flu-like symptoms

    c. Maintain blood studies as ordered such as CBC, platelet count, renal and hepatic function tests

    d. Assess nutritional status

    e. Encourage well-balanced meals with small frequent feedings

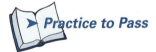

Practice to Pass

What learning objectives are appropriate for the nurse to develop for a client who will be receiving immunosuppressant agents?

11. Client education: educate client on the need for lab studies, prevention of infection, and all aspects of medication administration including action, side effects, and nursing implications

II. Immunizations

A. Vaccines

1. Action and use

   a. **Vaccines** are injectable or oral suspensions containing microorganisms that are live or weakened that when injected produce antibodies to fight against a disease

      b. Active immunity is the result of the introduction of a specific protein antigen by a way of a vaccine; the body responds by developing antibodies to confer a long lasting immunity to that organism

      c. Vaccines are used to prevent disease that may have high mortality and morbidity

2. Common medications (Figure 8-1)

3. Administration considerations

      a. Live vaccines should not be administered in less than 1 month of each other

      b. Hepatitis A is a 2-dose series for clients at risk

      c. Hepatitis B: initial dose followed by 2nd dose 1 month later, and 3rd dose is 6 months after the initial dose

      d. Measles, mumps, and rubella; total amount of reconstituted vial is administered SC

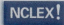

4. Contraindications

      a. Vaccines should not be administered during a moderate to severe febrile illness, pregnancy, cancer, leukemia, and while on immunosuppressive drug therapy

      b. Do not administer for 3 months after blood products have been administered

5. Significant drug interactions: immunosuppressive drug therapy

6. Significant food interactions: none reported

7. Significant laboratory studies: monitor antibody titer levels

8. Side effects

      a. Pain, swelling, or redness at injection site

      b. Flu-like symptoms

      c. Hypersensitivity (rarely noted)

9. Adverse effects/toxicity: rarely clients may experience a hypersensitivity reaction

10. Nursing considerations

      a. Determine administration guidelines and timing of immunization administration

      b. Adhere to individual vaccine storage recommendations to ensure vaccine potency

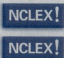

      c. Assess client for acute infection prior to administration

      d. Maintain documentation of immunization administration and client reaction to administration; provide client or caretaker with a record of immunizations administered

      e. Administer all vaccines for which client is eligible at different sites, using different syringes

      f. Observe client for manifestations of adverse reactions, and have epinephrine available in case of hypersensitivity reactions

Figure 8-1

Recommended Childhood and Adolescent Immunization Schedule—United States, January–June 2004.

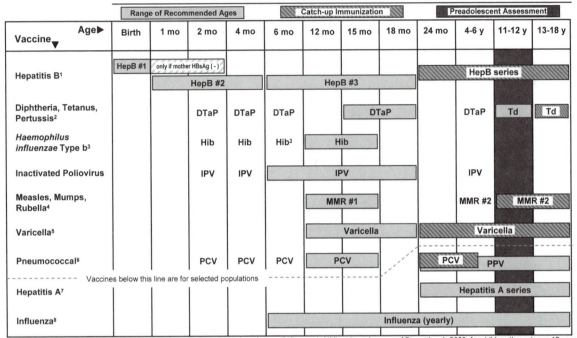

Vaccine ▼ / Age ►	Birth	1 mo	2 mo	4 mo	6 mo	12 mo	15 mo	18 mo	24 mo	4-6 y	11-12 y	13-18 y
Hepatitis B[1]	HepB #1	only if mother HBsAg (-)	HepB #2			HepB #3				HepB series		
Diphtheria, Tetanus, Pertussis[2]			DTaP	DTaP	DTaP		DTaP			DTaP	Td	Td
Haemophilus influenzae Type b[3]			Hib	Hib	Hib[3]	Hib						
Inactivated Poliovirus			IPV	IPV		IPV				IPV		
Measles, Mumps, Rubella[4]						MMR #1				MMR #2	MMR #2	
Varicella[5]						Varicella				Varicella		
Pneumococcal[6]			PCV	PCV	PCV	PCV			PCV	PPV		
Hepatitis A[7]									Hepatitis A series			
Influenza[8]					Influenza (yearly)							

Range of Recommended Ages / Catch-up Immunization / Preadolescent Assessment

Vaccines below this line are for selected populations

This schedule indicates the recommended ages for routine administration of currently licensed childhood vaccines, as of December 1, 2003, for children through age 18 years. Any dose not given at the recommended age should be given at any subsequent visit when indicated and feasible. ▧ Indicates age groups that warrant special effort to administer those vaccines not previously given. Additional vaccines may be licensed and recommended during the year. Licensed combination vaccines may be used whenever any components of the combination are indicated and the vaccine's other components are not contraindicated. Providers should consult the manufacturers' package inserts for detailed recommendations. Clinically significant adverse events that follow immunization should be reported to the Vaccine Adverse Event Reporting System (VAERS). Guidance about how to obtain and complete a VAERS form can be found on the Internet: http://www.vaers.org/ or by calling 1-800-822-7967.

1. Hepatitis B (HepB) vaccine. All infants should receive the first dose of hepatitis B vaccine soon after birth and before hospital discharge; the first dose may also be given by age 2 months if the infant's mother is hepatitis B surface antigen (HBsAg) negative. Only monovalent HepB can be used for the birth dose. Monovalent or combination vaccine containing HepB may be used to complete the series. Four doses of vaccine may be administered when a birth dose is given. The second dose should be given at least 4 weeks after the first dose, except for combination vaccines which cannot be administered before age 6 weeks. The third dose should be given at least 16 weeks after the first dose and at least 8 weeks after the second dose. The last dose in the vaccination series (third or fourth dose) should not be administered before age 24 weeks.

Infants born to HBsAg-positive mothers should receive HepB and 0.5 mL of Hepatitis B Immune Globulin (HBIG) within 12 hours of birth at separate sites. The second dose is recommended at age 1 to 2 months. The last dose in the immunization series should not be administered before age 24 weeks. These infants should be tested for HBsAg and antibody to HBsAg (anti-HBs) at age 9 to 15 months.

Infants born to mothers whose HBsAg status is unknown should receive the first dose of the HepB series within 12 hours of birth. Maternal blood should be drawn as soon as possible to determine the mother's HBsAg status; if the HBsAg test is positive, the infant should receive HBIG as soon as possible (no later than age 1 week). The second dose is recommended at age 1 to 2 months. The last dose in the immunization series should not be administered before age 24 weeks.

2. Diphtheria and tetanus toxoids and acellular pertussis (DTaP) vaccine. The fourth dose of DTaP may be administered as early as age 12 months, provided 6 months have elapsed since the third dose and the child is unlikely to return at age 15 to 18 months. The final dose in the series should be given at age ≥4 years. **Tetanus and diphtheria toxoids (Td)** is recommended at age 11 to 12 years if at least 5 years have elapsed since the last dose of tetanus and diphtheria toxoid-containing vaccine. Subsequent routine Td boosters are recommended every 10 years.

3. Haemophilus influenzae type b (Hib) conjugate vaccine. Three Hib conjugate vaccines are licensed for infant use. If PRP-OMP (PedvaxHIB or ComVax [Merck]) is administered at ages 2 and 4 months, a dose at age 6 months is not required. DTaP/Hib combination products should not be used for primary immunization in infants at ages 2, 4 or 6 months but can be used as boosters following any Hib vaccine. The final dose in the series should be given at age ≥12 months.

4. Measles, mumps, and rubella vaccine (MMR). The second dose of MMR is recommended routinely at age 4 to 6 years but may be administered during any visit, provided at least 4 weeks have elapsed since the first dose and both doses are administered beginning at or after age 12 months. Those who have not previously received the second dose should complete the schedule by the 11- to 12-year-old visit.

5. Varicella vaccine. Varicella vaccine is recommended at any visit at or after age 12 months for susceptible children (i.e., those who lack a reliable history of chickenpox). Susceptible persons age ≥13 years should receive 2 doses, given at least 4 weeks apart.

6. Pneumococcal vaccine. The heptavalent **pneumococcal conjugate vaccine (PCV)** is recommended for all children age 2 to 23 months. It is also recommended for certain children age 24 to 59 months. The final dose in the series should be given at age ≥12 months. **Pneumococcal polysaccharide vaccine (PPV)** is recommended in addition to PCV for certain high-risk groups. See MMWR 2000;49(RR-9):1-38.

7. Hepatitis A vaccine. Hepatitis A vaccine is recommended for children and adolescents in selected states and regions and for certain high-risk groups; consult your local public health authority. Children and adolescents in these states, regions, and high-risk groups who have not been immunized against hepatitis A can begin the hepatitis A immunization series during any visit. The 2 doses in the series should be administered at least 6 months apart. See MMWR 1999;48(RR-12):1-37.

8. Influenza vaccine. Influenza vaccine is recommended annually for children age ≥6 months with certain risk factors (including but not limited to children with asthma, cardiac disease, sickle cell disease, human immunodeficiency virus infection, and diabetes; and household members of persons in high-risk groups [see MMWR 2003;52(RR-8):1-36]) and can be administered to all others wishing to obtain immunity. In addition, healthy children age 6 to 23 months are encouraged to receive influenza vaccine if feasible, because children in this age group are at substantially increased risk of influenza-related hospitalizations. For healthy persons age 5 to 49 years, the intranasally administered live-attenuated influenza vaccine (LAIV) is an acceptable alternative to the intramuscular trivalent inactivated influenza vaccine (TIV). See MMWR 2003;52(RR-13):1-8. Children receiving TIV should be administered a dosage appropriate for their age (0.25 mL if age 6 to 35 months or 0.5 mL if age ≥3 years). Children age ≤8 years who are receiving influenza vaccine for the first time should receive 2 doses (separated by at least 4 weeks for TIV and at least 6 weeks for LAIV).

For additional information about vaccines, including precautions and contraindications for immunization and vaccine shortages, please visit the National Immunization Program Web site at www.cdc.gov/nip/ or call the National Immunization Information Hotline at 800-232-2522 (English) or 800-232-0233 (Spanish).

Approved by the Advisory Committee on Immunization Practices (www.cdc.gov/nip/acip), the American Academy of Pediatrics (www.aap.org), and the American Academy of Family Physicians (www.aafp.org).

g. Provide acetaminophen (Tylenol) after administration as needed

h. Apply heat to injection site as needed for comfort

11. Client education

a. Discuss with client and family risk of contracting vaccine-preventable illnesses as well as signs and symptoms

b. Instruct on treatment of flu-like symptoms using acetaminophen or nonsteroidal anti-inflammatory drugs (NSAIDs) such as ibuprofen

c. Instruct on the importance of keeping a record of immunizations and being up-to-date in immunization administration

d. Provide a copy of the Current Vaccine Information Statement for each vaccine administered; these are available from the Centers for Disease Control

e. Adults should be immunized against tetanus every 10 years

f. Woman of childbearing age should not become pregnant for 3 months after receiving a rubella immunization

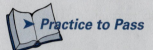

Practice to Pass

What client education should be implemented during a hepatitis A outbreak?

B. Immune sera

1. Action and use

a. **Immune sera** provide passive immunity to a disease

b. They can be used prophylactically to prevent disease following exposure

2. Common medications (Table 8-4)

3. Administration considerations (Table 8-4)

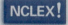

4. Contraindications: hypersensitivity to immune sera and use cautiously with thrombocytopenia and disorders affecting coagulation

5. Significant drug interactions: none reported

6. Significant food interactions: none reported

Table 8-4

Common Immune Sera

Generic/Trade Names	Usual Adult Dose	Actions
Cytomegalovirus immunoglobulin	72 hrs after renal transplant 150 mg/kg IV; 2-8 weeks after renal transplant 100 mg/kg IV	Treats cytomegalovirus in renal transplant clients
Hepatitis B immunoglobulin	0.06 mL/kg IM after exposure and repeat in 1 month	Prevents hepatitis B after exposure to hepatitis B
Immune serum globulin (Gammar)	See product literature	Provides immunoglobulin therapy after bone marrow transplant
Immune globulin (IGIM)	0.2-0.4 mL/kg IM with hepatitis A exposure; 0.25 mL/kg within 6 days after exposure to measles	Provides immunoglobulin therapy after exposure to hepatitis A or measles
Immune serum globulin IV	Gandimmune: 100 mg/kg IV one time per month Sandoglobulin: 200 mg/kg IV one time per month	Treats immunodeficiency syndrome
Respiratory syncytial virus (RSV) immune globulin	1.5 mL/kg/hr for 15 min., then 3 mL/kg/hr for 15 min., then 6 mL/kg/hr for 15 min.	Reduces severity of RSV in high risk infants

7. Significant laboratory studies: none reported

8. Side effects

   a. Allergic reaction

   b. Flu-like symptoms

   c. Irritation at injection site

9. Adverse effects/toxicity: anaphylaxis

10. Nursing considerations

    a. Monitor for signs and symptoms of hypersensitivity reaction following administration

    b. Provide comfort for flu-like symptoms

    c. Apply heat to irritated injection site

    d. Do not administer to clients with a history of coagulation disorders

    e. Document the medication administered, dosage, date, and response to medication

11. Client education

    a. Educate client and family on treatment of flu-like symptoms

    b. Educate client and family on signs and symptoms of anaphylaxis and to seek emergency care if noted

    c. Provide documentation to the client and family on the medication administered

C. Antitoxins and antivenins

1. Action and use: these are antibodies provided in immune sera for specific toxins that are released from invading pathogens

2. Common medications (Table 8-5)

3. Administration considerations: antirabies serum: can be applied to the animal bite wound

4. Contraindications: hypersensitivity to antitoxin, malignancy, and use cautiously with pregnancy

5. Significant drug interactions: immunosuppressive drug therapy

6. Significant food interactions: none reported

Table 8-5	Generic/Trade Names	Usual Adult Dose	Actions
Common Antitoxin Medications	Rabies immune globulin	1 mL for 5 doses IM; administer the initial dose and then 3, 7, 14, and 28 days later	Post-exposure prevention of rabies
	Antirabies serum, equine	55 units/kg IM	Horse serum used if human rabies immune globulin is unavailable
	Botulism antitoxin	See drug insert and test for hypersensitivity to the horse serum	Obtained from horses immunized against *Clostridium botulinum;* used to treat botulism

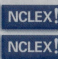
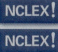

7. Significant laboratory studies: none reported

8. Side effects: irritation and pain at the injection site

9. Adverse effects/toxicity: hypersensitivity to the medication and severe pain at the injection site

10. Nursing considerations

    a. Monitor client response to medication

    b. Assess vital signs before and after administration

    c. Cleanse wound in the case of animal bite

    d. Document client's response to medication

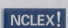

    e. Test sensitivity to horse serum and have epinephrine available

    f. Assess for neurological response to botulism antitoxin

11. Client education

    a. Educate client and family about the effect of medication administration

    b. Educate the client and family regarding adverse effects of medication

    c. Instruct client and family on the wound care of the client's animal bite

III. Medications to Treat Multiple Sclerosis

A. Action and use

1. The goal of medications administered for multiple sclerosis is to decrease inflammation, suppress the immune system to prevent nerve tissue destruction, and to decrease fatigue and ataxia

2. There are a wide variety of medications used to treat multiple sclerosis; they include the beta-adrenergic blockers, corticosteroids, anti-inflammatory agents, and interferon

B. Common medications (Table 8-6)

Table 8-6

Common Medications to Treat Multiple Sclerosis

Generic/Trade Names	Usual Adult Dose	Actions
Azathioprine (Imuran)	1 mg/kg PO 2 times per day, increasing dose in 6–8 weeks by 0.5 mg/kg per day, max 2.5 mg/kg/day	Decreases the severity of symptoms and the progress of the disease process
Beta 1a (Avonex)	30 mcg IM one time per week	Reduces the severity of acute exacerbations of multiple sclerosis; the drug decreases demyelination in the brain tissue
Beta 1b (Betaseron)	0.25 mg SC every other day	Reduces the severity of acute exacerbations of multiple sclerosis; the drug decreases demyelination in the brain tissue
Cyclophosphamide (Cytoxan)	40–50 mg/kg IV in divided doses for 2–5 days, then 1–5 mg/kg PO per day	Reduces the rate and progression of the disease by interfering with the replication of susceptible cells
Cyclosporine (Sandimmune)	2.5 mg/kg per day PO in divided doses	Reduces the severity of acute exacerbations of multiple sclerosis
Glatiramer acetate (Copaxone)	20 mg per day SC	Prevents the destruction of brain and nerve tissue

C. **Administration considerations:** Beta 1b (Betaseron) should be discontinued in 6 months if disease does not enter remission

D. **Contraindications**

1. These medications should be administered cautiously in the presence of hepatic or renal insufficiency and when the client has been diagnosed with a neoplasm

2. Contraindicated in pregnancy, lactation, and hypersensitivity to the drug

E. **Significant drug interactions**

1. Do not administer these medications with hepatotoxic or nephrotoxic medications

2. If azathioprine (Imuran) is administered with allopurinol, the azathioprine dose should be reduced

3. Do not administer cyclosporine (Sandimmune) with diltiazem, metoclopramide, or nicardipine due to the risk of toxicity

4. If cyclophosphamide (Cytoxan) is administered with digoxin, toxicity may result

F. **Significant food interactions**

1. Do not administer these medications with grapefruit juice or grapefruit

2. The effectiveness of the medication will be reduced if this occurs

G. **Significant laboratory studies**

1. AST/ALT

2. Blood glucose

3. BUN and creatinine

4. Calcium and phosphorus

5. Uric acid

H. **Side effects**

1. Azathioprine (Imuran): an increased risk of infection and renal or hepatic insufficiency; leukopenia and thrombocytopenia have also been noted

2. Beta 1a (Avonex): anorexia, nausea, vomiting, dizziness, and flu-like symptoms

3. Beta 1b (Betaseron): anorexia, confusion, dizziness, flu-like symptoms, and photosensitivity

4. Cyclophosphamide (Cytoxan): anorexia, nausea, vomiting, or hemorrhagic cystitis

5. Cyclosporine (Sandimmune): hepatotoxicity, hirsutism, and renal toxicity

6. Glatiramer acetate (Copaxone): anxiety, diarrhea, flu-like symptoms, hypertonia, and pain at the injection site

I. **Adverse effects/toxicity:** medications used to treat symptoms of multiple sclerosis has been noted to increase pulmonary edema leading to chest pain and shortness of breath

J. **Nursing considerations**

1. Assess the client for signs and symptoms of pulmonary edema, chest pain, and shortness of breath

2. Assess laboratory tests as ordered by physician

3. Provide comfort measures when the client experiences flu-like symptoms

4. Assess the injection sites for inflammation and pain

K. Client education

1. Educate the client and family regarding the side effects of the medication

2. Educate the client and family about the need for periodic laboratory studies

3. Educate the client and family to report any side effects to the health care provider

4. Educate the client and family about supportive care of flu-like symptoms, including adequate fluid intake, rest, and use of acetaminophen for relief of pain and fever

5. Educate the client and family about the signs and symptoms of pulmonary edema

IV. Medications to Treat Myasthenia Gravis

A. Action and use

1. The goal of anticholinesterase medications is to treat the symptoms of myasthenia gravis

2. These medications increase the concentration of acetylcholine at the neuromuscular junction

3. They are used to increase nerve impulses and strength

B. Common medications (Table 8-7)

C. Administration considerations

1. Edrophonium (Tensilon): the single dose is for diagnostic purposes only

2. Neostigmine (Prostigmine): it can be administered SC during an acute exacerbation of myasthenia gravis

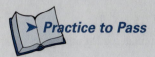

Practice to Pass

What nursing interventions should be implemented to relieve the flu-like symptoms that are side effects during administration of medications to treat multiple sclerosis?

NCLEX!

Table 8-7	Generic/Trade Names	Usual Adult Dose	Actions
Common Medications to Treat Myasthenia Gravis	Ambenonium (Mytelase)	5–30 mg PO 3 to 4 times daily	It is a long-acting medication to treat myasthenia gravis
	Edrophonium (Tensilon)	2–4 mg IV or 10 mg IM in one single dose	It is used for diagnostic purposes; clients who receive an injection of edrophonium and exhibit temporary relief of symptoms are diagnosed with decreased concentration of acetylcholine in the neuromuscular junction
	Neostigmine (Prostigmine)	15–30 mg PO every 2–4 hours while awake	Neostigmine has a duration of action of 2–4 hours and it increases acetylcholine concentration, facilitating neuromuscular function
	Physostigmine (Eserine)	0.5–2 mg IV or IM	It is anticholinesterase agent that crosses the blood brain barrier; it is used as an antidote for anticholinergic poisoning and for the treatment of glaucoma
	Pyridostigmine (Reganol, Mestinol)	60–120 mg PO every 3–4 hours while awake	Pyridostigmine increases acetylcholine concentration facilitating neuromuscular function; it is taken every 3–6 hours

   3. Physostigmine (Eserine): IV administration should be no faster than 1 mg per minute

   4. Pyridostigmine (Reganol, Mestinol): a timed-release preparation can be administered at bedtime; this medication can also be administered IM during periods of acute exacerbation

D. Contraindications

   1. Pregnancy and lactation

   2. Bradycardia and intestinal or urinary obstruction

   3. Use cautiously in clients with asthma, heart disease, Parkinson's disease, and seizure disorders

E. Significant drug interactions: the combination of myasthenia gravis medications and NSAID agents poses a threat of GI bleeding because of the increase in GI secretions

F. Significant food interactions: none reported

G. Significant laboratory studies

   1. ALT/AST

   2. BUN and creatinine

H. Side effects

   1. Bradycardia

   2. Hypotension

   3. Cardiac arrest

   4. Increased gastric secretions

   5. Diarrhea

   6. Increased urinary urgency

   7. Involuntary incontinence of stool

   8. Nausea and vomiting

NCLEX!

I. Adverse effects/toxicity: severe cholinergic reaction include excessive salivation, sphincter relaxation, diarrhea, and vomiting

J. Nursing considerations

NCLEX!

   1. Assess respiratory and general muscle strength including swallowing and heart rate prior to administration

   2. Administer medications with meals to enhance absorption and decrease GI irritation

NCLEX!

   3. Administer medications on time to prevent difficulty with respirations and swallowing caused by under medication or late medication administration

   4. Administer IV preparations slowly to prevent cholinergic reaction

5. Have atropine available to counteract cholinergic reaction

6. Assess the client's response to the medication and ability to perform activities of daily living

K. Client education

1. Instruct client on all aspects of medication administration

2. Instruct client on coordination of medication administration with the activities of daily living

3. Instruct that overmedication will result in cholinergic reaction

4. Instruct client on assessment of apical pulse

5. Instruct on side effects of medications

6. Instruct client to take medications with food to decrease GI irritation

V. Medications to Treat Rheumatoid Arthritis

A. Action and use

1. Management of rheumatoid arthritis in the early stages is accomplished with the used of NSAID agents

2. The latter stages of rheumatoid arthritis are treated with disease-modifying antirheumatic drugs (DMARDs)

3. These medications decrease the erythrocyte sedimentation rate, thus reducing inflammation, stiffness, swelling, and pain

4. Gold salts or gold compounds are also used to decrease the prostaglandin activity that contributes to joint destruction

B. Common medications (Table 8-8)

C. Administration considerations

1. Gold sodium thiomalate (Aurolate) should be injected into intragluteal muscle

2. Penicillamine (Depen): increase dose in 1 to 3 month intervals; continue increases at 2 to 3 month intervals; maintenance dose is 500 to 750 mg orally every day

D. Contraindications

1. Never administer medications to clients who have a known allergy to animal products

2. Contraindicated with pregnancy, lactation, liver disease, or renal disease

3. Penicillamine is contraindicated with a known hypersensitivity to penicillin

4. Gold salts are contraindicated with systemic lupus erythematosus or blood dyscrasias

E. Significant drug interactions

1. Do not administer these medications with any agents that are known to be hepatotoxic

2. Do not administer penicillamine with antacids

	Generic/Trade Names	Usual Adult Dose	Actions
Table 8-8	Auranofin (Ridaura)	6 mg PO QD	Decreases rheumatoid factor and immunoglobulins to suppress arthritic symptoms
Common Medications to Treat Rheumatoid Arthritis	Aurothioglucose (Solganal)	1st week 10 mg IM; 2nd and 3rd week 25 mg IM; 4th week and subsequent weeks 50 mg IM until 1 g given	Inhibits phagocytosis and lysosomal enzyme activity to decrease rheumatoid factor and decrease inflammation
	Etanercept (Enbrel)	25 mg SC 2 times per week	Tumor necrosis factor from Chinese hamsters that reacts with active lymphocytes to reduce signs and symptoms of rheumatoid arthritis
	Gold sodium thiomalate (Aurolate)	1st week 10 mg IM; 2nd week 25 mg IM; maintenance 25–50 mg IM	Suppresses the activity produced by prostaglandins, which contributes to the destruction of the joints
	Hylan G-F 20 (Synvisc)	2 mL intra-articular 1 time per week for 3 weeks	Lubricating hylan obtained from chicken combs is injected into the arthritic joint to provide lubrication
	Leflunomide (Arava)	100 mg PO 3 days then 20 mg QD	Produces the anti-inflammatory process by blocking the enzyme DHODH
	Methotrexate (Amethopterin)	7.5 mg per week PO	Inhibits DNA synthesis and folic acid reductase to reduce inflammation
	Penicillamine (Depen)	125–250 mg PO in a single dose	Lowers IgM rheumatoid factor
	Sodium hyaluronate (Hyalgan)	2 mg intra-articular injection 1 time per week for 5 weeks	Lubricating hylan injected into joint to provide cushioning

F. Significant food interactions: none reported

G. Significant laboratory studies

1. ALT/AST

2. BUN and creatinine

3. CBC and platelet count

H. Side effects

1. Alopecia

2. Colitis

3. Diarrhea

4. Dizziness

5. Itching

6. Rash

7. Stomatitis

    I. Adverse effects/toxicity

        1. Black furry tongue

        2. Hepatotoxicity, pericarditis

        3. Pulmonary edema

        4. Thrombosis, Stevens-Johnson syndrome, and death

    J. Nursing considerations

        1. Avoid the use of antacids for at least 2 hours following medication administration

        2. Assess for bone marrow suppression, pulmonary fibrosis and GI ulceration/bleeding with methotrexate

        3. Protect from exposure to sunlight

        4. Assess for side effects to medication

        5. Check for proteinuria and hematuria before giving initial dose and during therapy with gold drugs

        6. Inject gold preparations into the gluteal muscle

        7. Observe client for signs of allergic reaction for 30 minutes after gold injection for first 2 doses

        8. Inject etanercept into the abdomen, thigh or upper arm SC

        9. Assess for signs of infection with etanercept

    K. Client education

        1. Instruct client to protect self from infection when taking etanercept

        2. Instruct to use good oral hygiene to protect from stomatitis

        3. Instruct client taking gold preparations to report signs of gold toxicity, including metallic taste and pruritus

        4. Instruct client to monitor for and report bruising, petechiae, bleeding gums, or blood in stool

        5. Instruct client to monitor blood glucose and report elevations

        6. Instruct on all aspects of medication administration including side effects, action, use, and contraindications

VI. Medications to Treat Systemic Lupus Erythematosus

    A. Action and use

        1. Cytotoxic drugs or purine analogs are used along with NSAID agents and corticosteroids to treat the symptoms of systemic lupus erythematosus

        2. They provide immunosuppressive action to treat autoimmune diseases

    B. Common medications (Table 8-9)

    C. Administration considerations (Table 8-9)

NCLEX!

NCLEX!

NCLEX!

NCLEX!

NCLEX!

Table 8-9	Generic/Trade Names	Usual Adult Dose	Actions
Common Medications to Treat Systemic Lupus Erythematosus	Azathioprine (Imuran)	1 mg/kg PO 2 times daily, increase the dose in 6–8 weeks by 0.5 mg/kg daily, max. 2.5 mg/kg daily	Decreases the severity of symptoms and disease process
	Methotrexate (Amethopterin)	7.5 mg per week PO	Inhibits DNA synthesis and folic acid reductase to reduce inflammation

D. Contraindications

1. Do not administer with agents that are known to be hepatotoxic

2. Do not administer during pregnancy or lactation

E. Significant drug interactions: if azathioprine (Imuran) is administered with allopurinol (Zyloprim) the Imuran dose should be reduced

F. Significant food interactions: do not administer azathioprine with grapefruit juice

G. Significant laboratory studies

1. AST/ALT

2. Blood glucose

3. BUN and creatinine

4. CBC and platelet count

5. Calcium, phosphorus

6. Uric acid

H. Side effects

1. Alopecia

2. Diarrhea

3. Colitis

4. Dizziness

5. Itching or rash

6. Leukopenia or thrombocytopenia

7. Stomatitis

I. Adverse effects/toxicity

1. Black furry tongue

2. Hepatotoxicity

3. Pericarditis

4. Pulmonary edema

5. Stevens-Johnson Syndrome

6. Death

J. **Nursing considerations**

1. Assess for side effects of medications

2. Assess for pulmonary edema and shortness of breath

3. Assess laboratory tests as ordered by physician

K. **Client education**

1. Instruct client to protect self from infection

2. Instruct about good oral hygiene to protect from stomatitis

3. Instruct client to monitor blood glucose level and report elevations

4. Instruct on all aspects of medication administration, including side effects, actions, use, and contraindications

5. Instruct on signs and symptoms of pulmonary edema and to report to provider

Case Study

A 15-year-old girl is admitted to the pediatric gastrointestinal (GI) service following a severe nosebleed. Her ALT and AST levels are above 800. She is scheduled for a liver biopsy, which reveals cirrhosis of the liver. She is placed on the transplant list due to untreatable liver failure and esophageal varices with hemorrhage. Two weeks after her name was placed on the national transplant list she received a liver transplant. Prior to surgery and following surgery she stated she was anxious and depressed. Three weeks after surgery she was discharged on the following medications:

- Tacrolimus (Prograf) 3 mg bid
- Magnesium oxide 1 tablet bid
- Azathioprine (Imuran) 50 mg 2$\frac{1}{2}$ tablets qod
- Esomeprazole (Nexium)1 tablet bid
- Milk of Magnesia 30 cc qod

One week following her discharge, she fainted and experienced extreme abdominal pain. She was readmitted with signs of liver transplant rejection. A liver biopsy was performed and surgery was done to repair a closing portal vein. An order for methylprednisolone (SoluMedrol) 125 mg IVP every 8 hours was added to her medication list. Laboratory studies obtained included AST/ALT, CBC with platelets, chemistry profile, arterial blood gases, and serum bilirubin.

❶ What are the priority nursing diagnoses for this client both preoperatively and postoperatively?

❷ Prior to the administration of the above medications, what diagnostic studies and assessments should the nurse make?

❸ What should be included in a teaching plan for this client and her family?

❹ What nursing interventions should be implemented prior to discharge following the portal vein repair?

❺ What is the rationale for the administration of SoluMedrol following the portal vein repair?

For suggested responses, see pages 639–640.

Posttest

1 The preceptor assigned to a new graduate nurse has delegated him to administer filgrastim (Neupogen) to a client with cancer. The preceptor informs the graduate nurse to take which of the following actions related to administration of this medication?

(1) Administer the medication with IV normal saline.
(2) Never shake the bottle due to destruction of the protein.
(3) Assess the mobilization of stem cells.
(4) Administer before bone marrow transplant is done.

2 A client diagnosed with cancer who is receiving sargramostim (Leukine) should be instructed to do which of the following?

(1) Receive vitamin B$_6$ concurrently
(2) Use good oral hygiene
(3) Expect alopecia
(4) Assess blood glucose levels daily

3 A client with rheumatoid arthritis develops Type 1 or insulin-dependent diabetes mellitus (IDDM). The nurse should make it a priority to make which of the following client assessments?

(1) Response to corticosteroids
(2) Ability to fill syringes and give injections
(3) Ability to exercise
(4) Response to home environment

4 A client who underwent a liver transplant asks the nurse why it is necessary to do such frequent mouthcare. The best response by the nurse would be to state that it helps prevent the development of which of the following client problems?

(1) Dysphagia
(2) Halitosis
(3) Stomatitis
(4) Dental caries

5 A client diagnosed with cancer is receiving sargramostim (Leukine) prior to stem cell collection. The client asks the reason for the medication. Which of the following pieces of information would best be used in a response to the client?

(1) The medication diminishes the number of immature stem cells.
(2) The medication assists in the mobilization of stem cells, allowing for collection.
(3) The medication blocks the body's inflammatory response to an antigen.
(4) The medication suppresses T cell production.

6 Tacrolimus (Prograf) is being administered to a client to prevent transplant rejection following organ transplant. Which of the following laboratory studies is of great importance for the nurse to monitor?

(1) LDH and CPK
(2) Uric acid and bilirubin
(3) Alkaline phosphatase and albumin
(4) AST and ALT

7 During a well-baby visit, the nurse notes that a child is one year late for his third hepatitis B vaccine. What should the nurse do to correct this?

(1) Give the vaccine now
(2) Inform the parent that the series may need to be restarted and consult with the physician
(3) Inform the parent that vaccine will need to be given now and in one month
(4) Inform the parent that two vaccines are sufficient

8 An infant girl is brought to the clinic for a well-baby visit. She is scheduled to receive her second diphtheria, pertussis, and tetanus (DPT) and H-flu vaccines, along with her oral polio virus vaccine. While measuring the infant's weight, the nurse decides she feels warm, and assesses her temperature, which is 101° F. The nurse should take which of the following actions?

(1) Withhold the vaccines and reschedule her visit when she is not febrile.
(2) Instruct the mother on vaccine administration and have her give them tomorrow.
(3) Administer acetaminophen orally and give the immunizations.
(4) Obtain titers on the needed immunizations and withhold them until the results are obtained.

9 A client who has multiple sclerosis and receives cyclophosphamide (Cytoxan) and digoxin (Lanoxin) complains of nausea. The nurse would place highest priority on which of the following actions?

(1) Evaluate the cyclophosphamide level
(2) Administer an oral antiemetic daily
(3) Provide six small frequent meals
(4) Evaluate the digoxin level

10 A client is receiving cyclosporine (Sandimmune). The nurse will need to assess the client for evidence of which of the following nursing diagnoses?

(1) Disturbed body image
(2) Pain
(3) Deficient fluid volume
(4) Altered neurological status

See pages 326–327 for Answers and Rationales.

Answers and Rationales

Pretest

1 **Answer: 4** *Rationale:* Filgrastim (Neupogen) is contraindicated with a hypersensitivity to *E. coli* products. It is important for the nurse to assess for any contraindications prior to the administration of this medication because of the risk of allergic reaction. Option 1 constitutes changing a medication dosage and is unsafe. Options 2 and 3 do not provide for client safety.
Cognitive Level: Analysis
Nursing Process: Implementation; *Test Plan:* PHYS

2 **Answer: 3** *Rationale:* Adult respiratory distress syndrome can develop because of the toxicity of colony stimulating factors. The other options do not reflect concerns specific to this medication.
Cognitive Level: Application
Nursing Process: Assessment; *Test Plan:* PHYS

3 **Answer: 1** *Rationale:* Medications used to treat the symptoms of rheumatoid arthritis increase the client's susceptibility to infection. Fever accompanies infection and requires further assessment. Options 2 and 4 are incorrect because they do not reflect a concern related to this type of medication. Option 3 is incorrect because infection is harmful to the client and needs to be treated.
Cognitive Level: Analysis
Nursing Process: Analysis; *Test Plan:* PHYS

4 **Answer: 3** *Rationale:* Immune serum globulin will irritate tissues and the application of heat will reduce pain and discomfort. The other responses are unrelated to the issue of the question, which is local discomfort at the injection site.
Cognitive Level: Application
Nursing Process: Implementation; *Test Plan:* PHYS

5 **Answer: 1** *Rationale:* Anticonvulsant medications administered concurrently with cyclosporine will cause decreased therapeutic levels of the cyclosporine medication. For this reason, the cyclosporine dose will need to be increased. The anticonvulsant dose needs to be given at standard dosage to maintain therapeutic blood levels.
Cognitive Level: Analysis
Nursing Process: Implementation; *Test Plan:* PHYS

6 **Answer: 3** *Rationale:* The client and family should be instructed to assess for fluid retention and an irregular heart rate. However, with the client complaining of shortness of breath and edema 2 days after chemotherapy and administration of oprelvekin (Neumega), the nurse should suspect that the client is in cardiopulmonary insufficiency requiring medical attention. Options 1, 2, and 4 delay necessary medical attention and place the client at further risk for complications.
Cognitive Level: Application
Nursing Process: Implementation; *Test Plan:* PHYS

7 **Answer: 2** *Rationale:* The only food interaction of significance with cyclosporine (Sandimmune) is grapefruit. This combination will result in an increased serum cyclosporine level. The other options are completely false.
Cognitive Level: Application
Nursing Process: Implementation; *Test Plan:* PHYS

8 **Answer: 4** *Rationale:* Exposure to hepatitis A from a restaurant worker necessitates the administration of immune serum globulin to prevent hepatitis A following exposure. The other options do not address this concern and fail to address the client's need for protection against possible exposure.
Cognitive Level: Application
Nursing Process: Implementation; *Test Plan:* HPM

9 **Answer: 2** *Rationale:* Childhood illnesses possess a high rate of mortality and morbidity. The use of immunizations assists in the promotion of health and prevention of illness. Immunizations are begun shortly after birth and are absolutely required before a child can attend school. Option 3 is false. Options 1 and 4 are true but does not address the reason they need to be administered.
Cognitive Level: Application
Nursing Process Implementation; *Test Plan:* HPM

10 **Answer: 4** *Rationale:* Atropine (an anticholinergic medication) should be administered to counteract the cholinergic reaction of the medications used to treat myasthenia gravis. The other options are incorrect because they do not have anticholinergic activity.
Cognitive Level: Analysis
Nursing Process: Planning; *Test Plan:* PHYS

Posttest

1 **Answer: 2** *Rationale:* Shaking the vial of filgrastim (Neupogen) will result in destruction of the medication's protein. Option 1 is unnecessary, and options 3 and 4 are not actions related to the administration of this medication.
Cognitive Level: Application
Nursing Process: Implementation; *Test Plan:* PHYS

2 **Answer: 2** *Rationale:* The provision of good oral hygiene will reduce the chance of stomatitis, which is common in immunosuppressed clients with cancer, who are in need of this medication. There is no need to receive vitamin B_6 concurrently (option 1). Alopecia and elevated blood glucose levels (options 3 and 4) are not related to sargramostim.
Cognitive Level: Application
Nursing Process: Implementation; *Test Plan:* PHYS

3 **Answer: 2** *Rationale:* Monitoring strategies of care, particularly the ability to fill syringes and administer insulin, is a nursing priority. The diagnosis of rheumatoid arthritis may limit fine motor movements of the hands that are needed for self-administration of insulin, and this client may need further assistance from family or other caregivers. The assessments in the other options are also important, but the ability to manage medication therapy takes priority.
Cognitive Level: Analysis
Nursing Process: Evaluation; *Test Plan:* HPM

4 **Answer: 3** *Rationale:* Immunosuppressant agents reduce the client's ability to fight all infections, including inflammation and infection in the mouth

(stomatitis). The client is at risk of developing infection from organisms normally found in controlled numbers in the oral cavity. The other options do not relate to this particular effect of immunosuppressants.
Cognitive Level: Application
Nursing Process: Implementation; *Test Plan:* PHYS

5 **Answer: 2** *Rationale:* Sargramostim (Leukine) increases the production of granulocytes and macrophages. It also mobilizes stem cells to allow for stem cell collection. The information contained in the other options does not correctly describe the action of sargramostim.
Cognitive Level: Application
Nursing Process: Implementation; *Test Plan:* PHYS

6 **Answer: 4** *Rationale:* AST and ALT, which are liver enzymes, are of importance to monitor since tacrolimus (Prograf) and other immunosuppressants are hepatotoxic. The other responses do not relate as specifically to this adverse effect.
Cognitive Level: Application
Nursing Process: Evaluation; *Test Plan:* HPM

7 **Answer: 2** *Rationale:* Hepatitis B is administered in three doses. The second dose follows one month after the first dose and the third dose is given 6 months after the original dose. If too much time elapses between doses, as in this case, the series may need to be restarted. Options 1 and 4 may result in incomplete or insufficient vaccination. The nurse does not set up immunization schedules independently (option 3).
Cognitive Level: Application
Nursing Process: Implementation; *Test Plan:* HPM

8 **Answer: 1** *Rationale:* For all clients immunizations are contraindicated during a moderate to severe febrile illness. The nurse should withhold the vaccines and have the mother bring the infant in to receive them after the illness has subsided. The actions in the other responses are incorrect.
Cognitive Level: Application
Nursing Process: Implementation; *Test Plan:* PHYS

9 **Answer: 4** *Rationale:* Cyclophosphamide (Cytoxan) combined with digoxin (Lanoxin) may result in digoxin toxicity, thus the health care team must continually assess for signs and symptoms of toxicity. Nausea is an early sign of digoxin toxicity, making option 4 the best action. Option 1 does not help the situation; options 2 and 3 treat the symptom rather than the problem.
Cognitive Level: Analysis
Nursing Process: Assessment; *Test Plan:* HPM

10 **Answer: 1** *Rationale:* A side effect of cyclosporine (Sandimmune) is hirsutism, thus the nurse should assess for signs and symptoms that relate to the nursing diagnosis of Disturbed body image. Options 2 and 3 do not apply to the client with the information given in the question. Option 4 is not a nursing diagnosis.
Cognitive Level: Application
Nursing Process: Analysis; *Test Plan:* PHYS

References

Abrams, A. C. (2004). *Clinical drug therapy: Rationales for nursing practice* (7th ed.). Philadelphia: Lippincott.

Aschenbrenner, D. S., Cleveland, L. W., & Venable, S. J. (2002). *Drug therapy in nursing.* Philadelphia: Lippincott.

Aucker, R. S. & Lilley, L. L. (2001). *Pharmacology and the nursing process* (3rd ed.). St. Louis, MO: Mosby, Inc.

Karch, A. M. (2000). *Focus on nursing pharmacology.* Philadelphia: Lippincott.

Karch, A. M. (2002). *2002 Lippincott's nursing drug guide.* Philadelphia: Lippincott.

Kee, J. L., & Hayes, E. R. (2003). *Pharmacology: A nursing process approach* (4th ed.). Philadelphia: W. B. Saunders.

LeMone, P., & Burke, K. M. (2003). *Medical-surgical nursing: Critical thinking in client care* (3rd ed.). Upper Saddle River, NJ: Prentice-Hall, Inc.

Lutwick, S. M. (2000). Pediatric vaccine compliance. *The Pediatric Clinics of North America, 47* (2).

Malay, S., Tizer, K., & Lutwick, L. I. (2000). Current update of pediatric hepatitis vaccine use. *The Pediatric Clinics of North America, 47* (2).

Smeltzer, S. C., & Bare, B. G. (2003). *Brunner and Suddarth's textbook of medical-surgical nursing* (10th ed.). Philadelphia: Lippincott.

Taylor, C., Lillis, C., & LeMone, P. (2001). *Fundamentals of nursing: The art and science of nursing care* (4th ed.). Philadelphia: Lippincott.

Youngkin, E. Q., Sawin, K. J., Kissinger, J. F., & Israel, D. S. (1999). *Pharmacotherapeutics: A primary care clinical guide.* Stamford, CT: Appleton & Lange.

CHAPTER 9

Integumentary System Medications

Lynn Wemett Nicholls, RN, MSN

CHAPTER OUTLINE

General Agents
Protective Agents
Antipruritics

Antiinfectives
Corticosteroids
Keratolytics

Acne Medications
Burn Medications
Debriding Medications

OBJECTIVES

- Describe the principles related to skin absorption.
- Identify the general properties of topical dermatological medications.
- Describe the actions, purposes, and safe use of dermatological medications.
- Discuss the nursing considerations when administering medications for the integumentary system.
- Describe the general goals of therapy when administering integumentary medications.
- List the significant client education points related to integumentary medications.

 [Media Link]

Use the CD-ROM enclosed with this text, or log onto the address given to access the free, interactive Companion Website created for this series. The CD-ROM and Companion Website accompanying this book offer additional practice opportunities and information—NCLEX Review, Case Studies, Glossary, In Depth with NCLEX, and more.

www.prenhall.com/hogan

REVIEW AT A GLANCE

acne *most common chronic skin disease of adolescents and young adults that affects hair follicles and sebaceous glands; characterized by noninflammatory and inflammatory lesions that often involve the face, chest, and back*

antiseptics *chemical agents that inhibit growth of microorganisms but do not necessarily kill them*

creams *emulsions of oil in water, more complex preparations than ointments*

emollients *occlusive agents that make skin soft and pliable by increasing hydration of stratum corneum*

herpes simplex *an acute viral disease marked by groups of vesicles on the skin,*

often on the borders of the lips or the nares or on the genitals

lotions *liquid suspensions or dispersions intended for external use*

ointments *water-in-oil emulsions; semisolid preparations of medicinal substances in a base, such as petrolatum or lanolin*

papules *small, circumscribed, superficial, solid elevations of the skin*

pediculosis *parasitic infestation caused by lice; may involve hair, body, or pubic area*

powder *finely divided solid drug or mixtures of drugs*

pruritus *intense itching that is relieved fully by controlling the causative primary illness*

psoriasis *a chronic, genetically influenced skin disorder characterized by periodic exacerbation of erythematous papules and plaques covered by prominent, thick silvery-white scales*

scabies *parasitic infestation caused by a mite*

tinea pedis *a superficial fungal infection of the skin of the feet; also known as athlete's foot*

Pretest

1 The nurse is working with a client newly diagnosed with psoriasis. The client asks the nurse about this disorder. Which of the following responses by the nurse is best?

(1) "It is a chronic skin disorder characterized by whitish, scaling patches."
(2) "It is a disorder with reddish colored lesions of chest and trunk that usually do not recur."
(3) "It is a skin disease characterized by redness, tenderness, and edema."
(4) "It is a contact dermatitis that can involve any part of body."

2 A child has been diagnosed as having impetigo. The nurse anticipates that which topical agent will be prescribed?

(1) Ketoconazole (Nizoral)
(2) Mupirocin (Bactroban)
(3) Capsaicin (Capsin)
(4) Acyclovir (Zovirax) ointment

3 The nurse should teach a client to use which one of the following for a skin disorder in which the use of mild soap is needed?

(1) Dial™
(2) Safeguard™
(3) Dove™
(4) Ivory™

4 The nurse conducting a community health teaching session explains that sunscreen with an SPF of 6 means that the product has which of the following characteristics?

(1) Provides protection from sun's rays for 6 hours
(2) Is water-resistant but not waterproof
(3) Is waterproof for 6 immersions in the water
(4) Provides 6 times the sun exposure protection as use of no sunscreen

5 The nurse anticipates that which of the following agents would be used to treat pediculosis infestation in an adult client?

(1) Chlorhexidine (Hibiclens)
(2) Lindane (Kwell)
(3) Collagenase (Santyl)
(4) Terbinafine (Lamisal)

6 An adult client has scabies on the trunk. Permethrin (Elimite Cream) is prescribed. What instructions should be given to the client?

(1) "Apply the agent from the neck down. Leave on for 8 to 14 hours before washing it off."
(2) "Use this product with an agent such as lindane (Kwell)."
(3) "Apply the agent to the affected area; repeat application in 6 hours."
(4) "Treat the clothing rather than the body."

7 The nurse explains to a client with acne that which of the following products is one of the most effective topical agents for use in treating this condition?

(1) Mafenide (Sulfamylon)
(2) Benzoyl peroxide
(3) Chlorhexidine (Hibiclens)
(4) Cryotherapy

8 The nurse would provide instructions about how to take which of the following oral agents that can be used in treatment of acne?

(1) Adapalene (Differin)
(2) Tretinoin (Retin-A)
(3) Clindamycin (Cleocin T)
(4) Isotretinoin (Accutane)

9 Silver sulfadiazine (Silvadene) is used to prevent and treat sepsis in burns. The burn unit nurse explains to a new orientee that an important point about its mechanism of action is its:

(1) Facilitation of skin cell replication.
(2) Replacement of hydrogen bonding between DNA strands.
(3) Antifibrinolytic property.
(4) Small molecular size.

10 A client is to receive medication to treat external warts. The nurse would prepare instructions related to which of the following medications?

(1) Salicylic acid (Duofilm)
(2) Povidone-iodine (Betadine)
(3) Masoprocol (Actinex)
(4) Crotamiton (Eurax)

See pages 353–354 for Answers and Rationales.

I. General Agents

A. Soaps

1. Action and use

   a. Deodorant soaps are relatively harsh soaps that contain triclosan or triclocarban as topical antibacterial agents and are useful in decreasing body odor, preventing bacterial spread, and assisting in treatment of cutaneous infections

   b. True soaps mechanically remove bacteria and are effective at removing all sebum and environmental dirt

   c. Synthetic detergent bars are generally milder and compose a group of products known as beauty bars

   d. Allergic sensitization can occur to fragrances, dyes, antibacterial agents, or other additives in soaps

   e. Cleansing ingredients in shampoos are detergents that have different abilities to cleanse and lather

   f. Medicated shampoos may be used for dandruff, seborrheic dermatitis, or **psoriasis** (a chronic skin disorder characterized by periodic exacerbations of erythematous papules and plaques covered by prominent, thick silvery-white scales)

2. Common preparations (see Box 9-1)

3. Nursing considerations

   a. Assess any skin symptom, beginning with a history

Box 9-1	

Soaps and Shampoos	*Soaps*
	Deodorant Soaps: Harsh
	    Dial
	    Lever 2000
	    Safeguard
	True Soaps
	    Ivory
	Synthetic Detergent Soaps: Mild
	    Dove
	    Oil of Olay
	    Neutrogena
	    Tone
	
	Shampoos
	Unmedicated
	    Too numerous to list
	Medicated
	    Head & Shoulders Intensive Treatment Dandruff Shampoo (selenium sulfide 1%) and other related products
	    Selsun Blue Dandruff Shampoo and other related products

    b. Monitor for local adverse effects/irritation from use of selected soap(s) and/or shampoo(s)

    c. Read product literature carefully because some shampoos are not recommended for small children

  4. Client education

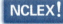

    a. Advise clients that soaps can be irritating to people with dry skin, especially in winter with low humidity

    b. Advise application of a moisturizing preparation after bathing if dry skin is a problem

    c. Teach client proper use of any prescribed shampoo

B. Cleansers

  1. Action and use

    a. Cleansers are used for preoperative cleansing of skin

    b. Cleansers may be used for treatment of wounds or abrasions

    c. May also be bacteriostatic or bactericidal depending on agent

  2. Common preparations (see Table 9-1)

  3. Nursing considerations

    a. Assess any skin symptom, beginning with a history

    b. Monitor for local irritation and/or drying as an adverse effect of these topical preparations

  4. Client education

    a. Teach client proper use of any prescribed cleanser

    b. If wounds or abrasions are present, explain inflammatory process and wound healing process

Table 9-1	Agent	Use
Cleansers	Povidone-iodine (Betadine, Betagen, Aerodine, Iodex, others)	Bactericidal
	Iodine (Iodine Topical, Iodine Tincture)	Cleansing action
	Benzalkonium chloride (Benza, Zephiran)	Bacteriostatic; can support growth of certain pseudomonas species; is inactivated by soap; do not cover with an occlusive dressing
	Alcohol	Bactericidal; is not as effective as povidone-iodine
	Hydrogen peroxide	Germicidal; has mechanical effectiveness; do not use after epithelium is formed because it will continue to debride newly growing cells
	Chlorhexidine gluconate (Hibiclens, Dyna-Hex, Exidine, Hibistat, Peridex)	Cleansing action
	Hexachlorophene (Phisohex, Septisol)	Cleansing action
	Oxychlorosene sodium (Clorpactin XCB, Clorpactin WCS-90)	Cleansing action
	Sodium hypochlorite (Dakin's)	Cleansing action

C. Lotions

1. Action and use

   a. **Lotions** historically were "shake lotions" or suspensions of a **powder** (finely divided solid drug or mixture of drugs) in water

   b. With a shake lotion, as the water in the lotion evaporates, a coating of powder is left on skin, producing a drying effect

   c. Today other types of liquid emulsions of thin, uniform consistency are also referred to as lotions

2. Common preparation: Calamine lotion (Calamox, Resinol, Clamatum); it is a preparation of calamine, zinc oxide, glycerin bentonite magma, calcium hydroxide, and others

3. Nursing considerations

   a. Shake the lotion before application to place the powder in suspension

   b. Monitor for local and systemic adverse effects of topical preparation

4. Client education

   a. Teach client proper use of any prescribed lotion

   b. Supervise initial use if appropriate to ensure correct application

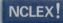

   c. Explain that some preparations of calamine lotion also contain diphenhydramine (Benadryl), which can cause drowsiness; use these products cautiously until effect of these agents is known

D. Emollients

1. Action and use

   a. **Emollients** are occlusive agents that make skin soft and pliable by increasing hydration of stratum corneum and by filling gaps in stratum corneum created by dry, contracted skin cells

    b. Include silicone oils, propylene glycol, isopropyl palmitate, and octyl stearate

    c. Can also function as skin protectants if they soothe the symptoms of **pruritus** (intense itching) due to exposed, traumatized nerve endings

    d. Moisturizers are intended to mimic function of sebum on skin; function is based on mechanisms of occlusion and humectancy

    e. The occlusion function employs petrolatum, lanolin, cocoa butter, or mineral oil to prevent evaporation of water from skin

    f. The humectancy function employs substances that attract moisture to skin, (e.g., glycerin, sorbitol, propylene glycol)

2. Common preparations (see Box 9-2)

3. Nursing considerations

    a. Assess any skin symptom, beginning with a history

    b. Unless otherwise directed by product instructions, apply to skin after bathing while skin is slightly moist

NCLEX!

4. Client education

    a. Explain to clients what contents to look for in over-the-counter (OTC) moisturizers that will indicate the product is of the highest quality

    b. Teach client proper use of any prescribed emollient

E. Protectants

1. Action and use

    a. Several preparations are designed to protect skin from wetness

    b. Help prevent and treat diaper rash, prickly heat, and/or chafing

2. Common preparations (see Box 9-3)

3. Nursing considerations

Box 9-2 **Emollients**	Aquaphor Cetaphil lotion Curel moisturizing lotion Dermasil lotion Eucerin crème or lotion Eucerin Plus crème Eucerin Plus lotion Eucerin Light lotion Keri lotion Lac-Hydrin cream Lac-Hydrin lotion 12% (prescription only) Lubriderm dry skin lotion Lubriderm sensitive lotion Lubriderm Bath & Shower Oil Moisturel lotion Neutrogena emulsion Penecare lotion White petrolatum

     a. Assess any skin symptom, beginning with a history

     b. Monitor skin for desired effect

  4. Client education

     a. Explain that powders should be kept away from face to avoid inhalation

     b. Explain some preparations should not be used on broken skin

     c. Explain if diaper rash or skin irritation worsens or does not improve within 7 days of beginning self-care, consult healthcare provider

F. Soaks and wet dressings

  1. Action and use

     a. General rule: acute lesions that are oozing, weeping, and crusting respond best to medication in aqueous, drying preparations

     b. General rule: scaling chronic lesions respond best to medication in moisturizing, lubricating preparations

     c. Open soaks are applied for 20 minutes, 3 times a day

     d. Closed soaks use a water-impermeable substance (occlusion) over a wet soak; this method causes heat retention, which is excellent for debridement but may lead to maceration; are applied for 1 to 2 hours 2 to 3 times a day

     e. Continuous closed soaks are left in place for 24 hours to treat thick crusts; it is important to rewet dressing 4-5 times a day

  2. Common preparations (Table 9-2)

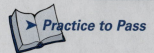

Practice to Pass

A 6-month-old infant has diaper rash. What would you include in a teaching plan for the mother?

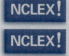

Table 9-2 **Soaks and Wet Dressings**	**Agent**	**Use**
	Burow's Solution (Bluboro Powder, Boropak Powder, Domeboro, Pedi-Boro Soak Paks): 5% aluminum acetate solution 1 Domeboro tablet or packet to 1 pint of tap water	Acts as astringent to decrease exudation by precipitation of protein
	Acetic Acid 0.1-1% solution: ½-cup white vinegar to 1 quart water	May be helpful for wound infected with *Pseudomonas* organisms
	Potassium Permanganate: 1:4,000-1:16,000 solution	Formerly considered to be useful for fungal infections, but use has decreased because of staining property
	Salt solution: 1 tbsp. of salt to 1 quart of water	Wetting action

3. Nursing considerations

    a. Assess any skin symptom, beginning with a history

    b. Monitor for achievement of intended effects

4. Client education

    a. In a healthcare institution, carry out prescribed soak procedure

    b. Teach procedure to clients for type of soak recommended or prescribed if scheduled for discharge

G. Rubs and liniments

1. Action and use: these are OTC preparations for temporary relief of minor aches and pains of muscles and joints associated with strains, bruises, sprains, sports injuries, simple backache, and arthritis

2. Common preparations (see Box 9-4)

3. Nursing considerations

    a. Assess symptom for which agent is to be used

    b. Monitor for achievement of intended effects

4. Client education

    a. Clean skin of all other **ointments** (water in oil emulsions), **creams** (more complex preparations of oil in water than ointments), sprays, or liniments before applying the product

    b. Apply to affected areas not more than 3 to 4 times daily

    c. Explain the some products have specific directions (i.e., BenGay should not be used with heating pad or tight bandage)

II. Protective Agents

A. Description

1. This section is limited to discussion of sunscreen preparations and protective dressings

2. For other preparations that can be defined as offering protection, see previous section on *Protectants*

NCLEX!

Practice to Pass

A client has osteoarthritis of both knees and does not want to take pills several times a day. Explain specific suggestions you could give to this client regarding a topical agent.

Box 9-4

Rubs and Liniments

Aspercreme External Analgesic Rub with Aloe
    Available as crème, lotion
    Contains trolamine salicylate, aloe vera gel, many others
BenGay External Analgesic Products
    Ointment, cream, arthritis formula cream
    Contains menthol in alcohol base gel, methyl salicylate, camphor, others
Sportscream External Analgesic Rub
    Available as crème, lotion
    Contains trolamine salicylate, acetyl alcohol, others
Therapeutic Mineral Ice, Pain Relieving Gel
    Menthol, others
Capsaicin (Capsin)
    Active ingredient from cayenne peppers

B. Sunscreen preparations

    1. Actions and use

        a. These are important because they can prevent skin cancer

        b. Chemical sunscreens absorb ultraviolet radiation in the spectrum of ultraviolet light (UVL) most responsible for sunburns

        c. Chemical absorbers formulated against ultraviolet B rays (UVB) include cinnamates, *p*-aminobenzoic acid (PABA) and PABA esters, or salicylates

        d. Chemical absorbers formulated against ultraviolet A rays (UVA) include benzophenones

        e. Physical sunscreens reflect or scatter light to prevent skin penetration

        f. Physical sunscreens contains ingredients such as titanium dioxide, zinc oxide, talc

        g. Effectiveness of a sunscreen is indicated by its sun protection factor (SPF); a SPF of 6 means product offers 6 times the protection as the use of no sunscreen

        h. A water-resistant sunscreen should continue to function after 40 minutes in water

        i. A waterproof sunscreen withstands 80 minutes in water

    2. Common preparations (see Table 9-3)

    3. Nursing considerations: assess skin for degree of burn if not used effectively

    4. Client education

        a. Advise clients who tend to sunburn easily to use products with SPF of 15 or greater

        b. Avoid contact between the products and the eyes

        c. Follow product directions

C. Protective dressings

NCLEX!

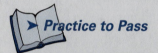

► Practice to Pass

Your cousin, who is fair-skinned, is planning to visit Florida for the first time. She has never seen the ocean and "can't wait to go to the beach." What would you discuss with her before she leaves?

Table 9-3	Brand Name	SPF	Active Ingredients
Sunscreen Preparations	Coppertone Broad Spectrum Lotion	25	Avobenzone, benzophenones, cinnamates
	DuraScreen	15	Benzophenones, cinnamates
	Johnson's Baby Sunblock Lotion	30	Benzophenones, cinnamates, salicylates
	Neutrogena Sunblock	30	Cinnamates, menthyl anthranilate, octocrylene
	Shade UVA/UVB	15, 25, 30, 45	Avobenzone benzophenones, cinnamates
	Sundown Sport	15	Titanium dioxide, zinc oxide
	Total Eclipse Lotion	15	Benzophenones, salicylates, PABA
	Water Babies UVA/UVB	12, 25, 30, 45	Benzophenones, cinnamates, ococrylene

1. Action and use

   a. Includes occlusive biosynthetic dressings for certain wound therapies

   b. As an example, DuoDERM as a hydrocolloid dressing hydrates wound surface; wound fluid interacts with wafer of the preparation and melts it, forming a moist jellylike substance that keeps the wound moist and promotes healing

2. Common dressings (see Table 9-4)

3. Nursing considerations

   a. Assess any skin wound, beginning with a history

   b. Inspect the dressing at least daily for leaks, dislodgment, wrinkling, or odor

   c. Change dressing when it becomes dislodged, leaks, or develops an odor

   d. If wound has substantial drainage, dressing might need to be changed every 24 to 48 hours, but generally is left in place for 3 to 7 days

   e. When changing dressing, leave residue that is difficult to remove; it will wear off in time; attempts to remove can irritate surrounding skin

4. Client education: teach client proper use of any prescribed occlusive biosynthetic dressing

III. Antipruritics

A. Description

1. Antipruritics are medications that stop the intense itching known as pruritis

2. Pruritus brings more clients to the healthcare provider than any other dermatological symptom

3. Pruritus has a multitude of causes and treatment needs to be tailored to specific cause

Table 9-4						
Common Protective Wound Dressings						
Dressing	**Transmits Oxygen**	**Transmits Water Vapor**	**Excludes Bacteria**	**Absorbs Fluids**	**Transparent**	**Adhesive**
Bioclusive	+	+	−	−	+	+
DuoDERM	−	−	+	+	−	+
Geliperm	+	+	+	+	+	+
Intrasite	−	−	+	+	−	+
Op-site	+	+	+	−	+	+
Replicare	−	−	+	−	−	+
Tegasorb	−	−	+	+	−	+
Tegaderm	+	+	?	−	+	+
Vigilon	+	−	−	+	+	−
Zenoderm	+	+	+	+	+	+

+ = has the stated action

− = does not have the stated action

? = may or may not have the stated action

4. Types of pruritis include winter pruritus, senior pruritus, lichen simplex chronicus, external otitis, pruritus ani (e.g., pinworm infestation in children), and genital pruritus

B. Action and use

1. Antipruritic medication therapy for some types of pruritis might include topical corticosteroids to decrease inflammation and/or methods to promote skin hydration

2. Antipruritic therapy may also necessitate use of a systemic antihistamine

C. Common medications (see Box 9-5)

D. Nursing considerations

1. Take a history of this systemic symptom and any associated skin symptoms

2. Monitor for local and systemic adverse effects of any topical preparation

3. Monitor for anticholinergic adverse reactions if systemic antihistamines of the anticholinergic type are used

E. Client education

NCLEX!

NCLEX!

1. Advise that general bathing be limited to once or twice a week and that only mild soaps should be used, and that any soap chosen is used in a sparing manner

2. Emphasize the negative effect of scratching and the need to interrupt any itch-and-scratch cycle

3. Recommend maintaining cool environment, especially in the bedroom for sleep

---

Box 9-5

Antipruritic Agents

Lotion or cream

Aveeno Anti-itch Lotion or Cream
Aveeno Moisturing Lotion or Cream
Eucerin Crème or Lotion
Sarna Topical Lotion (camphor, menthol, and phenol)
Zonalon Cream

Hydrating baths

Aveeno (colloidal oatmeal)
Aveeno Oil (colloidal oatmeal, mineral oil, glyceryl stearate, etc.)

Systemic H₁ Blockers or Combination

Hydroxyzine hydrochloride (Atarax)
Hydroxyzine pamoate (Vistaril)
Chlorpheniramine (Chlor-Trimeton)
Cyproheptadine hydrochloride (Periactin)

Unsafe

Benzocaine and other "-caine" derivatives
Antihistamines such as astemizole (Hismanal)

IV. Antiinfectives

A. Antibacterials

1. Action and use

   a. Certain topical antibiotics are used to inhibit growth of *Propionibacterium acnes* and reduce inflammatory lesions of acne

   b. Topical antibacterial therapy may be useful for prophylaxis of infections in wounds and injuries

2. Common medications (see Table 9-5)

3. Nursing considerations

   a. Assess any skin symptom, beginning with a history

   b. Assess for hypersensitivity to any ingredient in product to be used

   c. Monitor for skin irritation and superinfection

4. Client education

   a. Wash hands before using any topical antibacterial agent

   b. May wear gloves

   c. Generally these products are to be applied sparingly and gently to the affected area

   d. With some, a dressing should be applied and with some it should not; follow prescriber instructions

   e. Report worsening of condition or lack of healing

B. Antivirals

1. Action and use

   a. Used to treat cutaneous **herpes simplex** (an acute viral disease marked by groups of vesicles on the skin, often on the borders of the lips, nares, or on the genitals)

   b. May also be used to treat herpes zoster

   c. With some infections an oral agent may be needed instead of a topical agent

2. Common medication: acyclovir 5% ointment (Zovirax)

3. Nursing considerations

   a. Assess skin symptoms, beginning with a history

   b. Monitor for local adverse effects of topical product, such as mild pain, burning, stinging

4. Client education

   a. Wash hands before using topical antiviral

   b. Use gloves or finger cot when applying product to avoid autoinnoculation of other body sites

   c. Apply as soon as symptoms of herpes lesions begins

	Medication	Source	Mechanism of Action	Notes
Table 9-5 **Antibacterial Agents**	Bacitracin (Baciguent Topical)	*Bacillus subtilis*	Cell wall inhibitor	Effective against Gram-positive; staphylococci and streptococci; used with impetigo, furunculosis, pyodermas
	Bacitracin, polymyxin B, neosporin (Mycitracin Topical, Neomixin Topical, Neosporin Topical, Triple Antibiotic Topical)	*Bacillus subtilis, Streptomyces fradiae*	Cell wall inhibitor, 30S ribosome inhibition	Available as ointment to treat secondarily infected skin problems
	Chloramphenicol (Chloromycetin)	*Streptococcus venezuelae* or synthetic	50S ribosome inhibition	Used infrequently because dose-related bone marrow suppression has occurred following topical exposure
	Clindamycin phosphate (Cleocin T, Clinda-Derm Topical Solution	Semisynthetic	Binding to 50S ribosome and suppression of bacterial protein synthesis	Available as vaginal cream or suppositories, gel, solution, lotion; primarily for treatment of acne
	Erythromycin and benzoyl peroxide (Benzamycin)			Gel for acne vulgaris
	Gentamicin sulfate (G-myticin Topical)	Fermentation product from *Micromono-spora purpura*	Interferes with bacterial protein synthesis	Cream or ointment used following ear surgery to provide prophylaxis against otitis externa due to *Pseudomonas aeruginosa*
	Meclocycline sulfosa-licylate (Meclan Topical)	Semisynthetic	30S ribosome inhibition	Gram +/−; cream to be applied generously but contact with eyes, nose, and mouth to be avoided; do not cover; may stain fabric
	Metronidazole (MetroGel)		Unknown but may be due to antibiotic, antioxidant, and anti-inflammatory properties	Available as gel, topical treatment of rosacea
	Mupirocin (Bactroban)	*Pseudomonas fluorescens*	tRNA synthetase inhibitor	Topical treatment of impetigo caused by Gram-positives such as *Staphylococcus aureus,* beta-hemolytic *Streptococcus,* and *S. Pyogenes*
	Neomycin (Mycifradin Sulfate Topical)	*Streptomyces fradiae*	30S ribosome inhibition	Gram negative; cream or ointment used for prophylaxis against infection in abrasions, cuts, burns, but can cause allergic contact dermatitis
	Tetracycline (Achro-mycin Topical, Topicyc-line Topical)	Semisynthetic	30S ribosome inhibition	Gram positive/negative

    d. Apply sparingly and gently to the affected area

    e. Recommend wearing loose clothing and keeping area clean and dry

    f. Recommend avoiding sexual activity when skin lesions are present

C. Antifungals

1. Action and use

    a. Clients with limited disease and infection limited to glabrous (smooth, hairless) skin can be treated with topical antifungal agents

    b. Clients with extensive disease and infection of hair and nails are best treated with systemic therapy

    c. Advantages of topical use over systemic use: absence of serious adverse reactions, absence of drug interactions, over-the-counter availability of some preparations, ability to localize treatment to affected sites, no need to monitor laboratory tests

    d. New drugs have caused decrease in use of keratolytics and **antiseptics** (chemical agents that inhibit growth of microorganisms but do not necessarily kill them) used in the past

2. Common medications

    a. Topical agents (see Table 9-6)

    b. Oral agents include fluconazole (Diflucan), griseofulvin (Fulvicin, Grispeg), itraconazole (Sporanox), ketoconazole (Nizoral), and terbinafine (Lamisil)

3. Nursing considerations

    a. Assess any skin symptom, beginning with a history

    b. Assess for predisposing factors, such as trauma, general health, suppressed immune status, hygiene practices and exposure to infectious agent

    c. Monitor for local adverse effects of topical preparations, which often include irritation, burning, or stinging depending on specific product used

    d. Monitor for skin sensitization, noted by increased redness, swelling, weeping, or any burning or itching that were not present before treatment began

    e. Systemic effects of topical products are negligible, since absorption rates generally are only 3–6%

4. Client education

    a. Use products as directed for full course of therapy (may be prolonged); apply liberally to clean and dry skin

    b. Leave exposed to air; do not apply protective dressing unless specifically ordered

    c. To prevent such fungal infections as **tinea pedis** (a superficial fungal infection of the skin of the feet; athlete's foot)

        1) Wear shower shoes or thongs in public or communal showers and locker rooms

        2) Wear footwear of natural fibers (leather shoes, cotton or wool socks)

Table 9-6	Medication	Use
Topical Antifungals	***Allylamines***	
	Naftifine hydrochloride (Naftin): cream gel	Tinea pedis, tinea cruris, tinea corporis
	Terbinafine (Lamisal): cream	Tinea pedis, tinea cruris, tinea corporis, cutaneous candidiasis, tinea versicolor
	Imidazoles	
	Clotrimazole (Lotrimin, Mycelex): cream, solution, lotion, vaginal tablets, vaginal cream	Tinea pedis, tinea cruris, tinea corporis, cutaneous candidiasis, tinea versicolor, vulvovaginal candidiasis
	Econazole nitrate (Spectazole): cream	Tinea pedis, tinea cruris, tinea corporis, tinea versicolor, cutaneous candidiasis
	Ketoconazole (Nizoral): cream, shampoo	Tinea pedis, tinea cruris, tinea corporis, cutaneous candidiasis, tinea versicolor
	Miconazole nitrate (Monistat): cream, powder, spray, vaginal suppository, vaginal cream	Tinea pedis, tinea cruris, tinea corporis, cutaneous candidiasis, tinea versicolor, vulvovaginal candidiasis
	Oxiconazole (Oxistat): cream, lotion	Tinea pedis, tinea cruris, tinea corporis
	Sulfonazole nitrate (Exelderm): cream, solution	Tinea pedis, tinea cruris, tinea corporis, tinea versicolor
	Miscellaneous	
	Ciclopirox olamine (Loprox): cream, lotion	Tinea pedis, tinea cruris, tinea corporis, cutaneous candidiasis, tinea versicolor
	Triacetin (Fungoid) [includes triacetin, sodium propionate, benzalkonium chloride, cetylpyridium chloride, & chloroxylenol]: solution, cream	Tinea pedis and others
	Undecenoic acid, undecylenic acid (Desenex)	Tinea pedis, tinea corporis, except on nails or hairy sites; diaper rash, prickly heat, groin irritation
	Nystatin (Mycostatin, Nilstat): cream, ointment, powder, vaginal tablet	Cutaneous and mucocutaneous infections caused by candida species
	Tolnaftate (Tinactin): cream, solution, spray, liquid, spray powder; (Aftate) gel, powder, spray liquid	Tinea pedis, tinea cruris, tinea corporis, tinea versicolor

      3) Avoid going barefoot

      4) Change socks daily

   d. To avoid other fungal infections, practice adequate hygiene

      1) Keep affected areas clean, dry, and well ventilated (loose clothing)

      2) Use powders to keep skin dry and prevent maceration; these may or may not contain antifungal ingredients

  D. Antiparasitics

    1. Action and use

      a. Used to treat infestations such as **scabies** (parasitic infestation caused by the *Sarcoptes scabiei* mite) or **pediculosis** (parasitic infestation, caused by lice); may involve hair (tinea capitus), body (tinea corporis), or pubic area (tinea pubis)

      b. Recurrence of scabies is generally related to reinfection in incomplete treatment rather than resistance of mite

Table 9-7	Agent	Uses
Antiparasitics	Crotamiton (Eurax cream, lotion)	Scabies
	Malathion (Ovide lotion)	Pediculosis capitis and their ova
	Permethrin (Elimite cream, Nix liquid)	Pediculosis capitis, scabies
	Pyrethrin, piperonyl butoxide (liquid, Rid shampoo)	Pediculosis capitis, pediculosis corporis, pediculosis pubis
	Lindane (Kwell cream, lotion, shampoo)	Pediculosis capitis, pediculosis pubis, scabies

  c. Crotamiton can be used in clients with scabies and pediculosis capitis who are ragweed sensitive

2. Common medications (see Table 9-7)

3. Nursing considerations

  a. Assess any skin symptom, beginning with a history

  b. Monitor for local adverse effects, including irritation, pruritis, burning, or stinging

  c. Monitor for systemic effect of dizziness with lindane because it affects nervous system; avoid use in infants, children, and clients with known seizure disorders because of risk of convulsions

4. Client education

  a. For scabies

   1) Apply thin layer to dry skin from neck down and rub in thoroughly over entire body

   2) Permethrin and lindane: leave on 8 to 12 hours, remove thoroughly with washing

   3) Crotamiton: apply again after 24 hours, remove with washing 48 hours after initial application

  b. For pediculosis capitis

   1) Lindane lotion: apply lotion to dry hair, rub in thoroughly, leave on for 12 hours, remove thoroughly

   2) Lindane shampoo: apply shampoo to dry hair, lather with small amount water, work into hair for 4 minutes, rinse thoroughly

   3) Second treatment in 7 to 10 days may be needed with malathion, RID

V. Corticosteroids

A. Description

1. Topical corticosteroids may be used with skin disorders

2. Systemic corticosteroids may also be used with skin disorders

B. Action and use

1. Clinical effectiveness of corticosteroids relates to four properties

  a. Vasoconstriction; decreases erythema

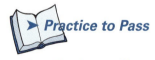

▶ Practice to Pass

A mother has an 8-year-old daughter who has come home from school with a note from the school nurse that says head lice have been noted on 2 children in her classroom. What would you include in a teaching plan for the mother?

     b. Antiproliferative effects; inhibits DNA synthesis and mitosis

     c. Immunosuppression; mechanism poorly understood

     d. Anti-inflammatory effects; inhibits formation of prostaglandins

  2. Responsiveness of diseases to topical corticosteroids varies: highly responsive diseases include psoriasis, atopic dermatitis in children, seborrheic dermatitis, intertrigo

  3. Penetration of preparation varies according to skin site

  4. Using these products on thin skin, on elderly or pediatric clients, or under occlusion will increase incidence of adverse reactions

  5. Adverse effects more common since introduction of higher potency preparations

  6. Local adverse reactions include atrophy, hypopigmentation, striae

NCLEX!

  7. Topical corticosteroids can cause systemic adverse reactions, including suppression of adrenal function

  8. Low-potency agents are best used for diffuse eruptions, those involving the face, those involving occluded areas such as axilla or groin, and chronic dermatoses

  9. Medium-potency agents are appropriate for acute flare-ups of chronic dermatoses and acute self-limited eruptions where they can be used for periods of 14 to 21 days

  10. High-potency agents best used for acute localized eruptions for a short time of 7 to 14 days

  11. High-potency agents should be avoided on areas susceptible to increased penetration and adverse reactions, such as face, intertriginous areas, perineum

  12. A twice-a-day application is usually sufficient; more frequent application does not appear to improve response

NCLEX!

  13. Abrupt discontinuation of mid- or high-potency corticosteroids may result in rebound flare-up of the disorder

C. Common medications (see Table 9-8)

D. Nursing considerations

  1. Assess any skin symptom, beginning with a history

  2. Generally these products are to be applied sparingly and gently in a thin film to the affected area

  3. At times, the preparation should be rubbed in thoroughly

NCLEX!

  4. Monitor for local adverse effects, which include acneiform skin eruptions, dryness, itching, burning, allergic contact dermatitis, hypopigmentation, and overgrowth of bacteria/fungi/viruses

NCLEX!

  5. Monitor for systemic adverse effects, which are more likely to include hirsutism (usually of the face), moon facies, alopecia (scalp area), and immunosuppression

NCLEX!

  6. These drugs, especially those of higher potency, should be tapered and not discontinued abruptly

	Potency Class	**Generic Name**	**Brand Name**
Table 9-8			
Corticosteroids	Lowest potency	Alclometasone 0.05% cream, ointment	Aclovate
		Desonide 0.05% cream, ointment, lotion	Desowen, Tridesilon
		Dexamethasone 0.04% aerosol	Decaspray
		Hydrocortisone 1% cream	Ala-Cort, Cort-Dome, Der-miCort, Hi-Cor-1.0, Hy-cort, Penecort, Synacort
		Hydrocortisone 1% lotion	Acticort 100, Cetacort, Cortizone-10, Dermacort, LactiCare-HC
		Hydrocortisone 1% ointment	Cortizone-10, Hycort, HydroSKIN, Hydro-Tex, Tegrin-HC
		Hydrocortisone 2.5% cream, ointment	
		Methylprednisolone acetate 0.25% ointment	Medrol
		Methylprednisolone acetate 1% ointment	Medrol
	Low potency	Betamethasone valerate 0.025% cream	Valisone
		Clocortolone 0.1% cream	Cloderm
		Fluocinolone acetonide 0.01% cream, solution	Synalar
		Flurandrenolide 0.025% cream, ointment	Cordran
		Hydrocortisone valerate 0.2% cream	Westcort
		Triamcinolone acetonide 0.025% cream, ointment	Kenalog
	Intermediate potency	Betamethasone benzoate 0.025% cream, gel, lotion	Uticort
		Betamethasone valerate 0.1% cream, ointment, lotion	Valisone
		Desoximetasone 0.05% cream, ointment	Topicort LP
		Fluocinolone acetonide 0.025% cream	Cutivate
		Halcinonide 0.025% cream, ointment	Halog
		Mometasone furoate 0.1% cream, ointment, lotion	Elocon
		Triamcinolone acetonide 0.1% cream, ointment	Kenalog
	High potency	Amcinonide 0.1% cream, ointment	Cyclocort
		Betamethasone dipropionate 0.05% cream, ointment, lotion	Diprosone
		Desoximetasone 0.25% cream, ointment	Topicort
		Flucinolone 0.2% cream	Synalar HP
		Flucinolone 0.05% cream, ointment	Lidex
		Halcinonide 0.1% cream, ointment, solution	Halog
		Triamcinolone acetonide 0.5% cream, ointment	Kenalog
	Very high potency	Augmented betamethasone dipropionate 0.05% ointment	Diprolene
		Clobetasol propionate 0.05% cream, ointment	Temovate
		Diflorasone 0.05% gel, ointment	Fluorone, Maxiflor, Psorcon
		Halobetasol propionate 0.05% cream, ointment	Ultravate

NCLEX!

E. Client education

1. Use exactly as directed; do not overuse

2. Do not apply to open wounds or weeping areas

3. Before using, wash and dry area gently

4. Report worsening of condition, signs of infection, or lack of healing

VI. Keratolytics

A. Description

1. These agents reduce thickness of hyperkeratotic stratum corneum

2. They reduce keratinocyte adhesion (remove or soften horny layer of skin)

B. Action and use

1. Used to treat disorders of keratinization (e.g., forms of ichthyosis that generally have genetic component)

2. Some are used to treat certain warts

3. They are available in different concentrations

4. Concentration necessary for keratolytic action differs among available agents

C. Common medications (see Table 9-9)

D. Nursing considerations

1. Assess any skin symptom, beginning with a history

2. Monitor for local adverse effects of topical preparations

E. Client education

1. Explain purpose, use, side effects, and anticipated length of treatment

2. Teach to use as directed; method will vary somewhat depending on condition for which it is used

VII. Acne Medications

A. Description

1. Generally a staged approach is used

2. Mild **acne** (noninflammatory and inflammatory lesions that most commonly involve face, chest, back), consisting of some comedones or few inflammatory lesions, is treated by topical therapy with agents such as salicylic acid, azelaic acid, benzoyl peroxide, and topical antibiotics

3. Moderate acne consisting of *comedones* (blackheads) and **papules** (small, circumscribed, superficial, solid elevations of the skin) can be managed by gradually increasing strength of topical tretinoin

> **➤ Practice to Pass**
>
> The client has two plantar warts on the ball of his left foot. What would you include in a plan of action for the client?

Table 9-9	Agent	Uses
Keratolytics	Salicylic acid	Warts, psoriasis, lichen simplex or chronicus, tinea of feet or palms when peeling desired, seborrheic dermatitis
	Resorcinol monoacetate (Resorcinol)	Acne vulgaris, rosacea, seborrheic dermatitis, psoriasis
	Urea	Black hairy tongue, removal of nails affected by fungal infection or psoriasis
	Sulfur (sulfur, precipitated)	Tinea of any area of body, acne vulgaris, rosacea, seborrheic dermatitis, pyodermas, psoriasis
	Alpha hydroxy acids (lactic, glycolic, citric, glucuronic, pyruvic acids)	Ichthyosis, hyperkeratotic eczema, photoaging, acne, hyperpigmentation
	Propylene glycol	Ichthyosis

4. Severe acne consisting of inflammatory papules and nodulocystic disease requires systemic antibiotics and isotretinoin (Accutane)

B. Action and use

1. Choice of vehicle for topical preparation depends on whether client has dry or oily skin

NCLEX!

2. Local adverse reactions to some topical preparations include erythema, burning or stinging, excessive dryness, and increased susceptibility to sunburn

3. Most clients will develop tolerance to local side effects within 3 to 4 weeks

C. Common medications (see Table 9-10)

D. Nursing considerations

Table 9-10

Acne Medications

Medication	Action or Use	Preparation
Adapalene (Differin)	Retinoid	Alcohol-free gel, cream; solution with alcohol
Benzoyl peroxide (Benzac)	Antibacterial, keratolytic; antibacterial activity against *Propionibacterium acnes*	Gel, wash
Benzoyl peroxide (Benzagel)	Antibacterial, keratolytic	Gel, wash
Benzoyl peroxide, erythromycin (Benzamycin)	Antibacterial, keratolytic; contains erythromycin and benzoyl peroxide	Gel
Azelaic acid (Azelex)	Antibacterial, keratolytic; competitively inhibits tyrosinase, antimicrobial against *Propionibacterium acnes,* inhibits comedone formation; may take 4 weeks until beneficial effect observed	Cream
Clindamycin (Cleocin T)	Antibacterial	Solution, pads, lotion, gel
Erythromycin (Emgel, Erycette, T-Stat)	Anti-inflammatory, antibacterial; Emgel is gel, Erycette is swabs, T-Stat is solution, pads	
Sodium sulfacetamide (Klaron)	Antibacterial	Lotion
Tazarotene (Tazorac)	Retinoid	Aqueous gel
Tetracycline (Monodox, Sumycin, Doryx, Vibramycin)	Antibacterial	Capsules
Tretinoin (Retin-A)	Retinoic acid derivative; increases mitotic activity and turnover of follicular epithelial cells; loosens keratin debris; promotes drainage of preexisting comedones; inhibits formation of new comedones; maximal results take up to 6 weeks; maintenance therapy may be necessary	Gel, liquid, aqueous gel, cream
Tretinoin (Avita)	Retinoid	Cream, gel
Isotretinoin (Accutane)	Retinoic acid derivative	Capsules

1. Assess skin lesions as baseline and periodically to evaluate effectiveness of therapy

2. Monitor for local adverse effects of topical preparations, such as excessive drying, erythema, and hypersensitivity

3. Monitor for systemic adverse effects as particular to individual product

E. Client education

1. Explain purpose, use, side effects, and anticipated length of treatment

2. Explain treatment is designed to control, not cure, therefore periodic breakouts (especially premenstrual flares) may still occur

3. With topical preparation, wash and dry skin; massage thin film gently into affected areas twice daily

4. Avoid getting product into eyes, mouth, and mucous membranes; wash hands after use

5. With certain preparations, minimize exposure to sun and UV light

6. If use of Accutane is needed, it is essential client understands it is a teratogen; females of child-bearing age must strictly avoid becoming pregnant; they should have negative pregnancy test within 2 weeks before starting therapy and monthly during therapy

VIII. Burn Medications

A. Description of burn therapy

1. Clients who have partial thickness burns greater than 5 to 10 % of body, full-thickness burns, burns associated with electrical current, burns of ears, eyes, face, hands, feet, and perineum need to be referred to a hospital prepared to handle burn clients

2. Remaining clients who have superficial thickness burns and partial thickness burns of less than 5 % of body should receive wound care and close follow-up

3. Goals of therapy are to decrease inflammation, prevent infection, relieve pain, and promote healing

B. Actions and use: topical agents are used to prevent infection in burn wounds, which could rapidly lead to sepsis

C. Common medications (see Table 9-11)

D. Nursing considerations

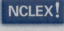

1. Agents are applied under sterile conditions once or twice daily to a thickness of approximately 1/16-inch to clean and debrided wound

2. If hospitalized, client may undergo hydrotherapy (bathing in whirlpool) to aid debridement prior to application

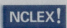

3. Client should be premedicated with analgesic whenever possible ½ hour prior to burn wound cleansing

4. Wound may be covered or left open

5. Monitor for adverse effects as outlined in Table 9-11

Table 9-11	Medication	Use	Notes
Burn Medications	Mafenide (Sulfamylon)	Bacteriostatic against *Pseudomonas aeruginosa* and *Clostridia*	Adverse reactions include pain, burning, or staining at application site for first 20–30 minutes after application In client with impaired renal function high blood levels of agent may lead to metabolic acidosis; watch for compensatory respiratory alkalosis as an indicator
	Silver sulfadiazine (Silvadene, Thermazene, SSD Cream)	Silver released from preparation in concentrations that are toxic to bacteria; silver prevents replication of *S. aureus, E. coli, Klebsiella, P. aeruginosa, P. mirabilis, Enterobacter, C. albicans*	Application is generally painless Watch for adverse reactions, including leukopenia, skin necrosis, erythema multiforme, skin discoloration, rashes Up to 10% may be absorbed; hazardous to use in clients with G6PD deficiency
	Nitrofurazone (Furacin)	Adjunctive therapy when bacterial resistance to other agents occurs	Must be used with caution in clients with impaired renal function because the polyethylene glycol in the preparation can be absorbed through denuded skin and may not be excreted normally by compromised kidney Watch for rash, itching, dermatitis, bacterial or fungal superinfection, and allergic reaction at site Drug darkens on exposure to light, but this does not affect potency

6. Watch for signs of infection and WBC count in clients receiving silver sulfadiazine because of leukopenic effect

E. Client education

1. Explain purpose, use, side effects, and anticipated length of treatment

2. Teach to use as directed if using preparation as an out-patient

IX. Debriding Medications

A. Description

1. Debriding agents are agents used to remove dirt, damaged tissue, and cellular debris from a wound to prevent infection and to promote healing

2. Their effectiveness in removing necrotic tissue, clotted blood, purulent exudates, or fibrinous accumulations has been questioned

B. Action and use

1. Appear most effective when wound base has collagen that must be removed before epithelialization can proceed

2. Specific indications may vary (e.g., collagenase is indicated for stage 3 and 4 decubitus ulcers)

C. Common medications (see Table 9-12)

D. Nursing considerations

1. Assess skin problem before use

	Agent	Action	Notes
Table 9-12 **Debriding Preparations**	Collagenase (Santyl)	Digests collagen; active at pH 6–8, takes 10-14 days	Active at pH 6–8, such enzymes tend to be inactivated by extremes of pH; also inactivated by hydrogen peroxide, heavy metals like silver, detergents, and by iodine, nitrofurazone, and hexachlorophene
	Sutilains (Travase)	Digests necrotic soft tissues by proteolytic action	See above
	Fibrinolysin and deoxyribonuclease (Elase)	Deoxyribonuclease attacks DNA; fibrinolysin attacks fibrin of blood clots and fibrinous exudates	Hypersensitivity reactions can occur; serious adverse reactions have been reported when using ointment preparation containing chloramphenicol
	Papain and urea (Panafil White)	Ointment source is papaya	Chlorophyll derivatives control wound odor
	Papain, urea, and chlorophyllin copper complex (Panafil)	Source is papaya	See above
	Trypsin, Balsam Peru, castor oil (Granulex)	Source of trypsin is bovine pancreas	Balsam Peru is capillary bed stimulant used to improve circulation; castor oil used to reduce premature epithelial cornification

    2. Monitor progress in wound healing

  E. Client education

    1. Explain purpose, use, and side effects of medications

    2. Assess client's understanding about anticipated length of treatment

Case Study

An 8-year-old female is brought to the physician's office by her mother. She is complaining of severe itching and a skin rash. Her legs show areas of erythema and small vesicles arranged linearly. The provider concludes the child has an allergic contact hypersensitivity reaction to poison ivy and orders specific therapy.

❶ You instruct the mother to apply dressings soaked in Burow's solution to the legs. How will this solution help this client?

❷ You instruct the mother also to thinly apply a corticosteroid twice a day. What are the possible adverse reactions associated with topical corticosteroids?

❸ The mother requested some medication to stop the itching. Which oral drug is most likely to be tried first?

❹ Why would the topical version of this same drug *not* be used?

❺ The child returns to the office a week later and now the rash and vesicles have spread over more of the body, including the hands and arms. On a Brownie scout outing the child had apparently had further contact with poison ivy. What would the healthcare provider suggest now?

For suggested responses, see page 640.

Posttest

1 The nurse would apply a closed soak to a client's skin to achieve which of the following benefits?

    (1) Cooling effect
    (2) Impermeability to air
    (3) Ability to change it once every 3 days
    (4) Heat retention

2 The nurse recommends the use of a topical cream to a client who needs which of the following ingredients in a skin product?

    (1) Emulsifying agent
    (2) Ointment
    (3) A drying agent
    (4) Lotion

3 The nurse teaches the client that which of the following skin cleansers is likely to stain the skin and/or clothing?

    (1) Benzalkonium (Zephiran)
    (2) Hexachlorophene (Phisohex)
    (3) Povidone-iodine (Betadine)
    (4) Hydrogen peroxide

4 The nurse would plan to use DuoDERM for a client with which of the following skin conditions?

    (1) An infected wound
    (2) An ulcer with heavy drainage
    (3) An ulcer with moderate amounts of necrotic material
    (4) An uninfected venous stasis ulcer

5 A client with acne is prescribed oral minocycline. The nurse would explain to the client that a disadvantage of this preparation includes which of the following?

    (1) Suppression of sebum production
    (2) Lupus-like syndrome and pigmentation changes
    (3) Lack of treatment efficacy
    (4) Occurrence of spontaneous abortions

6 The nurse who is using a very high-potency topical corticosteroid would generally plan to use it:

    (1) For any type of skin disorder.
    (2) For no longer than 2 weeks.
    (3) Under an appropriate dressing.
    (4) At least 4 times a day for best effect.

7 The client has moderate acne. After assessment, a topical preparation of benzoyl peroxide is recommended. The nurse will advise the client not to overuse the product because it could result in which of the following problems?

    (1) Excessive dryness
    (2) Extreme pruritus
    (3) Lack of healing of lesions
    (4) Localized infection

8 An 18-year-old female client has severe acne. There has been no improvement from the use of various preparations and isotretinoin (Accutane) is being prescribed. The nurse evaluates that the client understood medication instructions if the client stated to do which of the following?

    (1) Apply a thick layer of isotretinoin twice a day.
    (2) Increase exposure to the sun for added benefit.
    (3) Have a pregnancy test prior to beginning therapy and use contraception.
    (4) Have blood drawn for hormonal studies monthly for the first 6 months.

9 A client who experienced a burn injury is being treated with topical mafenide acetate (Sulfamylon). The client reports a stinging and burning sensation when the medication is applied. The nurse determines that it would be appropriate to do which of the following?

    (1) Withhold the medication and notify the physician
    (2) Wash off that dose of the medication
    (3) Explain that this is a normal sensation
    (4) Chill the preparation before using it next

10 A client has developed bacterial infection in skin damaged by thermal trauma. The nurse anticipates that wound culture will reveal the presence of one or both of which two most common causative agents?

(1) *Haemophilus influenzae* and *Haemophilus aegyptius*
(2) Herpes simplex and herpes zoster
(3) Tinea capitis and tinea pedis
(4) *Staphylococcus aureus* and *Streptococcus pyogenes*

See pages 354–355 for Answers and Rationales.

Answers and Rationales

Pretest

1 **Answer: 1** *Rationale:* Psoriasis is a common, chronically recurring skin disease with scaly patches of varying size most commonly seen on elbows, knees, and scalp. Pityriasis rosea is a common skin condition generally localized to chest and trunk of young adults and characterized by erythematous discrete lesions (option 2). Option 3 is a vague description unrelated to psoriasis. Contact dermatitis (option 4) develops after exposure to an irritant or allergen.
Cognitive Level: Application
Nursing Process: Implementation; *Test Plan:* PHYS

2 **Answer: 2** *Rationale:* Mupirocin is a topical antimicrobial agent effective against impetigo caused by *Staphylococcus aureus,* beta-hemolytic streptococci, and *Streptococcus pyogenes.* Ketoconazole is an antifungal agent; capsaicin is a topical agent that has been useful in certain painful syndromes; and acyclovir is an antiviral agent.
Cognitive Level: Analysis
Nursing Process: Planning; *Test Plan:* PHYS

3 **Answer: 3** *Rationale:* Synthetic detergent bars are milder on the skin. Dove is classified as synthetic detergent bar. Dial and Safeguard are deodorant soaps of a more harsh nature. Ivory is classified as a true soap.
Cognitive Level: Application
Nursing Process: Implementation; *Test Plan:* HPM

4 **Answer: 4** *Rationale:* The effectiveness of a sunscreen when compared to no use of sunscreen is usually indicated by its sun protection factor (SPF) (e.g., 6, 15, 30). Option 1 is a false interpretation. Sunscreens also may be classified as water-resistant (option 2) or waterproof (option 3), but the SPF number does not indicate this information.
Cognitive Level: Application
Nursing Process: Implementation; *Test Plan:* HPM

5 **Answer: 2** *Rationale:* Lindane has long been considered an appropriate treatment for pediculosis (lice).

Terbinafine is an antifungal agent for tinea infections. Collagenase is an enzyme used as a debriding preparation. Chlorhexidine is a skin and wound cleanser.
Cognitive Level: Analysis
Nursing Process: Analysis; *Test Plan:* PHYS

6 **Answer: 1** *Rationale:* Permethrin is preferred treatment for scabies at present time. A variety of treatment protocols are suggested, but the greatest success is reported when product is left on for at least 8 hours. If the treatment is repeated, it is repeated at 7 days, not 6 hours (option 3). Household articles in direct contact with the client need to be thoroughly washed or disinfected or both, but the human is the host for this parasite (option 4). Kwell can be used for pediculosis or scabies, but two similar agents would not be used together (option 2).
Cognitive Level: Application
Nursing Process: Implementation; *Test Plan:* PHYS

7 **Answer: 2** *Rationale:* Benzoyl peroxide has bactericidal activity against *Propionibacterium acnes.* It is available in over-the-counter and prescription formulations, including bar soaps, washes, gels, and lotions, in a variety of concentrations. Mafenide (option 1) is a preparation used in burn therapy. Chlorhexidine (option 3) is a skin and wound cleanser; it may be used for preoperative preparation of the skin. Cryotherapy (option 4) is a treatment used for some warts.
Cognitive Level: Analysis
Nursing Process: Implementation; *Test Plan:* PHYS

8 **Answer: 4** *Rationale:* Isotretinoin is available in capsule form. The other products are also used for acne, but are topical preparations.
Cognitive Level: Application
Nursing Process: Implementation; *Test Plan:* PHYS

9 **Answer: 2** *Rationale:* Silver sulfadiazine reacts with DNA and releases sulfadiazine. The silver replaces the hydrogen bonding between strands of DNA and prevents replication of the bacteria. It does not facilitate skin cell replication, and it is not of small

molecular size. It is not classified as an antifibri-
nolytic agent.
Cognitive Level: Comprehension
Nursing Process: Analysis; *Test Plan:* PHYS

10 **Answer: 1** *Rationale:* Salicylic acid preparations
are useful for the removal of common warts.
Povidone-iodine (option 2) is used to prepare or
cleanse skin preoperatively; masoprocol (option 3) is
indicated for actinic keratosis; and crotamiton (option
4) is an antiparasitic drug.
Cognitive Level: Application
Nursing Process: Planning; *Test Plan:* PHYS

Posttest

1 **Answer: 4** *Rationale:* Closed soaks lead to heat retention and are not used for a cooling effect. They are
typically applied for 1 to 2 hours at a time 2 to 3
times a day. They are not impermeable to air, but they
are water impermeable.
Cognitive Level: Application
Nursing Process: Planning; *Test Plan:* PHYS

2 **Answer: 1** *Rationale:* A cream is an emulsion of oil
in water; an ointment is considered to be a water-in-
oil product. Lotions are suspensions of powder in
water or a liquid emulsion of thin consistency. A
cream might or might not contain an antimicrobial
agent, and it is not a drying agent.
Cognitive Level: Application
Nursing Process: Implementation; *Test Plan:* PHYS

3 **Answer: 3** *Rationale:* Iodine preparations stain skin
and clothing. Benzalkonium, hexachlorophene, and
hydrogen peroxide do not cause staining.
Cognitive Level: Application
Nursing Process: Implementation; *Test Plan:* PHYS

4 **Answer: 4** *Rationale:* DuoDERM is indicated for ulcers with moderate drainage but which are unin-
fected. Agents like Iodosorb might be used for ulcers
with necrotic material (option 3) and Hydrasorb with
ulcers with heavy drainage (option 2). Antimicrobials
may be used to treat infected wounds.
Cognitive Level: Analysis
Nursing Process: Planning; *Test Plan:* PHYS

5 **Answer: 2** *Rationale:* Minocycline can lead to development of a lupus-like syndrome and also may cause
pigmentation changes. Minocycline does not suppress
sebum production (option 1), lead to spontaneous
abortions (option 4) or have low/lack of treatment efficacy (option 3).
Cognitive Level: Application
Nursing Process: Implementation; *Test Plan:* PHYS

6 **Answer: 2** *Rationale:* Potent topical steroid therapy
should be tapered within 2 weeks. Very high-potency
topical corticosteroids may induce atrophy, telangiectasia, and striae as early as 2 to 3 weeks following
daily application. High-potency topical corticosteroids and use of occlusion may induce hypothalamic-
pituitary-adrenal (HPA) axis suppression and adverse
reactions typically associated with chronic oral therapy. Dosing of topical corticosteroids more frequently
than two to three times daily is neither indicated nor
of proven benefit.
Cognitive Level: Application
Nursing Process: Planning; *Test Plan:* PHYS

7 **Answer: 1** *Rationale:* Adverse reactions of acne
preparations may include erythema, burning or
stinging, excessive dryness, and increased susceptibility to sunburn. Directions include using a thin application twice a day. Excessive use would be more
likely to result in evidence of adverse reaction than
would use as per product directions. Adverse reactions do not include extreme pruritus (option 2),
non-healing lesions (option 3), or localized infection
(option 4).
Cognitive Level: Application
Nursing Process: Implementation; *Test Plan:* PHYS

8 **Answer: 3** *Rationale:* Accutane is an oral preparation that is a known teratogen; strict adherence to
methods to prevent pregnancy is mandatory. Accutane is contraindicated in pregnancy because of the
occurrence of spontaneous abortions as well as major
abnormalities in the fetus at birth such as hydro-
cephalus. Elevated triglyceride levels might occur,
but changes in hormone functioning (option 4) are
not anticipated. The medication should be applied
thinly (option 1) and sun exposure provides no added
benefit (option 2).
Cognitive Level: Analysis
Nursing Process: Evaluation; *Test Plan:* PHYS

9 **Answer: 3** *Rationale:* Mafenide acetate is a water-
soluble cream that is used to treat burn injury. It may
cause a stinging or burning sensation after it is applied, and this is considered to be normal. Options 1
and 2 are inappropriate actions, while option 4 will
not prevent stinging of the medication.
Cognitive Level: Application
Nursing Process: Implementation; *Test Plan:* PHYS

10 **Answer: 4** *Rationale:* The two most common organisms causing infection are *Staphylococcus aureus*
and *Streptococcus pyogenes*. Herpes simplex and herpes zoster are members of the herpes virus family.
Dermatophytes cause fungal infections of the skin,

such as tinea capitis and tinea pedis. *Haemophilus aegyptius* causes pink eye. *Haemophilus influenzae* can cause meningitis, pneumonia, and serious throat and ear infections.
Cognitive Level: Application
Nursing Process: Analysis; *Test Plan:* PHYS

References

Anderson, K., Anderson, L., & Glanze, W. (2002). Mosby's medical, nursing & allied health dictionary (6th ed.). St. Louis, MO: Mosby, Inc.

Eisenhauer, L. A., Nichols, L. W., Spencer, R. T., & Bergan, F. W. (1998). *Clinical pharmacology and nursing management* (5th ed.). Philadelphia: Lippincott.

Freedberg, I. M., Eisen, A. Z., Wolff, K., Austen, K. Goldsmith, L. A., Katz, S. I., Fitzpatrick, T. B. (Eds.). (1999). *Fitzpatrick's dermatology in general medicine* (5th ed.). New York: McGraw-Hill.

Garner, S. E., Eady, E. A., Popescu, C., Newton, J., & Li Wan Po, A. (2000). Minocycline for acne vulgaris: efficacy and safety. (*Cochrane Review*). In: the Cochrane Library, 4, 2000. Oxford: Update Software.

McKenry, L., & Salerno, E. (2003). *Mosby's pharmacology in nursing* (21st ed revised update). St. Louis, MO: Mosby, Inc.

Turkoski, B. B., Lance, B. R., & Bonfiglio, M. F. (2000). *Drug information handbook for advanced practice nursing* (2nd ed.). Hudson, OH: Lexi-Comp Inc.

Youngkin, E. Q., Sawin, K. J., Kissinger, J. F., & Israel, D. S. (1999). *Pharmacotherapeutics: A primary care clinical guide.* Stamford, CT: Appleton & Lange.

Walker, G. J. A., & Johnstone, P. W. (2000). Interventions for treating scabies (*Cochrane Review*). In: the Cochrane Library, 4, 2000. Oxford: Update Software.

CHAPTER 10

Neurological and Musculoskeletal System Medications

Roni Ruhlandt, MSN, RN, CCRN, CNRN

CHAPTER OUTLINE

Analgesics
Anticonvulsants
Central Nervous System (CNS)
  Stimulants

Medications to Treat Parkinson's
  Disease
Medications to Treat Alzheimer's
  Disease

Centrally-Acting Skeletal Muscle
  Relaxants
Antianxiety, Sedative, and
  Hypnotics

OBJECTIVES

▌ Describe general goals of therapy when administering neurological and musculoskeletal system medications.

▌ Identify significant nursing considerations related to administering opioid analgesics.

▌ Describe side effects and adverse effects of acetylsalicylic acid (aspirin), acetaminophen (Tylenol), and nonsteroidal anti-inflammatory drugs (NSAIDs).

▌ Identify major anticonvulsant medication classifications.

▌ Discuss significant client education points related to the administration of anticonvulsants.

▌ Discuss nursing considerations related to the administration of central nervous system stimulants.

▌ Discuss nursing considerations related to the administration of medications commonly used to treat Parkinson's disease, Alzheimer's disease, narcolepsy, and attention-deficit hyperactivity disorder.

▌ Discuss primary uses, interactions, major side effects and adverse/toxic effects of the most commonly prescribed musculoskeletal relaxants.

▌ List significant client education points related to neurological and musculoskeletal system medications.

[Media Link]

Use the CD-ROM enclosed with this text, or log onto the address given to access the free, interactive Companion Website created for this series. The CD-ROM and Companion Website accompanying this book offer additional practice opportunities and information—NCLEX Review, Case Studies, Glossary, In Depth with NCLEX, and more.

www.prenhall.com/hogan

REVIEW AT A GLANCE

attention deficit disorder *also called ADD; a condition in which a child demonstrates inattention and impulsivity for more than a 6-month period*

attention deficit hyperactivity disorder *also called ADHD; a condition in which a child demonstrates inattention, impulsivity, and hyperactivity for more than a 6-month period*

anorexia *loss of appetite*

diplopia *double vision*

epilepsy *a chronic disorder characterized by recurring seizures in which there is a disturbance in some type of behavior (i.e., motor, sensory, autonomic, consciousness, or mentation)*

hepatotoxicity *a state in which liver damage has occurred; symptoms include: dark urine, clay-colored stools, yellowing of skin, sclera, itching, abdominal pain, fever, and diarrhea*

gamma-aminobutyric acid (GABA) *an excitatory neurotransmitter that is one of the amino acids*

gingival hyperplasia *increased growth of the gum tissue; an adverse effect of anticonvulsants, especially phenytoin (Dilantin)*

intracranial pressure *the pressure inside the skull; when increased may cause serious to disastrous sequelae*

level of consciousness *state of awareness that includes orientation (arousal and wakefulness) and cognition (sum of cerebral mental functions)*

narcolepsy *inability to stay awake during the day, regardless of amount of sleep or stimulation*

nystagmus *involuntary oscillation of the eye*

paresthesias *abnormal sensations, whether spontaneous or evoked*

psychomotor seizures *a term referring to complex partial (focal) seizures that cause the client to lose consciousness or black out for a few seconds; characteristic behavior may include lip smacking, patting, and picking at clothes*

reticular activating system *a diffuse system that extends from the lower brain stem to the cerebral cortex; controls the sleep-wakefulness cycle, consciousness, focused attention, and sensory perceptions*

spasms *involuntary contractions of large muscle groups (arms, legs, neck)*

spasticity *increased resistance to passive movement, often more pronounced at the extremes of range of motion and followed by a sudden or gradual release of resistance*

status epilepticus *a true neurological emergency, in which a seizure lasts more than 4 minutes or seizures are so frequently repeated or prolonged that they created a lasting condition (more than 30 minutes)*

Stevens-Johnson syndrome *an acute inflammatory disorder of the skin and mucous membranes (toxic epidermal necrolysis)*

tonic-clonic seizures *formerly grand mal seizures; tonic phase begins with a sudden loss of consciousness and a major tonic contraction (stiffening of body and extremities) that lasts for about one minute; clonic phase is characterized by violent, rhythmic, muscular contractions and hyperventilation that lasts from 30 seconds to a minute; postictal phase is a deep sleep followed by a period of confusion and lethargy can last minutes to hours*

Pretest

1 The client has been diagnosed with narcolepsy. The provider is considering prescribing methylphenidate (Ritalin). The nurse notes that the client has a history of which of the following prior medical conditions that would disqualify the client from using this medication?

(1) Congestive heart failure (CHF)
(2) Diabetes mellitus
(3) Glaucoma
(4) Hyperthyroidism

2 The client has just been diagnosed with a seizure disorder. The medication regimen has controlled the seizures for several days. Prior to discharge, the nurse should place highest priority on sharing which of the following information with the client?

(1) Seizure disorders will often eventually stop on their own.
(2) Adherence to medication therapy is essential to avoid recurrence of seizures.
(3) Urine will turn pink or brown from the medication.
(4) The client cannot drive a vehicle permanently.

3 The client with a history of cluster headaches should be taught which of the following information regarding use of ergotamine tartrate (Gynergen)?

(1) "Take the medication every 4 hours."
(2) "Take the medication with plenty of water."
(3) "You will feel energetic and warm after taking the medication."
(4) "Lie down in a darkened room after taking the medication."

4 The client is experiencing spasticity related to a spinal cord injury. The nurse anticipates that which of the following medications is most likely going to be added to the client's medication list?

(1) Dexamethasone (Decadron)
(2) Dantrolene (Dantrium)
(3) Dichlorphenamide (Daranide)
(4) Dobutamine (Dobutrex)

5 Which of the following are priority assessments by the nurse when administering opioid analgesics to a client?

(1) Pain intensity, respiratory rate, and level of consciousness
(2) Liver function studies, urine output, and pain intensity
(3) Seizure activity, mental status, and respiratory status
(4) Electrolytes, blood glucose, and pain intensity

6 The nurse is teaching a client about anti-inflammatory medications. Client education regarding taking aspirin, acetaminophen, or nonsteroidal anti-inflammatory drugs (NSAIDs) should include which of the following cautions?

(1) Radial pulse and temperature should be taken prior to medication administration.
(2) Consult provider before taking over-the-counter (OTC) medications, since many are combinations that may include more of the medication prescribed than is safe.
(3) Cholesterol levels must be measured prior to treatment with medication.
(4) Do not discontinue use of medication abruptly; medication must be tapered over a week.

7 The nurse is caring for a hospitalized client with diagnosis of seizure disorder. The client has an order for phenytoin (Dilantin). The nurse makes it a priority to assess which of the following parameters?

(1) Respiratory rate, and level of consciousness
(2) BUN, creatinine, and urine output
(3) Seizure activity, mental status, and respiratory status
(4) Electrolytes, serum osmolality, and leg edema

8 The client is prescribed carbamazepine (Tegretol) for a seizure disorder. The nurse cautions the client to avoid taking which of the following types of medications that could cause a fatal reaction with this medication?

(1) Nonsteroidal anti-inflammatory drugs (NSAIDs)
(2) Opioid analgesics
(3) Skeletal muscle relaxants
(4) Monoamine oxidase inhibitors (MAOIs)

9 A client with a seizure disorder has been started on medication therapy. The nurse should emphasize that which of the following types of medications should not be taking concurrently with anticonvulsants as they may lower the seizure threshold?

(1) Aspirin, acetaminophen, and nonsteroidal anti-inflammatory drugs (NSAIDs)
(2) Anorexiants and amphetamines
(3) Anticholinergics and dopamine agonists
(4) Hydantoins and benzodiazepines

10 The client with a spinal cord injury is taking dantrolene (Dantrium) for spasticity. The nurse should instruct client to notify the physician immediately if which of the following adverse effects of the medication occur?

(1) Twitching, diarrhea, or rash
(2) Change in blood or urine glucose levels
(3) Abdominal pain, jaundiced sclera, or clay-colored stools
(4) Urine changing to pink or brown or gingival hyperplasia

See pages 398–399 for Answers and Rationales.

I. Analgesics

A. Opioids

1. Action and use

a. Symptomatic relief of severe acute and chronic pain

    b. Most commonly used in the postoperative setting and to treat pain caused by malignancy

    c. Produce effects by binding to opioid receptors throughout the central nervous system (CNS) and peripheral tissues

    d. Considered controlled substances by FDA

    e. Classified by their ability to stimulate or block opioid receptors or by the severity of pain for which they are used

    f. Onset of action is immediate if given by intravenous (IV) route and rapid if given by intramuscular (IM) route or by mouth (PO)

    g. Peak action is from 1 to 2 hours and duration up to 7 hours

    h. These agents cross the blood–brain and placental barriers and also into breast milk

2. Common medications (Table 10-1)

3. Administration considerations

    a. Use caution if given to clients with addictive personality due to possibility of dependence

    b. Determine client's pattern of use if long-term; be aware that some opioids, such as Oxycontin, are used as street drugs

    c. May increase **intracranial pressure** (the pressure inside the skull)

    d. Clients with severe heart, liver or kidney disease, respiratory or seizure disorders should be closely monitored

    e. Decrease dosages for elderly or debilitated clients

    f. Double check dosages for neonates, infants, and children with physician/pharmacist

4. Contraindications

    a. Hypersensitivity reactions occur frequently

    b. Check for sensitivity prior to administration

    c. Do not use with clients who have acute bronchial asthma or upper airway obstruction, increased intracranial pressure, convulsive disorders, pancreatitis, acute ulcerative colitis, or severe liver or kidney insufficiency

5. Significant drug interactions

    a. Barbiturates, other narcotics, hypnotics, antipsychotics, or alcohol can increase CNS depression when combined with opiates

    b. Combined use with monoamine oxidase (MAO) inhibitors may precipitate hypertensive crisis

    c. Analgesia may be inhibited if used with phenothiazines

6. Significant food interactions: none reported

7. Significant laboratory studies: monitor liver and kidney function to determine ability to excrete medication and metabolites

Table 10-1	Type	Generic/Trade Names	Usual Adult Dose	Type of Pain
Common Opioid Analgesics	Pure agonists (No ceiling effect, increase in analgesia by increase in dose)	Codeine (Paveral) Dihydrocodeine, hydrocodone bitartrate (Vicodin) Oxycodone (Oxycontin) Propoxyphene (Darvon) Morphine sulfate (Duramorph)	15–60 mg IM/IV/PO 5–10 mg q4–6 h prn PO 5–10 mg q6h prn PO 65 mg q4h prn PO 10–30 mg q4h prn PO; 2.5–15 mg q4h IV	Moderate pain, most oral preparations combined with ASA or acetaminophen; dose frequently Severe pain, Short-acting Also sustained-release available for relief of constant pain
		Fentanyl citrate (Duragesic) Oxymorphone (Numorphan) Hydromorphone hydrochloride (Dilaudid) Meperidine (Demerol) Methadone hydrochloride (Dolophine) Levorphanal tartrate (Levo-dromoran)	Postoperative: 50–100 mcg q1–2 h IM Chronic pain: 25 mcg/h patch q3d 1–1.5 mg q4–6h prn SC/IM, 0.5 mg q4–6h IV 1–4 mg q4–6h prn PO/IM/IV/SC 50–150 mg q3–4h prn PO/IM/IV/SC 2.5–10 mg q3–4h prn PO/IM/SC 2–3 mg q6–8h prn PO/SC	 Potent, long-acting
	Mixed agonists-antagonists (Have ceiling effect)	Pentazocine hydrochloride (Talwin) Butorphanol tartrate (Stadol) Dezocine (Dalgan) Nalbuphine hydrochloride (Nubain)	50–100 mg q3–4h PO, 30 mg q3–4h IM/IV/SC 1–4 mg q3–4h prn IM, 0.5–2 mg q3–4h prn IV 2.5–10 mg q2–4h IV; 5–20 mg IM 10–20 mg q3–6h prn SC/IM/IV	Limited use for severe and chronic pain

NCLEX!

8. Side effects

   a. Nausea and vomiting

   b. **Anorexia** or loss of appetite

   c. Sedation

   d. Constipation, GI cramps, urinary retention, oliguria

   e. Pruritis, light-headedness, dizziness

NCLEX!

9. Adverse effects/toxicity

   a. Respiratory depression, respiratory arrest

   b. Circulatory depression

   c. Increased intracranial pressure

10. Nursing considerations

   a. Assess pain for type, intensity, and location of prior to administration (use pain scale)

   b. Assess for respiratory rate, depth, and rhythm; if less than 12 breaths per minute withhold medication

   c. Assess for CNS changes including **level of consciousness** (LOC), which is the state of awareness, as well as dizziness, drowsiness, hallucinations, and pupil size

   d. Assess client for the allergic reaction such as rash or urticaria

   e. Administer opiate for pain and antiemetic for nausea and vomiting

   f. Evaluate the therapeutic response and maintain comfort

   g. Monitor vital signs regularly

11. Client education

   a. Advise client to avoid alcohol and other CNS depressants while using opioids

   b. Advise client not to take over-the-counter (OTC) medications without approval by physician

   c. Warn client regarding ambulation, smoking, driving, or other activities without assistance after administration of medication until drug response is known

   d. Instruct client to report any CNS changes, allergic reactions, or shortness of breath

   e. Instruct client using medication on a long-term basis about withdrawal symptoms including nausea, vomiting, cramps, fever, faintness, and anorexia

B. Opioid antagonists

1. Actions and use

   a. Include naloxone (Narcan) and naltrexone (ReVia)

   b. Compete with opioids at the opiate receptor sites, blocking the effects of the opioids

   c. Used to reverse respiratory depression induced by overdose of opioids, pentazocine, and propoxyphene

   d. Onset of effect 1 to 2 minutes, duration 45 minutes

2. Side effects

   a. Reversal of analgesia

   b. Increased blood pressure (BP)

   c. Tremors, hyperventilation, drowsiness, nervousness, rapid pulse

   d. Nausea, vomiting, and hyperpnea

3. Adverse effects/toxicity

   a. Hypotension

   b. Ventricular tachycardia and fibrillation

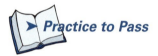

Practice to Pass

You are caring for a client with a patient-controlled analgesia (PCA) pump that has morphine sulfate as the medication. The client has been out of surgery for 1½ hours. He complains that his hands itch and he has a rash. What would you do first?

      c. Convulsions

      d. Hepatitis

      e. Pulmonary edema

  4. Nursing considerations

      a. Assess vital signs every 3 to 5 minutes

      b. Assess arterial blood gases (ABGs)

      c. Assess cardiac status: tachycardia, hypertension

      d. Monitor electrocardiogram (ECG)

NCLEX!

      e. Assess respiratory function (rate, rhythm) and LOC

      f. Administer only with resuscitative equipment nearby

NCLEX!

      g. Evaluate therapeutic response, LOC, and need for reversal of respiratory depression

C. Nonopioids

  1. Acetylsalicylic acid (Aspirin)

      a. Action and use

        1) Is a salicylate medication

        2) Inhibits prostaglandins involved in production of inflammation, pain and fever

        3) Blocks pain impulses in CNS

        4) Antipyretic action results from vasodilation of peripheral vessels

        5) Powerfully inhibits platelet aggregation

        6) Relieves mild to moderate pain, including pain caused by rheumatoid arthritis, osteoarthritis, acute rheumatic fever, systemic lupus erythematosus (SLE), bursitis, transient ischemic attacks (TIA), post myocardial infarction (MI), prophylaxis of MI, stroke and angina

NCLEX!

      b. Administration considerations

        1) Dosage varies depending on age of client and condition being treated

        2) Gastric irritation may be decreased by administering with full glass of water, milk, food, or antacid

        3) Pills can be crushed or chewed, but do not crush enteric-coated preparations

        4) Give 30 minutes prior to or 2 hours following meals

        5) Administer at least 30 minutes prior to physical therapy or planned exercise to minimize discomfort

      c. Contraindications

NCLEX!

        1) History of hypersensitivity to salicylates, or other non-steroidal anti-inflammatory drugs (NSAIDs), GI bleeding, bleeding disorders

NCLEX!

    2) Contraindicated in children younger than 12 years old because of risk of Reye's syndrome, children or teenagers with chicken pox or flu-like symptoms, pregnancy 3rd trimester, lactation

NCLEX!

    3) Contraindicated with vitamin K deficiency, peptic ulcer disease, anemia, renal or hepatic dysfunction

  d. Significant drug interactions

    1) Decreased effects of aspirin (ASA) with antacids (high-dose), and urinary alkalizers

NCLEX!

    2) Increased bleeding with anticoagulants and alcohol

NCLEX!

    3) Increased GI bleeding when taken concurrently with corticosteroids

    4) Increased effects of warfarin, insulin, thrombolytic agents, penicillins, phenytoin, valproic acid, oral hypoglycemics, and sulfonamides

    5) Increased salicylate levels (leads to toxicity) with ammonium chloride, urinary acidifiers, and nizatidine

    6) Decreased effects of probenecid, spironolactone, sulfinpyrazone, sulfonamides, NSAIDs, beta blockers

  e. Significant food interactions: increased risk of bleeding with horse chestnut and kelpware

  f. Significant laboratory studies

    1) Increases coagulation studies, liver function studies, serum uric acid, amylase, CO_2, and urinary protein

    2) Decreases serum potassium, cholesterol, and T_3 and T_4 concentrations

    3) Interference with urine catecholamines, pregnancy test, urine glucose tests (Clinistix, Tes-Tape)

  g. Side effects

NCLEX!

    1) Increased prothrombin time (PT), activated partial thromboplastin time (APTT), bleeding time

    2) Stimulation, drowsiness, dizziness, confusion, headache, hallucinations

    3) Nausea, vomiting, diarrhea, heartburn, anorexia

    4) Rash, urticaria, bruising

NCLEX!

    5) Tinnitis

  h. Adverse effects/toxicity

    1) Hematologic: thrombocytopenia, agranulocytosis, leukopenia, neutropenia, and hemolytic anemia

    2) Convulsion, coma

    3) GI bleeding, hepatitis

NCLEX!

    4) Reye's syndrome (children), characterized by encephalopathy and fatty liver degeneration

  i. Nursing considerations

1) Assess for allergy to salicylates prior to administration

2) Assess liver function tests, renal function tests (BUN, urine creatinine), and blood studies including complete blood count (CBC), hematocrit (Hct), hemoglobin (Hgb), PT if on long-term therapy

3) Assess for **hepatotoxicity** (state of liver damage): dark urine, clay-colored stools, yellowing of skin, sclera, itching

4) Abdominal pain, fever, diarrhea, especially if on long-term therapy

5) Evaluate for therapeutic responses such as decreased pain, inflammation, and fever

j. Client education

1) Instruct client to report any symptoms of hepatotoxicity or renal toxicity

2) Instruct client to report visual changes, tinnitus, allergic reactions, and bleeding

3) Advise client to take medication with 8 oz water, milk or food and sit upright for 30 minutes following dose

4) Advise client not to exceed recommended dose; acute salicylate poisoning may result

5) Instruct client not to combine with other OTC medications that also contain ASA

6) Inform client that therapeutic response can take up to 2 weeks

7) Instruct client to avoid alcohol ingestion to decrease chance of GI bleeding

8) Warn client that this medication should not be given to children or teens with flu-like or chickenpox symptoms (Reye's syndrome)

2. Acetaminophen (Tylenol)

a. Action and use

1) May block pain impulses peripherally that occur in response to inhibition of prostaglandin synthesis

2) Possesses weak anti-inflammatory properties

3) Antipyretic action results from inhibition of prostaglandins in the CNS resulting in peripheral vasodilation, sweating, and dissipation of heat

4) Used for mild to moderate pain or fever, especially when ASA or NSAIDs are not tolerated

b. Administration considerations

1) Usual dose is 325 to 600 mg q4–6h PO or PR; maximum dose is 4 grams per day

2) Oral forms may crushed or given as whole or chewable tablets

3) May give with food or milk to increase gastric tolerance

4) Co-administration with high-carbohydrate meal may significantly retard absorption rate

c. Contraindications

    1) Hypersensitivity to acetaminophen or phenacetin

    2) In children younger than 3 years unless directed by physician

    3) Repeated administration to clients with anemia or hepatic diseases, including alcoholism, malnutrition, or thrombocytopenia

d. Significant drug interactions

    1) Decreased effect and increased hepatotoxicity with barbiturates, alcohol, carbamazepine, hydantoins, rifampin, sulfinpyrazone

    2) Cholestyramine decreases absorption

    3) Hypoprothrombinemia may occur when used concurrently with warfarin

    4) Bone marrow suppression may occur with zidovudine

e. Significant food interactions: none reported

f. Significant laboratory studies: interference with Chemstrip G, Dextrostix, Visidex II (false increases in urinary glucose), 5-HIAA (false increases), blood glucose (false decreases), serum uric acid (false increases)

g. Side effects

    1) Negligible with recommended dosage

    2) Rash

h. Adverse effects/toxicity

    1) Anaphylaxis

    2) Hematology: leukopenia, neutropenia, hemolytic anemia, thrombocytopenia, pancytopenia

    3) GI: hepatotoxicity

    4) Angioedema

    5) Toxicity: cyanosis, anemia, neutropenia, jaundice, pancytopenia, CNS stimulation, delirium followed by vascular collapse, convulsions, coma, and death

i. Nursing considerations

    1) Assess liver function tests including aspartate aminotransferase (AST), alanine aminotransferase (ALT), bilirubin, creatinine, renal function tests (BUN, urine creatinine), blood studies (CBC, PT) if on long-term therapy

    2) May cause hepatotoxicity at doses greater than 4 g/day with chronic use

    3) Assess client for chronic poisoning; signs including rapid, weak pulse, dyspnea, cold, clammy extremities; report them immediately to physician

    4) Assess for hepatotoxicity: dark urine, clay-colored stools, yellowing of skin, sclera, itching, abdominal pain, fever, diarrhea, especially if on long-term therapy

NCLEX!

5) Be prepared to administer acetylcysteine (Mucomyst) as antidote for acetaminophen poisoning

6) Evaluate client for therapeutic response, such as decreased pain or fever

j. Client education

1) Instruct client not to exceed recommended dose; acute poisoning with liver damage may result

2) Instruct client about acute toxicity symptoms such as nausea, vomiting, abdominal pain; prescriber should be notified immediately

3) Advise client not to combine with other OTC medications that also contain acetaminophen

4) Instruct client to recognize signs of chronic overdose such as bleeding, bruising, malaise, fever, and sore throat

5) Instruct client to notify prescriber of pain or fever lasting longer than 3 days

3. Nonsteroidal anti-inflammatory drugs (NSAIDs)

a. Action and use

1) Nonsteroidal drugs decrease prostaglandin synthesis by inhibiting an enzyme needed for biosynthesis

2) They are used to treat mild to moderate pain, osteoarthritis, rheumatoid arthritis, and dysmenorrhea

b. Common medications (Table 10-2)

c. Administration considerations

1) Gastric irritation may be decreased by administering with full glass of water, milk, or food

2) Pills can be crushed or chewed

3) Capsules should not be crushed, dissolved or chewed

4) Give 30 minutes prior to or 2 hours following meals for best absorption

5) Administer at least 30 minutes prior to physical therapy or planned exercise to minimize discomfort

d. Contraindications

1) Hypersensitivity

2) Contraindicated with asthma, severe renal or hepatic disease, GI bleeding, bleeding disorders, peptic ulcer disease, or anemia

e. Significant drug interactions: see Table 10-2 for specific interactions for each medication

f. Significant food interactions: food may increase the peak, but not the overall absorption of nabumetone

g. Significant laboratory studies

1) Liver function tests

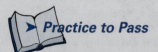

Practice to Pass

A client comes to the ambulatory care center complaining of nausea, vomiting, and abdominal pain. He has been taking acetaminophen for a headache (2 extra-strength) every 4 hours, as well as DayQuil and NyQuil every 4 hours for several days. What is the probable source of his nausea and vomiting?

Table 10-2	Medication	Usual Adult Dose	Significant Drug Interactions
Common Nonsteroidal Anti-inflammatory Agents	Celecoxib (Celebrex)	100–200 mg bid, or 200 mg qd PO	Increases effect of anticoagulants Decreases effect of ASA, ACE inhibitors, diuretics Increases adverse reactions of glucocorticoids, NSAIDS, ASA Increased toxicity: lithium, antineoplastics
	Diclofenac sodium (Voltaren)	150–200 mg/day in 3 to 4 divided doses PO	Decreases effect of β-blockers, diuretics Increases effect of anticoagulants, digoxin; increases toxicity of phenytoin, lithium, cyclosporin, methotrexate, ASA Hyperkalemia with potassium-sparing diuretics
	Etodolac (Lodine)	200–400 mg every 6–8 hours prn PO	Decreases effect of β-blockers, diuretics Increases effect of anticoagulants, digoxin Increases toxicity of phenytoin, lithium, cyclosporin, methotrexate, ASA; decreases effect of antacids
	Fenoprofen calcium (Nalfon)	200 mg every 4–6 hours prn PO	Phenobarbital decreases effect of fenoprofen Increases effects of oral anticoagulants and sulfonylureas Increased GI toxicity with ASA Decreased effect of diuretics Increased GI reactions with corticosteroids, alcohol
	Flurbiprofen sodium (Ansaid)	50–100 mg every 6–8 hours PO	Increased effects of oral anticoagulants, heparin, phenytoin, sulfonylureas, and sulfonamides Increased effect of flurbiprofen: phenytoin, sulfonylureas, sulfonamides
	Ibuprofen (Advil)	400 mg every 4–6 hours PO up to 1,200 mg/day	Decreases effect of antihypertensives, thyazides, furosemide Increased reactions: corticosteroids, ASA Increased toxicity: digoxin, lithium, oral anticoagulants, cyclosporine
	Indomethacin (Indocin)	25–50 mg bid or tid PO up to 200 mg/day	Decreases effect of antihypertensives Increases effect of digoxin, pencillamine, phenytoin Decreases effect of Indocin: ASA Increased toxicity: lithium, methotrexate, cyclosporin, aminoglycosides, ASA, corticosteroids, triamterene, alcohol Increased risk of bleeding with anticoagulants
	Ketoprofen (Actron)	12.5–50 mg PO every 6–8 hours	Increased toxicity: lithium, methotrexate, cyclosporin, phenytoin, alcohol Increases risk of bleeding: warfarin Increases effects of ketoprofen: ASA, probenecid Decreases effect of: diuretics, antihypertensives Increased GI reactions: corticosteroids, ASA
	Ketorolac (Toradol)	loading dose 30 mg IV; 30–60 mg loading dose, IM 15–30 mg q6h; 10 mg q6h PO	Increased toxicity: lithium, methotrexate Increased risk of bleeding: anticoagulants, salicylates Decreases effect of: diuretics, antihypertensives Increases renal impairment: ACE inhibitors
	Mefenemic acid (Ponstel)	500 mg loading dose, then 250 mg q6h prn PO	Increased toxicity: lithium, sulfanylureas, sulfonamides, phenytoin, warfarin Increased risk of bleeding: anticoagulants, heparin

(continued)

Table 10-2	Medication	Usual Adult Dose	Significant Drug Interactions
Common Nonsteroidal Anti-inflammatory Agents *(Continued)*	Nabumetone (Relafen)	1,000 mg/d as a single dose PO; may increase up to a max of 2,000 mg/d in 1–2 divided doses	Decreases effect of: diuretics, antihypertensives Increased adverse reactions: warfarin Increased risk of bleeding: anticoagulants, thrombolytics, valproic acid, cefamandole, cefotetan, cefoperazone Increased risk of hematologic reactions: antineoplastics, radiation Increased GI reactions: salicylates, NSAIDs, alcohol, potassium, corticosteroids
	Naproxen (Naprosyn)	500 mg followed by 200–250 mg PO q 6–8h prn up to 1250 mg/day	Increased toxicity: methotrexate, oral anticoagulants, sulfonylureas, probenecid, lithium Decreased effect of: diuretics, antihypertensives Increased GI reactions: ASA, alcohol, corticosteroids Possible renal impairment: ACE inhibitors Increased risk of bleeding: oral anticoagulants, heparin
	Piroxicam (Feldene)	10–20 mg 1–2 times/day PO	Increased toxicity: cyclosporine, methotrexate, lithium, alcohol, oral anticoagulants, ASA, corticosteroids Decreases effects of: antihypertensives, diuretics Hypoglycemia: oral antidiabetics; Increased risk of bleeding: oral anticoagulants, heparin Increased GI reactions: ASA, alcohol
	Sulindac (Clinoril)	150–200 mg bid up to 400 mg/day PO	Increased risk of bleeding: oral anticoagulants Increased nephrotoxicity: cyclosporine Decreases sulindac effect: diflunisal—**do not use together** Increased toxicity: methotrexate, sulfonamides, sulfonylureas, probenecid, lithium Increased GI reactions: ASA, NSAIDs

    2) Serum uric acid

    3) Urinary bilirubin, urinalysis, BUN, creatinine

    4) Bleeding time, PT, CBC

  h. Side effects

    1) Nausea, abdominal pain, anorexia

    2) Dizziness, drowsiness

  i. Adverse effects/toxicity

    1) Nephrotoxicity including dysuria, hematuria, oliguria, azotemia

    2) Blood dyscrasias, cholestatic hepatitis

  j. Nursing considerations

    1) Assess for renal and hepatic function, blood studies before treatment and periodically

    2) Audiometric, ophthalmic exam before, during, and after treatment

    3) Assess for ear and eye problems; blurred vision and tinnitus may indicate toxicity

    4) Evaluate for therapeutic response including decreased pain, stiffness in joints, decreased swelling in joints, ability to move more easily

NCLEX!

k. Client education

1) Instruct client to report blurred vision, ringing, roaring in ears, may indicate toxicity

2) Instruct client to avoid driving or other hazardous activities if dizziness and drowsiness occur, especially in elderly

3) Instruct client to report changes in urine pattern, increased weight, edema, increased pain in joints, fever, blood in urine indicating nephrotoxicity

4) Inform client that therapeutic effects may take up to one month

D. Medications to treat headaches

1. Action and use: aimed at prevention with prophylactic therapy and acute symptomatic treatment during attack

   a. Migraine headaches

   1) Acute therapy directed toward abolishing or limiting headache as it is beginning

   2) Ergot preparations are alpha-adrenergic agonists or antagonists that cause vasoconstriction or vasodilation, depending on state of vessel; they also block uptake of serotonin by platelets that can cause precipitous decline of serotonin leading to migraine attack

   3) Prophylaxis medications are beta-adrenergic blockers, serotonin antagonists, and anticonvulsants

   b. Tension-type headaches

   1) Therapy is directed toward rapid treatment of pain

   2) Prevention and reduction of occurrence is also a goal

   3) Mild analgesics and muscle relaxants are the first line medications; antidepressants may be used with counseling; ASA, acetaminophen, ibuprofen are used for pain; amitriptyline (Elavil) is helpful for muscle contraction pain

   c. Cluster headaches

   1) Treatment is directed at elimination of triggers

   2) Preventative therapies used may include high-dose calcium channel blockers, lithium, methysergide, or corticosteroids

2. Common medications (Table 10-3)

3. Administration considerations

   a. For abortive treatment medications, taking early in headache is imperative

   b. Taking dosage that was effective on last headache should be dosage to begin with for this headache

4. Contraindications

   a. Contraindicated in clients with hypersensitivity to ergot alkaloids

   b. Contraindicated during pregnancy

Table 10-3

Medications Used to Treat Headaches

Medications	Usual Adult Dose	Notes	Side Effects
Ergots Ergotamine tartrate (Ergostat)	1–2 mg followed by 1–2 mg q30 min PO until headache abates	Abortive treatment for headache unresponsive to nonnarcotic treatment Also used to treat cluster headaches	Have cumulative effect including numbness, tingling of fingers and toes, muscle pain, weakness
Dihydroergotamine mesylate (Migranal)	1 mg, may be repeated at 1 h intervals to a total of 3 mg IM or 2 mg IV Intranasal: 1 spray in each nostril	Parenteral treatment for established headache	Nausea is common; premedicate with antiemetics
Other Sumatriptan (Imitrex)	6 mg SC; may repeat 1 h after first injection 25 mg max 100 mg PO Intranasal: 5, 10 or 20 mg in one nostril	First-line abortive treatment Elective agonist for vascular serotonin receptors Causes vasoconstriction of cranial arteries Prompt relief of cluster headaches	Decreases blood pressure and heart rate

    c. Contraindicated in clients with cardiovascular disease, coronary artery disease, hypertension, sepsis, or severe pruritus

5. Significant drug interactions

    a. Beta blockers and calcium channel blockers are additive in effects with other cardiac medications

    b. May cause symptoms of ergot toxicity if given with erythromycin or other macrolides

6. Significant food interactions: none reported

7. Significant laboratory studies: see specific medications

8. Side effects: see Table 10-3

9. Adverse effects/toxicity: see Table 10-3

10. Nursing considerations

    a. Assess for medication-specific side effects as well as efficacy of treatment

    b. Planning for care must begin with careful history, including treatments that have been effective in the past

    c. Provide a quiet and low-light environment for client to relax

    d. Obtain an accurate dietary history form the client to determine if a relationship exists between onset of headache and certain foods

    e. Avoid prolonged use of the medication

    f. Beware of ergotamine rebound or an increase in frequency and duration of headache

  11. Client education

    a. Instruct client to identify type of headache: migraine, cluster, or tension

    b. Instruct client to identify triggers for headaches and how to ameliorate them

    c. Advise client to develop headache diary

    d. Educate client in stress reduction, stress management, lifestyle changes, including diet to minimize headaches

    e. Instruct client not to eat, drink, or smoke while the tablet is dissolving (using sublingual tablet)

    f. Instruct client to avoid exposure to cold weather for a long period of time; cold may increase the adverse reactions to the medication

    g. Warn client not to increase the dose of medication without consulting the physician

    h. Instruct client regarding comfort measures during attack, such as lying in darkened, quiet room with cold compresses applied to head

II. Anticonvulsants

A. Hydantoins

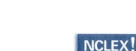

  1. Action and use

    a. Inhibit the spread of seizure activity in the motor cortex

    b. Used in general **tonic-clonic seizures** (grand mal seizures), **status epilepticus** (seizures that last longer than 4 minutes), and **psychomotor seizures** (complex focal seizures)

  2. Common medications (Table 10-4)

  3. Administration considerations

    a. Fosphenytoin should only be given IV for status epilepticus in emergency department or critical care area; respiratory rate, BP, and ECG should be monitored; loading dose given at 100 to 150 mg phenytoin equivalent (PE) per minute

    b. Do not interchange chewable phenytoin products with capsules

    c. Phenytoin readily binds with protein so should not be given with gastric feedings, which inhibit uptake

    d. Give ethosuximide, diazepam, and carbmazepine with food or milk to reduce GI symptoms

    e. Carbamazepine given via NG tube should be mixed with D_5W or NS and flush with at least 100 mL solution afterwards

    f. Do not crush tablets or capsules of valproate sodium; take whole

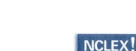

  4. Contraindications

    a. Hypersensitivity

Table 10-4	Medication	Usual Adult Dose	Significant Drug Interactions
Anticonvulsants	**_Hydantoins_** Fosphenytoin sodium (Cerebyx)	Loading dose: 15–20 PE/kg Maintenance dose: 4–6 mg PE/kg/day (PE-phenytoin sodium equivalents)	Decreased effects of fosphenytoin (FP): alcohol (chronic use), antihistamines, antacids, antineoplastics, CNS depressants, rifampin, folic acid, carbamazepine, reserpine, tricyclics; Increase fosphenytoin level: cimetidine, amiodarone, chloramphenicol, estrogens, H_2 antagonists, phenothiazines, salicylates, sulfonamides
	Phenytoin (Dilantin)	15–18 mg/kg or 1 gram loading dose PO; then 300 mg/day in 1–3 divided doses 15–18 mg/kg or 1 g loading dose IV; then 100 mg TID	Decreased effects of phenytoin: alcohol (chronic use), antihistamines, antacids, antineoplastics, CNS depressants, rifampin, folic acid Increased effect of phenytoin: low plasma albumin levels
	Barbiturates Phenobarbital sodium (Luminal)	100–300 mg/day, PO 200–300 mg up to 20 mg/kg IV/IM	Increased effects: CNS depression, alcohol, chloramphenicol, valproic acid, disulfiram, non-depolarizing skeletal muscle relaxants, sulfonamides Decreased effects: theophylline, oral anticoagulants, corticosteroids, metronidazole, doxycycline, quinidine Increased orthostatic hypotension: furosemide
	Succinimides Ethosuximide (Zarontin)	250 mg bid, may increase q4–7 days prn PO	Increased CNS depression: alcohol Increased hydantoin levels Decreased valproic acid levels
	Benzodiazepines Diazepam (Valium)	5–10 mg IM/IV 2–10 mg bid to qid PO	Increased effect of both: barbiturates Increased digoxin level Increased effect of benzodiazepine: cimetidine Decreased effects of benzodiazepine: oral contraceptives, rifampin, valproic acid, disulfiram, isoniazid, propranolol
	Lorazepam (Ativan)	0.1 mg/kg slow IV over 2–5 min	
	Clonazepam (Klonopin)	1.5 mg/day in 3 divided doses PO	Increased CNS depression: CNS depressants, alcohol
	Other Carbamazepine (Tegretol)	200 mg bid, gradually increased to 800–1200 mg/day PO in 3-4 divided doses	CNS toxicity: lithium Increased carbamazepine levels: cimetidine, clarithromycin, danazol, diltiazem, erythromycin, fluoxetine, fluvoxamine, isoniazid, propoxyphene, valproic acid, verapamil Decreased effects of: benzodiazepines, doxycycline, felbamate, haloperidol, oral contraceptives, phenobarbital, phenytoin, primidone, theophylline, thyroid hormones, warfarin Increased effects of: desmopressin, lithium, lypressin, vasopressin; **fatal reaction with MAOIs**
	Valproate sodium (Depakote)	15 mg/kg/day PO/IV in divided doses when total daily dose greater than 250 mg, increased at 1 wk intervals by 5–10 mg/kg/day	Increased effects: CNS depressants Increased toxicity of valproate: salicylates Increased toxicity of: warfarin Increased action of: phenytoin Increased CNS effects of: phenobarbital, primidone Increased sedation: benzodiazepines Decreased metabolism of valproate: cimetidine

   b. Contraindicated with psychiatric condition, pregnancy, bradycardia, SA and AV node block, Stokes-Adams syndrome, hepatic failure

5. Significant drug interactions: see Table 10-4

6. Significant food interactions: gastric feedings will compete at binding sites for drug; may need to withhold feedings 30–60 minutes before and after medication administration; check institutional policy and procedure manual

7. Significant laboratory studies: therapeutic phenytoin level

8. Side effects

   a. Drowsiness, dizziness, insomnia, **paresthesias** (abnormal sensations), depression, suicidal tendencies, aggression, headache, confusion, slurred speech

   b. Hypotension

   c. **Nystagmus** (involuntary oscillation of eye), **diplopia** (double vision), blurred vision

   d. Nausea, vomiting, constipation, anorexia, weight loss, hepatitis, jaundice, **gingival hyperplasia** (increased growth of gum tissue)

   e. Urine discoloration

   f. Rash, lupus erythematosus, hirsutism

   g. Hypocalcemia

9. Adverse effects/toxicity

   a. Ventricular fibrillation

   b. Hepatitis

   c. Nephritis

   d. Agranulocytosis, leukopenia, aplastic anemia, thrombocytopenia, megaloblastic anemia

   e. Lupus erythematosus, **Stevens-Johnson syndrome** (an acute inflammatory disorder of the skin)

   f. Toxicity: bone marrow suppression, nausea, vomiting, ataxia, diplopia, cardiovascular collapse, slurred speech, confusion

10. Nursing considerations

   a. Assess for seizure activity including type, location, duration, and character; provide seizure precautions

   b. Assess for mental status, mood, sensorium, affect, and memory (short and long term)

   c. Assess for respiratory depression, rate, depth, and character of respirations

   d. Assess for blood dyscrasias, fever, sore throat, bruising, rash, and jaundice

   e. Evaluate client for therapeutic responses such as decreases in severity of seizures and decreased ventricular dysrhythmias

11. Client education

    a. Instruct client about medication regimen including name, dose, schedule, side effects, and possible adverse effects

    b. Inform client that urine may turn pink

    c. Advise client not to discontinue medication abruptly or without consulting physician

    d. Instruct client about proper brushing of teeth with soft toothbrush, proper flossing to prevent gingival hyperplasia

    e. Advise client to carry Medic-Alert bracelet stating medication use

    f. Instruct client to avoid heavy use of alcohol as it may decrease effectiveness of medication

    g. Advise client not to change brands of medication once seizure activity has stabilized; bioavailability differs among formulations

B. Barbiturates

1. Action and use

    a. Decrease impulse transmission to the cerebral cortex

    b. Are used in all forms of **epilepsy,** a chronic disorder characterized by recurring seizures

2. Common medications (Table 10-4)

3. Administration considerations

    a. Administor IM injection into large muscle mass to prevent tissue sloughing

    b. Use less than 5 mL/site

    c. When ordered IV, give slowly (after dilution) at a rate of 65 mg or less per minute

4. Contraindications

    a. Hypersensitivity

    b. Contraindicated during pregnancy, porphyria, and liver disease

5. Significant drug interactions: see Table 10-4

6. Significant food interactions: none reported

7. Significant laboratory studies

    a. Increases serum phosphatase

    b. Affects bromsulphalein retention test which enhances hepatic uptake and excretion of dye

8. Side effects

    a. Paradoxical excitement (elderly), drowsiness, lethargy, hangover headache, flushing, hallucinations

    b. Nausea, vomiting, diarrhea, constipation

    c. Rash, urticaria, local pain, swelling, necrosis

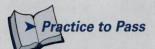

Practice to Pass

Your client is receiving continuous gastric feeding and receiving phenytoin (Dilantin) IV for seizures. The physician decides to change the phenytoin to oral suspension to be administered via the feeding tube. What precautions must you take to ensure that the client's level of anticonvulsant does not diminish due to the change in administration method?

9. Adverse effects/toxicity

   a. Coma

   b. Stevens-Johnson syndrome, angioedema, thrombophlebitis

10. Nursing considerations

    a. Assess for mental status changes such as mood, sensorium, affect, and memory (long and short term)

    b. Assess for respiratory status or depression including rate, rhythm, and depth

    c. Assess for blood dyscrasias, fever, sore throat, bruising, rash, and jaundice

    d. Assess for seizure activity including type, duration, and precipitating factors

    e. Blood studies and liver function tests are done routinely during long-term treatment

    f. Evaluate client for therapeutic responses such as decreased seizures or increased sedation

11. Client education

    a. Instruct client about medication regimen including name, dose, schedule, side effects, and possible adverse effects

    b. Instruct client to avoid other CNS depressants including alcohol

    c. Advise client not to discontinue medication abruptly or without consulting physician

    d. Advise client to avoid hazardous activities until stabilized on drug; drowsiness may occur

    e. Instruct client to carry Medic-Alert bracelet stating medication use

    f. Inform client that therapeutic effects may not be seen for 2 to 3 weeks

C. Succinimides

1. Action and use

   a. Inhibit spike, wave formation in absence seizures (petit mal), decrease amplitude, frequency, duration, and spread of discharges in minor motor seizures

   b. Used in absence seizures, partial seizures, and tonic-clonic seizures

2. Common medications (Table 10-4)

3. Administration considerations: give with food or milk to decrease GI symptoms

4. Contraindications: hypersensitivity

5. Significant drug interactions: see Table 10-4

6. Significant food interactions: none reported

7. Significant laboratory studies

   a. Increased liver function tests

   b. Direct Coomb's test: false positive

8. Side effects

    a. Drowsiness, dizziness, fatigue, euphoria, lethargy

    b. Nausea, vomiting, heartburn, anorexia

    c. Pink urine

    d. Urticaria, pruritic erythema

    e. Myopia, blurred vision

9. Adverse effects/toxicity

    a. Agranulocytosis, aplastic anemia, thrombocytopenia, leukocytosis, eosinophilia, pancytopenia

    b. Stevens-Johnson syndrome

    c. Toxicity: bone marrow depression, nausea, vomiting, ataxia, diplopia, and cardiovascular collapse

10. Nursing considerations

    a. Assess for mental status changes including mood, sensorium, affect, and behavioral changes

    b. Monitor renal studies including urine analysis, BUN, and creatinine

    c. Monitor blood studies including CBC, Hct, Hgb, reticulocyte counts every week for 4 weeks

    d. Monitor hepatic studies including AST, ALT, and bilirubin

    e. Assess for eye problems; may need regular ophthalmic exams

    f. Assess for allergic reactions such as red, raised rash or exfoliative dermatitis

    g. Assess for blood dyscrasias, fever, sore throat, bruising, rash, or jaundice

11. Client education

    a. Instruct client to carry ID card or Medic-Alert bracelet with medication, client's name, physician's name, and phone number

    b. Instruct client to avoid driving and other activities that require alertness

    c. Instruct client to avoid alcohol ingestion and other CNS depressants as they may increase sedation

    d. Advise client not to discontinue medication abruptly or without consulting physician

    e. Advise client to continue regular dental checkups to identify gingival hyperplasia

D. **Benzodiazepines**

1. Action and use

    a. Enhance the inhibitory neurotransmitter **GABA (gamma-aminobutyric acid)** to decrease anxiety and as an adjunct for seizure activity

    b. Relief of delirium tremens

2. Common medications (Table 10-4)

3. Administration considerations

   a. Give with food or milk to reduce GI symptoms

   b. IV injection should be given into large vein

   c. Administer IV medication at a rate of 5 mg or less per minute

4. Contraindications

   a. Hypersensitivity

   b. Contraindicated in acute narrow-angle glaucoma or psychosis

   c. Contraindicated in children younger than 6 months

   d. Do not give to clients with liver disease (clonazepam), or during lactation (diazepam)

5. Significant drug interactions: see Table 10-4

6. Significant food interactions: none reported

7. Significant laboratory studies

   a. Increases AST and ALT, serum bilirubin levels

   b. Increases 17-OHCS and decreases RAIU

8. Side effects

   a. Dizziness, drowsiness, confusion, headache, fatigue

   b. Orthostatic hypotension

   c. Blurred vision

   d. Constipation, dry mouth

   e. Rash, itching

9. Adverse effects/toxicity

   a. Neutropenia

   b. Respiratory depression

   c. ECG changes, tachycardia

10. Nursing considerations

   a. Assess BP (lying, standing), pulse; if systolic BP drops 20 mmHg, withhold drug, notify physician because of orthostatic hypotension

   b. Assess hepatic and renal function (AST, ALT, bilirubin, creatinine, high density lipoprotein), alkaline phosphatase

   c. Assess for mental status changes including mood, sensorium, affect, memory (long and short term)

   d. Assess respiratory status for depression including rate, rhythm, depth

   e. Assess for seizure activity including type, duration, and precipitating factors

   f. Evaluate client for therapeutic responses such as reduced or absent seizure activity, anxiety

11. Client education

 a. Instruct client about medication regimen including name, dose, schedule, side effects, and possible adverse effects

 b. Instruct client to avoid other CNS depressants, including alcohol

 c. Advise client not to discontinue medication abruptly or without consulting physician

 d. Instruct client to avoid hazardous activities until stabilized on drug; drowsiness may occur

E. Other anticonvulsants

 1. Carbamazepine (Tegretol)

 a. Action and use

 1) Inhibits nerve impulses by limiting influx of sodium ions across cell membrane in motor cortex

 2) Used in tonic-clonic, complex-partial, and mixed seizures

 b. For dosage see Table 10-4

 c. Administration considerations

 1) Give oral forms with food or milk to reduce GI symptoms

 2) Chewable pills must be chewed or crushed, should not be swallowed whole

 3) Medications administered via NG tube must be mixed with D_5W or NS and flushed with at least 100 mL solution afterwards

 d. Contraindications

 1) Hypersensitivity to carbamazepine or tricyclic antidepressants

 2) Contraindicated with bone marrow depression and concomitant use of MAOIs

 e. Significant drug interactions: see Table 10-4

 f. Significant food interactions: increased peak concentrations of carbamazepine with grapefruit

 g. Significant laboratory studies: increases false negatives for pregnancy tests

 h. Side effects

 1) Increased PT

 2) Syndrome of inappropriate anti-diuretic hormone (SIADH), mostly with elderly

 3) Drowsiness, dizziness, confusion

 4) Nausea, constipation, diarrhea, vomiting

 5) Rash, urticaria

 6) Tinnitis, dry mouth, blurred vision, nystagmus

 7) Hypotension

8) Fever, dyspnea, pneumonitis

9) Urinary frequency or retention, increased BUN

  i. Adverse effects/toxicity

1) Thrombocytopenia, agranulocytosis, leukocytosis, neutropenia, aplastic anemia, eosinophilia

2) Paralysis, worsening of seizures

3) Hepatitis

4) Stevens-Johnson syndrome

5) Hypertension, CHF, dysrhythmias, AV block

6) CNS toxicity with lithium

7) Fatal reaction with MAOIs

  j. Nursing considerations

1) Assess for seizure activity including type, duration, and precipitating factors

2) Monitor blood, hepatic, and renal studies including RBC, Hct, Hgb, reticulocyte count, AST, ALT, bilirubin, UA, BUN, creatinine

3) Assess mental status including mood, sensorium, affect, and memory (long- and short-term)

4) Assess for eye problems; may need regular ophthalmic exams

5) Assess for allergic reactions including purpura or red, raised rash

6) Assess for blood dyscrasias, fever, sore throat, bruising, rash, or jaundice

7) Evaluate client for therapeutic response such as decreased or absent seizure activity

  k. Client education

1) Instruct client about medication regimen including name, dose, schedule, side effects, and possible adverse effects

2) Instruct client to avoid other CNS depressants including alcohol

3) Advise client not to discontinue medication abruptly or without consulting physician

4) Instruct client to avoid hazardous activities until stabilized on drug, drowsiness may occur

5) Instruct client to carry Medic-Alert ID with name, drug, physician's name, phone number

6) Inform client that urine may turn pink to brown

  2. Valproate sodium

    a. Action and use

1) Increases levels of GABA in brain, which decreases seizure activity

2) Use in simple (petit mal), complex (petit mal) absence, or mixed seizures; manic episodes associate with bipolar disorder and migraine headaches

b. For dosage see Table 10-4

c. Administration considerations

   1) Do not crush tablets or capsules; take them whole

   2) Elixir forms should be given alone; do not dilute with carbonated beverage

   3) May give with food or milk to decrease GI symptoms

d. Contraindications

   1) Hypersensitivity

   2) Contraindicated during pregnancy and with hepatic disease

e. Significant drug interactions: see Table 10-4

f. Significant food interactions: none reported

g. Significant laboratory studies

   1) Increase the risk of false positive for ketones

   2) Interfere with thyroid function tests

h. Side effects

   1) Sedation, drowsiness

   2) Nausea, vomiting, constipation, diarrhea, heartburn

   3) Rash

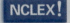

i. Adverse effects/toxicity

   1) Thrombocytopenia, leukopenia, lymphocytosis

   2) Hepatic failure, pancreatitis, toxic hepatitis

j. Nursing considerations

   1) Assess for seizure activity including type, duration, and precipitating factors

   2) Monitor blood, hepatic and renal studies including red blood cell (RBC), Hct, Hgb, serum folate, protime, platelets, vitamin D, reticulocyte count, AST, ALT, bilirubin, urine analysis, BUN, creatinine

   3) Assess mental status such as mood, sensorium, affect, and memory (long- and short-term)

   4) Assess respiratory status/depression including rate, rhythm, and depth

   5) Evaluate client for therapeutic response, such as decreased seizure activity

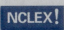

k. Client education

   1) Instruct client about medication regimen including name, dose, schedule, side effects, and possible adverse effects

   2) Instruct client to avoid other CNS depressants including alcohol

3) Instruct client not to discontinue medication abruptly or without consulting physician

4) Advise client to avoid hazardous activities until stabilized on drug; drowsiness may occur

5) Instruct client to carry medic alert ID with name, drug, physician's name, and phone number

6) Inform client that physical dependency may result from extended use

7) Advise client to report visual disturbances, rash, diarrhea, light colored stools, jaundice, or protracted vomiting to provider

III. Central Nervous System (CNS) Stimulants

A. Anorexiants

1. Action and use

   a. Most act similar to amphetamines, as indirect sympathomimetic amines with alpha- and beta-adrenergic activity

   b. Anorexigenic effect results from direct inhibition of lateral hypothalamic appetite center, as well as mood elevation

   c. Used for **narcolepsy** (inability to stay awake during day), **attention deficit disorder** (ADD), **attention deficit hyperactivity disorder** (ADHD) and in short-term adjunct to control obesity

2. Common medications (Table 10-5)

3. Administration considerations

   a. Anorexiant effects are temporary

   b. To avoid insomnia, take 6 hours prior to bedtime

   c. Do not abruptly discontinue medication

   d. Diethylproprion should be given on empty stomach; additional dose may be given mid-evening to control nighttime hunger; do not discontinue medication abruptly

4. Contraindications

   a. Hypersensitivity

   b. Contraindicated with angle-closure glaucoma, advanced cardiac disease, hyperthyroidism, agitated states, history of drug abuse, and children under 12 years of age

5. Significant drug interactions: see Table 10-5

6. Significant food interactions: none reported

7. Significant laboratory studies: none reported

8. Side effects

   a. Restlessness, insomnia

   b. Palpitations

Table 10-5	Medication	Usual Adult Dose	Significant Drug Interactions
Central Nervous System (Adrenergic) Stimulants	***Anorexiants*** Benzphetamine hydrochloride (Didrex)	25–50 mg 1–3 times/day PO	Decreased elimination of benzphetamine: acetazolamide, sodium bicarbonate Increased elimination of benzphetamine: ammonium chloride, ascorbic acid Decreased effects of: guanethidine, guanadrel Hypertensive crisis and intracranial hemorrhage may occur if given within 14 days of MAOIs or selegiline Decreased effectiveness of benzphetamine: tricyclic antidepressants
	Diethylpropion hydrochloride (Proprion)	25 mg tid, PO 30–60 min a.c. or 75 mg sustained-release QD midmorning	Increased BP effects: furazolidone Increased effects of: alcohol, other CNS depressants
	Sibutramine hydrochloride monohydrate (Meridia)	10 mg once daily PO; may be increased to 15 mg if inadequate weight loss (less than 4 lb in 4 weeks)	Increased BP effects: decongestants, cough, allergy medications; should not be taken with MAOIs Decreased clearance of sibutramine: ketoconazole
	Amphetamines		Decreased elimination of amphetamine: acetazolamide, sodium bicarbonate
	Amphetamine sulfate (Adderall)	Narcolepsy: 5–60 mg/day PO divided q4–6h in 2–3 doses Obesity: 5–10 mg PO 1 before meals	Increased elimination of amphetamine: ammonium chloride, ascorbic acid Decreased effects of: guanethidine, guanadrel Hypertensive crisis and intracranial hemorrhage may occur if given within 14 days of MAOIs or selegiline Decreased effectiveness of amphetamine: tricyclic antidepressants Increased BP effects: furazolidone Increased effects of: alcohol, other CNS depressants
	Methylphenidate hydrochloride (Ritalin)	Narcolepsy: 10 mg bid or tid PO, 30–45 min p.c. ADD (child): 5–10 mg before breakfast and lunch, with a gradual increase of 5–10 mg/wk	Hypertensive crisis: MAOIs within 14 days, or vasopressor Increased sympathomimetic effect: decongestants, vasoconstrictors Decreased effects of: warfarin, tricyclics, anticonvulsants
	Dextro-amphetamine sulfate (Dexadrine)	Narcolepsy 5–20 mg 1–3 times/day at 4–6h intervals PO ADD (child): 5 mg 1–2 times/day, PO; may increase by 5 mg at weekly intervals	Hypertensive crisis: MAOIs within 14 days; Delayed absorption: barbiturates, phenytoin Increased effect of dextroamphetamine: acetazolamide, antacids, $NaHCO_3$ Increased CNS effect: haloperidol, tricyclics, phenothiazines Decreased effect of dextroamphetamine: ascorbic acid, ammonium chloride Decreased effect of: adrenergic blockers, antidiabetics
	Pemoline (Cylert)	ADD: 37.5 mg/day PO; may be increased by 18.75 mg weekly	Increased CNS effect: other CNS stimulants

   c. Dysmenorrhea

 9. Adverse effects/toxicity

   a. Decrease in seizure threshold in epilepsy

   b. Tachycardia

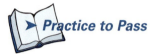

10. Nursing considerations

    a. Assess BP and pulse during treatment

    b. Current dosage of antihypertensives and antidiabetics may need to be adjusted

    c. Evaluate client for therapeutic response such as decrease in weight over time

11. Client education

    a. Discuss all medications currently taken (including OTC) with provider; serious or even fatal interactions can occur

    b. Instruct client to take medications exactly as prescribed

    c. Inform client that sustained-release tablets should be taken whole, not crushed

    d. Instruct client to avoid driving or other hazardous activities until reaction to medication is determined

B. Amphetamines

1. Action and use

    a. Increase release of norepinephrine and dopamine in cerebral cortex to **reticular activating system,** a diffuse system that extends from the lower brain stem to the cerebral cortex

    b. Used in treating narcolepsy, exogenous obesity, attention deficit disorder

2. Common medications (Table 10-5)

3. Administration considerations

    a. Give the first dose on awakening and give the last dose not closer than 6 hours to bedtime

    b. Administer on empty stomach 30 to 60 minutes prior to meal

4. Contraindications

    a. Hypersensitivity

    b. Contraindicated with hyperthyroidism, hypertension, glaucoma, severe arteriosclerosis, drug abuse, cardiovascular disease, anxiety, or lactation

5. Significant drug interactions: see Table 10-5

6. Significant food interactions: none reported

7. Significant laboratory studies: serum thyroxine (T_4) with high amphetamine doses

8. Side effects

    a. Hyperactivity, insomnia, restlessness, talkativeness

    b. Dry mouth, nausea, vomiting

> **▶ Practice to Pass**
>
> A female client has started taking an anorexiant as prescribed by her physician for weight reduction. If she has multiple medical diagnoses, what types of medications might need to be adjusted because of the addition of the anorexiant?

    c. Impotence, change in libido

    d. Palpitations, tachycardia

9. Adverse effects/toxicity: same as above

10. Nursing considerations

    a. Assess vital signs, especially BP, since anorexiants may reverse antihypertensive medication action

    b. Monitor CBC, urinanalysis, and in diabetics, monitor blood and urine glucose levels; changes in insulin may be required

    c. Assess mental status for mood, sensorium, and affect; stimulation, insomnia, or aggressiveness may occur

    d. Assess for withdrawal symptoms including headache, nausea, vomiting, muscle pain, weakness

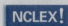

    e. Evaluate client for therapeutic responses such as decreased activity in ADHD, absence of sleeping during day in narcolepsy, decrease in weight

11. Client education

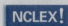

    a. Instruct client about medication regimen including name, dose, schedule, side effects, and possible adverse effects of the medication; if a dose is missed, do not take double dose

    b. Advise client to avoid or decrease caffeine consumption (coffee, tea, cola, chocolate), which may increase irritability or stimulation

    c. Advise client to avoid OTC preparations unless approved by provider and avoid alcohol consumption

    d. Instruct client not to discontinue medication abruptly or without consulting physician

    e. Advise client to avoid hazardous activities until stabilized on drug, drowsiness may occur

    f. Inform client about the importance of rest

    g. Inform client that seizure threshold is decreased in clients with seizure disorders

C. Medications to treat narcolepsy and attention deficit hyperactivity disorder (ADHD)

1. Action and use

    a. Increase release of norepinephrine, dopamine in cerebral cortex to reticular activating system

    b. Used in ADHD and narcolepsy

2. Common medications (Table 10-5)

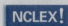

3. Administration considerations: administer medication at least 6 hours prior to bedtime

4. Contraindications

   a. Hypersensitivity

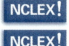

   b. Contraindicated with anxiety, history of Tourette's syndrome, children under 6 years of age, and glaucoma

5. Significant drug interactions: see Table 10-5

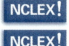

6. Significant food interactions

   a. Increased stimulation with caffeine

   b. Increased amine effect with caffeine

7. Significant laboratory studies: none reported

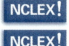

8. Side effects

   a. Hyperactivity, insomnia, restlessness, and talkativeness

   b. Dry mouth

   c. Palpitations and tachycardia

   d. Rash

9. Adverse effects/toxicity

   a. Dysrhythmias, thrombocytopenic purpura

   b. Exfoliative dermatitis

   c. Uremia

   d. Leukopenia or anemia

10. Nursing considerations

    a. Assess vital signs, especially BP, since reversal of antihypertensive medication effects may occur

    b. Monitor CBC, urinanalysis, and in diabetics, monitor closely blood and urine glucose levels; changes in insulin may be required

    c. Assess for mental status changes including mood, sensorium, and affect; stimulation, insomnia, and aggressiveness may occur

    d. Assess for withdrawal symptoms including headache, nausea, vomiting, muscle pain, weakness

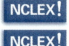

    e. Assess client for changes in appetite, sleep, speech patterns

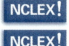

    f. Assess client for increased attention span and decreased hyperactivity

      g. Evaluate client for therapeutic responses such as decreased activity in ADHD, absence of sleeping during day in narcolepsy, or decrease in weight

  11. Client education

      a. Instruct client about medication regimen including name, dose, schedule, side effects, and possible adverse effects

      b. Instruct client to avoid or decrease caffeine consumption (coffee, tea, cola, chocolate), which may increase irritability or stimulation

      c. Advise client to avoid OTC preparations unless approved by provider and avoid alcohol consumption

      d. Advise client not to discontinue medication abruptly or without consulting physician

      e. Advise client to avoid hazardous activities until stabilized on drug; drowsiness may occur

      f. Inform client that seizure threshold is decreased in clients with seizure disorders

IV. Medications to Treat Parkinson's Disease

A. Anticholinergics

  1. Action and use

      a. Block or compete at central acetylcholine receptor sites in the autonomic nervous system

      b. Used to decrease involuntary movements in parkinsonism

  2. Common medications (Table 10-6)

  3. Administration considerations

      a. Parenteral dose of trihexyphenidyl is given with client in recumbent position to prevent postural hypotension

      b. Oral form of trihexyphenidyl is given with or after food to prevent GI upset; may give with fluids other than water

      c. Parenteral dose of benztropine is given slowly; keep client at least 1 hour after administering medication and monitor vital signs

      d. Monitor dosage of medication very carefully; even slight overdose can lead to toxicity

  4. Contraindications: clients with narrow-angle glaucoma, myasthenia gravis, or GI obstruction should not use

  5. Significant drug interactions: see Table 10-6

  6. Significant food interactions: none reported

  7. Significant laboratory studies: none reported

  8. Side effects

Table 10-6	**Medication**	**Usual Adult Dose**	**Significant Drug Interactions**
Medications Used to Treat Parkinson's Disease	***Anticholinergics*** Trihexyphenidyl hydrochloride (Artane)—*used in young clients with disabling tremors*	1 mg on day 1, 2 mg on day 2 PO, then increase by 2 mg q3–5d up to 6–10 mg/day	Increased anticholinergic effects: MAOIs, tricyclic antidepressants, amantadine Decreased effect of: phenothiazines, levodopa
	Benztropine mesylate (Cogentin)—*tremor treatment alone or in combination*	0.5–1 mg/day PO gradually increased as needed up to 6 mg/day	
	Antiviral Amantadine hydrochloride (Symmetrel)	100 mg 1–2 times/day PO	Increased anticholinergic effects: atropine, other anticholinergics Increased CNS stimulation: CNS stimulants Decreased renal excretion of amantadine: triamterene, hydrochlorothiazide
	Levodopa In combination as Sinemet, (L-dopa and Carbidopa)	500 mg to 1 gram daily PO in 2 or more equally divided doses, may be increased by 100–750 mg q3–7h	Hypertensive crisis: MAOIs, furazolidone Decreased effects of L-dopa: anticholinergics, hydantoins, methionine, papaverine, pyridoxine, benzodiazepines Increased effects of L-dopa: antacids, metoclopramide
	Dopamine agonists Bromocriptine mesylate (Parlodel)	1.25–2.5 mg/day PO up to 100 mg/day in divided doses	Decreased effects of bromocriptine: phenothiazines, oral contraceptives, progestins, estrogens, haloperidol, loxapine, methyldopa, metoclopramide, MAOIs, reserpine Increased effects of: antihypertensives, levodopa
	Pergolide (Permax)	Initiate with 0.05 mg daily for 2 days PO; then increase by 0.1 or 0.15 mg every 3 days for the next 12 days	Disulfiram-like reaction: alcohol Combination with levodopa: increase incidence of dyskinesias
	Monoamine oxidase B inhibitor Selegiline hydrochloride (Eldepryl)	5 mg bid PO	FATAL INTERACTION: opioids (esp. meperidine); do not give together Serotonin syndrome (confusion, seizures, fever, hypertension, agitation): fluoxetine, paroxetine, sertraline, fluvoxamine, (discontinue 5 wks prior to selegiline) Increased side effects of: levodopa/ carbidopa Do not use with tricyclics

       a. Dry mouth, constipation

       b. Urinary retention or hesitancy

       c. Headache or dizziness

   9. Adverse effects/toxicity: paralytic ileus

  10. Nursing considerations

       a. Monitor I & O; retention may cause decreased urinary output

       b. Assess client for urinary hesitancy and retention; palpate bladder if retention occurs

       c. Assess client for constipation; increase fluids, bulk, and exercise to counteract constipation

       d. If tolerance occurs during long-term therapy, dose may need to be increased or changed

       e. Assess mental status for affect, mood, CNS depression, worsening of mental symptoms during early therapy

       f. Evaluate client for therapeutic responses such as decreased tremors, secretions, absence of nausea and vomiting

  11. Client education

       a. Advise client to avoid driving or other hazardous activities; drowsiness may occur

       b. Advise client to avoid OTC medications such as cough and cold preparations with alcohol, and antihistamines unless prescribed by provider

B. Medications affecting the amount of dopamine in the brain

  1. Action and use

       a. These medications include amantadine, levodopa, dopamine agonists and MAO type B inhibitors

       b. Amantadine (an antiviral) promotes the synthesis and release of dopamine

       c. L-dopa is the immediate natural precursor of dopamine

       d. Dopamine agonists (DA) directly stimulate specific subclasses of dopamine receptors

       e. MAO type B inhibitors (MAOBI) increase dopamine activity by an incompletely understood mechanism

       f. DAs and MAOBIs are used to enhance the effects of L-dopa

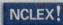

       g. All are used to increase the available dopamine; by having more dopamine available to the body, the parkinsonism symptoms are decreased

  2. Common medications (Table 10-6)

  3. Administration considerations

       a. Administer medication after meals for better absorption and to decrease GI symptoms

       b. Absorption of levodopa and selegiline is decreased with high protein meals

4. Contraindications

   a. Hypersensitivity

   b. Narrow-angle glaucoma

   c. Undiagnosed skin lesions

5. Significant drug interactions: see Table 10-6

6. Significant food interactions

   a. Decreased levodopa and selegiline absorption with high-protein foods

   b. With selegiline, tyramine-containing foods may increase hypertensive reactions

7. Significant laboratory studies

   a. Bromocriptine: increases growth hormone, AST, ALT, potassium, BUN, uric acid, alkaline phosphatase

   b. Pergolide suppresses prolactin levels

   c. Selegiline results in false positive of urine ketones and glucose; also results in false negative of urine glucose

8. Side effects

   a. Nausea, vomiting, dry mouth, and constipation

   b. Dizziness, headache, and depression

   c. Cough

   d. Cardiac dysrhythmias and orthostatic hypotension

   e. Sleep disturbance, "on-off" phenomenon

9. Adverse effects/toxicity

   a. Amantadine: convulsions, CHF, leukopenia

   b. Levodopa: hemolytic anemia, leukopenia, agranulocytosis

   c. DAs: convulsions, shock

   d. MAOBIs: tachycardia or sinus bradycardia

   e. Levodopa toxicity: mental, personality changes, increased twitching, grimacing, tongue protrusion

10. Nursing considerations

    a. Assess BP and respirations

    b. Assess mental status for affect, mood, behavioral changes, depression; complete a suicide assessment

    c. Monitor for involuntary movement, akinesia, tremors, staggering gait, muscle rigidity, and drooling

    d. Evaluate client for therapeutic responses such as a decrease in akathisia and increased mood

11. Client education

    a. Instruct client to change positions slowly to prevent orthostatic hypotension

    b. Advise client to report side effects such as twitching and eye spasm; may indicate overdose

    c. Instruct client to use drugs exactly as prescribed; never discontinue them abruptly since this may precipitate parkinsonian crisis

    d. Advise client to avoid alcohol use

    e. Advise client not to take foods high in protein

V. Medications to Treat Alzheimer's Disease

A. Action and use

    1. Cholinesterase inhibitors elevate acetylcholine concentrations in cerebral cortex

    2. They accomplish this by slowing degradation of acetylcholine released in cholinergic neurons

B. Common medications (Table 10-7)

C. Administration considerations

    1. Administer medication between meals; may be given with meal to reduce GI symptoms

    2. Dosage adjusted to response no more frequently than every 6 weeks

D. Contraindications

    1. Hypersensitivity to the drug

    2. Development of jaundice when taking drug

E. Significant drug interactions: see Table 10-7

F. Significant food interactions: none reported

G. Significant laboratory studies: none reported

H. Side effects

    1. Insomnia, headache, dizziness, confusion, ataxia, anxiety, depression, hostility, and abnormal thinking

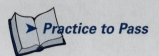

Practice to Pass

A client with Parkinson's disease is admitted to the nursing unit after a surgical procedure. What type of medication would you be careful not to administer because he takes selegiline, an MAOBI?

NCLEX!

NCLEX!

	Medication	Usual Adult Dose	Significant Drug Interactions
Table 10-7 **Medications Used to Treat Alzheimer's Disease**	Donepezil hydrochloride (Aricept)	5–10 mg PO, hs	Decreased activity of anticholinergics Synergistic effects: succinylcholine, cholinesterase inhibitors, cholinergic agonists Increased gastric acid secretions: NSAIDs Decreased donepezil effect: carbamazepine, dexamethasone, phenytoin, phenobarbital, rifampin
	Tacrine (Cognex)	10 mg qid, PO increase in 40 mg/day increments not sooner than q6 weeks to a maximum of 160 mg/day	Decreased activity of anticholinergics Increased levels of tacrine: cimetidine Increased elimination half-life of theophylline Synergistic effects: succinylcholine, cholinesterase inhibitors, cholinergic agonists

2. Nausea, vomiting, diarrhea, abdominal pain, and constipation

3. Urinary frequency and incontinence

4. Rash

5. Rhinitis or cough

I. Adverse effects/toxicity

1. Seizures

2. Hepatotoxicity

3. Urinary tract infection (UTI)

4. Atrial fibrillation

J. Nursing considerations

1. Assess BP for hypotension or hypertension

2. Assess mental status for affect, mood, behavioral changes, depression, hallucinations, confusion; complete a suicide assessment

3. Assess GI status for nausea, vomiting, anorexia, constipation, or abdominal pain

4. Assess client for urinary frequency and incontinence

5. Monitor liver function tests frequently

6. Evaluate client for therapeutic responses such as decrease in confusion, improved mood

K. Client education

1. Instruct client or caregiver to report side effects such as twitching, nausea, vomiting, sweating; they might indicate overdose

2. Instruct client or caregiver to use drug exactly as prescribed, at regular intervals, preferably between meals, may be taken with food to decrease GI upset

3. Advise client or caregiver to notify provider of nausea, vomiting, diarrhea (dose increase or beginning treatment) or rash

4. Advise client or caregiver not to increase or abruptly decrease dose; serious consequences may result

5. Inform client that drug is not a cure; it only relieves symptoms

VI. Centrally-Acting Skeletal Muscle Relaxants

A. Medications for spasticity

1. Action and use

   a. Decrease the synaptic responses at neurotransmitters to decrease frequency, severity of spasms

   b. Used to reduce **spasticity** (increased resistance to passive movement) after spinal cord injuries, strokes, and in cerebral palsy and multiple sclerosis

2. Common medications (Table 10-8)

3. Administration considerations: see Table 10-8

Table 10-8	**Medication**	**Usual Adult Dose**	**Significant Drug Interactions**
Skeletal Muscle Relaxants	Baclofen (Lioresal)	5 mg tid PO up to 5 mg/dose q3d prn; give with meals for GI symptoms; intrathecal, do not use IT solution for IM, IV, SC or epidural administration	Increased CNS depression: alcohol, tricyclic antidepressants, opiates, barbiturates, sedatives, hypnotics Dysrhythmias: verapamil IV Increased CNS depression: alcohol, tricyclic antidepressants, opiates, barbiturates, sedatives, hypnotics, antihistamines
	Dantrolene sodium (Dantrium)	25 mg once/day PO; increase to 25 mg bid to qid up to 100 mg; give with meals for GI symptoms	Increased action: warfarin, clofibrate Hepatotoxicity: estrogens Considered incompatible in syringe or solution
	Carisoprodol (Soma)	350 mg tid PO with meals for GI symptoms	Increased CNS depression: alcohol, tricyclic antidepressants, opiates, barbiturates, sedatives, hypnotics
	Cycloben-zaprine hydrochloride (Flexeril)	20–40 mg/day PO in 2–4 divided doses, up to 60 mg/day with meals for GI symptoms	Increased CNS depression: alcohol, tricyclic antidepressants, opiates, barbiturates, sedatives, hypnotics Do not use within 14 days of MAOIs
	Methocarbamol (Robaxin)	1.5 g qid PO for 2–3 days, then 4–4.5 g/day in 3–6 divided doses with meals for GI symptoms; 0.5–1 g q8h IM; 1–3 g/day IV in divided doses Give IV undiluted over 1 min. or more; give 300 mg or less/min Keep recumbent for 15 min after dose to prevent orthostatic hypotension Give IM deep in large muscle mass; rotate sites	Increased CNS depression: alcohol, tricyclic antidepressants, opiates, barbiturates, sedatives, hypnotics Considered incompatible in syringe or solution

4. Contraindications

   a. Hypersensitivity to medication

   b. Contraindicated in compromised pulmonary function, active hepatic disease, impaired myocardial function

5. Significant drug interactions: see Table 10-8

6. Significant food interactions: none reported

7. Significant laboratory studies: baclofen increases AST, alkaline phosphatase, and blood glucose levels

8. Side effects

   a. Dizziness, weakness, fatigue, drowsiness, disorientation

   b. Nausea, vomiting

9. Adverse effects/toxicity

   a. Seizures

   b. Eosinophilia, hepatic injury

10. Nursing considerations

    NCLEX!

    a. Monitor BP, weight, blood glucose level, and hepatic function

    b. Assess client for increased seizure activity; drugs decrease seizure threshold

    c. Monitor I & O, check for urinary frequency, retention, or hesitancy

    d. Monitor electroencephalogram (EEG) in epileptic clients due to poor seizure control

    e. Assess client for allergic reactions, fever, rash, or respiratory distress

    f. Monitor client for severe weakness or numbness in extremities

    NCLEX!

    g. Monitor client for CNS depression, dizziness, drowsiness, or psychiatric symptoms

    h. Monitor hepatic function (AST, ALT) and renal function (BUN, creatinine, CBC)

    NCLEX!

    i. Evaluate client for therapeutic responses such as decrease in pain and spasticity

    NCLEX!

11. Client education

    a. Advise client not to discontinue medication quickly; hallucinations, spasticity, tachycardia will occur; it should be tapered off gradually by provider

    b. Advise client to notify provider of abdominal pain, jaundiced sclera, clay-colored stools, or change in color of urine

    c. Advise client not to take alcohol or other CNS depressants

    d. Instruct client to avoid using OTC medications, cough preparations, or antihistamines, unless recommended by provider

    e. Advise client not to break, crush or chew capsules

B. Medications used for spasms

1. Action and use

    a. Depress multisynaptic pathways in the spinal cord, causing skeletal muscle relaxation and/or sedation

    b. Used for adjunct relief of **spasms** (involuntary contractions of large muscles) and pain in musculoskeletal conditions

2. Common medications (Table 10-8)

3. Administration considerations: see Table 10-8

4. Contraindications

    a. Hypersensitivity

    b. Contraindicated in children under age of 12, clients with intermittent por-phyria, acute recovery phase of MI, heart block, CHF, or thyroid disease

5. Significant drug interactions: see Table 10-8

6. Significant food interactions: none reported

7. Significant laboratory studies: methocarbamol results in false increased levels of VMA, urinary 5-HIAA

8. Side effects

    a. Dizziness, weakness, drowsiness

    b. Nausea

9. Adverse effects/toxicity

    a. Erythema multiforme

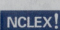

    b. Angioedema, anaphylaxis

    c. Dysrhythmias

    d. Seizures

10. Nursing considerations

    a. Blood studies including CBC, WBC with differentials

    b. During and after injection, assess for CNS effects, rash, conjunctivitis and nasal congestion

    c. Liver studies including AST, ALT, alkaline phosphatase

    d. EEG in clients with seizures

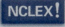

    e. Assess for allergic reactions including idiosyncratic reaction, anaphylaxis, rash, fever, or respiratory distress

    f. Assess client for severe weakness or numbness in extremities

    g. Assess for CNS depression, dizziness, drowsiness, and psychiatric symptoms

    h. Monitor client for psychological dependency, increased need for drug, and increased pain

    i. Evaluate client for therapeutic responses such as decreased pain, spasm, and spasticity

11. Client education

    a. Advise client not to discontinue medication abruptly; insomnia, nausea, headache, spasticity, tachycardia will occur

b. Advise client not to take with alcohol or other CNS depressants

c. Instruct client to avoid using OTC medications, cough preparations, antihistamines, unless recommended by provider

d. Instruct client to avoid hazardous activities if drowsiness/dizziness occurs

VII. Antianxiety, Sedative, and Hypnotics (refer to Chapter 11)

Case Study

T. P., a 48-year-old male client, is admitted to the Emergency Department (ED) after having a seizure while attending church. You are the admitting nurse in the ED. The client has a history of a seizure disorder. He is arousable but lethargic.

❶ What questions will you ask the client or the family upon arrival?

❷ What initial assessments will you make?

❸ What are the priorities of care for the client while he is in the ED?

❹ What education points are of highest priority prior to discharge home?

❺ Give examples of medications or foods that could interfere with T. P.'s prescribed seizure medications, phenytoin (Dilantin) and phenobarbital (Luminal).

For suggested responses, see page 640.

Posttest

1 The client is newly diagnosed with Parkinson's disease. The medication that has been prescribed is levodopa (Dopar). The nurse should place a high priority on teaching which of the following information prior to discharge?

(1) Side effects include cushingoid symptoms such as moon face and weight gain.
(2) There is a need to avoid vaccinations.
(3) Report any ulcerations or sores in the mouth to provider immediately.
(4) Avoid high-protein foods since they interfere with absorption of the medication.

2 Which of the following statements made by the client indicates an understanding of client teaching regarding anticonvulsant therapy?

(1) "After taking the medication, I should lie down."
(2) "I must be sure to have my cholesterol levels checked regularly."
(3) "It is essential for me to continue to take this medication to avoid recurrence of seizures."
(4) "Seizures will often stop without intervention, so I may not need this medication for long."

3 Which of the following statements made by the client with migraine headaches would indicate that she has understood client teaching regarding migraine medication?

(1) "I will be keeping a diary of my headaches so that I can see if there is a pattern."
(2) "I will be able to stop my exercise program since it has not helped my headaches."
(3) "I will take my headache medication every 4 hours."
(4) "I will never be able to drive again due to my headaches."

4 The client has been diagnosed with attention deficit hyperactivity disorder (ADHD), and the provider is considering prescribing methylphenidate (Ritalin). Which of the following past medical histories would be a contraindication for Ritalin?

(1) A history of chicken pox
(2) A history of diabetes
(3) A history of seizures
(4) A history of Tourette's syndrome

5 A female client is being medicated with a central nervous system (CNS) stimulant. The nurse should place highest priority on educating the client about adverse drug interactions with which type of medication she is presently taking?

(1) Nonsteroidal anti-inflammatory drug (NSAID)
(2) Skeletal muscle relaxant
(3) Antihypertensive
(4) Opioid analgesic

6 A client has begun taking an anticholinergic medication. The nurse plans to carefully assess which of the following client parameters?

(1) Pain intensity, respiratory rate, and level of consciousness
(2) Urinary retention, hesitancy and constipation
(3) Seizure activity, mental status, and respiratory status
(4) Electrolytes, blood glucose levels, and leg edema

7 The nurse is transcribing medication orders for a client taking selegiline (Eldepryl). The nurse makes it a priority to telephone the prescriber after noting an order for which of the following types of medications?

(1) Monoamine oxidase inhibitor (MAOI)
(2) Opioid analgesic
(3) Skeletal muscle relaxant
(4) Anticholinergic

8 A client has been given a prescription for a medication affecting the musculoskeletal system. Which of the following points would the nurse include as significant when teaching the client about this medication?

(1) To decrease risk factors by eating a low-fat diet, increasing exercise, and cessation of smoking
(2) The use of sunscreen, vitamins, and hats
(3) The history of the disease for which they are being medicated
(4) Name, dose, schedule, side effects, and possible adverse effects of the medication

9 A client with a seizure disorder is being medicated with IV phenytoin (Dilantin). The physician changes the mode of administration to feeding tube. Which of the following points does the nurse need to keep in mind so that the client's blood level of phenytoin does not decrease?

(1) The tube feeding should be stopped 30–60 minutes before and after administration of the medication to allow for proper absorption.
(2) The suspension of phenytoin is specially designed to be absorbed with tube feedings.
(3) The dose of IV phenytoin must be increased when given by the feeding tube.
(4) No specific requirements are needed to ensure the drug level stays steady.

10 The client has a back injury. The provider orders cyclobenzaprine (Flexeril) for the muscle spasms. What significant educational point does the nurse need to share with the client?

(1) "Do not take this medication with alcohol or cough preparations, and do not drive during its use."
(2) "It is important for you to have your cholesterol levels checked regularly."
(3) "An apical pulse must be taken prior to taking this medication."
(4) "The medication must be finished even if symptoms improve or cease."

See pages 399–400 for Answers and Rationales.

Answers and Rationales

Pretest

1 Answer: 3 *Rationale:* Methylphenidate is a central nervous system stimulant. It increases releases of norepinephrine and dopamine in cerebral cortex to reticular activating system. Ritalin is contraindicated in clients with glaucoma. Congestive heart failure, diabetes mellitus, and hyperthyroidism do not represent contraindications to the use of methylphenidate.
Cognitive Level: Application
Nursing Process: Planning; *Test Plan:* PHYS

2 Answer: 2 *Rationale:* Medication must be taken to maintain therapeutic blood levels, even if there is no seizure activity. The urine may turn pink or brown, but that is not the most important item to teach. Options 1 and 4 are incorrect. After 6 months with no seizures, a client can often drive again.
Cognitive Level: Analysis
Nursing Process: Implementation; *Test Plan:* HPM

3 Answer: 4 *Rationale:* The client needs to give the medication opportunity to work without aggravating the headache. Ergotamine should be given orally 1 to 2 mg followed by 1 to 2 mg every 30 minutes until the headache abates or until the maximum dose of 6 mg/24 hours (option 1). It is unnecessary to drink large amounts of fluids (option 2) and increased warmth and energy are not associated with this medication (option 3).
Cognitive Level: Application
Nursing Process: Implementation; *Test Plan:* PHYS

4 Answer: 2 *Rationale:* Dantrolene is a central-acting skeletal muscle relaxant. This medication may be used to control spasticity after spinal cord injury. Dexamethasone is a corticosteroid used to decrease swelling, especially cerebral edema. Dichlorphenamide is a carbonic anhydrase inhibitor used to treat glaucoma by decreasing production of aqueous humor and thereby lowering intraocular pressure. Dobutamine is a medication used to treat hypotension by increasing cardiac output.
Cognitive Level: Application
Nursing Process: Analysis; *Test Plan:* PHYS

5 Answer: 1 *Rationale:* Because opioid analgesics relieve pain, the nurse needs to assess the client's pain intensity before and 30 minutes after administering a dose. The respiratory rate and level of consciousness need to be assessed because respiratory depression and sedation are two adverse effects of this drug class. The items in the each of the other options are only partially correct. Urine output, liver function studies, seizure activity, electrolytes and blood glucose are not ongoing assessments directly related to opioid administration.
Cognitive Level: Application
Nursing Process: Assessment; *Test Plan:* PHYS

6 Answer: 2 *Rationale:* Clients may take more aspirin, acetaminophen, and NSAIDs than prescribed by their providers if they are not aware that many OTC medications are combined with these medications. The other answers are cautions for other a variety of other types of medications.
Cognitive Level: Application
Nursing Process: Implementation; *Test Plan:* PHYS

7 Answer: 3 *Rationale:* The client should be assessed for seizure activity, changes in mental status, and respiratory status as highest priority. Assessing kidney function (BUN and creatinine) and urine output are not the priority nursing considerations when the client is taking anticonvulsants. The assessments in the other options are pertinent for a variety of other types of medications.
Cognitive Level: Application
Nursing Process: Assessment; *Test Plan:* PHYS

8 Answer: 4 *Rationale:* Tegretol is contraindicated within 14 days of taking MAOIs because this can lead to a fatal reaction. The other drug classes listed do not have this interactive effect with carbamazepine. NSAIDs are used to treat inflammation and pain, while opioid analgesics and skeletal muscle relaxants are drug classes that exert an effect on the central nervous system.
Cognitive Level: Application
Nursing Process: Implementation; *Test Plan:* PHYS

9 Answer: 2 *Rationale:* The seizure threshold is decreased when anorexiants or amphetamines are used concurrently with anticonvulsants because of changes in the brain chemicals caused by the anorexiants and amphetamines. The medications listed in options 1 and 3 listed do not change the seizure threshold. The medications listed in option 4 may be used to treat seizures, which may raise the seizure threshold.
Cognitive Level: Application
Nursing Process: Implementation; *Test Plan:* PHYS

10 Answer: 3 *Rationale:* Dantrolene is a skeletal muscle relaxant. Hepatotoxicity is an adverse reaction

for dantrolene, which may be manifested by abdominal pain, jaundiced sclera, or clay colored stools. The items in the other options do not address this adverse effect.
Cognitive Level: Application
Nursing Process: Implementation; *Test Plan:* PHYS

Posttest

1   **Answer: 4** *Rationale:* The client needs to understand that high-protein foods must be avoided so that the medication can be absorbed properly. Side effects do not include cushinguid symptoms (option 1) or oral ulcerations (option 3). There is no need to avoid vaccinations (option 2).
Cognitive Level: Application
Nursing Process: Planning; *Test Plan:* PHYS

2   **Answer: 3** *Rationale:* Medication must be taken to maintain therapeutic blood levels, even with no seizure activity. If the client understands that adherence is important, he or she is more likely to be compliant with the medication regimen. The client does not need to lie down after a dose (option 1) or have cholesterol levels checked (option 2). Anticonvulsant therapy is prescribed for long-term or lifelong use (option 4).
Cognitive Level: Analysis
Nursing Process: Evaluation; *Test Plan:* PHYS

3   **Answer: 1** *Rationale:* If the client understands the importance of the finding the triggering factors, she or he will be more willing to be involved in decreasing the triggers, including lifestyle changes that may be necessary. The client should continue to exercise for general health and stress management (option 2). Medication may not be needed every 4 hours (option 3) and driving is permitted (option 4).
Cognitive Level: Analysis
Nursing Process: Evaluation; *Test Plan:* PHYS

4   **Answer: 4** *Rationale:* A history of Tourette's syndrome is a contraindication for Ritalin. There would be other medications that could be used for treatment of ADHD, such as pemoline (Cylert) or dextroamphetamine (Dexedrine). The medications listed in the other options are not contraindications for methylphenidate.
Cognitive Level: Application
Nursing Process: Assessment; *Test Plan:* PHYS

5   **Answer: 3** *Rationale:* The dose of an antihypertensive medication usually needs to be adjusted when a CNS stimulant is added to a client's medication regi-

men. The other options are incorrect because NSAIDs, skeletal muscle relaxants, and opioids are less affected than antihypertensives.
Cognitive Level: Analysis
Nursing Process: Planning; *Test Plan:* PHYS

6   **Answer: 2** *Rationale:* Anticholinergic medications cause decreased stimulation in the GI and urinary tract systems that lead to urinary and bowel problems such as urinary retention, hesitancy, and constipation. Other side effects of the anticholinergic medications are dry mouth and constipation. The items in options 1, 3, and 4 do not represent particular concerns when administering an anticholinergic medication.
Cognitive Level: Application
Nursing Process: Assessment; *Test Plan:* PHYS

7   **Answer: 2** *Rationale:* Potentially fatal interactions occur between selegiline and opioids, especially meperidine (Demerol). Therefore, nurses should be aware of all medications that a client routinely takes when selegiline is ordered concurrently. The other classifications may have interactions, but none are potentially fatal.
Cognitive Level: Analysis
Nursing Process: Implementation; *Test Plan:* PHYS

8   **Answer: 4** *Rationale:* The medications used to treat disorders of either the neurological or musculoskeletal system are complex and require the client to understand how they work. When the client is informed, he or she is more likely to take the medication correctly. Options 1 and 2 may not apply, and option 3 is of lesser importance than option 4.
Cognitive Level: Application
Nursing Process: Implementation; *Test Plan:* PHYS

9   **Answer: 1** *Rationale:* Phenytoin binds with the protein in the tube feedings, which decreases the medication absorption into the blood. The tube feedings may need to be shut off for 30 minutes to an hour before and after the dose. The other answers are incorrect statements.
Cognitive Level: Application
Nursing Process: Planning; *Test Plan:* PHYS

10   **Answer: 1** *Rationale:* The effects of muscle relaxants are intensified when taken in combination with other central nervous system (CNS) depressants such as alcohol or cough preparations. The client should consult with the provider before taking other medications. Cholesterol levels do not need to be checked (option 2). Apical pulse measurement is

unnecessary (option 3), and it is antibiotics, not cyclobenzaprine, that must be finished even if symptoms improve (option 4).
Cognitive Level: Application
Nursing Process: Implementation; *Test Plan:* PHYS

References

Abrams, A. (2004). *Clinical drug therapy: Rationales for nursing practice* (7th ed.). Philadelphia: Lippincott, Williams, & Wilkins, pp. 182–219.

Aschenbrenner, D., Cleveland, L., & Venable, S. (2002). *Drug therapy in nursing.* Philadelphia: Lippincott, Williams, & Wilkins, pp. 297–355.

Hickey, J. (2001). *The clinical practice of neurological and neurosurgical nursing.* Philadelphia: Lippincott, pp. 192–688.

Karch, A. (2003). *Focus on pharmacology* (2nd ed.). Philadelphia: Lippincott, Williams, & Wilkins, pp. 302–341.

Lehne, R. (2004). *Pharmacology for nursing care* (5th ed.). St. Louis, MO: Mosby, Inc., pp. 181–220.

McKenry, L., & Salerno, G. (2003). *Mosby's pharmacology in nursing* (21st ed.). St. Louis, MO: Mosby, Inc., pp. 491–519.

Skidmore-Roth, L. (2001). *2001 Nursing drug reference.* St. Louis, MO: Mosby, pp. 6–983.

Wilson, B.A., Shannon, M.T., Stang, C.L. (2003). *Nurses drug reference 2003.* Upper Saddle River, NJ: Prentice Hall.

Youngkin, E.Q., Sawin, K.J., Kissinger, J.F., & Israel, D.S. (1999). *Pharmacotherapeutics: A primary care clinical guide.* Stamford, CT: Appleton & Lange, p. 622.

CHAPTER 11

Psychiatric Medications

Lee Murray, MSN, RN, CS, CADAC

CHAPTER OUTLINE

Antipsychotics

Antidepressants

Antimania Medications

Sedative-Hypnotic and Anxiolytic
 Medications

Substance Misuse

OBJECTIVES

- Describe the general goals of therapy when administering medications to treat psychiatric disorders.

- Discuss the indications for use of an antipsychotic medication.

- Identify the signs and symptoms and nursing management of extrapyramidal adverse effects that can occur with the administration of antipsychotic medications.

- List the classifications of antidepressant medications.

- Describe dietary restrictions associated with the use of monoamine oxidase inhibitors.

- Identify the indications for the use of lithium.

- Describe the signs and symptoms and nursing management of the adverse/toxic effects associated with the use of lithium.

- Discuss client teaching points related to safety and the use of sedative-hypnotics and anxiolytics.

- Identify the signs associated with substance misuse.

- Identify specific client education points related to disulfiram (Antabuse) therapy.

- Discuss significant client education points related to the administration of medications to treat psychiatric disorders.

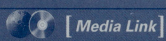

[Media Link]

Use the CD-ROM enclosed with this text, or log onto the address given to access the free, interactive Companion Website created for this series. The CD-ROM and Companion Website accompanying this book offer additional practice opportunities and information—NCLEX Review, Case Studies, Glossary, In Depth with NCLEX, and more.

www.prenhall.com/hogan

REVIEW AT A GLANCE

agranulocytosis *an acute disease marked by deficit or absolute lack of granulocytic white blood cells*

akathisia *a subjective sense of restlessness with a need to move or pace continuously*

antagonists *chemicals that inhibit activity at a receptor site.*

anticholinergic effects *effects caused by drugs that block acetylcholine receptors*

dystonia *rigidity in muscles that control posture, gait or ocular movements*

extrapyramidal side effects (EPSE) *involuntary muscle movements resulting from the effects of neuroleptic medications on the extrapyramidal system of the body; they include akathisia, akinesia, dystonia, drug-induced parkinsonism, and neuroleptic malignant syndrome*

metabolite *the results of the biotransformation of a drug; most tend to be pharmacologically inactive; there are exceptions including many of the benzodiazepines, fluoxetine and ethanol*

neuroleptics *antipsychotic medications*

neuroleptic malignant syndrome (NMS) *a disorder associated with sudden high fever, rigidity, tachycardia, hypertension and decreased level of consciousness*

parkinsonism *masked facies, muscle rigidity, and shuffling gait; extrapyramidal side effects related to dopamine blockade*

serotonin syndrome *a state (agitation, sweating, confusion, fever, hyperreflexia, tachycardia, hypotension, muscle rigidity, and ataxia) that occurs when SSRIs are given concurrently with other serotonin*

enhancing drugs, causing an excess of serotonin in the system

synesthesia *a condition in which stimulation to one sense causes a reaction in another sense, such as smelling a flavor or tasting an odor*

tardive dyskinesia (TD) *an extrapyramidal syndrome that includes movements such as grimacing, buccolingual movements, and dystonia (impaired muscle tone); usually are late-onset side effects of antipsychotic agents; may be irreversible*

tolerance *the need for an increased amount of an agent to achieve the same effects*

Pretest

1 The psychiatrist is prescribing chlorpromazine (Thorazine) 50 mg IM as an initial dose for a client hospitalized with psychosis. The nurse's initial concern is to monitor:

(1) Blood pressure and pulse.
(2) A decrease in psychotic symptoms.
(3) The client's ability to walk.
(4) The client's ability to eat lunch.

2 The home care nurse is visiting a client discharged yesterday from an inpatient unit. The client is taking olanzapine (Zyprexa) 10 mg daily. The client states that he needs more medication because what he was given yesterday is all gone. He was given a 10-day supply upon discharge. The nurse would then assess for which of the following signs?

(1) Headache and psychosis
(2) Lightheadedness and diarrhea
(3) Slurred speech and drowsiness
(4) Diarrhea and vomiting

3 A female client reports during an initial interview that she has been prescribed to take trazodone (Desyrel). The nurse questions her about a history of which of the following problems?

(1) Insomnia
(2) Panic attacks
(3) Mania
(4) Anxiety

4 A client is discharged taking a monoamine oxidase inhibitor (MAOI). Which of the following are the most important client teaching objectives?

(1) Give the client written and oral instructions on how to take daily doses of the medication.
(2) Instruct family members how to notify the appropriate health care professional after discharge.
(3) Give client written and oral instructions about medication administration, side effects, adverse effects, and food interactions.
(4) Instruct the client's family about the administration of medication.

5 Keeping in mind that few benzodiazepines are safe for use with the elderly, the nurse would anticipate that which of the following would be the most effective for use with a 74-year-old client?

(1) Diazepam (Valium)
(2) Chlordiazepoxide (Librium)
(3) Trazadone (Desyrel)
(4) Lorazepam (Ativan)

6 The client is being discharged today on lithium. Which of the following would be the most likely reason the client will be readmitted to the inpatient unit?

(1) There will be a crisis in the client's family.
(2) The client will begin a diet regime to lose weight.
(3) The client will stop taking lithium as prescribed.
(4) The client's spouse will become seriously ill.

7 The nurse is working in the emergency department when a client is brought in vomiting profusely and smelling of alcohol. The client keeps repeating, "It's the medicine that's doing it, if I live through this I'll never drink again." Based on what the client is saying, you begin your assessment by *first* asking the client:

(1) "When was the last time you drank alcohol?"
(2) "Are you taking antihypertensive medications?"
(3) "Have you eaten today?"
(4) "Are you taking disulfiram (Antabuse)?"

8 The client states, "Before I came to the hospital this time I used to take Tofranil for my depression. The doctor said he thought it was time for me to change to a newer medicine but I can't remember what he said about why this Zoloft would be better for me." The nurse's *best* response to this client would be which of the following?

(1) "Maybe the physician didn't think the Tofranil was working anymore."
(2) "I know there are fewer side effects with Zoloft than with Tofranil."
(3) "Did you always take the Tofranil as prescribed?"
(4) "Would you like me to get the physician so you can talk with him about this?"

9 The client is visiting the clinic today after taking fluoxetine (Prozac) 20 mg PO daily in the morning for 3 weeks. He is complaining of weight loss of 10 pounds in the last 2 weeks but states he has not changed his diet at all. The nurse would draw which of the following conclusions from this assessment data?

(1) The client will need to have a change in medication.
(2) The nurse will need to instruct the client on how to increase his daily fluid intake.
(3) This is a normal effect for clients taking fluoxetine.
(4) The physician needs to decrease the dosage of the medication.

10 A client is experiencing recurrent hiccups. The nurse telephones the physician, anticipating an order for which of the following phenothiazines that is also used as an antipsychotic agent?

(1) Risperidone (Risperdal)
(2) Molindone (Moban)
(3) Chlorpromazine (Thorazine)
(4) Thioridazine (Mellaril)

See pages 451–452 for Answers and Rationales.

I. Antipsychotics

A. Phenothiazines

1. Action and use

a. The phenothiazines are **neuroleptics** (medications used to treat psychosis); they are also known as typical (traditional) antipsychotic agents

b. They are divided into three chemical sub-classes: the aliphatics, the piperidines and the piperazines; see Table 11-1 for a complete list of neuroleptic medications

Table 11-1

Typical Neuroleptic Drugs and Atypical Antipsychotic Drugs

| Chemical Class & Generic Name (Trade Name) | Route | Total Daily Dose | |
		Short-Term	Maintenance
Traditional Agents			
Phenothiazine: aliphatic			
Chlorpromazine (Thorazine)	PO, IM, L, R	200–1000 mg	50–400 mg
Triflupromazine (Vesprin)	IM	30–150 mg	20–100 mg
Phenothiazine: piperidine			
Mesoridazine (Serentil)	PO, IM	100–400 mg	25–200 mg
Thioridazine (Mellaril)	PO	200–800 mg	50–400 mg
Phenothiazine: piperazine			
Acetophenazine (Tindal)	PO	60–150 mg	40–80 mg
Fluphenazine (Prolixin)	PO, IM, LA	5–50 mg	1–15 mg
Perphenazine (Trilafon)	PO, IM	12–64 mg	8–24 mg
Trifluoperazine (Stelazine)	PO, IM	10–60 mg	4–30 mg
Thioxanthene			
Thiothixene (Navane)	PO, IM	10–60 mg	6–30 mg
Butyrophenone			
Haloperidol (Haldol)	PO, IM, LA	5–50 mg	1–15 mg
Dihydroindolone			
Molindone (Moban)	PO	40–225 mg	15–100 mg
Dibenzoxazepine			
Loxapine (Loxitane)	PO	20–160 mg	10–60 mg
Atypical Agents			
Dibenzodiazepine			
Clozapine (Clozaril)	PO	300–900 mg	200–400 mg
Benzisoxazole			
Risperidone (Risperdal)	PO, L	4–8 mg	2–8 mg
Thiobenzodiazepine			
Olanzapine (Zyprexa)	PO	10 mg	5–20 mg

PO = oral tablets, capsules, IM = intramuscular injection, R = rectal (suppository), L = oral liquid, suspension, concentrate, LA = long-acting injectable preparations.

c. The typical antipsychotics are predominantly dopamine (DA) **antagonists** (which produce their effect by preventing receptor activation by endogenous regulatory molecules and drugs); thus they block postsynaptic D_2 receptors in several DA tracts in the brain, although they have other synaptic effects as well; their 2 main effects are:

1) A decrease in the positive symptoms of schizophrenia (see Box 11-1 for a listing of positive and negative symptoms of schizophrenia)

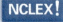

2) The production of **extrapyramidal side effects** (EPSE): a variety of neurological disturbances that result from dysfunction of the extrapyramidal system; this may occur as a reversible side effect of certain psychotropic drugs, particularly antipsychotics; see Table 11-2 for a list of EPSE manifestations and their management

d. Psychosis is a phenomenon of brain activity; therefore the sought-after effects of antipsychotic medications occur in the central nervous system (CNS)

Positive Symptoms

Hallucinations

Delusions

Disordered thinking

Combativeness

Agitation

Paranoia

Grandiosity

Illusions

Insomnia

Negative Symptoms

Social withdrawal

Emotional withdrawal

Lack of motivation

Poverty of speech

Alogia

Anergia

Anhedonia

Attention deficits

Blunted affect

Poor insight

Poor judgment

Poor self-care

e. Selected agents are also used as antiemetics and antihistamines; chlorpromazine is also used in the treatment of intractable hiccups

f. Typical antipsychotics are most effective in treating the "positive" symptoms of schizophrenia, but are less effective in treating the "negative" symptoms of schizophrenia (symptoms that develop over an extended period of time); refer again to Box 11-1 for positive and negative symptoms of schizophrenia

g. The typical antipsychotics are not different from each other in terms of overall clinical response at equivalent doses; thus selection of a drug is determined by the extent, type and severity of side effects produced, as well as effect of the drug in a first-degree relative (see Box 11-2 for a list of antipsychotics by potency classification)

  1) A low-potency drug such as chlorpromazine can reduce the risk of EPSEs, while a high-potency drug such as haloperidol can minimize postural hypotension, sedation, and anticholinergic effects

  2) These drugs are equally effective in treating the positive symptoms of schizophrenia but are less effective in treating the negative symptoms

h. Tolerance to antipsychotic medications is very uncommon; they are also the most toxic drugs used in psychiatry

	Side Effects	Nursing Interventions
Table 11-2 **Extrapyramidal Side Effects (EPSE)**	*Peripheral Nervous System Effects*	
	Constipation	Increase fluid intake, encourage high dietary intake, provide laxatives as necessary.
	Dry mouth	Advise client to use sugarless hard candy or gum, sips of water frequently.
	Nasal congestion	Suggest over-the-counter nasal decongestants that are safe for use with antipsychotic agents.
	Blurred vision	Ask client to avoid dangerous tasks. This symptom will usually last only a short time at the beginning of treatment. Eye drops should be used for the short-term need.
	Mydriasis	Advise client to report any eye pain immediately.
	Photophobia	Advise client to wear sunglasses when in sunlight.
	Orthostatic hypotension	Advise client to get out of chair or bed slowly, to sit before standing, and rise slowly. Observe to see if change to another antipsychotic is advisable.
	Tachycardia	This is usually a reflex response to hypotension. When intervention for hypotension is effective, reflex tachycardia usually decreases. With clozapine, hold the dose if pulse rate is > than 140.
	Urinary retention	Encourage client to void when urge is present and void frequently. Catheterize for residual urine. Client should closely monitor output. Older men with benign prostatic hyperplasia are particularly susceptible to urinary retention.
	Urinary hesitation	Provide privacy, encourage client to take the time to void, run water in sink or pour warm water over perineum.
	Sedation	Help client to get up, get dressed and begin the day early.
	Weight gain	Advise client to maintain appropriate diet.
	Agranulocytosis	There is a high incidence of agranulocytosis for clients who are taking clozapine. White cell counts need to be monitored weekly. If the WBC < 3500 cells/mm^3 prior to therapy, no treatment should begin. After treatment has begun a WBC < 3000 cells/mm^3 and a granulocyte count of < 1500 cells/mm^3 indicate that treatment should be interrupted to monitor for infection. If WBC is < 2000 cells/mm^3, and granulocyte count is < 1000 cells/mm^3, halt therapy and do not begin treatment with the drug again. If infection develops, antibiotics should be prescribed.
	Central Nervous System Effects	
	Akathisia	Usually develops within the first 2 months. There is an uncontrollable need to move. Occurs most often with high-potency antipsychotics. Treatment is usually with beta-blockers, benzodiazepines, and anticholinergic drugs. The antipsychotic agent should be changed to a lower potency agent. It is important to distinguish between akathisia and exacerbation of psychosis. If akathisia is confused with anxiety or psychotic agitation, it is likely that antipsychotic dosage would be increased, thereby making akathisia more intense.
	Dystonias	Acute: Usually occur early in treatment, and are dangerous and severe. Oculogyric crisis or torticollis are the most common occurrences. Treatment includes antiparkinson drug or antihistamine immediately and offer reassurance. Obtain an order for IM administration when client begins treatment with antipsychotics or if in acute state of dystonia, call physician immediately.

(continued)

Table 11-2 **Extrapyramidal Side Effects (EPSE) (Continued)**		For less acute dystonias, notify the physician when an order for an antiparkinson drug is warranted.
	Drug-induced parkinsonism	A chronic nervous disease characterized by a fine, slowly spreading tremor, muscular, weakness and rigidity, and a peculiar gait induced by some antipsychotic medications. Assess for three major symptoms: tremors, rigidity, and bradykinesia. Report to physician immediately. Antiparkinson drugs will be indicated.
	Tardive dyskinesia (TD)	Develops in 15 to 20% of clients during long-term therapy. The risk is related to duration of treatment and dosage size. For many clients symptoms are irreversible. Assess for signs using the Abnormal Inventory Movement Scale (AIMS). Anticholinergic agents will worsen TD, so use is contraindicated.
	Neuroleptic malignant syndrome	This is a fatal side effect of antipsychotic medications. Routinely take client's temperature and encourage adequate water intake. Also routinely assess for rigidity, tremor, and similar symptoms.
	Seizures	Occur in approximately 1% of clients taking antipsychotic medications. Clozapine causes an even higher rate, up to 5% of clients taking 600–900 mg/day. For dosages of clozapine greater than 600 mg/day a normal EEG should be performed. If a seizure occurs, it may be necessary to discontinue clozapine.

2. Common medications (refer again to Table 11-1)

    a. Chlorpromazine (Thorazine) and the other antipsychotic drugs are used primarily to treat psychotic disorders, specifically, schizophrenia and other chronic mental illnesses; treatment of schizophrenia has three goals:

      1) Suppression of acute episodes

      2) Prevention of acute exacerbations

      3) Maintenance of the highest possible level of functioning

Box 11-2 **Classification of Traditional Antipsychotics by Potency**	*High-Potency Antipsychotic Drugs* • Fluphenazine (Prolixin) • Haloperidol (Haldol) • Thiothixene (Navane) • Trifluoperazine (Stelazine) *Moderate-Potency Antipsychotic Drugs* • Loxapine (Loxitane) • Molindone (Moban) • Perphenazine (Trilafon) *Low-Potency Antipsychotic Drugs* • Chlorpromazine (Thorazine) • Mesoridazine (Serentil) • Thioridazine (Mellaril)

b. Selection of traditional antipsychotic drugs is based largely on side effect profile

c. The client should not be given a drug that, because of its side effects, is likely to cause discomfort, inconvenience, or harm; for example, if a client has a history of prostatic hyperplasia or glaucoma, or is sensitive to anticholinergic drugs, a low-potency neuroleptic should not be prescribed

3. Administration considerations

a. Typical antipsychotics effectively suppress symptoms during acute psychotic episodes, and when taken chronically, can greatly reduce the incidence of relapse (a major risk in the treatment of clients with schizophrenia); but since the etiology of psychotic illness is entirely unknown, the relationship of receptor blockade to therapeutic effects can only be estimated

b. Medication effects can usually be seen in 1 to 2 days, but substantial improvement usually takes 2 to 4 weeks and full effects may not develop for several months

c. Dosage requirements vary considerably for each client and must be adjusted as the target symptom changes and side effects are monitored; initially, depending on the drug dosage recommendations, the client receives several doses per day and the daily dose can be titrated slowly until a safe, effective dose is reached

d. The half-life of antipsychotic drugs is greater than 24 hours, so the client usually can be dosed once a day after the safe, effective dose is reached

e. Dosing for elderly clients requires small doses, typically 30 to 50 percent of those taken by younger clients; also poorly responsive clients may need larger doses than highly responsive clients (although very large doses are generally avoided)

f. Positive symptoms of schizophrenia respond better than negative symptoms

g. Antipsychotic drugs do not alter the underlying pathology of schizophrenia; the treatment is not curative, it offers only symptomatic relief

h. A thorough baseline evaluation should be done, including laboratory tests and electrocardiogram (ECG), for clients beginning treatment

i. Antipsychotic medications can also be used for clients with bipolar disorder (used to reduce the acute symptoms of psychosis); they are also used with clients who have Tourette's syndrome (specifically, haloperidol can reduce the severe symptoms of the disease); neuroleptics suppress emesis in clients by blocking dopamine receptors in the chemoreceptor trigger zone of the medulla

j. Depot antipsychotic preparations such as haloperidol and fluphenazine are long-acting injectable preparations used for long-term maintenance therapy of schizophrenia; with this form of treatment the rate of relapse is usually reduced and therefore is more favorable if a client needs to have long-term therapy

4. Contraindications

a. Hypersensitivity

b. Cross-sensitivity may exist among phenothiazines

c. Use with caution in clients with narrow-angle glaucoma, adynamic ileus, prostatic hyperplasia, cardiovascular disease, hepatic or renal dysfunction, and seizure disorders

d. Should not be used in clients who have CNS depression

e. Contraindicated for comatose or severely depressed clients

f. Also contraindicated for clients with Parkinson's disease, prolactin-dependent carcinoma of the breast, bone marrow depression, and severe hypotension or hypertension

5. Significant drug interactions

   a. May decrease the therapeutic response to levodopa

   b. May be at increased risk for **agranulocytosis**, a low white blood cell (WBC) count, when also taking antithyroid agents

   c. See Table 11-3 for additional adverse drug-drug interactions and effects

6. Significant food interactions: are not usually of concern with typical antipsychotics

7. Significant laboratory studies

   a. Before treatment is started, clients should have a complete evaluation including blood profile and ECG

   b. Ongoing monitoring is indicated to assess for decreases in WBC counts

8. Side effects (refer back to Table 11-2)

   a. D_2 receptor blockade is known to be responsible for many of the side effects of the typical antipsychotics

   b. Dopamine blockade can lead to gynecomastia, galactorrhea, amenorrhea (occasionally), and weight gain

9. Adverse effects/toxicity (refer back to Table 11-2)

   a. The most common adverse effects are sedation, orthostatic hypotension, and **anticholinergic effects** (dry mouth, blurred vision, urinary retention, photophobia, constipation, tachycardia); others include **akathisia** (an uncontrollable need to move), and **parkinsonism** (a set of symptoms that resembles Parkinson's disease),

   b. Photosensitivity occurs; clients should take measures to protect eyes when exposed to sunlight

   c. Agranulocytosis is a rare effect that must be watched for; it is an acute process marked by a deficit or absolute lack of granulocytic white blood cells (neutrophils, basophils, and eosinophils)

   d. **Neuroleptic malignant syndrome (NMS)** is characterized by catatonia, rigidity, stupor, unstable blood pressure, hyperthermia, profuse sweating, dyspnea, and incontinence; it sometimes occurs as a toxic reaction to the use of potent neuroleptic agents in therapeutic doses and condition lasts 5 to 10 days after discontinuation of the drug; the mortality rate may be as high as 20 percent; bromocriptine (Parlodel) and dantrolene (Dantrium)

Table 11-3	Drug	Effect of Interaction
Adverse Interactions of Antipsychotics with Other Drugs	Alcohol, antihistamines, opioids, antidepressants, sedative/hypnotics or analgesics	Additive CNS depression with other CNS depressants
	Alcohol, nitrates or antihypertensives	Additive hypotension with acute ingestion
	Amoxapine, fluoxetine	Increased extrapyramidal side effects
	Amphetamines	Decreased antipsychotic effect
	Antacids	May decrease absorption
	Anticholinergic/antiparkinson drugs	Increased anticholinergic effects; delayed onset of the effects of oral doses of antipsychotics; potentially increased risk of hyperthermia
	Barbiturates, nonbarbiturate hypnotics	Respiratory depression and increased sedation; decreased antipsychotic serum levels; hypotension
	Benzodiazepines	Increased sedation; respiratory depression with lorazepam and loxapine
	Beta-adrenergic blocking agents (propranolol)	Effects of either or both drugs increased
	Cimetidine	Chlorpromazine absorption decreased; increased sedation with chlorpromazine
	Diazoxide	Can cause severe hyperglycemia
	Dopaminergic antiparkinson drugs (e.g., bromocriptine)	Antagonizes the antipsychotic effect
	Guanethidine	Control of hypertension is decreased
	Insulin, oral hypoglycemics	Control of diabetes is weakened
	L-dopa	Decreased antiparkinson effect; may exacerbate psychosis
	Lithium	May decrease blood levels and effectiveness of phenothiazines
	Phenobarbital	May increase metabolism and decrease the effectiveness of the drug
	Phenytoin	May increase phenytoin toxicity; decreased antipsychotic blood serum levels
	Trazodone	Additive hypotension with phenothiazines
	Tricyclics	Possible ventricular dysrhythmias with thioridazine; possible increased blood serum levels of both; hypotension; sedation; anticholinergic effect; increased risk of seizures

have been used to treat NMS if the usual treatment for hyperthermia is ineffective; antipsychotic drug withdrawal is mandatory

NCLEX!

e. The low-potency drugs are more likely to cause sedation and hypotension, while the high-potency drugs cause more EPSEs

f. Overdoses of antipsychotic drugs are not usually fatal and treatment for attempted overdose is supportive (e.g., gastric lavage to empty the stomach); it can cause severe CNS depression (somnolence to coma, hypotension, EPSEs); also reported are restlessness or agitation, convulsions (lowered seizure threshold), hyperthermia, increased anticholinergic symptoms, and dysrhythmias

10. Nursing considerations

NCLEX!

a. While in an inpatient setting, clients need to be observed while taking their medication so that they are swallowing medications and not "cheeking" them; clients have a difficult time with some of the "clouding" and sedating effects noted with their antipsychotic medications

b. Client teaching (see section below) is a major aspect of nursing care

c. Refer once more to Table 11-2 for more specific nursing care and teaching considerations

11. Client education

NCLEX!

a. Clients need to understand the importance of taking medication as prescribed; the major relapse factor for clients with schizophrenia is discontinuing medications, which then leads to relapse and re-hospitalization

b. Clients need education and monitoring with powerful antipsychotic medications; teaching should include family members involved in the client's care and should be done at a level that the client/family is able to grasp and demonstrate the knowledge acquired; written instructions should also be provided, as well as other resources, including phone contacts, if problems should arise

c. Teach clients to take PO meds with food, milk or a full glass of water to decrease gastric irritation

NCLEX!

d. Teach clients to dilute most concentrates in 120 mL of distilled or acidified tap water or fruit juice just before administration

e. Teach client about other medications that may be prescribed to treat ESPEs (see Box 11-3)

B. Atypical antipsychotic drugs

1. Action and use

a. The atypical antipsychotics exert both dopamine receptor sub-type 2 (D_2) and serotonin receptor sub-type 2 ($5HT_2$) receptor-blocking action (are DA and 5HT antagonists)

b. Blockage of serotonin receptors is thought to liberate dopamine in the cortex and may explain some of the reduction in negative symptoms

NCLEX!

c. Atypical agents cause few or no extrapyramidal symptoms, including **tardive dyskinesia** (dyskinesia is the inability to perform voluntary movement, while tardive indicates late onset—usually seen as a serious side effect of antipsychotic agents)

NCLEX!

d. They are used to treat the positive and negative symptoms of schizophrenia and other mental illnesses with psychotic features, and to treat the mood symptoms, hostility, violence, suicidal behavior, and cognitive impairment seen in schizophrenia

Box 11-3

Medications Used to Treat Extrapyramidal Side Effects

Anticholinergic
- Benztropine (Cogentin)
- Trihexyphenidyl (Artane)

Antihistamine
- Diphenhydramine (Benadryl)

Dopamine Agonist
- Amantadine (Symmetrel)

e. They provide new hope for clients with psychosis, particularly those who are experiencing their first episode, who have not responded well to typical antipsychotics, or who have suffered dose-limiting side effects from the traditional neuroleptics

2. Common medications (refer back to Table 11-1 for drug names, doses, and routes)

    a. The following are some atypical antipsychotic medications commonly used at present: clozapine (Clozaril), risperidone (Risperdal), and olanzapine (Zyprexa)

    b. Clozapine

        1) Was the first new antipsychotic agent to be introduced in the United States in 40 years when released in 1990

        2) Because of its serious side effect, agranulocytosis, it was released with a very rigid set of protocols including weekly blood analysis

        3) Clients are not prescribed more than a one-week supply of medication to enforce compliance with weekly blood analysis

        4) The beneficial effects of clozapine are usually very positive for most and remarkable for others

        5) Clozapine has a greater affinity for dopamine-D_1, dopamine-D_4, and serotonin ($5HT_2$) as well as dopamine D_2 receptors

    c. Risperidone (Risperdal)

        1) Was FDA approved in 1994 and is currently the most frequently prescribed antipsychotic agent

        2) It has a greater affinity for dopamine D_2 receptors and a similar antagonism of serotonin $5HT_2$

        3) Its lack of serious side effects makes it a very well-tolerated agent

        4) It has little affinity for muscarinic (i.e., cholinergic receptors), so anticholinergic side effects are minimized; neither does it appear to cause agranulocytosis, EPSEs, tardive dyskinesia, or NMS

        5) Side effects include orthostatic hypotension, insomnia, agitation, headache, anxiety, and rhinitis

    d. Olanzapine (Zyprexa)

        1) Is also a newer atypical antipsychotic agent, being released for use in 1996

        2) It is comparable to risperidone in efficacy of treating both positive and negative symptoms and has a comparable side effects profile; it does not cause agranulocytosis; early clinical trials indicate few incidents of EPSE

3. Administration considerations

    a. Clozapine is usually given 1 to 2 times daily and should not exceed 900 mg/day; because of the strict protocol, blood testing is done weekly; if client does not comply, the drug will not be continued

    b. Risperidone is usually administered PO in 1 to 2 daily doses; for debilitated or elderly clients or for those with renal or hepatic impairment, dosage should be reduced at onset of treatment

c. Olanzapine is usually administered PO as well; dosage should not exceed 15 mg/day; for debilitated or nonsmoking female clients > 65 years, therapy should be initiated at 5 mg/day

d. Refer back to Table 11-1 for generic and trade names, dosages and route of administration for antipsychotics

4. Contraindications

NCLEX!

a. Clozapine, risperidone and olanzapine are all contraindicated for clients with hypersensitivity to the drug; other considerations include cautious use in clients with bone marrow depression, severe CNS depression/coma, and during lactation

b. Clozapine should be used cautiously with clients who have a depressed bone marrow, prostatic enlargement, narrow-angle glaucoma, malnourished state, or in clients with cardiovascular, hepatic or renal disease; it should also be used cautiously in clients with diabetes, seizure disorder, or for children < 16 years (safety is not yet established)

c. Risperidone should be used cautiously for elderly or debilitated clients, those with renal or hepatic impairment, cardiovascular disease, or history of seizures, suicide attempts or drug abuse; safety has not been established for use during pregnancy or lactation, or for use with children

d. Olanzapine should be used cautiously with clients with liver disease or during pregnancy or lactation; safety for use with children has not yet been established

NCLEX!

e. For elderly or debilitated clients, or clients with known liver, renal, or cardiovascular disease, initial dosing should be lowered and ongoing monitoring should be emphasized

5. Significant drug interactions

a. Effects may be decreased by concurrent use of carbamazepine (Tegretol), omeprazole (Prilosec), or rifampin (Rifadin); additive hypotension may occur with concurrent use of antihypertensive agents; additive CNS depression may occur with concurrent use of alcohol or other CNS depressants; atypical antipsychotics may antagonize the effects of levodopa or other dopamine agonists

b. Risperidone may decrease the antiparkinson effects of levodopa or other dopamine agonists; carbamazepine increases metabolism and may decrease effectiveness of risperidone; clozapine decreases metabolism and may increase the effects of risperidone; additive CNS depression may occur with other CNS depressants including alcohol, antihistamines, sedative/hypnotics or opioids

c. Olanzapine effects may be decreased by concurrent use of carbamazepine, omeprazole, or rifampin; there may be additive CNS depression with concurrent use of alcohol or other CNS depressants; olanzapine may also antagonize the effects of levodopa or other dopamine agonists

6. Significant food interactions: none

7. Significant laboratory studies: for clients prescribed clozapine, there is a mandatory need for weekly blood tests (WBC counts) to prevent/detect agranulocytosis

8. Side effects

   a. Seizure incidence for clients taking clozapine is 3 percent; this is one reason that the maximum dose should not exceed 900 mg/day

   b. See Table 11-4 for common side effects of the atypical antipsychotics discussed in this chapter

9. Adverse effects/toxicity

   a. Some of the more serious adverse/toxic effects listed for clozapine have been discussed in the section above on side effects; other considerations include neuroleptic malignant syndrome (NMS)

   b. For clients prescribed risperidone, monitor for NMS

   c. For clients taking olanzapine, monitor for NMS and seizures

10. Nursing considerations

    a. Because of the risk of fatal agranulocytosis, clozapine is reserved for clients with severe schizophrenia who have not responded to traditional antipsychotic drugs (40 to 60 percent success rate for treatment in this group)

    b. The nurse works with clients to assist them to adjust to the changes experienced (the improvement in positive and negative symptoms, the ability to become more animated, and to have behavior that is more socially acceptable)

    c. Usually with clients who respond well to clozapine, there is a decreased need for rehospitalization as well

11. Client education: clients will still need help with psychoeducation, social skills training, group support, and other rehabilitative interventions to improve their overall level of functioning and quality of life while incorporating the atypical antipsychotic medications into their life pattern

II. Antidepressants

A. Tricyclics

1. Action and use

   a. Imipramine (Tofranil) was the first antidepressant medication used to treat depression (1950s) and is still used effectively today

   b. Tricyclic antidepressants (TCAs) such as imipramine block monoamine reuptake, which indicates that TCAs intensify the effects of the norepineph-

Practice To Pass

A client taking an antipsychotic medication asks, "What is neuroleptic malignant syndrome?" How would the nurse describe the syndrome and its management?

Table 11-4		Clozapine	Risperidone	Olanzapine
Common Side Effects of Atypical Antipsychotics	Extrapyramidal	None	+	+
	Cardiac	+++	++	+
	Sedation	++++	++	+
	Anticholinergic	++++	+	++
	Weight gain	+++	++	++++

Occurrence: + = least, ++++ = greatest

rine and serotonin; TCAs can elevate mood, increase activity and alertness, decrease a client's preoccupation with morbidity, improve appetite, and regulate sleep patterns

c. The initial mechanism of the TCAs takes about 1 to 3 weeks to develop while the maximum response is achieved in approximately 6 to 8 weeks

d. Other uses for the TCAs are to treat clients with chronic insomnia, attention-deficit/hyperactivity disorder and panic disorder

2. Common medications (Table 11-5)

a. Nine TCAs are available that are all are equally effective; major differences can be found in side effects

b. For example, doxepin has sedative effects and could be more effectively used with clients who experience insomnia

c. Elderly clients and clients with glaucoma, constipation, or prostatic hyperplasia can be especially sensitive to the anticholinergic effects of the TCAs; therefore, a TCA such as desipramine with weak anticholinergic effects would be more appropriate with these clients

3. Administration considerations

a. Dosing with TCAs is individualized and based on clinical response or plasma drug levels (which must be above 225 ng/ml for antidepressant effects to occur)

b. The normal route for TCAs is by mouth; amitriptyline and imipramine may be given by intramuscular (IM) injection; intravenous (IV) administration is not usually used

c. TCAs have long half-lives, so they can be taken daily in a single dose; because the half-life of the individual drugs varies, client dosing is also individualized

d. Once-a-day dosing at bedtime has several advantages, such as ease of taking as part of daily routine, promoting sleep by its sedative effect, and reducing the intensity of the daytime side effects

4. Contraindications: a major consideration for clients at risk for suicide is availability of large amounts of TCA medication; therefore, clients at risk for suicide who are taking TCAs should not have access to a large quantity of the medication and should always be hospitalized until the danger of suicide has been ruled out

5. Significant drug interactions

a. The combination of TCAs and a MAOI can lead to severe hypertension from excessive adrenergic stimulation of the heart and blood vessels

b. TCAs potentiate responses to direct-acting sympathomimetics (i.e., drugs such as epinephrine and norepinephrine that produce their effects by direct interaction with adrenergic receptors); sympathetic nervous system (SNS) stimulation by these drugs can be increased because TCAs block uptake of these drugs into the adrenergic terminals, which prolongs their presence in the synaptic space

NCLEX!

NCLEX!

NCLEX!

Drug Class and Name: Generic (Trade)	Usual Adult Dosage Range (mg/day)	Nursing Responsibilities
Tricyclic Antidepressants (TCAs)		
Amitriptyline (Elavil)	75–300	• Educate the client early about potential side effects.
Clomipramine (Anafranil)	75–300	• Inform client that side effects will diminish with time and if necessary there are management alternatives that can be implemented.
Desipramine (Norpramin)	75–300	• Advise client that response will take some time and continued use is essential.
Doxepin (Senequin)	75–300	
Imipramine (Tofranil)	50–150	• Inform client that first-time treatment for major depression should continue for 6 to 12 months.
Maprotiline (Ludiomil)	50–100	• Warn client of a possible significant weight gain.
Nortriptyline (Pamelor)	25–100	• Monitor for improvement. If no change or minimum change after 2 to 4 weeks it may be necessary to change the medication.
Protriptyline (Vivactil)	10–60	
Trimipramine (Surmontil)	50–150	
Selective Serotonin Reuptake Inhibitors (SSRIs)		
Fluoxetine (Prozac)	20–80	• Inform client to take medication as prescribed. Abrupt discontinuation of the drug is contraindicated.
Fluvoxamine (Luvox)	50–100	• Continuously monitor client for side effects or adverse effects, particularly in the area of sexual dysfunction. Client may be reluctant to discuss.
Paroxetine (Paxil)	20–50	
Sertraline (Zoloft)	50–200	
Monoamine Oxidase Inhibitors (MAOIs)		
Phenelzine (Nardil)	45–75	• Educate client concerning a tyramine-restricted diet.
Tranylcypromine (Parnate)	20–30	• Caution client about side effects and adverse effects of the MAOIs.
		• Educate client about careful use of over-the-counter or other prescription medications and be sure client understands the seriousness of the effects.
		• Monitor efficacy of drugs and continuously re-educate client to avoid abruptly discontinuing medication or not taking medications as prescribed.
Atypical Antidepressants		
Bupropion (Wellbutrin)	200	• Instruct client about the side effects and adverse effect of the medication, especially seizure risks at higher drug doses.
		• Instruct client concerning the importance of taking this and all medication as prescribed.
Trazodone (Desyrel)	150	• Instruct client to take medication as prescribed and monitor for any adverse or side effects.
		• Instruct client to report any signs of sexual dysfunction, especially priapism, immediately.

    c. TCAs decrease responses to indirect-acting sympathomimetics (i.e., drugs such as ephedrine and amphetamine that produce their effects by promoting release of transmitter from adrenergic nerves) because TCAs block uptake of these agents into adrenergic nerves, which prevents them from reaching their site of action within the nerve terminal

    d. TCAs exert anticholinergic actions of their own; therefore, TCAs will intensify the effects of other medications that have anticholinergic actions, such as antihistamines and certain over-the-counter (OTC) sleep aids; these products should be avoided while taking TCAs

    e. CNS depression caused by TCAs will add to CNS depression caused by other drugs; therefore clients taking TCAs should avoid CNS depressants, including alcohol, antihistamines, opioids and barbiturates

6. Significant food interactions: none

7. Significant laboratory studies: in order for antidepressant effects to occur, serum drug levels need to be maintained within a specified therapeutic range

8. Side effects

    a. The most common undesirable effects of the TCAs are orthostatic hypotension, sedation, and anticholinergic effects

    b. Instruct client to move slowly when changing position (lying to sitting, sitting to standing or turning) to avoid injury; monitor blood pressure both lying and sitting if client is hospitalized

9. Adverse effects/toxicity

    a. The most serious adverse effect of the TCAs is cardiac toxicity; in the absence of overdose or pre-existing cardiac impairment, serious cardiotoxicity is rare

    b. To avoid adverse cardiac effects, clients over the age of 40 and those with heart disease should undergo baseline ECG and then every 6 months

    c. Adverse effects of each drug are indicated in Table 11-5

10. Nursing considerations

    a. Clients should be advised early of potential side effects and that therapeutic response will take some weeks to be established once medications are begun; clients and families often become impatient when the client is experiencing medication side effects while still having the original symptoms

    b. Refer back to Table 11-5 for nursing responsibilities with TCAs and see Table 11-6 for manifestations of common adverse effects

11. Client education

    a. Compliance is often enhanced when the nurse discusses expectations regarding medications with clients and families; explain that side effects will diminish with time and symptoms will be lessened as the medication regime is followed

    b. Encourage the client and family to utilize other available therapies as well

    c. Refer back to Tables 11-5 and 11-6 for specific teaching points

	Effect	Manifestations
Table 11-6 **Most Common Adverse Effects from Antidepressant Medications**	1. Orthostatic hypotension 2. Anticholinergic	Major decrease in blood pressure with body position changes Block muscarinic cholinergic receptors, which produces: • Dry mouth • Blurred vision • Photophobia • Constipation • Urinary hesitancy • Tachycardia
	3. Sedation	Sleepiness and difficulty maintaining arousal are common responses to TCAs. The cause is blockade of histamine receptors in the CNS.
	4. Cardiac toxicity	TCAs can adversely affect the heart's function. • Decreasing vagal influence (secondary to muscarinic blockade) • Acting directly on the bundle of His to slow conduction
	5. Seizures	Lower seizure threshold
	6. Hypomania	Mild mania can occur
	7. Sexual dysfunction	• Anorgasm • Delayed ejaculation • Decreased libido
	8. Hypertensive crisis from dietary tyramine	Although MAOIs normally produce hypotension these drugs can be the cause of severe hypertension if client eats tyramine-rich foods.
	9. Drug interactions	Always teach clients the importance of preventing adverse drug effects/drug interactions. See individual classifications for specific nursing responsibilities.

B. Monoamine oxidase inhibitors (MAOIs)

1. Action and use

   a. Because of potentially fatal food and drug interactions, this class of antidepressant is usually not a first choice to treat clients with depression unless the client suffers from atypical depression

   b. Monoamine oxidase (MAO) is an enzyme present in the liver, intestinal wall, and the terminals of monoamine-containing neurons; the function of MAO in neurons is to convert monoamine transmitters (norepinephrine, serotonin, and dopamine) into inactive products; in the liver and intestine, MAO serves to inactivate tyramine and other biogenic amines in food

   c. MAOIs decrease the amount of monoamine oxidase in the liver that breaks down the amino acids tyramine and tryptophan

   d. There is an antidepressant effect of MAOIs because of MAO-A in nerve terminals along with other enzymatic and chemical actions; the biochemical action of MAOIs takes place rapidly, whereas the clinical response (relief of depression) develops slowly; in the interval between, additional as-yet-unknown neurochemical events are presumed to be taking place to cause the beneficial response to treatment

   e. MAOIs have been used with some success to treat bulimia and obsessive-compulsive disorders and to treat panic attacks in clients with panic disorder

2. Common medications: refer again to Table 11-5 and 11-6 for MAOIs commonly used

3. Administration considerations: route of administration is usually PO; see Table 11-5 for details

4. Contraindications: clients over the age of 60 or those with pheochromocytoma, congestive heart failure, liver disease, severe renal impairment, cerebrovascular defect, cardiovascular disease, or hypertension

5. Significant drug interactions

   a. Use with caution for clients taking other TCAs

   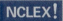

   b. Taking SSRIs with MAOIs can cause **serotonin syndrome** (agitation, sweating, confusion, fever, hyperreflexia, tachycardia, hypotension, muscle rigidity, and ataxia); avoid this combination

   c. Antihypertensive drugs will potentiate the hypotensive effects of MAOIs

   d. Meperidine can produce hyperthermia in clients taking MAOIs and should be avoided

   e. Instruct the client to avoid all medications (prescription and nonprescription) that have not been specifically approved by the physician

6. Significant food interactions

   a. Dietary tyramine, some other dietary constituents, and indirect-acting sympathomimetics (e.g., amphetamine, methylphenidate, ephedrine, cocaine) can precipitate a hypertensive crisis in clients taking MAOIs

   b. See Box 11-4 for lists of foods to avoid and to use cautiously while taking an MAOI

7. Significant laboratory studies: in order for antidepressant effects to occur, serum drug levels need to be maintained within a specified therapeutic range

---

Box 11-4

Foods to Avoid with Monoamine Oxidase Inhibitors

Foods to Avoid

- All cheeses except cream or cottage cheese
- Meats and fish: aged/cured
- Fruits and vegetables: broad bean pods, tofu, soy bean extracts
- Alcohol: draft beer
- Other: sauerkraut, soy sauce, yeast extracts, soups (especially miso), and any non-fresh foods
- Drugs: other antidepressant drugs, nasal and sinus decongestants, allergy, hay fever and asthma remedies, narcotics (especially meperidine), epinephrine, stimulants, cocaine, amphetamines

Consume with Caution

- Cheeses: mozzarella, cottage, ricotta, cream, processed
- Meats and fish: chicken liver, meats, liver, herring
- Fruits and vegetables: raspberries, bananas, small amounts only of avocado, spinach
- Alcohol: wine
- Other: monosodium glutamate, pizza, small amounts only of chocolate, caffeine, nuts, dairy products
- Drugs: insulin, oral hypoglycemics, oral anticoagulants, thiazide diuretics, anticholinergic agents, muscle relaxants

8. Side effects

a. Orthostatic hypotension is a common initial and sometimes persistent side effect of MAOIs

b. Edema, sexual dysfunction, and weight gain are also common and can lead to drug discontinuation

c. Complaints of insomnia occur with all MAOIs

9. Adverse effects/toxicity: in contrast to TCAs, MAOIs cause direct CNS stimulation, which in excess can produce anxiety, agitation, hypomania, and even mania

10. Nursing considerations

a. Give clients and families oral and written instructions of how to avoid adverse effects of the MAOIs; there are many factors that need to be considered with client's safe use of and appropriate treatment for major depression because of the side effects and adverse effects of MAOIs

b. Assess the client for ability to adhere to a strict dietary regime

c. Consult with the primary physician with changes in vital signs to avoid potentially fatal hypertensive crisis

d. Instruct the client not to take any prescribed or OTC medication without first consulting or notifying the physician who prescribed the MAOI

11. Client education

a. Familiarize the client with the symptoms of orthostatic hypotension and how to avoid injury when rising from bed or chair slowly

b. If client is hospitalized, blood pressure needs to be monitored regularly

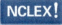

c. Educate the client orally and in writing or provide a dietary consultation if appropriate for the client and family in order to avoid hypertensive crisis

d. Teach the client to avoid all medications (prescribed or OTC) that have not been specifically approved by the physician

C. Selective serotonin reuptake inhibitors (SSRIs)

1. Action and use

a. The mechanism of action for SSRIs is to block the reuptake of serotonin and intensify the transmission at serotonergic synapses; the effects can usually be seen after 1 to 3 weeks and are equivalent to those produced from TCAs

b. SSRIs have the same efficacy as TCAs, exhibit fewer side effects than either TCAs or MAOIs, and have a decreased time between the initial dose and the beginning of reduced signs and symptoms of the depression

c. All SSRIs have been found to be effective in the treatment of obsessive-compulsive disorder (OCD), panic disorder, and bulimia nervosa

2. Common medications (refer again to Table 11-5)

3. Administration considerations

a. The SSRIs are administered orally in liquid or pulvules; elderly clients or those with impaired renal function should be given a low dosage with increases made cautiously

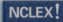

b. Evaluate client frequently for safety and desired effects of the medication

4. Contraindications

a. Most SSRIs should not be prescribed for clients with a hypersensitivity to the drug or those with severe hepatic or renal disease

b. Caution should be used for debilitated clients or those with a history of seizure disorder or diabetes mellitus

c. Lowered drug doses or longer dosing interval may be needed in elderly clients, clients with impaired hepatic function or those receiving multiple drug therapy

5. Significant drug interactions

a. SSRIs should not be administered with MAOIs to prevent serotonin syndrome, a hyperserotonergic state (confusion, autonomic dysfunction, muscle rigidity, ataxia) that occurs when an SSRI is given concurrently with other serotonin-enhancing drugs, causing an excess of serotonin in the system

b. If a client is on an MAOI and is transferred to fluoxetine, at least five weeks should elapse before beginning the fluoxetine; to transfer from fluoxetine to MAOIs, at least two weeks should elapse before beginning the MAOI

c. A client who is taking fluoxetine and warfarin should have warfarin level monitored closely because fluoxetine is highly bound to plasma proteins and may displace other highly-bound drugs such as warfarin

d. Fluoxetine can elevate plasma levels of TCAs and lithium and should be given cautiously when prescribed along with these other agents

6. Significant food interactions

a. Each SSRI is individual for effect with food; fluoxetine, paroxetine, and fluvoxamine can be taken with or without food, while sertraline is slowly absorbed following oral administration; food increases the extent of absorption for sertraline; yet, if there is gastric upset, the literature recommends administration of paroxetine with food

b. When administering a newer SSRI, the nurse should consult the literature for the individual agent

7. Significant laboratory studies

a. Serum drug levels are not clinically useful to determine dose or monitor for toxicity

b. Monitor CBC, differential, and bleeding time periodically throughout treatment for signs of leukopenia, anemia, or thrombocytopenia or for increased bleeding time

8. Side effects

a. The side effect profile of SSRIs is relatively mild compared with that of other antidepressants; there is minimal cardiac toxicity, eliminating the need for ECGs

b. Common initial side effects of SSRIs include nausea, drowsiness, dizziness, headache, sweating, anxiety, insomnia, anorexia, and nervousness; these are generally milder and better tolerated than the side effects of TCAs

9. Adverse effects/toxicity

    a. Most SSRIs on the market today are relatively safe in overdose; when taken as a single agent, SSRI overdoses are serious and can cause seizures, but complete recovery is common

    b. Sexual dysfunction, experienced by 20 to 40 percent of clients taking SSRIs, is an adverse effect that needs to be discussed with the client by the healthcare provider

10. Nursing considerations

    a. Monitor mood changes; notify physician if client demonstrates an increase in anxiety, nervousness, or insomnia

    b. Assess for suicidal tendencies, especially during early drug therapy

    c. Restrict the amount of drug available to the client to prevent overdose

    d. Monitor appetite, nutritional intake and weight

11. Client education

    a. Encourage client to comply with diet recommendations of healthcare professionals; give written and oral instructions to client and family

    b. Instruct client to notify healthcare professional if a rash occurs, which may indicate hypersensitivity

    c. Emphasize the importance of follow-up exams to evaluate progress

    d. See also Tables 11-5 and 11-6 for points on specific SSRIs

D. Other antidepressants

1. Action and use

    a. Trazodone (Desyrel) and bupropion (Wellbutrin) are newer antidepressant agents that have varied chemical structures and modes of action; they are not easily collapsed into a group and are thus discussed individually here

    b. Bupropion (Wellbutrin)

        1) Is similar in structure to amphetamines and can suppress appetite; it does not have cardiotoxic, anticholinergic, and anti-adrenergic side effects and can therefore be used more readily with elderly clients; it can also be used for smoking cessation

        2) It has a somewhat different mechanism of action in that it blocks the reuptake of dopamine while having only minimal reuptake effects on norepinephrine

    c. Trazodone (Desyrel)

        1) Is a second-line agent for the treatment of depression; it is usually used in combination with another antidepressant and is usually prescribed to treat insomnia because of its very pronounced sedative effect

        2) Trazodone alters the effects of serotonin in the CNS; its antidepressant action may develop only over several weeks

2. Common medications: both of these are listed in Table 11-5

3. Administration considerations

   a. The starting dose of bupropion should be no greater than 75 mg TID; because of dose-related seizure risk, never give more than 150 mg at one time; when the maximum dose is required, the recommended regimen is 150 mg TID

   b. The initial dose of trazodone is usually 150 mg/day in two or three divided doses, and may be gradually increased to a maximum of 400 mg/day (outpatients) and 600 mg/day (hospitalized clients); also, a majority of the medication dose may be given at bedtime to decrease daytime drowsiness and dizziness

4. Contraindications

   a. Bupropion can cause dose-related seizures

   b. Trazodone is contraindicated for clients with hypersensitivity, those recovering from myocardial infarction, or those who are using concurrent electroconvulsive therapy; it should be used cautiously in clients with cardiovascular disease or who exhibit suicidal behavior; dosage should be reduced in elderly clients or those who have severe hepatic or renal disease

5. Significant drug interactions

   a. With bupropion there is an increased risk of adverse reactions when used with levodopa or MAOIs; there is also an increased risk of seizures with phenothiazines, antidepressants, theophylline, corticosteroids, OTC stimulants/anorexiants, or cessation of alcohol or benzodiazepines

   b. Trazodone may increase digoxin or phenytoin serum levels; additive CNS depression can occur with alcohol, opioids, and sedative/hypnotics; additive hypotension can occur with antihypertensive agents, acute ingestion of alcohol or use of nitrates; concurrent use with fluoxetine increases levels and risk of toxicity from trazodone

6. Significant food interactions: none

7. Significant laboratory studies

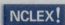

   a. Monitor hepatic and renal function closely in clients with kidney or liver impairment to prevent elevated serum and tissue bupropion concentrations

   b. For trazodone, assess CBC, renal and hepatic functioning before and periodically during treatment; slight, clinically insignificant decrease in leukocyte and neutrophil counts may occur

8. Side effects (refer again to Tables 11-5 and 11-6)

   a. The most common side effects of bupropion are agitation and insomnia

   b. Common side effects of trazodone are sedation, orthostatic hypotension, nausea, and vomiting; in contrast to tricyclic agents, it lacks anticholinergic actions and is not cardiotoxic; it may cause priapism

9. Adverse effects/toxicity

   a. The major adverse effect of bupropion is seizure activity; other adverse effects include headache, mania, psychoses, dry mouth, nausea, vomiting, change in appetite, weight gain, weight loss, photosensitivity, hyperglycemia, hypoglycemia, and syndrome of inappropriate ADH secretion (SIADH)

b. Overdose with trazodone is considered safer than with TCAs or MOAIs; death from overdose with trazodone alone has not been reported; adverse effects include drowsiness, confusion, dizziness, fatigue, hallucinations, headache, insomnia, nightmares, slurred speech, syncope, weakness, blurred vision and tinnitus; also reported are hypotension, arrhythmias, chest pain, hypertension, palpitations, tachycardia, dry mouth, altered taste, constipation, diarrhea, excess salivation, flatulence, nausea, vomiting, rash, hematuria, impotence, priapism, urinary frequency, anemia, leukopenia, myalgia, and tremors

10. Nursing considerations

a. Individuals with a history of bipolar disorder taking bupropion need to be assessed for symptoms of mania

b. Monitor blood pressure and pulse rate before and during initial therapy with trazodone; clients with pre-existing cardiac disease should have ECG monitored before and periodically during therapy to detect dysrhythmias

c. Assess mental status and mood changes frequently; assess for suicidal tendencies, especially during early therapy; restrict amount of drug available to client

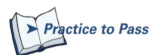
Practice to Pass

d. Give bupropion with food to decrease GI side effects; give trazodone immediately after meals to minimize side effects (nausea, dizziness) and allow for maximum absorption

11. Client education: as described in Tables 11-5 and 11-6

Describe the most common adverse effects that should be discussed with a client taking fluoxetine (Prozac).

III. Antimania Medications

A. Lithium

1. Action and use

a. Lithium is the drug of choice for controlling manic episodes in clients with bipolar disorder and is also used for long-term prophylaxis against recurrent mania and depression

b. Lithium is an inorganic ion that carries a single positive charge; it occurs naturally in animal tissue but has no known physiologic function; it is well-absorbed following oral administration and is distributed evenly to all tissue and body fluids

c. The exact mechanism of action of lithium is not fully understood, but it alters many neurotransmitter functions; it may correct an ion exchange abnormality in the neuron and/or may play a role in normalizing neurotransmission of norepinephrine, serotonin, dopamine, and acetylcholine

d. Lithium is used to treat a variety of psychiatric disorders, particularly to treat the effects of bipolar disorders (treatment of acute manic episodes and prophylaxis against recurrence)

2. Common medications: see Table 11-7

3. Administration considerations

a. Precise dosing is based on serum lithium levels; 300 mg lithium carbonate contains 8–12 mEq lithium; refer to Table 11-7 for dosing ranges of adults and children

Table 11-7					
Commonly Used Mood-Stabilizing Drugs	**Name: Generic (Trade)**	**Usual Adult Dosage Range (mg/day)**	**Preparations**	**Half-life (hr)**	**Peak Plasma Levels (hr)**
	Lithium carbonate (Eskalith, Lithobid, lithium citrate, etc.)	600–2400 mg; in children 15–20 mg (0.4–0.5 mEq/kg/ day in 2–3 divided doses; dosage may be adjusted weekly	PO, SR, L	18–36	1–4
	Carbamazepine (Tegretol)	200–1600 mg	PO, Ch	25–65; 8–29	1.5–6
	Valproic acid (Valproate, Depakote, Divalproex, others)	750$^+$ mg	PO, L	9–16	

PO, oral tablet/capsule; SR, oral slow-release tablets; L, liquid; Ch, chewable tablets.

   b. Lithium reduces euphoria, hyperactivity, and other symptoms of mania but does not cause sedation; antimanic effects are usually seen in 5 to 7 days after initial doses, but full effect does not usually occur for 2 to 3 weeks

   c. For many clients using lithium, adjunctive therapy with a benzodiazepine can be used to provide the sedation clients need

   d. Antipsychotic medications can also be used short term to rapidly decrease the symptoms of psychoses

4. Contraindications

   a. Lithium is contraindicated for clients who have a sensitivity to the drug, for those who are debilitated or elderly, or who have dehydration, or severe cardiovascular or renal disease; it should only be used where therapy (including blood levels) may be closely monitored; some products contain alcohol or tartrazine and should be avoided in clients with known hypersensitivity or intolerance

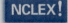

   b. Use cautiously in elderly or debilitated clients (decrease the initial dose); also use cautiously with clients who have any degree of cardiac, renal or thyroid disease, or with diabetes mellitus

5. Significant drug interactions

   a. Lithium may prolong the action of neuromuscular blocking agents

   b. Neurologic toxicity may occur with haloperidol or molindone

   c. Diuretics, methyldopa, probenecid, fluoxetine, and NSAIDs may increase the risk of toxicity

   d. Blood levels may be increased by angiotensin-converting enzyme (ACE) inhibitors

   e. Lithium may decrease the effects of chlorpromazine, and chlorpromazine may mask early signs of lithium toxicity

f. Hypothyroid effects may be additive with potassium iodide or antithyroid agents

g. Aminophylline, phenothiazines, and drugs containing large amounts of sodium increase renal elimination and may decrease effectiveness

6. Significant food interactions: large changes in sodium intake may alter the renal elimination of lithium; increasing sodium intake will increase renal excretion

7. Significant laboratory studies

a. It is essential that serum lithium levels be monitored frequently because of danger of lithium toxicity, especially since the therapeutic level and the toxic levels are very close; therapeutic range is 0.8 to 1.4 mEq/L, while the toxic dose is 1.5 mEq/L or greater

b. Pre-lithium work-up

    1) Renal: urinalysis, blood urea, nitrogen (BUN), creatinine, electrolytes, 24-hour creatinine clearance

    2) Thyroid: thyroid-stimulating hormone (TSH), T_4 (thyroxine), T_3 resin uptake, T_4I (free thyroxine index)

    3) Other: fasting blood glucose, complete blood count (CBC), ECG

c. Maintenance lithium dosing: lithium level every 3 months (for the first 6 months); every 6 months reassess thyroid function and ECG; assess more often if client is symptomatic

8. Side effects

a. Seizures, fatigue, headache, impaired memory, ataxia, confusion, dizziness, drowsiness, psychomotor retardation, restlessness, stupor

b. Also aphasia, blurred vision, dysarthria, tinnitus, arrhythmias, ECG changes, edema, hypotension

c. Others include abdominal pain, anorexia, bloating, diarrhea, nausea, dry mouth, metallic taste in the mouth; also polyuria, glycosuria, nephrogenic diabetes insipidus, and renal toxicity

d. Dermatological signs include alopecia, diminished sensation, and pruritis

e. Also reported are hypothyroidism, goiter, hyperglycemia and hyperthyroidism, hyponatremia, leukocytosis, weight gain, muscle weakness, hyperirritability, rigidity, and tremors

9. Adverse effects/toxicity

a. Lithium has a short half-life and high toxicity; it is excreted by the kidneys; sodium depletion will decrease renal excretion of lithium, which in turn will cause the drug to accumulate and lead to lithium toxicity

b. Other adverse effects reported by clients on therapeutic doses include fine hand tremors, GI upset, thirst, muscle weakness; at toxic levels more adverse effects are seen, such as persistent GI upset, coarse hand tremor, confusion, hyperirritability of muscles, ECG changes, sedation, incoordination; at serum levels greater than 2.5 mEq/L, death may result

10. Nursing considerations

a. Assess mood, ideation, and behaviors frequently; initiate suicide precautions if indicated

b. Monitor intake and output ratios; report significant changes in totals

c. Unless contraindicated, provide fluid intake of at least 2000 to 3000 mL/day

d. Monitor weight at least every 3 months

e. Assess client for signs and symptoms of lithium toxicity (vomiting, diarrhea, slurred speech, decreased coordination, drowsiness, muscle weakness, or twitching); if these occur, report before administration of the next dose

11. Client education

a. Instruct client to take medication exactly as directed, even if feeling well; take a missed dose as soon as remembered unless within 2 hours of next dose (6 hours if extended release)

b. Medication may cause dizziness or drowsiness; caution client to avoid driving, operating heavy machinery, or other activities requiring alertness until client's response to medication is known

c. Low sodium levels may predispose client to toxicity; advise client to drink 2000 to 3000 mL fluid each day and eat a diet with consistent and moderate sodium intake

d. Instruct client to avoid excessive amounts of coffee, tea, and cola (because of their diuretic effect); instruct client to avoid activities that cause excess sodium loss; notify healthcare professional of fever, vomiting, and diarrhea, which also cause sodium loss

e. Advise client that weight gain may occur; review with client the principles of a low-calorie diet

f. Instruct client to consult with healthcare professional before taking any OTC medications, before use of contraception, or if pregnancy is suspected

g. Review side effects and toxicity effects of medication and instruct client to report any of these to a health care professional promptly

h. Explain to clients with cardiovascular disease or over 40 years of age the need of ECG evaluation before and periodically during therapy; instruct client to report any irregular pulse or difficulty breathing, or if fainting occurs

B. Other antimania medications

1. Action and use

a. Growing evidence indicates that a variety of anticonvulsant drugs have beneficial effects in the treatment of bipolar disorder when lithium is ineffective, although they do not have FDA approval for this use

b. The two such medications presented here include carbamazepine (Tegretol) and valproic acid (e.g., Valproate, Depakote); these are the best studied of these agents and have acute antimanic and long-term mood-stabilizing effects in some clients with bipolar disorder; they are also better than lithium in treating mixed or dysphoric bipolar states and in clients who are rapid cyclers

      c. When given to clients who have failed to respond to lithium, carbamazepine has had a success rate of about 60 percent; for treatment of acute manic episodes the mechanism by which carbamazepine stabilizes mood is unknown

      d. Clinical studies indicate that valproic acid can control symptoms in acute manic episodes of mania and depression; it alters GABA-mediated neurotransmission, and this action may underlie the drug's mood-stabilizing effects

  2. Common medications (refer again to Table 11-7)

  3. Administration considerations

      a. Carbamazepine should be started using low initial dose (200 mg to 400 mg/day) and then gradually increased to as much as 1.6 to 2.2 grams/day

      b. Valproic acid for treatment of acute mania is 500 to 1000 mg/day in 2 to 4 divided doses initially; maintenance dosages range from 250 to 500 mg/day

  4. Contraindications

      a. Carbamazepine is contraindicated with hypersensitivity to the drug or bone marrow depression; it should be used only in pregnancy if potential benefits outweigh risks to the fetus; it should be used cautiously in clients with cardiac or hepatic disease, prostatic hyperplasia, or increased intraocular pressure

      b. Valproic acid is contraindicated in clients with hypersensitivity or with hepatic impairment; it should not be used with products containing tartrazine; it should be used cautiously by clients who have bleeding disorders, history of liver disease, organic brain disease, bone marrow depression, renal impairment and by children (because of increased risk of hepatotoxicity); safe use in pregnancy has not been established

  5. Significant drug interactions

      a. Carbamazepine may decrease the levels and effectiveness of corticosteroids, doxycycline, flebamate, quinidine, warfarin, oral contraceptives, barbiturates, cyclosporine, benzodiazepines, theophylline, lamotrigine, valproic acid, bupropion and haloperidol; danazol increases blood levels; concurrent use (within 2 weeks) of MAO inhibitors may result in hyperpyrexia, hypertension, seizures, and death; verapamil, diltiazem, propoxyphene, erythromycin (should not be prescribed), clarithromycin, SSRI antidepressants, or cimetidine increases levels and may cause toxicity; may increase risk of hepatotoxicity from isoniazid; felbamate decreases carbamazepine levels but increases levels of active metabolite

      b. Carbamazepine may decrease the effectiveness and increase the risk of toxicity from acetaminophen, increase the risk of CNS toxicity from lithium, and decrease the duration of action of nondepolarizing neuromuscular blocking agents

      c. The significant drug–drug interactions for valproic acid include an increased risk of bleeding with antiplatelet agents (including aspirin, NSAIDs, tirofiban, eptifibatide, and abciximab), cefamandole, cefoperazone, cefotetan, heparin and heparin-like agents, thrombolytic agents, or warfarin; there is a decreased metabolism of barbiturates and primidone, which increases the risk for toxicity; blood levels and toxicity may be increased by carbamazepine, cimetidine, erythromycin, or felbamate; additive CNS depression with other CNS depressants, including alcohol, antihistamines, antidepressants, opioids, MAOIs, and sedative/hypnotics

    d. Large doses of salicylates (in children) increase the effects of valproic acid; it may also increase or decrease effects and toxicity of phenytoin; MAOIs and other antidepressants may also lower seizure threshold and decrease effectiveness of valproates

    e. Carbamazepine, rifampin, or lamotrigine may decrease valproic acid blood levels; valproic acid may increase toxicity of carbamazepine, ethosuximide, lamotrigine, or zidovudine

6. Significant food interactions: none reported for either agent

7. Significant laboratory studies

    a. For clients receiving carbamazepine, target trough plasma levels are 6 to 12 μg/ml

    b. Routine CBC, including platelet count, reticulocyte count, and serum iron should be checked weekly during the first 2 months and yearly thereafter for evidence of potentially fatal blood cell abnormalities; drug should be discontinued if bone marrow depression occurs

    c. The target plasma drug level of valproic acid is 50 to 125 μg/mL; clients receiving near the maximum recommended 60 mg/kg/day should be monitored for toxicity

    d. Also monitor hepatic function (LDH, AST, ALT, and bilirubin) and serum ammonia concentrations prior to and periodically throughout therapy with valproic acid; the drug may cause hepatotoxicity; therapy should be discontinued if ammonia level becomes elevated

8. Side effects

    a. Common side effects for carbamazepine include sedation, GI disturbance, tremor, leukopenia, and hepatotoxicity

    b. Reported side effects for valproic acid include sedation, nausea, tremor, hepatotoxicity, and hair loss; nausea can be reduced by using delayed-release tablets or by applying the "sprinkle" formulation to food

9. Adverse effects/toxicity

    a. Some of the adverse effects for carbamazepine include ataxia, drowsiness, agranulocytosis, aplastic anemia, thrombocytopenia, chills, fever and lymphadenopathy

    b. For valproic acid some of the reported adverse effects include confusion, dizziness, headache, hepatotoxicity, indigestion, nausea, vomiting, prolonged bleeding time, thrombocytopenia, ataxia, and paresthesia

10. Nursing considerations

    a. Assess client frequently for seizure activity when taking carbamazepine and assess for facial pain because of the possibility of trigeminal neuralgia

    b. Perform liver function tests, urinalysis, and BUN routinely and measure serum ionized calcium levels at least every 6 months or if seizure frequency increases

NCLEX!

    c. Implement seizure precautions as indicated; administer medication with food to minimize gastric irritation; tablets may be crushed if client has difficulty swallowing—except for extended-release tablets

11. Client education

NCLEX!

    a. Instruct client to take carbamazepine around the clock, exactly as directed; if a dose is missed, take as soon as possible but not just before next dose is due; medication should be gradually decreased to prevent seizures

NCLEX!

    b. Instruct client taking carbamazepine to report fever, sore throat, mouth ulcers, easy bruising, petechiae, unusual bleeding, abdominal pain, chills, rash, pale stools, dark urine, or jaundice to the healthcare professional immediately

NCLEX!

    c. Caution client to use sunscreen and protective clothing to prevent photosensitivity reactions with carbamazepine

    d. Advise female clients to use a nonhormonal form of contraception while taking carbamazepine

NCLEX!

    e. Instruct client to avoid activities requiring alertness; carbamazepine and valproic acid may cause dizziness or drowsiness

    f. Client should not concurrently use alcohol, other CNS depressants or OTC drugs with either of these medications without consulting a healthcare professional first

    g. Advise client to carry information describing disease and medication regimen at all times such as a Medic-Alert tag/bracelet

    h. Instruct client to notify healthcare professional of medication regimen before any treatment or surgery

    i. Emphasize the importance of follow-up lab tests, eye exams, and ECGs

    j. For valproic acid, instruct client to take medication exactly as directed; if a dose is missed on a once-a-day schedule, take it as soon as remembered that day; if on a multiple-dose schedule, tell client to take it within 6 hours of the scheduled time, then space the remaining doses throughout the remainder of the day; abrupt withdrawal may lead to seizures

    k. Also advise clients taking valproic acid to notify healthcare professional if anorexia, severe nausea and vomiting, yellow skin or eyes, fever, sore throat, malaise, weakness, facial edema, lethargy, unusual bleeding or bruising, pregnancy or loss of seizure control occurs; children less than two years of age are especially at risk for fatal hepatotoxicity

IV. Sedative-Hypnotic and Anxiolytic Medications

A. Benzodiazepines

1. Action and use

    a. Benzodiazepines (BZ), the most widely prescribed medications in the world, are thought to reduce anxiety because they are powerful potentiators (receptor agonists) of the inhibitory neurotransmitter GABA

▶ *Practice to Pass*

The client is being discharged on lithium carbonate. What would be included in the teaching plan related to the client's medication regimen when at home?

b. A postsynaptic receptor site specific for the BZ molecule is located next to the GABA receptor; the BZ molecule and GABA bind to each other at the GABA receptor site, resulting in an *inhibition* of neurotransmission that results in a clinical decrease in the person's anxiety level

c. Most BZs are well absorbed following oral administration; because of their high lipid solubility, BZs readily cross the blood-brain barrier to reach sites within the CNS; most BZs undergo extensive metabolic alterations; with few exceptions, the **metabolites** (the result of biotransformation of a drug) are pharmacologically active so drug effects persist long after the parent drug is gone from the plasma (thus there may be a poor correlation between the plasma half-life of the parent drug and duration of pharmacological effect)

NCLEX!

d. Major indications for use of the BZs are anxiety, insomnia (sedative-hypnotic effect), and seizure disorders

e. Other uses include alcohol withdrawal, anxiety associated with medical disease, skeletal muscle relaxation, preoperative anxiety and apprehension, substance-induced (except for amphetamines) and psychotic agitation in emergency departments or in other crisis situations; in higher doses alprazolam and clonazepam may effectively treat panic disorder and social phobia; other uses are to induce general anesthesia and to manage seizure disorders and muscle spasm

2. Common medications: see Table 11-8 for generic and trade names, dosage, half-life, metabolite status, speed of onset, and approved use indications

   a. Benzodiazepines differ significantly from one another with regard to time course of action; specifically, they differ in onset of action, duration of action, and tendency to accumulate with repeated dosing

   b. Because all the BZs have essentially equivalent pharmacologic actions, selection among these agents is based in large part on differences in time course

3. Administration considerations

   a. Benzodiazepines should be started at low doses and gradually increased as needed to achieve the desired clinical response; there is a rapid onset of clinical action once an appropriate dose is achieved

   b. In anxiety disorders, some anxiety reduction may be apparent almost immediately; the antianxiety effect with initial dosing may not last as long as the serum half-life would suggest because of the drug redistributing out of the brain; with continued dosing, steady-state brain levels and sustained efficacy are achieved; for the treatment of anxiety, BZs are usually dosed at bedtime or BID; only occasionally is TID dosing required

   c. For use as a hypnotic, BZs are rapidly absorbed, have a short onset of action and a short elimination half-life, so that next-day sedation and impaired cognition are minimized (although individuals may experience some sedation or "hangover effect" the next day)

NCLEX!

   d. Treatment for insomnia should occur for as short a time as possible (not longer than 7 to 10 days), and should be used as an adjunct to help clients establish a regular sleep pattern along with improved sleep hygiene

Table 11-8

Sedative-Hypnotic and Anxiolytic Medications

Drug Class and Name: Generic (Trade)	Usual Adult Dosage Range (mg/day)	Dosage Forms	Half-Life (hr)	Speed of Onset (PO)	Approved Use Indication
Barbiturates					
Amobarbital (Amytal)	100–200	C	8–42	Short to intermediate	Hypnotic
Butabarbital (Butisol)	50–100	C	34–42	Short-to intermediate	Hypnotic
Pentobarbital (Nembutal)	100–200	C	15–48	Long-acting	Hypnotic
Phenobarbital (Luminal)	100–200	C	80–120	Long-acting	Hypnotic
Secobarbital (Seconal)	100–300	C	15–40	Short to intermediate	Hypnotic
Benzodiazepines					
Alprazolam (Xanax)	0.75–4 (A)	T	12–15	Intermediate	A, AD, P
Chlordiazepoxide (Librium)	25–200	C, T, I	5–30	Intermediate	A, AW, PS
Clonazepam (Klonopin)	1–6 1–20 (LGS)	T	20–50	Intermediate	LGS
Clorazepate (Tranxene)	7.5–90	C, T, T-SR	20–80	Fast	A
Diazepam (Valium)	2–40	C-SR, T, L, I	20–80	Very fast	A, PS, SE
Lorazepam (Ativan)	0.5–10	T, I	10–20	Intermediate	A, PS
Oxazepam (Serax)	30–120	C, T	5–20	Intermediate to slow	A, AD, AW
Nonbarbiturate/ nondiazepines					
Buspirone (Buspar)	10–60	T	2–4	Intermediate	A
Zolpidem (Ambien)	5–10	T	1.5–4	Fast	Hypnotic
Benzodiazepine Antagonist					
Flumazenil (Romazicon)	0.2–1 (adult) 0.01–0.2 (child)	I	—	Fast	Reversal of conscious sedation or general anesthesia

Approved Use Indicators: A = anxiety; AD = anxiety associated with depression; AW = alcohol withdrawal; LGS = Lennox-Gastaut syndrome/seizures; P = panic disorder; PS = psychotic disorder; SE = status epilepticus
Dosage Forms: C = capsule; C-SR = capsule, sustained-release; I = injection; L = oral, liquid; T = tablet; T-SR = tablet, sustained release.

techniques; clients are at risk for rebound insomnia and anxiety if the drugs are used longer periods of time

4. Contraindications

   a. BZs are contraindicated with drug sensitivity or during pregnancy or lactation because they do cross the blood-brain barrier and enter breast milk with ease (and develop quickly to toxic levels)

   b. BZs should not be used with clients who have pre-existing CNS depression, severe uncontrolled pain, or for clients with narrow-angle glaucoma

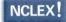

c. BZs are readily absorbed after oral ingestion; however, intramuscular (IM) injection produces slow and inconsistent absorption for most of these drugs

d. A convenient way of categorizing BZs is to divide them into those with short half-lives (less than 20 hours) and long half-lives (more than 20 hours) (see Table 11-8 for details); BZs with short half-life are usually preferable for use with elderly clients

e. Because hepatic metabolism is the primary mechanism for drug disposition, drugs that interfere with liver metabolism (e.g., alcohol) dangerously compound the effect of benzodiazepines

5. Significant drug interactions

NCLEX!

a. The CNS depressant actions of BZs are additive to those of other CNS depressants (e.g., alcohol, barbiturates, opioids), so although BZs are very safe when used alone, they can be extremely hazardous in combination with other depressants

   1) A combined overdose of a benzodiazepine with another CNS depressant can lead to profound respiratory depression, coma, and death

   2) Clients should be warned against use of alcohol and all other CNS depressants

b. BZs are poorly absorbed when taken with antacids; disulfiram and cimetidine use increases the plasma level of BZs that are oxidized; befazodone inhibits metabolism of alprazolam and trizolam while phenytoin increases anticonvulsant serum level; use of BZs with TCAs increases sedation, confusion, and impairs motor function; when used with MAOIs, CNS depression occurs, and succinylcholine decreases neuromuscular blockade

NCLEX!

c. With prolonged use of benzodiazepines, **tolerance** (an increased need of the drug in order to achieve the same effect) develops to some effects but not to others

   1) No tolerance develops to anxiolytic effects, and tolerance to hypnotic effects is generally low

   2) In contrast, significant tolerance develops to antiseizure effects

   3) Clients tolerant to barbiturates, alcohol, and other general CNS depressants show some cross-tolerance to benzodiazepines

   4) BZ can cause physical dependence, but the incidence of substantial dependence is low (especially for clients taking alprazolam)

6. Significant food interactions: none

7. Significant laboratory studies: none unless a client is on long-term therapy with the benzodiazepines; then CBC, liver, and renal function should be monitored

8. Side effects

NCLEX!

a. The most common side effect is decreased mental alertness; caution clients against driving or using heavy or hazardous equipment

b. Tolerance to most side effects quickly develops

NCLEX!

c. Monitor blood pressure of inpatients routinely, withhold the drug dose and report to the prescriber a drop of 20 mm Hg (systolic) while standing

NCLEX!

d. Other side effects include dry mouth, ataxia, dizziness, drowsiness, nausea and withdrawal symptoms (increased anxiety, flu-like symptoms, tremors)

9. Adverse effects/toxicity: as stated earlier, use of benzodiazepines with other CNS depressants can cause fatal results; signs and symptoms of overdose include somnolence, confusion, coma, diminished reflexes, and hypotension

10. Nursing considerations

    a. Assess degree and manifestation of anxiety before client begins therapy

    b. Assess client for drowsiness, light-headedness, and dizziness periodically during treatment; these usually disappear as therapy progresses

    c. Always caution client about driving or operating hazardous machinery especially in early treatment with benzodiazepines

    d. Monitor blood pressure, pulse, and respirations and provide supportive care as indicated

    e. Prolonged therapy may lead to psychological or physical dependence; risk is greater with larger doses of the medication; restrict amount of drug available to client

    f. Most BZs can be taken with food or crushed and put in food if client has difficulty swallowing

11. Client education

    a. Instruct client to take medications exactly as prescribed and not to skip or double up on missed doses; if a dose is missed, take within 1 hour or skip the dose and return to the regular schedule

    b. If medication is less effective after a few weeks, check with prescriber; do not increase the dose

    c. Abrupt withdrawal of the medication may cause sweating, vomiting, muscle cramps, tremors, and convulsions

    d. Advise client to avoid the use of alcohol or other CNS depressants concurrently with benzodiazepine therapy

B. **Benzodiazepine antagonist**

1. Action and use

    a. Flumazenil (Romazicon) is a BZ antagonist (receptor blocker); it selectively blocks BZ receptors but does not block adrenergic or cholinergic receptors

    b. In other words, it can reverse the *sedative* effects of BZs but may not reverse BZ-induced *respiratory depression*

    c. Because it does not stimulate the CNS and does not block other receptors, it can be given when BZ overdose is suspected and can also be used to reverse the effects of BZs following general anesthesia

    d. A reaction occurs within 30 to 60 seconds after administration

2. Common medications: flumazenil is the only drug in this class

3. Administration considerations

    a. It does not speed up the metabolism or excretion of BZs and has a short duration of action, which poses a clinical management problem; if the client responds to flumazenil, then BZs are present, but the client may need vigilant, ongoing dosing and monitoring as the client's body eliminates the BZs

  b. Administration is IV: inject dose slowly over 30 seconds and repeat every minute as needed; the first dose is 0.2 mg, the second is 0.3 mg, and all subsequent doses are 0.5 mg; effects fade in approximately one hour, so additional dosing may be needed

  c. In children, 0.01 mg/kg (up to 0.2 mg); if the desired level of consciousness (LOC) is not obtained after waiting an additional 45 seconds, further injections of 0.01 mg/kg can be given and repeated at 60-second intervals when necessary (up to a maximum of four additional times)

4. Contraindications

  a. Flumazenil is contraindicated for clients who have hypersensitivity to it; clients receiving BZs for life-threatening medical problems, including status epilepticus or increased intracranial pressure, should not be given flumazenil; clients with serious TCA overdose should not be given flumazenil

  b. Use the drug cautiously in clients with mixed CNS depressant overdose, with history of seizures, or clients with head injury; safety has not been established for use during pregnancy, lactation, or in children less than 2 years old

5. Significant drug interactions: none noted

6. Significant food interactions: none noted

7. Significant laboratory studies: none

8. Side effects: minor side and adverse effects include dizziness, agitation, confusion, nausea, vomiting, hiccups, paresthesia, rigors, and shivering

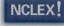

9. Adverse effects/toxicity: the principle adverse effect is precipitation of convulsions/seizures, which is most likely to occur in clients taking BZs to treat epilepsy and in clients who are physically dependent on BZs

10. Nursing considerations

  a. Assess LOC and respiratory status before and throughout therapy

  b. Establish that the client has a patent airway before administration of flumazenil

  c. Observe IV site frequently for redness or irritation; give drug through a free-flowing IV infusion into a large vein to minimize pain at the injection site

  d. Institute seizure precautions; seizures are more likely to occur in clients who are experiencing sedative/hypnotic withdrawal, who have recently received repeated doses of BZs, or who have a previous history of seizure activity; seizures may be treated with BZs, barbiturates, or phenytoin (larger than normal doses of BZs may be required)

  e. For suspected BZ overdose: if no effects are seen after giving flumazenil, consider other causes of decreased LOC (alcohol, barbiturates, opioid analgesics)

  f. Observe client for at least 2 hours after giving last dose for the appearance of resedation; hypoventilation may occur

NCLEX!

11. Client education

    a. Flumazenil does not consistently reverse the amnesic effects of BZs; provide client and family with written instructions for postprocedure care

    b. Inform family that client may appear alert at the time of discharge but the sedative effects of the BZ may reoccur; instruct client to avoid driving or other activities requiring alertness for at least 24 hours after discharge

NCLEX!

    c. Instruct client not to take *any* alcohol or nonprescription drugs for at least 18 to 24 hours after discharge

    d. Client should resume usual activities only when no residual effects of BZs remain

C. Barbiturates

  1. Action and use

    a. Like BZs, barbiturates bind to the GABA receptor-chloride channel complex to enhance inhibitory actions of GABA and directly mimic the actions of GABA; since barbiturates can directly mimic GABA, there is no ceiling to the degree of CNS depression they can produce and, unlike BZs, they can readily cause death when taken in overdose

    b. Barbiturates cause relatively nonselective depression of CNS function and are prototypes of the general CNS depressants; because they depress multiple aspects of CNS function, barbiturates can be used for daytime sedation, induction of sleep, suppression of seizures, and general anesthesia

NCLEX!

    c. Barbiturates can cause tolerance and dependence, have a high abuse potential, and are subject to multiple drug interactions; they are powerful respiratory depressants that can readily prove fatal in overdose as well; because of these effects, they have been often been replaced by safer drugs such as the BZs

    d. Barbiturates can be grouped into three classes, based on duration of action: (1) ultrashort-acting agents, (2) short- to intermediate-acting agents, and (3) long-acting agents; the duration of action is inversely related to their lipid solubility; barbiturates with the highest lipid solubility have the shortest duration of action; conversely, barbiturates with the lowest lipid solubility have the longest duration

  2. Common medications (see Table 11-8)

  3. Administration considerations

    a. Barbiturates are administered orally usually for daytime sedation and to treat insomnia; for general anesthesia and emergency treatment of convulsions, they are usually given by IV injection; barbiturates solutions are highly alkaline and can cause pain and necrosis when injected IM, so this route is generally avoided

    b. The ability to cause generalized CNS depression underlies both the therapeutic effects and their adverse effects; as the dosage is increased, responses progress from *sedation* to *sleep* to *general anesthesia*

    c. Most barbiturates can be considered nonselective CNS depressants; exceptions are phenobarbital and other barbiturates used to control seizures

    d. At hypnotic doses, barbiturates may reduce BP and heart rate; by contrast, toxic doses can cause profound hypotension and shock (from direct depressant effects on both myocardium and vascular smooth muscle)

    e. Barbiturates stimulate synthesis of hepatic microsomal enzymes, the principal drug-metabolizing enzymes of the liver; as a result, barbiturates can accelerate their own metabolism as well as the metabolism of many other drugs

    f. Tolerance develops over the course of repeated drug use; when taken regularly, tolerance develops to many (but not all) CNS effects; specifically, tolerance develops to sedative and hypnotic effects and to other effects that underlie barbiturate abuse

4. Contraindications: clients who have hypersensitivity, or who have overt or latent porphyria, severe hepatic/renal/respiratory dysfunction, or previous addiction to sedative/hypnotics

5. Significant drug interactions

NCLEX!

    a. Drugs with CNS-depressant properties (e.g., barbiturates, benzodiazepines, alcohol, opioids, antihistamines) intensify each other's effects; if these drugs are combined, the degree of CNS depression can be hazardous or even fatal; warn clients emphatically not to combine barbiturates with alcohol and other CNS depressants

    b. Because barbiturates stimulate synthesis of hepatic drug-metabolizing enzymes and accelerate metabolism of other drugs, doses of *warfarin* (an anticoagulant), *oral contraceptives,* and *phenytoin* (an antiseizure agent) should be increased to account for accelerated degradation; once drug dosages are increased, they need to be gradually re-regulated once barbiturate treatment ends to their pre-barbiturate amounts; barbiturates must be tapered and not stopped abruptly

6. Significant food interactions: none

7. Significant laboratory studies: clients on prolonged therapy (e.g., antiseizure therapy) should have hepatic and renal function and CBC evaluated periodically; also see individual agents for specific laboratory tests

8. Side effects

    a. Barbiturates have long half-lives and therefore can produce residual effects (hangover) when taken to treat insomnia; hangover can manifest as sedation, impaired judgment, and reduced motor skills; another possible effect is paradoxical excitement (especially the elderly and debilitated); the mechanism of this response is not known

    b. Barbiturates can intensify sensitivity to pain and may cause pain directly; their use has produced muscle pain, joint pain, and pain along nerves

9. Adverse effects/toxicity

    a. Acute intoxication with barbiturates is a medical emergency; left untreated, overdose can be fatal; poisoning is often the result of attempted suicide, although it can also occur by accident (usually in children or drug abusers)

NCLEX!

    b. Acute barbiturate overdose produces a classic triad of symptoms: *respiratory depression, coma,* and *pinpoint pupils,* which are frequently accompanied by *hypotension* and *hypothermia;* death is likely to result from pulmonary complications and renal failure

NCLEX!

c. Proper management usually requires admission to an intensive care unit; barbiturate poisoning has no specific antidote, so treatment usually includes gastric lavage, induction of emesis, and use of a cathartic (to reduce absorption by accelerating drug transit through the intestine); hemodialysis can remove drug that is already absorbed; forced diuresis and alkalinization of urine may facilitate drug removal via the kidneys

10. Nursing considerations

NCLEX!

a. With clients taking barbiturates, *always monitor respiratory status, pulse, and blood pressure frequently*

b. Prolonged therapy may lead to psychological or physical dependence; restrict amount of drug available to client, especially if depressed, suicidal, or with a history of addiction

c. Always monitor client for safety, alertness, and need for help with ambulation or self-care

11. Client education

NCLEX!

a. Always advise client to take medication exactly as prescribed and not to discontinue medication without consulting prescriber

NCLEX!

b. Medication may cause daytime drowsiness; caution client to avoid driving and other activities requiring alertness until response to medication is known

c. Advise female clients using oral contraceptives to use an additional non-hormonal contraceptive during therapy

d. Advise client to contact prescriber immediately if any adverse or toxic signs or symptoms occur

D. Other sedative-hypnotics and anxiolytics

1. Action and use

a. Buspirone (BuSpar) and zolpidem (Ambien) are 2 sedative-hypnotics/anxiolytics that are not barbiturates or BZs

b. Buspirone is indicated for management of anxiety; it binds to serotonin and dopamine receptors in the brain and increases norepinephrine metabolism in the brain; 95 percent of the drug is bound to plasma proteins; it is extensively metabolized by the liver and 20 to 40 percent is excreted in feces

c. Buspirone is quite different from other anxiolytics because it reduces anxiety while producing even less sedation than the BZs; its mechanism of action is unknown; major advantages are that it does not cause sedation, has no abuse potential, and does not enhance CNS depression caused by BZs, alcohol, barbiturates, and related drugs; its major disadvantage is that the onset of anxiolytic effects is delayed

d. Zolpidem is used for the short-term treatment of insomnia; it produces CNS depression by binding to GABA receptors; it has no analgesic properties, but produces sedation and induction of sleep; it is rapidly absorbed following oral administration and 92 percent binds to protein; zolpidem is metabolized by being converted to inactive metabolites that are excreted by the kidneys

2. Common medications (refer again to Table 11-8)

3. Administration considerations

    a. Buspirone is well absorbed following oral administration but undergoes extensive first-pass metabolism in the liver; giving it with food delays absorption but enhances bioavailability (by reducing first-pass metabolism)

    b. Zolpidem is rapidly absorbed following oral administration and is usually given orally just before bedtime because of its rapid onset of action

4. Contraindications

    a. Buspirone and zolpidem are contraindicated for clients with a hypersensitivity to the drug

    b. Buspirone is also contraindicated in severe hepatic or renal impairment and should be used cautiously in clients receiving other antianxiety agents; slowly withdraw other agents to prevent rebound phenomenon; use cautiously for clients receiving other psychoactive drugs or who are pregnant or lactating; also use cautiously with children because safety has not yet been established

    c. Zolpidem should not be used for clients with apnea; it should be used cautiously in clients with a history of previous psychiatric illness, suicide attempt, drug or alcohol abuse, impaired hepatic function or pulmonary disease, the elderly, pregnant or lactating women, and children (safety has not yet been established)

5. Significant drug interactions

    a. Buspirone interacts with MAOIs, which may result in hypertension; there may also be an increased risk for hepatic effects when used with trazadone; blood levels are increased with concurrent use with itraconazole or erythromycin; avoid concurrent use with alcohol

    b. For zolpidem, additive CNS depression can occur with concurrent use of other sedative/hypnotics, alcohol, phenothiazines, TCAs, opioids, or antihistamines

6. Significant food interactions: none reported with buspirone while food decreases and delays absorption of zolpidem

7. Significant laboratory studies: none since they are indicated for short-term use only

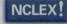

8. Side effects

    a. Buspirone is generally well tolerated; the most common reactions are dizziness, nausea, headache, nervousness, lightheadedness and excitement

    b. Zolpidem has a side effect profile like that of the BZs; daytime drowsiness and dizziness are most common, but only occur in about 1 to 2 percent of clients

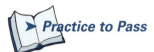

9. Adverse effects/toxicity

   a. Buspirone is non-sedating and does not interfere with daytime activities and poses little to no risk of suicide; the drug does not enhance the depressant effects of alcohol, barbiturates, and other general CNS depressants

   b. Zolpidem is not usually associated with tolerance, dependence, or abuse because it is used for short-term treatment only, but (like other sedative-hypnotics) it can intensify the effects of CNS depressants; warn clients not to combine zolpidem with alcohol or other CNS depressants

10. Nursing considerations

   a. Assess degree and manifestations of anxiety before and periodically throughout therapy with buspirone

   b. Buspirone does not appear to cause physical or psychological dependence or tolerance; however, clients with a history of drug abuse should be assessed for tolerance or dependence, and the amount of drug available to these clients should be restricted

   c. Clients changing from other antianxiety agents should receive gradually decreasing doses; buspirone will not prevent withdrawal symptoms

   d. With zolpidem, there may be a potential for physical or psychological dependence if used longer than 7 to 10 days; limit the amount of drug available to the client

   e. For clients taking zolpidem, assess alertness at time of peak effect; notify prescriber if desired sedation does not occur

   f. Assess client who has pain and medicate as needed; untreated pain decreases sedative effects of zolpidem

11. Client education

   a. As with all medications, instruct client to take exactly as prescribed

   b. Buspirone and zolpidem may cause dizziness or drowsiness; caution client to avoid driving or other activities requiring alertness until response to the medication is known

   c. Advise client to avoid concurrent use of buspirone and zolpidem and alcohol or other CNS depressants

   d. Advise client not to take OTC medications without consulting prescriber

   e. Instruct the client taking buspirone to report any chronic abnormal movements such as **dystonias** (muscle rigidity), motor restlessness, involuntary movements of facial or cervical muscles, or if pregnancy is suspected

   f. For clients taking zolpidem, advise the client to go to bed immediately after taking the medication because of the rapid onset of action

   g. Always stress the importance of follow-up exams to determine effectiveness of medication

V. Substance Misuse

A. Alcohol and disulfiram (Antabuse) therapy

1. Action and use

   a. Alcohol is a CNS depressant and like barbiturates, it causes general (relatively nonselective) depression of CNS function

   b. Alcohol appears to affect the CNS primarily by enhancing the actions of GABA

   c. The effect of alcohol on the CNS is dose-dependent

      1) When dosage is low, the higher brain centers (cortical areas) are primarily affected

      2) As the dosage is increased, more primitive brain areas (e.g., medulla) become depressed

      3) With depression of cortical function, thought processes and learned behaviors are altered, inhibitions are released, and self-restraint is replaced by increased sociability and expansiveness; cortical depression also results in significant impairment of motor function; as CNS depression deepens, reflexes diminish greatly and consciousness becomes impaired

      4) At very high doses, alcohol produces a state of general anesthesia

   d. Tolerance to alcohol increases with alcohol use; abuse and addiction progress over time

   e. Management of withdrawal depends on the degree of alcohol dependence; when dependence is mild, withdrawal can be accomplished on an outpatient basis; when dependence is great, the risks of withdrawal can be fatal if medical intervention is not carried out

   f. The major objective of medically supervised withdrawal is safe and effective removal of alcohol and/or other drugs from the individual; most medical treatment includes use of BZs—chlordiazepoxide (Librium), diazepam (Valium) and lorazepam (Ativan) have been used safely; a regime of atenolol (a beta-adrenergic blocking agent) used in conjunction with BZs decreases the amount of BZs necessary for safe detoxification

   g. Disulfiram is an inhibitor of the enzyme *alcohol dehydrogenase,* which catalyzes a major step in the breakdown of alcohol

      1) When the enzyme is inhibited and an individual drinks alcohol, blood concentrations of the toxic metabolite *acetaldehyde* increase significantly

      2) Acetaldehyde produces unpleasant symptoms of flushing, tachycardia, nausea, vomiting, and hypotension

      3) In medically fragile individuals, these symptoms may rarely prove life-threatening; because of associated risks, disulfiram is used only with highly selected individuals who have good physical health

2. Common medications: disulfiram (Antabuse) is the only alcohol antagonist in use

3. Administration considerations

   a. Studies show that disulfiram maintenance can significantly reduce drinking; the dose is typically 500 mg daily for 1 to 2 weeks; maintenance

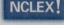

NCLEX!

dosages range from 125 to 500 mg a day, usually taken as a single dose in the morning

    b. At least 12 hours should elapse from the time of last alcohol intake and the initial dose of disulfiram

    c. The relatively long half-life of disulfiram ensures that several days must elapse between stopping the medication and safely drinking alcohol; this long half-life probably decreases the likelihood of impulsive relapse

  4. Contraindications: because of the severity of the acetaldehyde syndrome, candidates for therapy must be carefully chosen; those who lack the determination to stop drinking should not be given disulfiram

  5. Significant drug interactions

    a. Disulfiram causes irreversible inhibition of aldehyde dehydrogenase, the enzyme that converts acetaldehyde to acetic acid

    b. The adverse effects caused by alcohol plus disulfiram are collectively known as the *acetaldehyde syndrome*

  6. Significant food interactions: none

  7. Significant laboratory studies: none

  8. Side effects: in the absence of alcohol, disulfiram rarely causes significant effects; drowsiness and skin eruptions may occur during initial drug use but these responses diminish with time

  9. Adverse effects/toxicity: acetaldehyde syndrome is manifested by marked respiratory depression, cardiovascular collapse, cardiac dysrhythmias, myocardial infarction, acute congestive heart failure, convulsions, and death

  10. Nursing considerations

    a. As with all medications advise client to take medication as prescribed

    b. Advise client that simultaneous use with alcohol can precipitate the acetaldehyde syndrome

    c. Advise client that the effects of disulfiram may persist for about 2 weeks after the last dose is taken; alcohol must not be consumed until this interval is over

  11. Client education

    a. Warn client to avoid all forms of alcohol, including alcohol found in sauces and cough and cold syrups, and alcohol applied to the skin in aftershave lotions, colognes, and liniments

    b. Encourage client to adhere to all forms of self-help groups, individual and group therapies while using disulfiram therapy to establish a recovery program

B. Opioids

  1. Opioids (e.g., morphine, heroin) are major drugs of abuse and are usually Schedule II substances

2. Opioid abuse may be found in all segments of American society

3. For most abusers, initial exposure to opioids occurs either socially (illicitly) or in the context of pain management in a medical setting; only an exceedingly small percentage of individuals who develop an addictive pattern begin use therapeutically

NCLEX!

4. Opioid abuse by healthcare providers deserves special consideration; physicians, nurses, and pharmacists, as a group, abuse opioids to a greater extent than all other groups with similar educational backgrounds, and this is believed to be primarily the result of drug access

5. Tolerance develops with prolonged opioid use; persons tolerant to one opioid are cross-tolerant to other opioids; however, there is no cross-tolerance between opioids and general CNS depressants (e.g., barbiturates, benzodiazepines, alcohol)

6. Physical dependence is substantial with long-term use, but although opioid withdrawal syndrome can be extremely unpleasant, it is rarely dangerous

NCLEX!

7. Opioid toxicity produces a classic triad of symptoms: respiratory depression, coma, and pinpoint pupils; withdrawal symptoms begin 6 to 8 hours after the last dose and reach peak intensity within 48 to 72 hours, including craving, chills, sweating and piloerection (gooseflesh), abdominal pain and cramps, diarrhea, runny nose, and irritability

8. Naloxone (Narcan), an opioid antagonist, is the treatment of choice; it rapidly reverses all signs of opioid poisoning; dosage must be titrated carefully, however, because if too much naloxone is given, the client will swing from a state of intoxication to one of withdrawal; because of its short half-life, naloxone must be given again every few hours until the opioid has dropped to a nontoxic level

9. Nalmefene (Revex), a long-acting opioid antagonist, is an alternative to naloxone; because of its long half-life, nalmefene does not require repeated dosing; however, if the dose is excessive in an opioid-dependent person, then nalmefene will put the client into prolonged withdrawal

10. Methadone, an oral opioid with a long duration of action, is the agent most commonly used for easing opioid withdrawal and preventing abstinence syndrome; once stabilized on methadone, withdrawal is accomplished by administering it in gradually smaller doses; the resultant abstinence syndrome is mild, with symptoms resembling those of moderate influenza; the entire process of methadone substitution and withdrawal takes about 10 days; the objective of maintenance therapy is to avoid withdrawal and the need to procure illicit drugs; methadone maintenance is most effective when done in conjunction with non-drug measures directed at altering patterns of drug use

C. Cocaine

1. Cocaine, extracted from the coca plant, is a fine, white, odorless powder; cocaine and its offspring crack have caused major drug problems in the United States

2. Cocaine passes the blood-brain barrier readily, which causes an instantaneous high; when administered IV (mainlining) it is rapidly metabolized by the liver, so the exhilarating "rush" does not last long; cocaine exerts both CNS and peripheral nervous system (PNS) effects because of its ability to block

norepinephrine and dopamine reuptake into presynaptic neurons; it depletes these neurotransmitters

3. Cocaine can be taken orally but is poorly absorbed and has little effect by this route; it is also "snorted" (absorbed through nasal mucosa) or mixed with baking soda and ether and smoked (called freebasing, probably the most dangerous method of ingesting cocaine); crack is a less expensive way of using cocaine than snorting or mainlining, primarily because it is sold and marketed in smaller packages ($10 or $20 "rocks"); crack is used at every level in society, is reported to be the most addictive drug on the streets today, and the risk for overdose is extremely high; although physical dependence is less than with opioid abuse, psychological dependence is intense

4. Death from cocaine is linked to metabolic and respiratory acidosis and hyperthermia associated with prolonged seizures; tachyarrhythmias have also led to death

5. Although cocaine is highly addictive, physical withdrawal is relatively mild; psychological withdrawal is severe because the drug is so pleasurable and causes an intense craving for the drug; treatment is aimed at restoring the depleted neurotransmitters; amino acid catecholamine precursors (such as tyrosine and phenylalanine), TCAs, and the dopamine agonist bromocriptine are three approaches used to increase the availability of neurotransmitters

D. Cannabis (marijuana/hashish)

1. Marijuana, the most widely used illegal drug in the United States, is derived from the Indian hemp plant *Cannabis sativa,* which has separate male and female forms; the two most common cannabis derivatives are marijuana and hashish; the major psychoactive substance in *Cannabis sativa* is delta-9-tetrahydrocannabinol (THC), which is an oily chemical with high lipid solubility

2. THC has several possible mechanisms, including activation of specific cannabinoid receptors found in various brain regions; when marijuana or hashish is smoked, about 60 percent of the THC content is absorbed; absorption from the lungs is rapid; subjective effects begin in minutes and peak in 20 to 30 minutes; effects from a single marijuana cigarette may persist 2 to 3 hours; with oral administration, absorption is only 6% to 20%

3. Marijuana produces three principal subjective effects: euphoria, sedation, and hallucinations; no other psychoactive drug produces all three of these; because of this singular pattern of effects, marijuana is in a class by itself

   a. Responses to low doses of THC are variable and depend on several factors including dosage size, route of administration, setting of drug use, and expectations and previous experience of the user

   b. Some of the more common effects of low-dose THC include euphoria and relaxation; gaiety and a heightened sense of humor; an increased sensitivity to visual and auditory stimuli; enhanced sense of touch, taste, and smell; increased appetite and a more intense appreciation of the flavor of food; distortion of time (times seems to move more slowly)

   c. Some of the undesirable effects of low-dose THC include impairment of short-term memory; decreased capacity to perform multiple tasks; decreased ability to drive or operate machinery; inability to distinguish time (past, present, and future); depersonalization (a sense of feeling strange about self); a decreased ability to distinguish the emotions of others and reduced interpersonal interactions

    d. In higher doses, marijuana can have some serious adverse psychological effects including hallucinations, delusions, and paranoia; euphoria may be replaced by intense anxiety and a dissociative state in which the user feels "outside of himself/herself"

    e. In extremely high doses, marijuana can produce a state resembling toxic psychosis, which may persist for weeks; also dangerous is the use of marijuana with alcohol or other CNS depressants

4. Chronic use of marijuana can produce a syndrome known as *amotivational syndrome,* characterized by apathy, dullness, poor grooming, reduced interest in achievement, and disinterest in the pursuit of conventional goals

5. Other effects of marijuana include change in heart rate, orthostatic hypotension, pronounced reddening of the conjunctivae and, when used acutely, respiratory bronchodilation; when smoked chronically, effects such as bronchitis, sinusitis, and asthma can be seen; scientists believe that the carcinogens in marijuana smoke are more potent than the tar from cigarettes

6. When used in extremely high doses, marijuana is able to produce tolerance and physical dependence; symptoms brought on by abrupt discontinuation of marijuana include irritability, restlessness, nervousness, insomnia, reduced appetite, and weight loss; tremor, hyperthermia, and chills may also occur but these symptoms usually subside in 4 to 5 days and no symptoms of withdrawal are noted

7. Cannabinoids are sometimes used to treat nausea and vomiting (more effectively than traditional anti-emetics) that occur as severe side effects of cancer chemotherapy; THC was recently approved for stimulating appetite in clients with AIDS

E. Hallucinogens

1. Use of hallucinogens, also called psychedelics or psychomimetics, is on the rise again, especially among young people; these drugs alter perception; there are 2 basic groups of hallucinogens—natural and synthetic; see Table 11-9 for examples of hallucinogens

2. In general, hallucinogens can heighten awareness of reality or cause a terrifying psychosis-like reaction; users report distortions in body image, a sense of depersonalization, and/or a frightening loss of the sense of reality; individuals have also reported seeing grotesque creatures; emotional consequences are panic, anxiety, confusion, and paranoid reactions; individuals have experienced frank psychotic reactions after minimal use, sometimes referred to as a "bad trip"; two most commonly used hallucinogens, LSD and PCP, are discussed here

    a. LSD causes a phenomenon known as **synesthesia**, a blending of senses (such as smelling a color or tasting a sound); it can cause increases in blood pressure, tachycardia, trembling, and dilated pupils; CNS effects include a sense of unreality, perceptual alteration, distortions, and impaired judgment

    b. LSD users can experience flashbacks (frightening episodes that can heighten a sense of "going crazy"); bad trips from LSD cause anxiety, paranoia, and acute panic; some individuals who have experienced psychotic

Category	Examples
General CNS depressants	Alcohol Barbiturates: the three most widely abused are *secobarbital, pentobarbital,* and *amobarbital.* Benzodiazepines: diazepam (Valium) is the most widely abused.
Opioids	Heroin Morphine Meperidine Hydromorphone
Stimulants	Cocaine Amphetamines Nicotine
Marijuana/hashish	Can sometimes be classified with hallucinogens because of hallucination effect but is in a class by itself
Hallucinogens	LSD (lysergic acid diethylamide-25) PCP (phencyclidine) Mescaline (peyote from cactus) MDA (3,4-methylenedioxyamphetamine)
Inhalants	Anesthetics (nitrous oxide, ether) Nitrites (amyl nitrite, butyl nitrite, isobutyl nitrite) Organic solvents (toluene, gasoline, lighter fluid, paint thinner, nail-polish remover, benzene, acetone, chloroform, and model-airplane glue)
Anabolic (androgenic) steroids	Testosterone Dantrolene (Durabolin) Stanozolol (Winstrol)

Table 11-9 Categories and Examples of Drugs of Abuse

"breaks" from LSD have never fully recovered and a number of individuals have killed themselves while under the influence of LSD

c. PCP, a synthetic drug, traditionally has been used as an animal tranquilizer; the main safety risk for users is the unpredictable behavior (progressing from coma to violent behavior without warning); PCP can be taken orally, IV, smoked, or snorted; it is well absorbed by all routes and effects last from 6 to 8 hours

d. With PCP the user experiences a high; euphoria and peaceful feelings are the effects sought after; undesired effects of PCP can be serious; BP and heart rate are elevated; other peripheral nervous system effects include ataxia, salivation, and vomiting; a catatonic type of muscular rigidity alternating with violent outbursts may be frightening to others; psychological symptoms include hostile, bizarre behavior, a blank stare, and agitation

e. LSD and PCP deaths may be caused by overdose but are more likely to be linked to perceptual disorientation and unresponsiveness to environmental stimuli; hallucinogens do not produce physical dependence, so there are no withdrawal symptoms

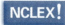 f. The nurse should provide a safe, calm, reassuring environment for clients detoxifying from hallucinogens

F. Inhalants

1. Inhalants are a varied group of drugs that are all taken by inhalation; they can be divided into three classes: anesthetics, volatile nitrites, and organic solvents (see Table 11-9 for examples)

2. Anesthetics produce subjective effects similar to those of alcohol—euphoria, exhilaration, and loss of inhibitions; the anesthetics most abused are nitrous oxide—"laughing gas"—and ether; these drugs may be popular because of ease of administration (neither requires difficult-to-obtain equipment); for nitrous oxide, ready availability also promotes use (small cylinders of the drug, marketed for aerating whipping cream, can be purchased without restrictions)

3. The nitrites (refer again to Table 11-9) are subject to abuse most often by homosexual males because of an ability to relax the anal sphincter, and by males in general because of a reputed ability to prolong and intensify sexual orgasm; the most pronounced effect of the nitrites is venodilation, which in turn causes a profound drop in systolic BP; the result is dizziness, light-headedness, palpitations, and possibly pulsatile headache; the effect of the drug begins seconds after inhalation and fades rapidly; the primary toxicity is methemoglobinemia, which can be treated with methylene blue and supplemental oxygen

4. A wide assortment of organic solvents have been inhaled to induce intoxication (see Table 11-9 for examples); these are used primarily by children and the very poor; they are administered by three processes

   a. "Bagging": pouring solvent in a plastic bag and inhaling the vapor

   b. "Huffing": pouring the solvent on a rag and inhaling the vapor

   c. "Sniffing": inhaling the solvent directly from its container

5. The acute effects of organic solvents are somewhat like those of alcohol (euphoria, impaired judgment, slurred speech, flushing, and CNS depression); they can also cause visual hallucinations and disorientation to time and place; high doses can cause sudden death, possibly from anoxia, respiratory depression, vagal stimulation (which slows heart rate), and dysrhythmias; prolonged use can cause multiple toxicities; gasoline can cause lead poisoning; chloroform is toxic to heart, liver, and kidneys; and toluene can cause severe brain damage and bone marrow depression; many of these solvents can cause damage to the heart

6. Management of acute toxicity is strictly supportive; the objective is to stabilize vital signs because there are no antidotes for these agents

G. Anabolic (androgenic) steroids

1. Androgens are frequently abused to enhance athletic performance; most are now regulated by the Controlled Substances Act; the most widely used androgen is testosterone; there are substantial benefits for the athletes as well as many risks

2. Steroids increase muscle mass in young males and in females of all ages and significantly increase muscle mass and strength in sexually mature males; the potential for adverse effects of androgens is significant; salt and water retention can lead to hypertension; when athletes take high doses there can be an increase in LH and FSH, resulting in testicular shrinkage and sterility; acne is common; reduction of HDL-cholesterol and elevation of LDL-cholesterol may accelerate development of atherosclerosis; there are potentially harmful effects to the liver as well; in females, androgens can cause menstrual irregularities and virilization (growth of facial hair, deepening of the voice, decreased breast size, uterine atrophy, clitoral enlargement, and male-pattern baldness); hair loss, and irreversible voice change

3. Long-term androgen use can lead to abuse or "addiction" syndrome; characteristics include preoccupation with androgen use and difficulty in stopping use; when it is discontinued an abstinence syndrome can develop similar to that produced by withdrawal from alcohol, opioids, and cocaine

H. CNS depressants

1. Refer back to previous section on sedative-hypnotic and anxiolytic medications

2. Benzodiazepines are not likely to produce abuse in clients who do not have a history of substance dependence; they are usually abused in combination with alcohol and/or barbiturates, which leads to CNS depression and may cause death; tolerance in individuals with substance dependence is rapid for sedative and euphoric effects and negligible for antianxiety effects

3. Barbiturates are frequently abused drugs among young or middle-aged users who abuse prescription drugs because they are legitimately manufactured and are available in many forms; the usual route of administration is oral or IV; barbiturates have a cross-tolerance to other chemically similar drugs, including alcohol, BZs, and heroin; IV users experience a sudden warm "rush," followed by a prolonged drowsy feeling

4. Mild barbiturate intoxication is exhibited by sluggishness in coordination, emotional lability, aggressive impulses, slowness of speech, thought disorders, and faulty judgment; neurologic signs include nystagmus (involuntary eye oscillations), diplopia (double vision), strabismus (deviation of the eye), ataxic gait, positive Romberg's sign (swaying of the body when standing with the feet close together and eyes closed), hypotonia, dysmetria (disturbance to control range of movement in muscular acts), and decreased superficial reflexes; intoxication with barbiturates is confirmed by blood tests

5. Barbiturates have potentially fatal effects; they are used frequently in accidental overdose and suicide attempts; death occurs as a result of deep coma, which progresses to respiratory arrest and cardiovascular failure; lethal doses vary widely from person to person; there is a narrow therapeutic index for sedative effects with the therapeutic dose being very close to the lethal dose

6. Tolerance and withdrawal are similar to alcohol because they are both CNS depressants

I. Central nervous system stimulants

1. The CNS stimulants that will be discussed here are amphetamines; discussion of cocaine, another CNS stimulant, can be found in a previous section

2. Amphetamines are also discussed in Chapter 10; the family of amphetamines includes dextroamphetamine, methamphetamine; when used for abuse, they are usually taken by mouth or IV; in addition, a form of dextroamphetamine known as "ice" or "crystal meth" can be smoked

3. The effects from amphetamine abuse include arousal and elevation of mood, euphoria, talkativeness, a sense of increased physical strength and mental capacity, increased self-confidence, and little or no desire for food or sleep (thus the term "uppers"); sexual orgasm is delayed, intensified, and more pleasurable

4. Some adverse effects of amphetamines can be fatal, including production of a psychotic state characterized by hallucinations and paranoid ideation; also, because of their sympathomimetic actions, they can cause vasoconstriction and excessive stimulation of the heart, leading to hypertension, angina pectoris, and dysrhythmias; overdose may also cause cerebral and systemic vasculitis

and renal failure; vasoconstriction can be relieved by phentolamine—an alpha-adrenergic blocker; cardiac stimulation can be reduced with a beta blocker (e.g., labetalol); drug elimination can be accelerated by giving ammonium chloride to acidify the urine

5. Extended use of amphetamines produces a tolerance to mood elevation, appetite suppression, and cardiovascular effects; physical dependence is moderate while psychological addiction is intense; amphetamine withdrawal can produce dysphoria and a strong sense of craving; other symptoms include fatigue, prolonged sleep, excessive eating, and depression

6. A stimulant drug that is becoming more and more unacceptable is nicotine; it is the only pharmacologically active drug in tobacco smoke apart from carcinogenic tars; it exerts powerful effects on the brain, spinal cord, peripheral nervous system, heart and various other body structures; nicotine stimulates specific acetylcholine receptors in the CNS including the cerebral cortex, producing increases in psychomotor activity, cognitive function, sensorimotor performance, attention and memory consolidation; as with all stimulant drugs, a period of depression follows withdrawal

7. Nicotine does not appear to induce any pronounced degree of biological tolerance; smokers seem to learn how to dose themselves so as to maintain a blood level of nicotine within a reasonably narrow range; nicotine induces both physiological and psychological dependence

8. Nicotine exerts a potent reinforcing action, especially in the early phases of drug use; in the veteran smoker, the reinforcing action of repeated smoking is primarily to relieve or avoid withdrawal symptoms; in addition to CNS effects, normal doses of nicotine can increase heart rate, blood pressure, and cardiac contractility; withdrawal from cigarettes is characterized by an abstinence syndrome, including a craving for nicotine, irritability, anxiety, anger, difficulty in concentrating, restlessness, impatience, increased appetite, and insomnia; the period of withdrawal may last many months

9. See Chapter 10 for discussion of other specific CNS stimulants

▶ Practice to Pass

The client is admitted to the unit for detoxification from alcohol. He states that his last drink was 12 hours ago. What are 4 major nursing priorities related to withdrawal from alcohol for the client?

Case Study

A 22-year-old, single male client is being discharged home today after detoxification from alcohol and cocaine. He will be taking disulfiram (Antabuse) 250 mg PO. He is scheduled to meet with the aftercare nurse tomorrow at 9:00 AM.

❶ Briefly describe the mechanism of action of disulfiram (Antabuse).

❷ Describe the teaching plan the nurse will use to reinforce the adverse effects of disulfiram and alcohol use.

❸ What is the purpose of taking disulfiram (Antabuse)?

❹ With disulfiram (Antabuse) therapy, identify at least three other recommendations the nurse will make for inclusion in a recovery plan for the client.

❺ What is the usual length of time a client will take disulfiram (Antabuse)?

For suggested responses, see pages 640–641.

Posttest

1 The client is taking haloperidol (Haldol) 2 mg TID. The nurse plans to assess the client frequently for dystonia, parkinsonism, and akathisia as adverse effects of this:

(1) Relative-potency antipsychotic.
(2) High-potency antipsychotic.
(3) Medium-potency antipsychotic.
(4) Low-potency antipsychotic.

2 A client who has been taking bupropion (Wellbutrin) 100 mg twice daily for 2 weeks is returning to the clinic. As part of the nursing evaluation, you ask the client which of the following priority questions regarding adverse effects of the medication?

(1) "Have you experienced a decrease in appetite?"
(2) "Have you experienced a change from your depressed mood?"
(3) "Have you had any episodes of dizziness, drowsiness, headache, or insomnia?"
(4) "Are you still hearing voices?"

3 A client with major depression is on suicide precautions since being admitted 2 days ago. While formulating the care plan the nurse includes which of the following interventions pertaining to safe medication administration?

(1) Always crush the medication and put in applesauce.
(2) Ask the nursing assistant to watch the client drink all of the water given with the medication.
(3) Observe the same safety precautions of medication administration as for all clients.
(4) Remain with the client at least 5 minutes after medication administration.

4 The client taking lithium carbonate (Eskalith) is having a difficult time walking, is confused, agitated and is complaining of blurred vision. The nurse checks the lithium level drawn earlier in the day, expecting the level to be within which of the following ranges?

(1) 0.5 to 0.8 mEq/L
(2) 1.2 to 1.5 mEq/L
(3) 1.5 to 1.8 mEq/L
(4) 2.0 to 3.0 mEq/L

5 The client is taking an antidepressant medication. She arrives at the clinic for a six-week follow-up visit. The nurse evaluates the medication as being effective if the client:

(1) Reports going back to work 2 hours/day and sleeping 12 hours each night and 3 hours after coming home from her office job.
(2) Is talking about vacation plans for the following month, reports sleeping 9 hours each night, working a full time job, and feeling less tired and anxious than 2 weeks ago.
(3) Reports working a full-time job and being able to work at least 3 or 4 hours/week overtime, sleeping 6 hours each night, and only feeling depressed after working 10 hours/day.
(4) Is complaining of weight gain, but obtains 3 extra hours of sleep per night.

6 You have admitted a client who is undergoing withdrawal from heroin. You expect the client to exhibit which of the following during the *initial* phase of withdrawal?

(1) Irritability and insomnia
(2) Drug craving, lacrimation, rhinorrhea, yawning, and diaphoresis
(3) Tremors, agitation, anxiety, diaphoresis
(4) Hallucinations, delusions, and increases in blood pressure and pulse

7   An adult client has been taking alprazolam (Xanax) 2 mg for generalized anxiety for the last 2 weeks. Today he is in the clinic and states, "I can't believe how dry my mouth is since I have been taking this stuff. And sometimes I get so dizzy and lightheaded but otherwise it works great. I don't feel all anxious anymore." The priority response by the nurse will be which of the following?

(1) "You can use gum or hard candy or sugarless gum to relieve some of those symptoms."
(2) "You will need to have the dosage of your medication lowered today so that you will not experience the side effects you are describing."
(3) "You feel dizzy and lightheaded, which is a side effect of the medication. Don't participate in activities that require you to be alert or operate heavy equipment, which could be a safety hazard, until you no longer have these side effects or are not taking the medication anymore."
(4) "You will need to take this medication with food from now on."

8   A client is beginning treatment with an antidepressant medication. The nurse will include appropriate teaching strategies and precautions in the care plan, knowing that there is a high risk for successful suicide with medications in which of the following antidepressant classes?

(1) Selective serotonin reuptake inhibitors (SSRIs)
(2) Monoamine oxidase inhibitors (MAOIs)
(3) Tricyclic antidepressants (TCAs)
(4) Anxiolytics

9   A 46-year-old client newly diagnosed with schizophrenia is being discharged to home in 5 days. The client lives in a two-bedroom apartment with his elderly mother who is frail but self-sufficient. The nursing care plan *must* include which of the following to promote compliance with medication administration?

(1) Teaching client and his mother about the prescribed medication and why compliance is so important to the client's ongoing recovery process.
(2) Teaching the client's mother the importance of regular meals so the client can take his medication after breakfast.
(3) Instructing the mother to be sure that the client is taking his medication daily as prescribed.
(4) Teaching the client about his medication regime and how taking his medication as prescribed will help him remain symptom-free indefinitely.

10   An adult client is in the clinic today for a follow-up 2-week visit. Diazepam (Valium) 10 mg was prescribed during the client's last visit. In order to evaluate that there are positive effects from the medication the nurse would need which of the following pieces of evidence?

(1) Hear the client saying that she is feeling much calmer now.
(2) See a change from the very anxious person documented at the last visit to a calmer and more focused person at present.
(3) None; there are probably no observable changes in the client's behavior after only 2 weeks
(4) Hear the client describe her increased appetite and how much more she is able to do since taking the medication.

See pages 452–453 for Answers and Rationales.

Answers and Rationales

Pretest

1 Answer: 2 *Rationale:* Because the client is hospitalized and is receiving an IM dose of thorazine, the primary concern should be to monitor for a decrease in the psychosis. Blood pressure and pulse should be monitored as a general measure for initial treatment with thorazine whether IM or PO. Ability to walk

and eat lunch are not significant to the issue of initial concern.
Cognitive Level: Analysis
Nursing Process: Assessment; *Test Plan:* PHYS

2 Answer: 3 *Rationale:* The only correct option is slurred speech and drowsiness. Olanzapine is a relatively new drug approved for schizophrenia and other

psychotic disorders. This agent is generally well tolerated and appears devoid of serious adverse effects.
Cognitive Level: Analysis
Nursing Process: Evaluation; *Test Plan:* PHYS

3 **Answer: 1** *Rationale:* The only correct answer is option 1. Trazodone is an atypical antidepressant used more often for insomnia than for depression. It is not used for panic attacks or anxiety.
Cognitive Level: Application
Nursing Process: Implementation; *Test Plan:* PSYC

4 **Answer: 3** *Rationale:* The most important person to instruct is the client (not the family member, as indicated in option 4). With MAOIs it is important to give the client not only oral but also complete written instructions concerning medication administration, food interactions, etc. It is good to instruct the client how to notify the appropriate health care professional, but it is not a major objective to teach the family how to contact an appropriate health care professional.
Cognitive Level: Application
Nursing Process: Implementation; *Test Plan:* HPM

5 **Answer: 4** *Rationale:* Diazepam and chlordiazepoxide are contraindicated for use with elderly clients (options 1 and 2) while trazadone is an atypical antidepressant, not a benzodiazepine. Lorazepam is the only appropriate benzodiazepine listed that is good for use with elderly clients.
Cognitive Level: Analysis
Nursing Process: Planning; *Test Plan:* PHYS

6 **Answer: 3** *Rationale:* The primary reason for re-hospitalization is that a client with bipolar disorder stops taking medication (option 3). There will always be other problems in families and in life (options 1 and 4), but these do not necessarily bring the client back to the hospital. If the client decides to lose weight, this in itself does not indicate that the client will need to be hospitalized.
Cognitive Level: Analysis
Nursing Process: Analysis; *Test Plan:* HPM

7 **Answer: 4** *Rationale:* The nurse should ask if the client is taking disulfiram because this medication causes the adverse reactions noted above when alcohol is also ingested. Option 1 is not highest priority because the smell of alcohol indicates that the time of the last intake was relatively recent. Options 2 and 3 are not the first questions that the client should be asked in this situation because they do not relate to the issue of vomiting and drug interactions.
Cognitive Level: Analysis
Nursing Process: Assessment; *Test Plan:* PHYS

8 **Answer: 4** *Rationale:* The nurse should refer the client back to the physician for clarification rather than try to second-guess the physician's thoughts or speak for the physician. Option 1 is not appropriate because there is no basis for the statement. Option 2 is only one aspect of the difference between a tricyclic antidepressant and a selective serotonin reuptake inhibitor, but it does not address the client's concern. Option 3 is accusatory and therefore inappropriate.
Cognitive Level: Application
Nursing Process: Implementation; *Test Plan:* PSYC

9 **Answer: 3** *Rationale:* Clients taking fluoxetine usually demonstrate a weight loss. The client needs to weigh him- or herself daily and adjust nutritional intake as necessary. The client will need to increase the caloric intake (option 2) not the fluid intake. The client does not necessarily need a change in medication (option 1). Option 4 is incorrect; it will take 3 to 4 weeks for the effect of the medication to be seen.
Cognitive Level: Analysis
Nursing Process: Analysis; *Test Plan:* PHYS

10 **Answer: 3** *Rationale:* Chlorpromazine (Thorazine) is not only the oldest of the antipsychotic medications, it can also used for relief of intractable hiccups. Risperidone (option 1), molindone (option 2) and thioridazine (option 4) do not have this effect.
Cognitive Level: Application
Nursing Process: Analysis; *Test Plan:* PHYS

Posttest

1 **Answer: 2** *Rationale:* Haloperidol is a high potency antipsychotic. Option 1 is not a classification of antipsychotics. Options 3 and 4 are valid classifications of antipsychotics, but they do not describe haloperidol.
Cognitive Level: Comprehension
Nursing Process: Planning; *Test Plan:* PHYS

2 **Answer: 3** *Rationale:* Dizziness, drowsiness, headache, and insomnia are some of the common CNS adverse effects of bupropion. Decreased appetite (option 1) is not a concern. Option 2 is incorrect because it asks about depression, while bupropion is used to treat anxiety. Option 4 indicates that the client has had hallucinations, which are not associated with bupropion.
Cognitive Level: Analysis
Nursing Process: Evaluation; *Test Plan:* PHYS

3 **Answer: 3** *Rationale:* The nurse should observe the same safety standards of medication administration as with all clients. Crushing a medication and placing

it in applesauce is not necessary for a client on suicide precautions unless there is a problem with swallowing or taking tablets or capsules (option 1). Option 2 is incorrect because it is not the responsibility of the nursing assistant to remain with a client taking medications. Staying with the client for 5 minutes (option 4) is not necessary for safe medication administration.
Cognitive Level: Application
Nursing Process: Implementation; *Test Plan:* SECE

4 **Answer: 4** *Rationale:* The symptoms listed are those of lithium toxicity, and are seen when the serum level is 2 to 3 mEq/L. The other options indicate lesser serum concentrations that would not produce these manifestations.
Cognitive Level: Analysis
Nursing Process: Analysis; *Test Plan:* PHYS

5 **Answer: 2** *Rationale:* In option 2, the client is demonstrating progress in returning to usual living. She is working a reasonable amount of the day, sleeping regularly, and making plans with others. In option 1, the client is sleeping too many hours each day. She is reporting very little activity outside of sleeping. She remains withdrawn and demonstrates no change in mood or activities. Option 3 indicates that the client is overworking, sleeping only 6 hours each night and still reporting feelings of depression. Option 4 alone shows no signs of change.
Cognitive Level: Analysis
Nursing Process: Evaluation; *Test Plan:* PHYS

6 **Answer: 2** *Rationale:* Clients undergoing withdrawal from heroin exhibit drug craving, lacrimation, rhinorrhea, yawning, and diaphoresis. Option 1 is incorrect because irritability and insomnia are seen with withdrawal from marijuana. The manifestations listed in options 3 and 4 pertain to withdrawal from alcohol.
Cognitive Level: Application
Nursing Process: Assessment; *Test Plan:* PHYS

7 **Answer: 3** *Rationale:* Option 3 is the priority because of the need for safety when using a benzodiazepine, given the side effects the client described. Option 1 is true for the symptoms of dry mouth, but it is not the priority response because it does not fully address the information provided by the client. Op-

tion 2 is incorrect. The client is describing expected side effects of the medication ordered to decrease anxiety, so the dosage should not be changed. Option 4 will serve no benefit to treat or help with the described side effects.
Cognitive Level: Analysis
Nursing Process: Implementation; *Test Plan:* HPM

8 **Answer: 3** *Rationale:* TCAs account for 70 percent of all deaths from intentional drug overdose. SSRIs are not usually fatal if overdose is taken. MAOIs can be fatal if the client experiences a hypertensive crisis but MAOIs are not usually that widely prescribed because of their numerous side effects, especially with tyramine-rich foods and drug-drug interactions. Anxiolytics are not a class of antidepressants.
Cognitive Level: Application
Nursing Process: Planning; *Test Plan:* HPM

9 **Answer: 1** *Rationale:* Option 1 is the only correct answer; you can teach the client and his mother about the medication and why compliance is very important. Option 2 is incorrect because it is placing responsibility for eating and taking medications on the mother, not on the client, which is inappropriate. Option 3 is incorrect because it is the client's responsibility to take prescribed medications. Family members should know about the medications and be able to support the client and remind the client of the benefits of taking the prescribed medication, but it is ultimately the client's responsibility. Option 4 is inappropriate because there is no guarantee for the client that he will remain symptom-free indefinitely.
Cognitive Level: Analysis
Nursing Process: Assessment; *Test Plan:* HPM

10 **Answer: 2** *Rationale:* Option 2 is an objective evaluation and uses both previous data and present facts to evaluate the client's condition. Option 1 is subjective data only and should not be the sole data for the nurses' evaluation of the effects of the anxiolytic medication. Option 3 is false; there should be a change observed with an anxiolytic after two weeks, and option 4 does not address the primary effects desired for use of anxiolytics (decrease of the anxiety).
Cognitive Level: Analysis
Nursing Process: Evaluation; *Test Plan:* PSYC

References

American Psychiatric Association (2000). *Diagnostic and statistical manual of mental disorders, Fourth Edition, Text Revision* (DSM-IV-TR). Washington, DC: American Psychiatric Association.

Aschenbrenner, O., Cleveland, L., & Venable, S. (2002). *Drug therapy in nursing.* Philadelphia: Lippincott Williams & Wilkins, pp. 227–296.

Carpenito, L.J. (1999). *Nursing care plans & documentation: Nursing diagnoses and collaborative problems* (3rd ed.). Philadelphia: Lippincott, pp. 426–433.

Deglin, J.H. & Vallerand, A.H. (2003). *Davis's drug guide for nurses* (9th ed.). Philadelphia: F.A. Davis, pp. C8-C12, 23-24, 131-132, 149-152, 417-419, 427, 464, 918.

Fontaine, K.L. & Fletcher, S.J. (2003). *Mental health nursing.* (5th ed.). Menlo Park, CA: Addison-Wesley, pp. 145-166, 169-200, 233-351.

Hagerty, B. (2000). Mood disorders: Depression and mania. In K. Fortinash, & P. Holoday-Worret (Eds.), *Psychiatric mental health nursing* (2nd ed.). St. Louis, MO: Mosby, Inc, pp. 258–292.

Jefferson, L.V. (2001). Chemically mediated responses and substance-related disorders. In G. Stuart, & M. Laraia (Eds.), *Principles and practice of psychiatric nursing* (7th ed.). St. Louis, MO: Mosby, Inc., pp. 485–525.

Laraia, M. (2001). Psychopharmacology. In G. Stuart & M. Laraia (Eds.), *Principles and practice of psychiatric nursing* (7th ed.). St. Louis, MO: Mosby, Inc., pp. 572-607.

Lefever Kee, J. & Harpi, E. (2003). *Pharmacology: A nursing process approach* (4th ed.). Philadelphia: Elsevier Science, pp. 231–316.

Lehne, R. (2004). *Pharmacology for nursing care* (5th ed.). Philadelphia: W.B. Saunders, pp. 279–390, 666–672.

McKenry, L. & Salerno, G. (2003). Mosby's pharmacology in nursing. (Revised and updated 21st ed.). St. Louis: Elsevier Science, pp. 325–349, 392–429.

Moller, M.D. & Murphy, M.F. (2001). Neurobiological responses and schizophrenia and psychotic disorders. In G. Stuart, & M. Laraia (Eds.), *Principles and practice of psychiatric nursing* (7th ed.). St. Louis, MO: Mosby, Inc., pp. 402–437.

Riggin, O.Z. & Redding, B.A. (2000). Substance-related disorders. In K.M. Fortinash & P.A. Holoday-Worret (Eds.), *Psychiatric mental health nursing* (2nd ed.). St. Louis, MO: Mosby, Inc., pp. 354–384.

Sherr, J. (2000). Psychopharmacology and other biologic therapies. In K. Fortinash & P. Holoday-Worret (Eds.), *Psychiatric mental health nursing* (2nd ed.). St. Louis, MO: Mosby, Inc., pp. 536–572.

Stuart, G.W. (2001). Anxiety responses and anxiety disorders. In G. Stuart, & M. Laraia (Eds.), *Principles and practice of psychiatric nursing* (7th ed.) St. Louis, MO: Mosby, Inc., pp. 274–98.

Stuart, G.W. (2001). Emotional responses and mood disorders. In G. Stuart, & M. Laraia (Eds.), *Principles and practice of psychiatric nursing* (7th ed.) St. Louis, MO: Mosby, Inc., pp. 345–380.

Videbeck, S.L. (2001). *Psychiatric mental health nursing.* Philadelphia: Lippincott, pp. 260–381.

Youngkin, E. Q., Sawin, K.J., Kissinger, J.F. & Israel, D.S. (1999). *Pharmacotherapeutics: A primary care clinical guide.* Stamford, CT: Appleton & Lange, pp. 747–799, 1181–1182, 1204–1205, 1209.

Renal System Medications

Julie A. Adkins, RN, MSN, FNP-C

CHAPTER OUTLINE

Diuretics
Potassium Supplements
Antihypertensives
Antihypotensives
  (Sympathomimetics)

Urinary Tract and Bladder
  Medications
Medications to Treat Benign
  Prostatic Hyperplasia (BPH)
Medications to Treat Renal Failure

Hematopoietic Growth Factor
Medications to Prevent Organ
  Rejection

OBJECTIVES

▪ Describe general goals of therapy when administering renal system medications.

▪ Describe actions, side effects, and adverse effects of commonly used diuretics.

▪ Discriminate between potassium-losing and potassium-sparing diuretics.

▪ Identify significant laboratory values to monitor in the client taking a diuretic.

▪ Discuss client compliance issues related to self-administration of diuretic and other urinary medications.

▪ Describe actions, side effects, and adverse effects of commonly used urinary anti-infectives, antispasmodics, and analgesics.

▪ Identify client teaching points related to medications prescribed for benign prostatic hyperplasia.

▪ Describe rationale for medications prescribed to treat acute and chronic renal failure.

▪ Identify significant client education points related to renal system medications.

[Media Link]

Use the CD-ROM enclosed with this text, or log onto the address given to access the free, interactive Companion Website created for this series. The CD-ROM and Companion Website accompanying this book offer additional practice opportunities and information—NCLEX Review, Case Studies, Glossary, In Depth with NCLEX, and more.

www.prenhall.com/hogan

REVIEW AT A GLANCE

anuria *absence of urination and urine production (less than 400 mL/day)*

benign prostatic hyperplasia *a symptom complex defined as benign adenomatous hyperplasia of the periurethral prostate gland*

bactericidal *destroying or killing bacteria*

baceriostasis *inhibition of the growth of bacteria without destruction*

conductivity *amount of force and pressure to pump blood out of the ventricles*

diuretic *an agent that increases the amount of urine excreted*

hypertension *high blood pressure*

orthostatic hypotension *a blood pressure fall of more than 10 to 15 mmHg of the systolic pressure or a fall of more than 10 mmHg of the diastole pressure and a 10 to 20% increase in heart rate*

renin-angiotensin system *the complex system in which renin, released by the juxtaglomerular cells of the kidney, changes angiotensin from the liver to angiotensin I; angiotensin I is converted in the lungs to angiotensin II, a powerful*

vasoconstrictor that increases peripheral resistance and thereby increases blood pressure

shock *severe disturbance of hemodynamics in which the circulatory system fails to maintain adequate perfusion of vital organs*

vasoconstriction *narrowing of the blood vessels in response to an internal stimulus such as the nervous system or an external stimulus, such as cold*

Pretest

1 A client is beginning medication therapy with furosemide (Lasix) once daily. The nurse should instruct the client to take the medication at which of the following optimal times?

(1) 8:00 A.M.
(2) 12 noon
(3) 6:00 P.M.
(4) At bedtime

2 The nurse is assessing the blood pressure (BP) of a client diagnosed with primary hypertension. The nurse explains to the client that the basis for the diagnosis of hypertension should be established by:

(1) Five readings one month apart.
(2) At least 3 readings with average blood pressure of 140/90.
(3) One reading of blood pressure greater than 140/90.
(4) Three blood pressure readings taken on the same day in different positions

3 The physician prescribes losartan (Cozaar) for a client with hypertension. The nurse carrying out the order teaches the client that this medication promotes vasodilation by:

(1) Inhibiting calcium influx.
(2) Promoting catecholamines.
(3) Promoting release of aldosterone.
(4) Inhibiting conversion of angiotensin I to angiotensin II.

4 After beginning an antihypertensive medication, the client returns for a follow-up visit and complains of a dry, nonproductive cough. The nurse knows that this side effect is mostly caused by which type of antihypertensive medication?

(1) Beta blocker
(2) Angiotensin converting enzyme (ACE) inhibitor
(3) Calcium channel blocker
(4) Diuretic

5 The nurse is teaching a newly diagnosed client with hypertension about her medications. The client has a history of chronic obstructive pulmonary disease (COPD). The nurse informs the client that she should avoid which antihypertensive medication?

(1) Angiotensin converting enzyme (ACE) inhibitors
(2) Calcium channel blockers
(3) Diuretics
(4) Beta blockers

6 A 45-year-old female comes to the clinic with complaints of leg cramps. She has hypertension and has been taking indipamide (Lozol) 2.5mg daily. Her blood pressure is 126/70 upon arrival. After completion of assessment, the nurse plans to:

(1) Stop the indipamide (Lozol).
(2) Evaluate the electrolytes.
(3) Switch to furosemide (Lasix).
(4) Give her a nonsteroidal, anti-inflammatory drug (NSAID).

7 A hypertensive male client presents to the clinic with complaints of a red, painful toe. In addition to treating the client for gout, the nurse concludes that this may be due to:

(1) A thiazide diuretic.
(2) Obesity.
(3) Diabetes.
(4) Alcohol intake.

8 The nurse practitioner has prescribed oxybutynin (Ditropan) for a 65-year-old female with urinary frequency and urgency. The nurse teaching the client about the side effects of this medication should explain that which of the following manifestations is associated with this medication?

(1) Dizziness
(2) Increased bruising
(3) Diarrhea
(4) Dry mouth and increased thirst

9 A 25-year-old female presents to the office with complaints of burning, frequency, and urgency. The most appropriate intervention taken by the nurse is to:

(1) Increase fluid.
(2) Dipstick urine for leukocytes.
(3) Order phenazopyridine (Pyridium).
(4) Start antibiotic therapy.

10 A 45-year-old man has been prescribed finasteride (Proscar) for his enlarged prostate. The nurse plans to include which of the following points in the teaching session?

(1) Abstain from sex
(2) Use contraceptives
(3) Increase fluid intake
(4) Take only for 3 days

See pages 499–500 for Answers and Rationales.

I. Diuretics

A. Loop diuretics

1. Action and use

    a. Diuretics (agents that increase the amount of urine excreted) inhibit electrolyte reabsorption in the thick ascending loop of Henle, thereby promoting the excretion of sodium, water, chloride, and potassium

    b. The antihypertensive action involves renal **vasodilation** (dilation or widening of vessels), to provide a temporary increase in the glomerular filtration rate (GFR) and a decrease in peripheral vascular resistance

    c. Loop diuretics are more potent than thiazide diuretics, causing rapid diuresis; this results in decreasing vascular fluid volume, cardiac output, and blood pressure

    d. They are used in clients with low GFR and hypertensive emergencies

    e. They are also used in clients with edema, pulmonary edema, congestive heart failure (CHF), chronic renal failure (CRF), and hepatic cirrhosis

    f. They may be used as treatment in drug overdose to increase renal elimination

2. Common medications (Table 12-1)

3. Administration considerations

    a. Take early in the day to avoid nocturia

Table 12-1	Generic/Trade Names	Usual Adult Dose	Side Effects
Common Loop Diuretics	Bumetanide (Bumex)	0.5–2 mg PO daily, 0.5–1 mg IV QD	Dehydration Dizziness
	Ethacrynic acid (Edecrin)	50 mg or 0.5–1 mg/kg IV, 50–200 mg/day	Headache Abdominal pain
	Furosemide (Lasix)	20–80 mg/day IV, 20–40 mg/day PO	Orthostatic hypotension Nocturia
	Toresemide (Demedex)	10–20 mg/day PO, IV	Excessive urination Elevated lipids Photosensitivity

    b. Give intravenous (IV) doses slowly over 1 to 2 minutes; rapid injection may cause hypotension

    c. For IV infusion, dilute in 5% dextrose in water, 0.9% NaCl, or lactated ringers; use infusion fluids within 24 hours

    d. Administer IV furosemide (Lasix) slowly, as hearing loss can occur if injected rapidly

  4. Contraindications: anuria, electrolyte depletion

  5. Significant drug interactions

    a. Interact with aminoglycosides causing ototoxicity

    b. Interact with digitalis (increase digitalis induced arrhythmias), indomethacin, lithium, ethacrynic acid, salicylates and nonsteroidal anti-inflammatory drugs (NSAIDS), which may decrease efficacy of loop diuretic, tubocurarine, succinylcholine, other antihypertensives

    c. An additive effect with thiazide diuretics and thiazide-like diuretics

    d. Interact with anticoagulants (increase anticoagulant activity), propranolol (increase plasma levels of propranolol), sulfonylureas (hyperglycemia), cisplatin (ototoxicity), and probenecid

  6. Significant food interactions: taking ethacrynic acid (Edecrin) with food or milk will increase urination

  7. Significant laboratory studies

    a. Monitor for electrolyte imbalance especially sodium and potassium

    b. Monitor hemoglobin and hematocrit as these may be increased due to hemoconcentration

    c. Monitor for blood dyscrasias, liver, or kidney damage

    d. Monitor blood glucose levels and lipids for possible drug interaction

  8. Side effects

    a. CNS: dizziness, headache, orthostatic hypotension, weakness

    b. GI: nausea, vomiting, abdominal pain, elevated lipids with decreased high density lipoprotein (HDL), pancreatitis, anorexia, constipation

    c. GU: excessive urination, nocturia, urinary bladder spasms

    d. Photosensitivity, sulfonamide allergy, and ototoxicity (tinnitus, hearing impairment, deafness, vertigo and sense of fullness in ears)

    e. Skin: dermatitis, urticaria, pruritis, and muscle spasm

    f. Severe watery diarrhea is the side effect of ethacrynic acid

9. Adverse effects/toxicity

    a. Electrolyte imbalances: hyponatremia, hypochloremia, hypokalemia, hypomagnesemia, hypocalcemia, and hyperuricemia

    b. Thrombocytopenia, systemic vasculitis, interstitial nephritis, thrombophlebitis, agranulocytosis, and aplastic anemia

10. Nursing considerations

NCLEX!

    a. Monitor vital signs for hypotension and tachycardia

    b. Monitor serum electrolytes, calcium, and uric acid levels

NCLEX!

    c. Monitor and record body weight at regular intervals at the same time of day and same scale

NCLEX!

    d. Monitor intake and output (I & O)

    e. Assess indicators of dehydration: thirst, poor skin turgor, coated tongue

    f. Assess for inadequate tissue perfusion and weakness, decreased muscle strength, restlessness, anxiety and agitation

11. Client education

    a. Instruct client to eat food high in potassium to prevent hypokalemia

NCLEX!

    b. Instruct client to restrict sodium intake; instruct client not to not use salt substitutes if taking potassium supplement

    c. Advise client to avoid dehydration by avoiding alcohol and caffeine beverages and replacing fluids during exercise or hot weather

    d. Advise client to avoid exposure to intense heat as with baths, showers and electric blankets

    e. Instruct client to take small frequent amounts of ice chips or clear liquids if vomiting

    f. Instruct client with diarrhea to replace fluids with fruit juice or bouillon

    g. Inform client that diuretics increase the amount and frequency of urination, therefore taking the medication in the morning and afternoon will avoid nighttime urination

    h. Warn client of photosensitivity while taking a loop diuretic

NCLEX!

    i. Instruct client to change position slowly to avoid dizziness and **orthostatic hypotension** (a blood pressure fall of more than 10 to 15 mmHg of the systolic pressure or a fall of more than 10 mmHg of the diastolic pressure and a 10 to 20% increase in heart rate)

    j. Instruct client to weigh daily and report sudden weight gains or losses

NCLEX!

    k. Report ringing in ears immediately

    l. Loop diuretics should not be used while breastfeeding

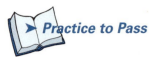

B. Thiazide diuretics

1. Action and uses

   a. Increased urinary excretion of sodium and water by inhibiting sodium reabsorption in the cortical diluting tubule of kidney

   b. Its hypotensive effect may be due to direct arteriolar vasodilation and decreased total peripheral resistance

   c. Used for edema and **hypertension** (persistent elevation of the systolic blood pressure above 140 mmHg and the diastolic BP above 90 mmHg)

   d. Not effective for immediate diuresis

2. Common medications (Table 12-2)

3. Administration considerations

   a. Take the medication early in the day to avoid nocturia

   b. Thiazide diuretics are ineffective if creatinine clearance level is less 30mL/min

   c. Allow 2 to 4 weeks for maximum antihypertensive effect

   d. Metolazone is not recommended in children because safety has not been established

4. Contraindications

   a. Hypersensitivity to thiazide diuretics or sulfonamide derivatives

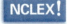

Table 12-2	Generic/Trade Names	Usual Adult Dose	Side Effects
Common Thiazide Diuretics	Bendroflumethiazide (Naturetin)	5–20 mg/day PO	Dizziness Vertigo
	Benzothiazide (Exna, Diucardin)	50–200 mg/day PO	Headache Weakness
	Chlorothiazide (Diuril, Microzide)	12.5–100 mg/day PO	Dehydration Orthostatic hypotension
	Chlorthalidone (Hygroton, Thalitone)	50–100 mg/day or 100–200 mg PO qod for edema 25–50–100 mg/day PO for HTN	Nausea and vomiting Abdominal pain Rash Electrolyte imbalance
	Hydrochlorothiazide (Esidrix, Hydrodiuril)	25–100 mg/day PO	Muscle cramps Jaundice
	Indapamide (Lozol)	1.25–2.5 mg/day PO	Impotence
	Methyclothiazide (Enduron)	2.5–10 mg/day PO	Hyperuricemia
	Metolazone (Zaroxylin)	2.5–20 mg/day	Frequent urination Constipation
	Polythiazide (Minizide, Renese)	1–2 mg PO bid to tid	
	Quinethazone (Hydromox)	50–100 mg/day PO	
	Trichlormethiazide (Diurese)	2–4 mg/day PO	

    b. Clients with anuria

    c. Use cautiously in client with severely impaired renal or hepatic function

    d. Contraindicated in pregnancy; women who breast feed should not use thiazide diuretics

  5. Significant drug interactions

    a. Concomitant use with lithium will increase serum lithium levels

    b. Thiazide diuretics decrease the effectiveness of hyperuricemic agents, sulfonylureas and insulin

    c. There is an additive effect if used with loop diuretics

    d. NSAIDs cause a decreased thiazide diuretic effect

    e. Bile acid resins decrease absorption of thiazide diuretics

    f. Thiazide diuretics may increase the hypersensitivity to allopurinol

  6. Significant food interactions: none reported

  7. Significant laboratory studies

    a. May alter serum electrolytes, especially lowering potassium

    b. May increase serum urate, glucose, cholesterol, and triglycerides

    c. May interfere with tests for parathyroid function

  8. Side effects

    a. Dizziness, vertigo, headache and weakness

    b. Dehydration, orthostatic hypotension, nausea and vomiting, abdominal pain, diarrhea, constipation, and frequent urination

    c. Dermatitis and rash

    d. Electrolyte imbalance, impaired glucose tolerance, jaundice, muscle cramps, photosensitivity, impotence, and hyperuricemia

  9. Adverse effects/toxicity: renal failure, aplastic anemia, agranulocytosis, thrombocytopenia, and anaphylactic reaction

 10. Nursing considerations

    a. Monitor vital signs for hypotension and tachycardia

    b. Monitor serum electrolytes, calcium, and uric acid levels

    c. Monitor and record body weight at regular intervals at the same time of day and same scale

    d. Monitor intake and output (I & O)

    e. Assess indicators of dehydration: thirst, poor skin turgor, coated tongue

    f. Assess for inadequate tissue perfusion and weakness, decreased muscle strength, restlessness, anxiety and agitation

 11. Client education

    a. Instruct client to eat foods high in potassium to prevent hypokalemia

NCLEX!

  b. Instruct client to restrict sodium intake; instruct client not to not use salt substitutes if taking potassium supplement

  c. Advise client to avoid dehydration by avoiding alcohol and caffeine beverages and replacing fluids during exercise or hot weather

  d. Advise client to avoid exposure to intense heat as with baths, showers, and electric blankets

  e. Instruct client to take small frequent amounts of ice chips or clear liquids if vomiting

  f. Instruct client with diarrhea to replace fluids with fruit juice or bouillion

NCLEX!

  g. Inform client that diuretics increase the amount and frequency of urination, therefore taking the medication in the morning and afternoon will avoid nighttime urination

NCLEX!

  h. Instruct client to change position slowly to avoid dizziness and orthostatic hypotension

NCLEX!

  i. Instruct to weigh daily and report sudden weight gains or losses

  j. Instruct the diabetic clients to have blood glucose checked periodically

 C. Potassium-sparing diuretics

  1. Action and use

   a. Act directly on the distal convoluted tubule to increase sodium excretion and decrease potassium secretion

   b. Used for hypertension and edema associated with heart failure

   c. Spironolactone is also used for detection of primary hyperaldosteronism, hirsutism, and premenstrual syndrome

  2. Common medications (Table 12-3)

  3. Administration considerations

   a. Take with food or milk

NCLEX!

   b. Avoid salt substitutes

NCLEX!

   c. Avoid excessive ingestion of foods high in potassium

Table 12-3

Common Potassium-Sparing Diuretics

Generic/Trade Names	Usual Adult Dose	Side Effects
Amiloride (Midamor)	5–20 mg/day PO	Headache Weakness
Spironolactone (Aldactone)	25–200mg/day PO	Dizziness Orthostatic hypotension
Triamterene (Dyrenium)	100 mg bid up to 300 mg/day PO	Urticaria Gynecomastia Dry mouth, impotence

       d. When administering spironolactone to children, crush tablet and mix in flavored syrup as oral suspension

   4. Contraindications

       a. Serum potassium levels greater than 5.5 mEq/mL

       b. Concomitant use with other potassium-sparing diuretics

       c. Fluid and electrolyte imbalances

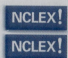

       d. Anuria, acute and chronic renal insufficiency, diabetic nephropathy, hypersensitivity, and impaired hepatic function

       e. Caution in client with diabetes mellitus

   5. Significant drug interactions

       a. May potentiate hypotensive effects of antihypertensive medications

       b. Increased risk of hyperkalemia with other potassium-sparing diuretics

       c. May increase serum blood levels of lithium due to decreased renal clearance

       d. Digitalis may decrease renal clearance

       e. Aspirin may slightly decrease response of spironolactone

       f. Antidiabetic drugs may need adjustment as triamterene may increase blood glucose levels

       g. Corticosteroids may increase electrolyte depletion

   6. Significant food interactions: administering spironolactone with food increases its absorption

   7. Significant laboratory studies

       a. Monitor electrolytes especially potassium and creatinine

       b. Digoxin level

       c. Triamterene may interfere with enzyme assays

   8. Side effects

       a. CNS: headache, weakness, dizziness, and orthostatic hypotension

       b. GI: nausea, vomiting, diarrhea, and constipation

       c. Impotence, muscle cramps, urticaria, gynecomastia, and breast soreness

       d. Dry mouth, photosensitivity, transient elevated blood urea nitrogen (BUN) and creatinine

   9. Adverse effects/toxicity

       a. Aplastic anemia and thrombocytopenia

       b. Hyperkalemia

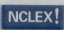

  10. Nursing considerations

       a. Monitor vital signs

       b. Monitor urine output

     c. Discontinue potassium supplements

     d. Observe closely elderly and debilitated clients for drug-induced diuresis and hyperkalemia

     e. Monitor for dehydration and electrolyte imbalance

     f. Monitor periodic serum electrolytes such as BUN and creatinine

  11. Client education

     a. Instruct client to take medication with food to avoid GI upset except with triamterene

     b. Avoid consumption of large quantities of foods high in potassium

     c. Report any mental confusion or lethargy immediately

     d. Instruct client to monitor for signs and symptoms of hyperkalemia such as nausea, diarrhea, abdominal cramps, and tachycardia followed by bradycardia

     e. Explain that side effects usually disappear after the drug is discontinued except gynecomastia may persist

     f. With spironolactone, maximal diuresis may not occur until day 3 of therapy and diuresis may continue 2 to 3 days after the drug is stopped

     g. Inform client that triamterene may turn the urine blue

     h. Instruct client to avoid salt substitutes because they contain potassium

     i. Instruct client to avoid exposure to direct sunlight

D. Carbonic anhydrase inhibitors

  1. Action and use

     a. Noncompetitive reversible inhibition of the enzyme carbonic anhydrase, which promotes excretion of bicarbonate, sodium, potassium, and water

     b. Used for treatment of edema caused by CHF

     c. Used for open angle glaucoma to decrease intraocular pressure

     d. Used for treatment of epilepsy

     e. Used to treat metabolic alkalosis

  2. Common medications (Table 12-4)

Table 12-4	Generic/Trade Names	Usual Adult Dose	Side Effects
Common Carbonic Anhydrase Inhibitors	Acetazolamide (Diamox)	5 mg/kg PO, may be given 500 mg IV	Confusion Drowsiness Paresthesias
	Dichlorphenamide (Daranide)	Initial:100–200mg followed by 100 mg q 12h; then 25–50 mg/day to TID, PO	Hearing dysfunction Transient myopia Renal calculus Photosensitivity
	Methazolamide (Neptazane)	50–100 mg bid to tid daily, PO	Rash Electrolyte imbalance

3. Administration considerations

    a. Increasing the dose does not appear to increase diuresis

    b. Do not administer with high dose aspirin

    c. Intramuscular administration is not recommended

4. Contraindications

    a. Contraindicated in narrow angle or acute glaucoma

    b. Contraindicated in any situation with decreased sodium and/or potassium levels

    c. Marked kidney or liver dysfunction

    d. Cautionary use in client with chronic obstructive pulmonary disease (COPD)

5. Significant drug interactions

    a. Aspirin may cause accumulation and toxicity of acetazolamide

    b. May increase levels of cyclosporine and decreased levels of primidone

6. Significant food interactions: none reported

7. Significant laboratory studies

    a. Obtain platelet and complete blood cell counts (CBC) prior to and periodically during therapy

    b. Monitor serum electrolytes

    c. May cause false positive proteinuria

    d. May decrease thyroid iodine uptake

8. Side effects

    a. Confusion, drowsiness, and paresthesias

    b. Hearing dysfunction, GI upset, polyuria, and transient myopia

    c. Electrolyte imbalance, fever, rash, renal calculus, and photosensitivity

9. Adverse effects/toxicity

    a. Metabolic acidosis

    b. Anaphylaxis

    c. Bone marrow depression

    d. Thrombocytopenia purpura, hemolytic anemia, leukopenia, pancytopenia, and agranulocytosis

    e. Severe reactions to sulfonamides including Stevens-Johnson syndrome, toxic epidermal necrolysis, fulminant hepatic necrosis, coma and death have occurred

10. Nursing considerations

    a. Monitor for signs and symptoms of dehydration, I & O

    b. Assess for alterations in skin integrity

    c. Assess for edema

    d. Assess vital signs and daily weight

    e. Assess cardiovascular and respiratory status

    f. Assess changes in level of consciousness and activity level

    g. Dietary assessment of high salt-containing foods

    h. Fluid restriction as ordered

11. Client education

    a. Advise client not to take aspirin or aspirin-containing medications

    b. Instruct client to report symptoms of anorexia, lethargy, or tachypnea

    c. Warn client to use caution while driving or performing tasks that require alertness, coordination or physical dexterity because they can cause drowsiness

    d. Instruct client to monitor for signs of renal calculi

    e. Stress the importance of follow-up scheduled lab tests

    f. Instruct to weigh daily at the same time of day and report any acute weight gain or loss

    g. Teach client about high sodium containing foods and beverages

E. Osmotic diuretics

1. Action and use

    a. Increase osmotic pressure of glomerular filtrate in proximal tubule and loop of Henle inhibiting reabsorption of water and electrolytes, thus promoting diuresis

    b. Used to prevent and manage acute renal failure (ARF) and oliguria

    c. Used to decrease intracranial or intraocular pressure

    d. Mannitol is used with chemotherapy to induce diuresis

2. Common medications (Table 12-5)

3. Administration considerations

    a. Medications are administered IV by slow infusion

    b. Urea turns to ammonia if left standing

    c. Do not infuse with blood or blood products

Table 12-5	Generic/Trade Names	Usual Adult Dose	Side Effects
Common Osmotic Diuretics	Mannitol	0.5–1.5 g/kg 30% sol, IV over 30 minutes to 2 hr	Syncope Nausea and vomiting Blurred vision
	Urea	0.5–1.5 g/kg 30% sol, IV over 30 minutes to 2 hr	Urine retention Hypotension Headache

d. Mannitol crystallizes at low temperatures

  4. Contraindications

      a. Contraindicated in clients with severely impaired renal function, marked dehydration, breast feeding, hepatic failure, active intracranial bleed, and anuria

      b. Contraindicated in client with severe pulmonary congestion and severe congestive heart failure

  5. Significant drug interactions

      a. Decrease serum lithium levels

      b. Use with cardiac glycosides may cause an increased possibility of digitalis toxicity

      c. Increase the effects of other diuretics

  6. Significant food interactions: none reported

  7. Significant laboratory studies: monitor BUN and electrolytes frequently

  8. Side effects

      a. Headache, syncope, and hypotension

      b. Nausea, vomiting, dry mouth, urine retention, electrolyte imbalance, and urticaria

  9. Adverse effects/toxicity

      a. Seizures

      b. Thrombophlebitis

      c. Congestive heart failure

      d. Cardiovascular collapse

  10. Nursing considerations

      a. Maintain adequate hydration

      b. Monitor fluid and electrolyte balance

      c. Monitor BUN

      d. Indwelling catheter should be used in comatose clients for accurate I & O

      e. Monitor I & O and vital signs hourly while on Mannitol

      f. Daily weight

      g. Monitor renal function, fluid balance, serum and urinary sodium and potassium levels

      h. Assess for signs of decreasing intracranial pressure if appropriate

      i. Monitor lung and heart sounds for signs of pulmonary edema

  11. Client education

      a. Advise client to monitor weight

      b. Instruct client to report immediately pain in chest or legs, shortness of breath or apnea

c. Advise client to change position slowly to prevent dizziness or orthostatic hypotension

d. Stress importance of drinking only fluids ordered even though thirsty and/or experiencing dry mouth

e. Monitor neuro status such as decreased level of consciousness (LOC)

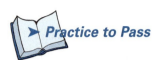

Practice to Pass

Potassium supplementation has been ordered along with furosemide (Lasix) to initially treat the client with acute renal failure. The nurse teaching the client should inform her that what medications should be avoided while on Lasix?

II. Potassium Supplements

A. Action and use

1. Potassium is the main cation in body cells

2. Acts to maintain intracellular tonicity, maintain balance with sodium across cell membranes, transmit nerve impulses, and maintain cellular metabolism

3. Help contracting cardiac and skeletal muscle, maintaining acid-base balance and maintaining normal renal function

4. Potassium is well absorbed from the GI tract and excreted largely by the kidneys

5. Used to prevent and treat hypokalemia

B. Administration considerations

1. Tablet form should be taken with a full glass of water

2. Tablets are not to be crushed, chewed, or sucked; if difficulty swallowing, the tablet may be broken and dissolved in water

3. Powder preparations should be mixed with 4 ounces of water or other liquid

4. Potassium supplements should be taken with meals to decrease GI irritation

5. Tablets in wax matrix sometimes lodge in the esophagus and cause ulceration; in cardiac clients who have esophageal compression due to enlarged left atrium, use liquid form

6. Enteric coated tablets are not recommended because of the potential for GI bleeding and small bowel ulcerations

7. Parenteral potassium should be given slowly and in diluted form

C. Contraindications

1. Severe renal impairment with oliguria, **anuria** (absence of urine), or azotemia

2. Untreated Addison's disease

3. Acute dehydration and heat cramps

4. Hyperkalemia and form of familial periodic paralysis, as well as conditions associated with extensive tissue breakdown

5. Use cautiously with cardiac and renal disease

D. Significant drug interactions

1. Anticholinergics may increase the chance of GI irritation and ulceration

2. Potassium-containing agents increase risk for hyperkalemia

3. Potassium is not recommended in clients with severe or complete heart block taking digitalis due to potential for arrhythmias

4. Use with potassium-sparing diuretics, angiotensin converting enzyme (ACE) inhibitors or salt substitutes containing potassium salts can cause severe hyperkalemia

5. May decrease absorption of Vitamin B_{12} in the GI tract

E. Significant food interactions

1. Foods high in potassium

2. Examples include apple juice, grapefruit, bananas, oranges, peaches, pears, raisins, broccoli, peas, tomatoes, eggplant, chicken, liver, turkey, salmon, beef, low-fat yogurt, milk, and chocolate milk

F. Significant laboratory studies: none reported

G. Side effects

1. Paresthesia of extremities, restlessness, confusion, weakness, or heaviness of legs

2. Hypotension and electrocardiogram (EKG) changes

3. Nausea, vomiting, abdominal pain, and diarrhea

4. Hyperkalemia

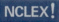

H. Adverse effects/toxicity

1. Arrhythmias

2. Cardiac arrest

3. Respiratory paralysis

I. Nursing considerations

1. Monitor serum potassium, BUN, and creatinine

2. Monitor I & O

3. Monitor EKG for arrhythmias

4. Monitor for side effects such as weakness, feeling of heaviness in legs, confusion, hypotension (signs of hyperkalemia)

5. Potassium should not be given immediately postoperatively until urine flow is established

6. Attempt to identify cause of hypokalemia

7. Assess parenteral infusion site frequently for signs of pain and inflammation

J. Client education

1. Instruct client on foods high in potassium

2. Instruct client to avoid salt substitutes while taking potassium supplements

3. Instruct client to contact the provider if swallowing problems

4. Instruct client to monitor stools for the evidence of GI bleed

5. Advise client to notify the provider of any other prescription or over-the-counter (OTC) medications

6. Instruct client to report the presence of diarrhea or vomiting due to increased risk for hypokalemia

7. Advise client to report immediately any confusion, irregular heartbeat, numbness of feet, fingers or lips, shortness of breath, anxiety, excessive tiredness, or weakness of legs

8. Instruct client to take potassium supplement with meals to decrease GI irritation

9. Instruct client to take only the prescribed amount of potassium as other doses may cause severe reactions

10. Instruct client to dissolve powder, soluble tablets, or granules completely in at least 4 ounces of water or juice before drinking

11. Instruct client to not crush or chew sustained-release capsules but the contents can be opened and sprinkled onto soft foods

12. Inform client that expelling a whole tablet in the stool (sustained-release tablet) is normal as the body eliminates the shell after absorbing the potassium

III. Antihypertensives

A. Stepped care management

1. The Joint National Commission (JNC) VI guidelines direct the practitioner to individualize each client's management of lowering blood pressure to the desired range using blood pressure measurements, risk factors and target organ disease

2. Hypertension is not diagnosed on the basis of a single blood pressure reading but is defined as a sustained elevation of systolic and/or diastolic blood pressure

3. Consideration must be given to cost, ease of following the treatment regimen, the potential for drug-drug interactions, and the profile of side effects

B. Diuretics

1. Reduce blood pressure and edema by increasing urine production, enhancing water and sodium excretion

2. The most common diuretics used for hypertension are thiazide diuretics and loop diuretics (see previous discussion)

3. Other diuretics that may be used are potassium-sparing, osmotic, and carbonic anhydrase inhibitors (see previous discussion)

C. Adrenergic inhibitors (alpha and beta-blockers)

1. Action and use

   a. Alpha-adrenergic blocking agents decrease vasomotor tone to cause vasodilation and thus reduce BP

   b. Beta-blockers reduce BP by preventing stimulation of the beta receptors in the heart by epinephrine and norepinephrine, thereby decreasing heart rate and cardiac output (CO)

   c. Beta-blockers also interfere with the release of renin by the kidneys to decrease the **renin-angiotensin** mechanism resulting in reduced BP

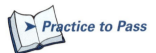
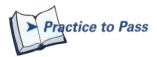

Practice to Pass

A client has just been diagnosed with hypertension. Besides instructions regarding medication, what modifiable factors should be discussed?

Practice to Pass

What routine labs need to be monitored for the hypertensive client?

    d. Alpha-blockers are used for peripheral vascular disorders, hypertension and **benign prostatic hyperplasia (BPH)** (a symptom complex defined as benign adenomatous hyperplasia of the periurethral prostate gland)

    e. Beta-blockers are used for hypertension, angina, arrhythmia, glaucoma, myocardial infarction (MI), and migraine

2. Common medications (Tables 12-6 and 12-7)

3. Administration considerations

    a. Alpha-blockers may cause syncope within 30 minutes to 1 hour after the first dose; the effect is transient and may be diminished by giving at bedtime

    b. To avoid first dose syncope, begin with a small dose

    c. Beta-blockers: monitor apical pulse for increased risk of bradycardia; signs of hypoglycemia may be masked

    d. Cautionary use of B_2 blockage due to increased risk of bronchospasm

    e. Do not stop drug abruptly

    f. Metoprolol and propranolol should be taken with food to increase absorption

    g. Absorption is decreased when sotalol is taken with food

4. Contraindications

    a. Alpha blockers: hypersensitivity to drug

    b. Beta blockers: hypersensitivity to drug, symptomatic bradycardia, greater than first degree heart block, class IV heart failure, and asthma

5. Significant drug interactions

    a. Alpha blockers

      1) Decrease antihypertensive effect of clonidine

      2) Prazosin and indomethacin (Indocin): decreased antihypertensive effect

      3) Prazosin and verapamil (Calan): increase serum prazosin concentration

      4) Prazosin and beta blockers: increase first dose syncope

    b. Alpha and beta blockers

      1) Additive effects with other antihypertensive medications

Table 12-6

Common Alpha Blocker Medications

Generic/Trade Names	Usual Adult Dose	Side Effects
Prazosin (Minipress)	1 mg bid to tid up to 20 mg/day, PO	First-dose syncope
Terazosin (Hytrin)	1–5 mg/day up to 20 mg/day, PO	Headache Drowsiness
Doxazosin (Cardura)	1 mg at bed time, up to 16 mg/day, PO	Hypotension Palpitations Impotence
Labetalol (Trandate/Normodyne)	200–400 mg bid, PO	Nasal congestion Nausea and vomiting Tachycardia
Carvedilol (Coreg)	6.25 mg bid up to 50 mg/day, PO	

	Generic/Trade Names	Usual Adult Dose	Side Effects
Table 12-7 **Common Beta Blocker Medications**	Atenolol (Tenormin)	50–100 mg/day PO	Insomnia
	Betaxolol (Kerlone)	10–20 mg/day PO	Fatigue
	Metoprolol (Lopressor)	50 mg bid up to 400 mg/day PO	Dizziness
	Acebutolol (Sectral)	400 mg/d up to 1,200 mg/day PO	Edema
	Propranolol (Inderal)	40 mg bid or 80 mg/day up to 640 mg/day PO	Increased airway resistance Muscle pain
	Nadolol (Corgard)	40 mg/d up to 320 mg/day PO	Joint pain
	Pindolol (Visken)	5 mg bid up to 60 mg/day PO	Bradycardia
			Abdominal pain

      2) Coreg/digoxin: increase digoxin levels

      3) Coreg or labetalol/cimetidine: increase Coreg or labetalol levels

      4) Coreg/rifampin: decrease Coreg level

   c. Beta blockers

      1) Additive effects with other antihypertensives

      2) Metoprolol/cimetidine: increase effect

      3) Metoprolol may increase bradycardia of cardiac glycosides

      4) Bile acid resins/propranolol: decrease absorption of propranolol

      5) May alter insulin and oral hypoglycemic agents

 6. Significant food interactions: none reported

 7. Significant laboratory studies

   a. Alpha blockers

      1) May cause false positive urine assays for pheochromocytoma

      2) Liver function tests, CBC, serum uric acid, and BUN

   b. Alpha/beta blockers: may cause increased urine free and total catecholamines

   c. Beta blockers

      1) May increase or decrease serum glucose levels

      2) Monitor potassium levels, transaminase, uric acid, and alkaline phosphatase

      3) BUN and creatinine

 8. Side effects

   a. Alpha blockers: first dose syncope, headache, drowsiness, hypotension, palpitations, impotence, nasal congestion, nausea and vomiting, tachycardia

   b. Alpha/beta blockers: fatigue, orthostatic hypotension, dizziness, nausea and vomiting, diarrhea, bronchospasm, muscle spasm, transient scalp tingling, hyperglycemia, upper respiratory infections, impotence, and arthralgias

   c. Beta blockers: insomnia, fatigue, dizziness, nervousness, edema, increased airway resistance, muscle pain, joint pain, diarrhea, rash, bradycardia, hypotension, nausea and vomiting, and abdominal pain

9. Adverse effects/toxicity

    a. Alpha blockers: leukopenia, neutropenia, thrombocytopenia, myelosuppression, anaphylaxis, bronchospasm, and arrhythmia

    b. Alpha/beta blockers: ventricular arrhythmias, AV block, bradycardia, thrombocytopenia, and sudden death

    c. Beta blockers: heart failure, agranulocytosis, bronchospasm

10. Nursing considerations

    a. Monitor client for the past medical history

    b. Monitor vital signs especially BP and heart rate

    c. Monitor for manifestations of CHF such as edema

    d. Monitor peripheral circulation

    e. Monitor diabetic clients for manifestations of hypoglycemia

    f. Abrupt discontinuance of medication may exacerbate angina or precipitate MI

    g. Hypotensive effects may be more pronounced in the elderly

    h. Maintain safety when the client is changing positions

    i. Monitor for first dose syncope (alpha and alpha/beta blockers); give the first dose at bedtime to minimize risk

11. Client education

    a. Instruct client to take the drug exactly as prescribed

    b. Explain the rationale of therapy

    c. Instruct client to change position slowly to prevent dizziness and falls

    d. Advise client to report any side effects to the health care provider

    e. Instruct client to monitor blood glucose levels and BP more frequently if taking insulin or oral antidiabetic medications

    f. Monitor weight daily and report weight gain over 5 pounds (lb) per week

    g. Instruct client to avoid hazardous activities at the beginning of therapy

    h. Advise client not to stop medications without notifying the physician

    i. Instruct client to seek medical approval before taking any OTC medications

    j. Explain that therapeutic effect may take 3 to 4 weeks

    k. Advise client to avoid alcohol use, excessive exercise, prolonged standing and exposure to heat due to increased risk of side effects

D. Angiotensin-converting enzyme (ACE) inhibitors

1. Action and use

    a. Inhibit the renin-angiotensin-aldosterone mechanism by blocking conversion of angiotensin I to angiotensin II and prevent peripheral vasoconstriction

    b. Used to treat hypertension; they are preferred drug for hypertensive clients with diabetic nephropathy

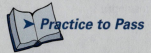
Practice to Pass

The client with hypertension asks if it is all right to use salt substitute. How should the nurse respond?

Table 12-8	Generic/Trade Names	Usual Adult Dose	Side Effects
Common Angiotensin-Converting Enzyme Inhibitors	Captopril (Capoten)	Initial 12.5 mg tid Max. 50 mg/day, PO	Persistent dry cough Dyspnea
	Lisinopril (Prinivil)	Initial 10 mg/day Max. 40 mg/day, PO	Fatigue Insomnia
	Enalapril (Vasotec)	Initial 5 mg/day Max. 40 mg/day, PO	Anxiety Dizziness
	Ramipril (Altace)	Initial 2.5 mg/day Max. 20 mg/day, PO	Headache Rash
	Benzapril (Lotensin)	Initial 10 mg/day Max. 40 mg/day, PO	Hypotension Arthralgia
	Fosinopril (Monopril)	Initial 10 mg/day Max. 80 mg/day, PO	Constipation Abdominal pain
	Quinapril (Accupril)	Initial 10 mg/day Max. 80 mg/day, PO	Palpitation Impotence
	Moexipril (Univasc)	Initial 7.5 mg/day Max. 30 mg/day, PO	Nausea Vomiting
	Trandolapril (Mavik)	Initial 1mg/day, then 2–4 mg/day, PO	Nervousness

2. Common medications (Table 12-8)

3. Administration considerations

   a. Discontinue as soon as possible if pregnancy detected

   b. Moexipril and captopril should be taken on an empty stomach due to decreased absorption with food

4. Contraindications

   a. Hypersensitivity to angiotensin converting enzyme inhibitors

   b. Avoid use with potassium supplements and potassium-sparing diuretics

5. Significant drug interactions

   a. Potassium-sparing diuretics or potassium supplements: hyperkalemia

   b. Increased lithium concentration

   c. Increased risk of hypersensitivity with allopurinol

   d. May increase digoxin concentration

   e. Antacids may decrease absorption of captopril and fosinopril

6. Significant food interactions: none reported

7. Significant laboratory studies

   a. Agranulocytosis and bone marrow depression

   b. May increase serum BUN and creatinine

   c. May increase liver enzymes, serum bilirubin, uric acid and blood glucose

   d. Captopril may cause false positive urinary acetone

8. Side effects

    a. Headache, dizziness, anxiety, fatigue, insomnia, nervousness, hypotension, and palpitations

    b. Nausea, vomiting, abdominal pain, constipation, persistent dry nonproductive cough, and dyspnea

    c. Rash, arthralgia, impotence, and dysgeusia (altered taste)

9. Adverse effects/toxicity

    a. Angioedema, leukopenia, agranulocytosis, pancytopenia, thrombocytopenia

    b. Cerebrovascular accident (CVA), MI, and hypertensive crisis

10. Nursing considerations

    a. Administer 1 hour before meals to increase absorption

    b. Tablets may be crushed

    c. Do not administer to pregnant or lactating women

    d. Monitor labs for increased potassium, liver enzymes, bilirubin, BUN and creatinine, and decreased sodium levels

    e. Take BP before giving dose and monitor regularly

    f. Monitor for rashes or hives

    g. Assess for peripheral edema

    h. If the client has renal disease, monitor urine protein on a regular basis by dipstick method

    i. Diuretics should be discontinued 2 to 3 days before ACE inhibitor therapy

    j. Monitor white blood cells (WBC) and differential counts periodically

    k. BP is lowered within 1 hour of fosinopril with peak at 2 to 6 hours

11. Client education

    a. Instruct client to report peripheral edema, signs of infection, facial swelling, loss of taste, or difficulty breathing

    b. Instruct client to change position slowly to prevent dizziness and falls

    c. Instruct client not to skip doses or stop taking the drug; it may cause serious rebound BP

    d. Advise client to seek medical approval before taking OTC medications

    e. Instruct client to notify the provider if a persistent, dry cough occurs

    f. Instruct client to take antacids 2 hours before or after dose of fosinopril and captopril

    g. Advise client to avoid potassium-containing salt substitutes

    h. Instruct client to monitor for bruising, petechiae, or bleeding with captopril

    i. Instruct client that the taste of food may be diminished during the first month of therapy

    j. Instruct client to take captopril 20 minutes to 1 hour before a meal

E. Angiotensin II antagonists

1. Action and use

   a. Antagonist at angiotensin II receptor of vascular smooth muscle blocking vasoconstriction and aldosterone-secreting effects

   b. Used for hypertension

2. Common medications (Table 12-9)

3. Administration considerations: discontinue as soon as pregnancy is detected

4. Contraindications

   a. Pregnancy

   b. Hypersensitivity

   c. Caution in clients with renal or hepatic disease

5. Significant drug interactions

   a. Losartan and phenobarbital: decreased losartan levels

   b. Losartan and cimetidine (Tagamet): increased losartan levels

   c. Diuretics may increase the risk for hypotension

6. Significant food interactions: none reported

7. Significant laboratory studies

   a. WBC for neutropenia

   b. Electrolytes for hyperkalemia

NCLEX!

8. Side effects

   a. Hypotension and dizziness

   b. Cough, GI upset, insomnia, nasal congestion, and myalgia

9. Adverse effects/toxicity

   a. Hypotension

   b. Tachycardia or bradycardia

10. Nursing considerations

NCLEX!

   a. Monitor client taking diuretics for increased hypotension

   b. Regularly assess renal function

   c. Do not administer to pregnant or lactating women

Table 12-9	Generic/Trade Names	Usual Adult Dose	Side Effects
Common Angiotensin II Antagonist Medications	Losartan (Cozaar)	Initial 50 mg/day, then 30–100 mg/day, PO	Hypotension Dizziness, cough
	Valsartan (Diovan)	Initial 80 mg/day, then 80–320 mg/day, PO	GI upset Insomnia Nasal congestion

     d. Monitor potassium levels

     e. Monitor regularly BP and apical pulse

     f. Monitor WBC and differential periodically

NCLEX!

11. Client education

     a. Instruct client not to discontinue medication abruptly

     b. Advise client to avoid salt substitutes

     c. Advise client to notify the physician immediately if pregnancy is suspected

     d. Advise client on alternative birth control methods

     e. Instruct client to report any side effects to healthcare provider

     f. Instruct client to change positions slowly to avoid dizziness

F. Calcium channel blockers

  1. Action and use

     a. Class IV antiarrhythmics drugs that inhibit calcium ion influx through slow channels into cell of myocardial and arterial smooth muscle (both cardiac and peripheral blood vessels)

     b. Intracellular calcium remains below levels needed to stimulate cell

     c. Dilates coronary arteries and arterioles and prevents coronary artery spasm

     d. Myocardial oxygen (O_2) delivery is increased, preventing angina

     e. Slow the conduction through the sinoatrial (SA) node and atrioventricular (AV) node, resulting in a lower heart rate and a decrease in the strength of the heart muscle contraction (negative inotropic effect)

     f. Decrease the automaticity and **conductivity** (which is the amount of force and pressure to pump blood out of the ventricles) by blocking the flow of calcium into the cell

     g. Decrease systemic vascular resistance (SVR) and thus afterload by dilating peripheral arterioles

     h. Reduce arterial BP (antihypertensive effect) and heart rate

     i. They are used for vasospastic angina (Prinzmetal s variant or angina at rest), chronic stable (classic and activity induced) angina, and essential hypertension; the IV form is useful in treating atrial fibrillation, atrial flutter, and supraventricular tachycardia

  2. Common medications (Table 12-10)

  3. Administration considerations

     a. Administer oral diltiazem before meals and at bedtime and oral verapamil with food to reduce gastric irritation

     b. Evaluate BP and EKG before initiation of therapy

     c. Monitor for headache; an analgesic may be required

     d. Intravenous forms of diltiazem: undiluted IV push over 2 minutes and repeated in 15 minutes or diluted in 5% dextrose of water (D_5W), normal

	Generic/Trade Name	Usual Adult Dose	Side Effects
Table 12-10 **Common Calcium Channel Blockers**	Amlodipine (Norvasc)	2.5–10 mg daily	Hypotension Peripheral edema
	Diltiazem (Cardizem, Dilacor XR, Tiazac)	Regular release: 30–120 mg tid or QID Sustained-release: 60–240 mg bid	Tachycardia Flushing Headache
	Nifedipine (Adalat, Procardia)	Regular release: 10–20 mg tid or qid SR: 30–120 mg daily	GI upset
	Verapamil (Calan, Covera HS, Verelan, Isoptin)	Regular release: 40–160 mg tid SR: 120–480 mg daily	

saline (NS) or $D_5W/0.45\%NaCl$; continuous infusion may be given via infusion pump at a rate of 5 to 15 mg/hr; infusion over 24 hours and greater than 15 mg/hr are not recommended

    e. Intravenous verapamil may be given via direct IV diluted in 5 ml of sterile water for injection at a rate of 10 mg/min

    f. Withhold medication if BP less than 90/60

4. Contraindications

    a. Avoid use when there is known hypersensitivity to drug

    b. Sick sinus syndrome (unless pacemaker is in place)

    c. Second- or third-degree heart blocks

        1) Second degree Type I or Wenckebach: progressive PR prolongation until a QRS is dropped

        2) Second-degree Type II: P waves march out until a QRS is dropped

        3) Third-degree heart block: no association between P waves and QRS, usually heart rate is between 20 to 40 bpm

    d. Severe hypotension, BP less than 90/60

5. Significant drug interactions

    a. Beta blockers and digoxin may have an additive effect on prolongation of the AV node conduction

    b. They may increase digoxin or quinidine levels leading to toxicity

    c. Cimetidine may increase serum levels of calcium channel blockers

    d. Calcium channel blockers may increase serum levels of cyclosporine (an immunosuppressant)

    e. Furosemide is incompatible in IV solution

6. Significant food interactions: do not take with grapefruit

7. Significant laboratory studies

    a. Do not alter total serum calcium levels

    b. Monitor baseline and periodic lab tests of hepatic and renal function

c. Monitor diabetics closely; it may induce hyperglycemia

d. Cyclosporine levels may become elevated

e. Digoxin and quinidine levels may become elevated

8. Side effects

a. Headache

b. Fatigue

c. Constipation (especially with oral and sustained-release forms)

d. Postural hypotension

9. Adverse effects/toxicity

a. Heart block and profound bradycardia, CHF, profound hypotension with syncope, palpitations, and fluid volume overload

b. Dizziness, nervousness, insomnia, confusion, tremor, and gait disturbance

c. Nausea, vomiting, and impaired taste

d. Skin rash

10. Nursing considerations

a. Evaluate BP and EKG before the initiation of treatment and monitor them closely during medication adjustment

b. Monitor hepatic and renal lab test results

c. Monitor for headache

d. May induce hyperglycemia; monitor diabetic clients closely

e. Advise client to report gradual weight gain and evidence of edema

11. Client education

a. Inform client about the importance of taking radial pulse before each dose (especially verapamil); an irregular pulse or one slower than base level should be reported

b. Encourage client to change position slowly to prevent postural hypotension

c. Caution client to avoid driving if dizziness or faintness is noted; these symptoms should be reported immediately

d. Advise client to take medication exactly as prescribed

e. Instruct client not to crush or chew sustained-release tablets

f. Stress the importance of follow-up care

g. Inform client to avoid OTC medications and herbal supplements without consulting physician

h. Encourage client to stop smoking

i. Encourage client to avoid alcohol consumption

j. Instruct client to report easy bruising, petechiae, or unexplained bleeding

G. Vasodilators

1. Action and use

   a. Reduce BP by relaxing vascular smooth muscle thereby decreasing peripheral vascular resistance

   b. Increase renal blood flow directly

   c. Used to treat hypertension

2. Common medications (Table 12-11)

3. Administration considerations

   a. Taking hydralazine with food increases absorption

   b. Allow 3 days before titrating dose

4. Contraindications

   a. Hypersensitivity

   b. Coronary artery disease (CAD), rheumatic mitral valve disease, pheochromocytoma, and acute MI

5. Significant drug interactions

   a. Hydralazine/metoprolol or propranolol: increase the concentration

   b. Hydralazine/indomethacin: decrease effect of hydralazine

   c. Minoxidil/guanethidine: profound orthostatic hypotension

6. Significant food interactions: none reported

7. Significant laboratory studies

   a. Electrolytes

   b. Liver function tests, BUN, creatinine

   c. CBC

   d. EKG

8. Side effects

   a. Reflex tachycardia, peripheral edema, headache, dizziness, and palpitations

   b. GI upset, hirsutism, and lupus-like syndrome

   c. Pericardial effusion and tamponade, rash, breast tenderness, and weight gain

Table 12-11	Generic/Trade Name	Usual Adult Dose	Side Effects
Common Peripheral Vasodilators	Hydralazine HCL (Alazine, Apresoline)	10 mg PO qid up to 300 mg/day in divided doses	Dizziness Hypotension Headache Palpitations
	Nitroprusside (Nipride, Nitropress)	IV 0.5 to 10 mcg/kg/min	Tachycardia Peripheral edema
	Prazosin (Minipress)	1 mg bid to tid up to 20 mg/day	Orthostatic hypotension First dose syncope with prazosin

NCLEX!

9. Adverse effects/toxicity

    a. Agranulocytosis, cardiac arrhythmias, **shock** (failure of heart to pump adequately resulting in low CO and compromising tissue perfusion), CHF

    b. Stevens-Johnson syndrome

10. Nursing considerations

    a. Headache and palpitations may occur 2 to 4 hours after the first dose and should subside spontaneously

    b. Food enhances absorption and decreases gastric irritation

    c. Monitor BP and apical pulse regularly

    d. Observe for signs of weight gain and edema

    e. Monitor client for manifestations of CHF, fluid retention, and angina

    f. In renal dialysis clients, minoxidil is removed by dialysis; drug administration times should be altered

11. Client education

    a. Instruct client to monitor weight

    b. Instruct client to change position slowly to prevent dizziness and possible falls

    c. Advise client to report muscle, joint aches, and fever immediately

    d. Inform client that headache, palpitations, and rapid pulse may occur but should be gone in about 10 days

    e. Advise client to not discontinue medications without discussing with the healthcare provider

    f. Explain adverse effects and side effects and instruct to report any unusual side effects

    g. Advise client to avoid alcohol

    h. Advise client to avoid hazardous activities until tolerance develops

    i. Advise client to notify physician before taking OTC medications

    j. Instruct client to report increased heart rate, shortness of breath, chest pain, severe indigestion, dizziness, or fainting

    k. Assure client that hypertrichosis will disappear 1 to 6 months after stopping the drug

H. Other antihypertensives

1. Action and use

    a. Centrally acting sympatholytics

        1) Stimulate the alpha 2 receptors in the central nervous system (CNS) to inhibit the sympathetic cardio-accelerator and vasoconstrictor centers

        2) Decrease sympathetic outflow from the CNS resulting in decrease the arterial pressure

    b. Peripheral anti-adrenergics

1) Deplete catecholamine stores in the peripheral nervous system and perhaps in the CNS

2) Decrease total peripheral resistance, heart rate, and CO

2. Common medications (Table 12-12)

3. Administration considerations

NCLEX!

    a. Abrupt discontinuance may result in rebound hypertension

    b. Guanabenz: allow 1 to 2 weeks before adjusting dose

    c. Guanfacine: administer at bedtime to decrease daytime somnolence; allow 3 to 4 weeks before adjusting dose

    d. Methyldopa: allow 2 days for maximum response before adjusting dose

4. Contraindications

    a. Hypersensitivity for all drugs from this group

    b. Active hepatitis or cirrhosis

    c. Co-administration with monoamine oxidative (MAO) inhibitors (methyldopa)

    d. If signs of heart failure occur, discontinue methyldopa

    e. History of mental depression, active peptic ulcer disease, ulcerative colitis, CHF, asthma, and bronchitis (reserpine)

5. Significant drug interactions

    a. Clonidine/beta blockers: paradoxical hypertension

    b. Clonidine/tricyclic antidepressants: may block antihypertensive effect

    c. Methyldopa may increase effects of levodopa, lithium, haloperidol, MAO inhibitors, and sympathomimetics

    d. Methyldopa/propranolol: paradoxical hypertension

Table 12-12	**Generic/Trade Names**	**Usual Adult Dose**	**Side Effects**
Common Centrally and Peripherally Acting Anti-Adrenergic Medications	***Centrally Acting Antiadrenergics***		
	Clonidine (Catapres)	Initial 0.1 mg bid, PO and patch; maint. 0.2 to 0.8 mg/day	Headache Weakness
	Guanabenz (Wytensin)	Initial 4 mg bid, PO Max. 32 mg bid	Dizziness Depression
	Guanfacine (Tenex)	Initial 1 mg/day, PO, then 1–2 mg/day	Nightmares Parkinsonism
	Methyldopa (Aldomet)	Initial 250 mg bid to tid, PO Then 500–3,000 mg/day	Bradycardia Rash
	Peripherally Acting Antiadrenergics		
	Reserpine (Serpasil)	0.1–0.25 mg/day, PO	Sedation, involuntary choreo-athetoid movements, parkinsonism, edema
	Guanadrel (Hylorel)	Initial 5 mg bid, PO then 20–75 mg/day	Weight gain, dry mouth, galactorrhea, amenorrhea

    e. Guanadrel/phenothiazines, sympathomimetics and tricyclic antidepressants: inhibit antihypertensive effect

    f. Reserpine/tricyclic antidepressants: block antihypertensive effect

6. Significant food interactions: none reported

7. Significant laboratory studies

    a. Blood glucose levels

    b. A positive Coomb's test

    c. May decrease serum cholesterol and total triglycerides slightly but does not alter HDL

    d. May cause nonprogressive elevation of liver enzymes

    e. Methyldopa alters urine uric acid, serum creatinine, and aspartate aminotransferase (AST) and alanine aminotransferase (ALT); it may cause falsely elevated levels of urine catecholamines interfering with the diagnosis of pheochromocytoma

8. Side effects

    a. Sedation, headache, weakness, dizziness, and decreased mental acuity

    b. Involuntary choreoathetoid movements, parkinsonism, depression, nightmares

    c. Bradycardia, orthostatic hypotension, aggravation of angina, edema

    d. GI disturbance, rash, gynecomastia, galactorrhea, amenorrhea, impotence, dry mouth, weight gain

9. Adverse effects/toxicity

    a. Myocarditis, hemolytic anemia, thrombocytopenia

    b. Hepatic necrosis

    c. Severe rebound hypertension

10. Nursing considerations

    a. Administer orally; tablets may be crushed

    b. They do not need to be given with food unless GI upset occurs

    c. Intravenous methyldopa should be given over 30 to 60 minutes; do not give subcutaneously or IM

    d. Transdermal systems (Clonidine) are applied to dry, hairless areas of the skin of chest or upper arm

    e. Assess areas for rash

    f. Monitor labs for elevated AST, ALT, alkaline phosphatase, bilirubin, BUN, creatinine, potassium, sodium, and uric acid

    g. May prolong prothrombin times

    h. Obtain baseline BP, apical pulse, and monitor weight regularly

    i. Assess client for peripheral edema

j. Dry mouth may contribute to development of dental caries, periodontal disease, oral candidiasis, and discomfort

k. Do not discontinue the medications abruptly

11. Client education

a. Stress importance of diet and possible need for sodium restriction and weight reduction; report weight gain of greater than 5 lb per week

b. Instruct client to relieve dry mouth by sipping water or chewing sugarless gum

c. Instruct client to treat nausea by eating unsalted crackers, non-cola beverages or dry toast

d. Advise client to change position slowly to prevent dizziness and possible falls

e. Instruct client to report mental acuity changes to healthcare provider

f. Inform client that some drugs cause the urine to become darker

g. Advise client to not drive a car or perform hazardous activities if the medications cause drowsiness

h. Instruct client to take medication as prescribed

i. Instruct client to consult the physician before taking OTC medications

j. Avoid alcohol or other CNS depressants medications

k. Advise client not to stop drug abruptly

I. Medications for hypertensive emergencies

1. Action and use

   a. Relax arteriolar smooth muscle causing vasodilation

   b. Reduce peripheral vascular resistance thus decreasing BP

   c. Used to treat hypertensive crisis

2. Common medications (Table 12-13): other medications used that have been previously discussed include: hydralazine, labetalol, enalapril, furosemide and nicardipine

3. Administration considerations

   a. Infusion pump must be used for administration

   b. Intravenous infusion titrated to BP

   c. Protect solutions from light, heat or freezing

Table 12-13	Generic/Trade Names	Usual Adult Dose	Side Effects
Common Emergency Antihypertensive Medications	Nitroprusside (Nipride)	0.3 to 10 mcg/kg/min, IV Max. 10 mcg/kg/min for 10 minutes	Dizziness, weakness, headache, malaise, flushing, insomnia, arrhythmia, hypotension, angina
	Nitroglycerin	5–100 mcg/min, IV	Hyperglycemia, rash
	Diazoxide (Hyperstat)	1–3 mg/kg every 5–15 minutes Max. 150 mg, IV	Diaphoresis, GI disturbance, sodium and water retention

    d. Do not administer solutions that have darkened or contain particle matter

    e. Intravenous diazoxide is given undiluted by rapid direct IV injection over 10 to 30 seconds

    f. Client should be recumbent while receiving IV and should remain in bed for a at least 30 minutes following administration

    g. A diuretic should be prescribed to prevent CHF after administering diazoxide since it causes sodium and water retention

  4. Contraindications

    a. Hypersensitivity to thiazide

    b. Compensatory hypertension, inadequate cerebral circulation, severe anemia, angle-closure glaucoma, and CHF

  5. Significant drug interactions

    a. Epinephrine may potentiate effects of other antihypertensive medications; it may displace highly protein bound substances from protein binding sites

    b. Diuretics may potentiate hypoglycemia, hyperuricemia, and antihypertensive effects

    c. Concomitant use of nitroglycerin (NTG) with alcohol, antihypertensive drugs, or phenothiazines may cause additive hypotensive effects

  6. Significant food interactions: none reported

  7. Significant laboratory studies

    a. Increase serum creatinine clearance

    b. Falsely decreased cholesterol levels

    c. Diazoxide inhibits glucose stimulated insulin release and may cause false negative insulin response to glucagons

    d. May cause decrease in hemoglobin or hematocrit

  8. Side effects

    a. Dizziness, weakness, headache, malaise, flushing, palpitations, insomnia, paresthesia, arrhythmia, tachycardia, hypotension, angina, diaphoresis

    b. Sodium and water retention, visual disturbances, GI disturbances, azotemia, decreased urinary output, rash

    c. Ketoacidosis, hyperuricemia, hyperglycemia

  9. Adverse effects/toxicity

    a. Seizures, paralysis, cerebral ischemia, arrhythmias, shock, MI

    b. Thrombocytopenia, increased intracranial pressure, thiocyanate toxicity, methemoglobinemia, cyanide toxicity

 10. Nursing considerations

    a. Monitor BP every 5 minutes for 15 to 30 minutes, then hourly until client is stable

    b. Discontinue if severe hypotension develops or BP continues to fall 30 minutes after drug infusion

    c. Monitor IV site for infiltration

    d. Monitor I & O carefully

    e. Monitor blood glucose levels, electrolytes, and daily weight

    f. Check serum uric acid frequently

    g. Monitor for headache and other side effects

    h. Check thiocyanate levels every 72 hours

11. Client education

    a. Instruct client to monitor blood glucose levels, especially diabetic clients

    b. Instruct client to avoid sudden position changes due to dizziness and orthostatic hypotension

    c. Advise client to report adverse effects immediately including pain or redness at injection site

    d. Teach client about signs and symptoms of CHF

    e. Instruct client to monitor I & O and daily weight

    f. Instruct client to weigh daily and report weight gain greater than 5 lb per week

    g. Inform client to take Tylenol for a headache if needed

IV. Antihypotensives (Sympathomimetics)

A. Action and use

1. Mimic the fight or flight response of the sympathetic nervous system, selectively stimulating alpha-adrenergic and beta-adrenergic receptors

2. Stimulation of alpha-adrenergic receptors results in vasoconstriction and increase systemic BP

3. Stimulation of beta-adrenergic receptors increases the force and rate of myocardial contraction

4. Used to treat shock

B. Common medications (Table 12-14)

Table 12-14	Generic/Trade Names	Usual Adult Dose	Side Effects
Common Sympathomimetic Medications	Norepinephrine (Levophed)	8–12 mcg/min, IV, then 2–4 mg/min	Anxiety, weakness, dizziness, tremor
	Metaraminol (Aramine)	0.5 to 5 mg, IV	Restlessness, bradycardia
	Dopamine (Intropin)	1–5 mcg/kg/min increasing to 50 mcg/kg/min	Shortness of breath, nausea, vomiting, flushing
	Dobutamine (Dobutrex)	2.5–10 mcg/kg/min increasing to 40 mcg/kg/min, IV	Diaphoresis, azotemia
	Isoproterenol (Isuprel)	0.5 to 5 mg/min, IV infusion 0.02 to 0.06 mg, IV bolus 0.2 mg, IM or SC	Sloughing upon extravasation Bronchospasm Palpitation

NCLEX!
NCLEX!
NCLEX!
NCLEX!
NCLEX!
NCLEX!

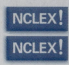

C. Administration considerations

   1. Drug must be diluted before administration

   2. Client should be attended constantly during drug administration

D. Contraindications

   1. Uncorrected arrhythmias, mesenteric or peripheral vascular thrombosis

   2. Profound hypoxia, hypercapnia, hypotension due to blood volume deficit

   3. Cautionary use with those receiving MAO inhibitors or imipramine-type antidepressants

E. Significant drug interactions

   1. Norepinephrine interacts with general anesthesia, tricyclic antidepressants, and MAO inhibitors

   2. Beta blockers may increase potential for hypertension

   3. Diuretics decrease arterial response

   4. Atropine enhances pressor effects

   5. Metaraminol/MAO inhibitors: increase vasopressor effects

F. Significant food interactions: none reported

G. Significant laboratory studies

   1. Monitor serum electrolytes

   2. Monitor blood glucose levels

   3. Isoproterenol decreases sensitivity of spirometry in the diagnosis of asthma

H. Side effects

   1. Anxiety, weakness, dizziness, tremor, restlessness

   2. Bradycardia, tachycardia, palpitations

   3. Nausea and vomiting, flushing, diaphoresis, sloughing upon extravasation

   4. Azotemia, shortness of breath, and bronchospasm

I. Adverse effects/toxicity

   1. Severe hypertension, anaphylaxis

   2. Arrhythmias, cardiac arrest, ventricular tachycardia

   3. Stokes-Adams seizures, asthmatic episodes

J. Nursing considerations

   1. Reevaluate if 3 to 5 treatments in 6 to 12 hours provide minimal to no relief

   2. Carefully monitor vital signs, EKG, and I & O

   3. Monitor for rebound hypertension

   4. Constant infusion pump prevents sudden infusion of excessive amounts of drugs

   5. Correct blood volume depletion first

6. Antidote for extravasation: 5 to 10 mg phentolamine mesylate (Regitine) in 10 to 15 mL of normal saline

7. Monitor infusion site frequently

8. Client should be attended constantly during administration

9. Protect solution from light

10. Sympathomimetics are incompatible with sodium bicarbonate

K. Client education

1. Instruct client to report adverse reactions and side effects immediately

2. Inform client that vital signs will be monitored frequently

3. Instruct client to report anginal pain while on dobutamine

V. Urinary Tract and Bladder Medications

A. Anti-infectives

1. Action and use

   a. Act as **bacteriostatic** (inhibition of the growth of bacterial without destruction) and **bactericidal** (destroying bacteria) actions

   b. Act as disinfectants within the urinary tract

   c. Used to treat urinary tract infections

2. Common medications (Table 12-15)

3. Administration considerations

   a. May take with food or milk to decrease GI upset

   b. Check renal and hepatic function before administering

   c. Oral suspension may stain teeth

   d. Complete full course of therapy

4. Contraindications

   a. Hypersensitivity

Table 12-15	Generic/Trade Names	Usual Adult Dose	Side Effects
Common Urinary Tract Anti-infectives	Methenamine (Hiprex, Mandelamine)	1 g bid, PO	Drowsiness Weakness
	Nalidixic acid (NegGram)	1 g qid for 7–14 days, then 2 g daily for long-term use, PO	Headache Dizziness
	Nitrofurantoin (Macrodantin)	50–100 mg qid, PO	Photosensitivity Blurred vision
	Trimethoprim (Proloprim)	100 mg every 12 hrs	GI distress Pruritis
	Sulfisoxazole and Phenazopyridine (Azo-Gantrisin)	Initial 2–4 g/day, then 4–8 g daily in divided doses, PO	Rash Arthralgia

    b. Megaloblastic anemia and folate deficiency, renal insufficiency, and severe hepatic insufficiency

    c. Severe dehydration, anuria, oliguria, and seizure disorder

5. Significant drug interactions

    a. Hiprex/sulfonamides: may cause formation of an insoluble precipitate in the urine

    b. Nalidixic acid/warfarin: increase the effect of warfarin

    c. Sulfonamides may increase the effects of methotrexate, phenytoin, sulfonylureas, and warfarin

    d. Trimethoprim increases the effects of phenytoin

6. Significant food interactions: none reported

7. Significant laboratory studies

    a. May increase liver function enzymes and renal function

    b. May cause false positive urinary glucose test

8. Side effects

    a. Drowsiness, weakness, headache, dizziness

    b. Sensitivity to light, blurred vision

    c. GI distress, pruritis, rash, arthralgia

9. Adverse effects/toxicity

    a. Seizures, increased intracranial pressure

    b. Leukopenia, thrombocytopenia, angioedema

10. Nursing considerations

    a. Drugs work best if client is well (but not overly) hydrated

    b. Administer with meals to decrease GI distress

    c. Monitor renal and liver function

    d. Check urine pH before administration as some drugs work best in acidic urine

    e. Cranberry juice or vitamin C may be added to acidify the urine

    f. Monitor CNS side effects

    g. If using an oral suspension nitrofurantoin, instruct the client to rinse mouth to avoid staining of the teeth

    h. Ingestion of large amount of fluid while taking methenamide will reduce antibacterial effects by diluting the medication and raising the urinary pH

11. Client education

    a. Inform client that long term therapy is common even if feeling fine

    b. Advise client to drink at least 8 glasses of water daily

    c. Instruct client to take medications with meals to decrease GI distress

NCLEX!

       d. Advise client to avoid alkalizing fluids such as milk, fruit juices or sodium bicarbonate

       e. Advise client to notify physician of any new medications

NCLEX!

       f. Instruct client to use sunscreen to avoid excessive exposure to sunlight

       g. Instruct client to notify physician of any CNS side effects

NCLEX!

       h. Inform client that the medication may discolor the urine and assure this is not harmful and will disappear after the drug is discontinued

B. Antispasmodics

    1. Action and use

       a. Relax smooth muscles of the urinary tract

       b. Decrease bladder muscle spasms

NCLEX!

       c. Used to manage the disorders of the lower urinary tract associated with hypermotility: dysuria, urgency, nocturia, suprapubic pain, frequency and incontinence

    2. Common medications (Table 12-16)

    3. Administration considerations: administer 1 hour before antacids or antidiarrheals

    4. Contraindications

       a. Glaucoma

       b. Obstructive breathing, obstructive GI disease, severe ulcerative colitis, and myasthenia gravis

NCLEX!

       c. Hypersensitivity to anticholinergics, paralytic ileus, unstable cardiovascular (CV) status

    5. Significant drug interactions

       a. Amantadine increases adverse anticholinergic effects

       b. Phenothiazines or haloperidol will result in decreased antipsychotic effect

       c. Antacids and antidiarrheals result in decreased absorption of hyoscamine

       d. Additive effect with other anticholinergic drugs

    6. Significant food interactions: none reported

Table 12-16	Generic/Trade Names	Usual Adult Dose	Side Effects
Common Antispasmodic Medications	Hyoscyamine (Cystospaz)	0.125–0.25 mg qid and HS, PO	Headache, insomnia Drowsiness
		0.25–0.5 mg bid to qid, IM, SC, IV	Dizziness Confusion
	Tolterodine tartrate (Detrol)	2 mg bid, PO	Excitement Blurred vision
	Oxybutynin chloride (Ditropan)	5 mg bid to tid, PO Max. 20 mg/day	Dry mouth GI distress, urinary retention
	Flavoxate (Urispas)	100–200 mg tid to qid, PO	Urinary hesitancy

7. Significant laboratory studies: none reported

NCLEX!

8. Side effects

   a. Headache, insomnia, drowsiness, dizziness, confusion, excitement, palpitations

   b. Blurred vision

   c. Dry mouth, GI distress, urinary hesitancy, urine retention, urticaria

9. Adverse effects/toxicity: leukopenia

10. Nursing considerations

NCLEX!

NCLEX!

   a. Monitor effect of medication

   b. Monitor for CNS manifestations

   c. Monitor I & O

11. Client education

   a. Warn client that drowsiness and blurred vision may occur and caution should be used with driving or operating machinery

   b. Instruct client to use hard sugarless candy for dry mouth

   c. Instruct client to avoid alcohol, which increases drowsiness

   d. Instruct client to swallow pill whole and do not chew or crush

   e. Inform client that the shell of the medication may appear in the stool

   f. Inform client of side effects and to report them to the provider

C. Urinary analgesic

1. Action and use

   a. Has a local anesthetic effect on the urinary tract mucosa

   b. Used to relieve pain with urinary tract infections or irritation

2. Common medication: phenazopyridine (Pyridium): 100 to 200 mg tid

3. Administration considerations

NCLEX!

   a. Drug colors the urine red or orange and may stain fabrics

   b. May be used with antibiotics and should be discontinued after 2 days of antibiotic use

4. Contraindications

   a. Hypersensitivity

   b. Contraindicated in renal or hepatic diseases

5. Significant drug interactions: none reported

6. Significant food interactions: none reported

7. Significant laboratory studies: may alter the results of urinary Dipstix

8. Side effects

   a. Headache and vertigo

   b. Nausea and GI distress

9. Adverse effects/toxicity

    a. Anaphylaxis

    b. Methemoglobinemia

    c. Renal and hepatic failure

10. Nursing considerations

    a. Assess for presence of urinary tract infection (UTI)

    b. Assess urinary function and output

    c. Monitor I & O

    d. Monitor sclera for yellow tinge

    e. Ensure renal function before administering

    f. Use only as an analgesic

11. Client education

    a. Instruct client to maintain a good hygiene to prevent UTI

    b. Advise client of possible side effects

    c. Advise client that the drug colors the urine red/orange and may stain clothing

    d. Instruct client not to double the dose if a dose is missed

    e. Instruct client to take medication with food to decrease GI distress

    f. Encourage client to increase fluids

    g. Inform client that it may not be effective for more than 24 to 48 hours

    h. Instruct client to notify provider if notices yellowing of the eyes

    i. Advise client to report symptoms that worsen or do not resolve

VI. Medications to Treat Benign Prostatic Hyperplasia (BPH)

A. Action and use

1. Block alpha 1 receptors in the prostate leading to relaxation of smooth muscles, improving urine flow and decreasing BPH symptoms

2. Used to increase urine flow and decrease symptoms of BPH

B. Common medications (Table 12-17)

C. Administration considerations

1. Do not handle crushed tablets if pregnant

2. Not indicated for females or pediatric use

3. Postural effects may occur 2 to 6 hours after dose

4. If treatment is interrupted for several days, restart medication at initial dose

D. Contraindications

1. Hypersensitivity

2. Caution in clients with impaired hepatic function

Table 12-17	Generic/Trade Names	Usual Adult Dose	Side Effects
Common Medications to Treat Benign Prostatic Hyperplasia	Doxazosin (Cardura)	Initial 1 mg/day, increase if needed 1, 4, and 8 mg with 1–2 week intervals, PO	Impotence Decreased volume of ejaculate Decreased libido
	Tamsulosin (Flomax)	0.4 mg/day increase to 0.8 mg/day if needed, PO	Asthenia Dizziness
	Terazosin (Hytrin)	1 mg/d slowly increase to 2, 5, 10 mg/day, PO	Postural hypotension Nasal congestion
	Finasteride (Proscar)	5 mg/day, PO	Peripheral edema, diarrhea

E. Significant drug interactions

    1. May increase theophylline clearance (finasteride)

    2. Concomitant use with other antihypertensive agents/diuretics (terazosin)

    3. Do not use with alpha adrenergic blockers

    4. Cimetidine may decrease clearance

    5. Use cautiously with warfarin

F. Significant food interactions: none reported

G. Significant laboratory studies

    1. Decrease WBC and neutrophil counts with doxazosin

    2. Decreased hematocrit, WBC, hemoglobin, total protein and albumin levels with terazosin

    3. Decreased prostate-specific antigen (PSA), even in prostate cancer with finasteride

H. Side effects

    1. Impotence, decreased volume of ejaculate, decreased libido, asthenia

    2. Dizziness, headache, nervousness, palpitations, peripheral edema, postural hypotension, nasal congestion, myalgia

    3. Diarrhea and nausea

I. Adverse effects/toxicity: hypotension, shock, and arrhythmias

J. Nursing considerations

    1. Assess client for the severity of symptoms

    2. Provide treatment options

    3. Monitor for decreased BP

    4. Rule out cancer of the prostate before initiating therapy

    5. Monitor for concomitant medications for interactions

    6. Monitor urine volume

K. Client education

1. Instruct client to change position slowly to prevent orthostatic hypotension

2. Instruct client to avoid driving and hazardous tasks for the first 12 to 24 hours or after increasing the dose due to drowsiness and somnolence

3. Instruct client to report side effects to provider

4. Advise client to take medication at the same time each day

5. Advise women who are or may become pregnant not to handle crushed tablets of finasteride due to risk of adverse effect to male fetus

6. Instruct male client whose sexual partner is or may become pregnant to avoid exposing her to his semen or else discontinue finasteride

7. Inform client that the volume of ejaculate may be decreased but does not impair fertility

VII. Medications to Treat Renal Failure

A. Action and use

1. The primary focus of pharmacologic management of renal failure is to restore and maintain renal perfusion and to eliminate drugs that are directly nephrotoxic

2. Diuretics to improve urinary outflow and antihypertensive have been previously discussed and are not covered in this category

3. Dopaminergic receptors cause vasodilation in the renal, mesenteric, coronary and intracerebral vascular beds

4. Are used to increase urine flow

B. Common medications: dopamine (Intropin), 2 to 5 mcg/kg/min to increase renal perfusion; may increase to 50 mcg/kg/min IV to raise blood pressure

C. Administration considerations

1. Administered IV using an infusion device to control the rate of flow

2. Administered into a large vein to prevent possibility of extravasation

3. Hypovolemia should be corrected before initiation of dopamine therapy

4. Decrease dose as soon as hemodynamic condition is stabilized

5. Do not mix with other medications

6. Discard solutions after 24 hours

D. Contraindications

1. Uncorrected tachyarrhythmias, pheochromocytoma, or ventricular fibrillation

2. Caution in use with occlusive vascular disease, cold injuries, diabetic endarteritis, and arterial embolism

E. Significant drug interactions

1. MAO may prolong and intensify the effect of dopamine

2. Beta blockers antagonize cardiac effects

3. General anesthetics may cause ventricular arrhythmias and hypertension

4. Diuretics may result in increased diuretic effects

F. Significant food interactions: none reported

G. Significant laboratory studies

1. Increased catecholamines

2. Increased serum glucose levels

H. Side effects

1. Headache, tachycardia, angina, palpitations, hypotension, bradycardia, vaso-constriction, widening of QRS complex

2. Nausea and vomiting, piloerection, azotemia

I. Adverse effects/toxicity

1. Anaphylaxis

2. Asthmatic episodes

3. Severe hypertension

J. Nursing considerations

1. Carefully monitor I & O

2. Assess infusion site frequently for extravasation; use 5 to 10 mg phentolamine mesylate (Regitine) in 10 to 15 mL of normal saline as an antidote

3. Monitor vital signs, cardiac output and EKG frequently

4. Monitor for side effects

K. Client education

1. Instruct client to report side effects

2. Inform client to monitor vital signs and I & O

VIII. Hematopoietic Growth Factor

A. Action and use

1. Used to stimulate red blood cell (RBC) production

2. Reverses anemia associated with chronic renal failure (CRF)

B. Common medication: epoetin alfa (Epogen, Procrit), SC/IV 300–500 U/kg/dose 3 times/wk

C. Administration considerations

1. Initial effects can be seen within 1 to 2 weeks

2. Hematocrit (Hct) reaches normal levels (30 to 33%) in 2 to 3 months

3. Do not shake solution

4. IV administration: Epoetin alfa may be given undiluted by direct IV as a bolus dose

D. Contraindications

1. Uncontrolled hypertension

2. Known hypersensitivity to mammalian cell-derived products and albumin

E. Significant drug interactions: none reported

F. Significant food interactions: none reported

G. Significant laboratory studies

1. CBC with differential and platelet count

2. Monitor BUN, creatinine, phosphorus, and potassium

3. Monitor partial thromboplastin time (APPT)

4. Evaluate transferrin and serum ferritin prior to initiation of therapy

H. Side effects

1. Hypertension

2. Headache, seizure

3. Iron deficiency, sweating

I. Adverse effects/toxicity

1. Thrombocytosis, clotting of AV fistula

2. Bone pain, arthralgias

J. Nursing considerations

1. Blood pressure may rise during early therapy as the Hct increases; notify physician of a rapid rise in Hct greater than 4 points in 2 weeks

2. Do not give with any other drug solution

3. Use only one dose per vial, and do not reenter vial

4. Inspect solution for particulate matter prior to use

5. Monitor for hypertensive encephalopathy in clients with CRF during period of increasing Hct

6. Client may require additional heparin during dialysis to prevent clotting of the vascular access

K. Client education

1. Instruct client to monitor vital signs, especially BP

2. Inform client that headache is a common adverse effect; it should be reported if it is severe

3. Inform client to avoid driving or being involved in other hazardous activity because of possible seizure activity especially during the first 90 days of therapy

4. Stress importance of keeping all follow-up appointments

IX. Medications to Prevent Organ Rejection

A. Cyclosporine (Neoral)

1. Is an immunosuppressant

2. Acts on T lymphocytes to suppress production of interleukin-2

3. Used to prevent rejection of allogenic kidney transplant

4. Oral administration is preferred

5. Blood levels should be monitored frequently

6. Administer prednisone concurrently

7. Client should be instructed to monitor for signs of infection

8. Grapefruit juice can raise cyclosporine levels, thus increasing the risk of toxicity

9. Client should be instructed to mix the concentrated medication solution with milk, chocolate milk, or orange juice just before administration

10. Side effects: nausea and vomiting, hypertension, tremor, hirsutism, depression, and anaphylactic shock

11. Dose: oral route, 14 to 18 mg/kg beginning 4 to 12 hours before transplantation and continued for 1 to 2 weeks after surgery

B. Azathioprine (Imuran)

1. Is a cytotoxic medication

2. Suppresses cell-mediated and humoral immunity

3. Used with cyclosporine to help suppress transplant rejection

4. Can cause neutropenia

5. Side effects: nausea and vomiting, bone marrow depression, agranulocytosis, and secondary infection

6. Dose: PO, 3 to 5 mg/kg/d initially, may reduce to 1 to 3 mg/kg/day

C. Muromonab-CD3 (Orthoclone OKT3)

1. Is an antibody

2. Used to prevent acute allograft rejection of kidney transplants

3. Side effects: nausea and vomiting, chest pain, and dyspnea

4. Dose: IV, 5 mg/d administered in less than 1 minute for 10 to 14 days

---

Case Study

T. S. is a 40-year-old male recently diagnosed with uncomplicated hypertension. He started taking metoprolol (Lopressor) 100 mg daily 2 weeks ago and has returned for a follow-up visit. He states that he feels fine.

❶ What additional subjective data should the nurse collect?

❷ What type of medication is metoprolol and what are the common side effects?

❸ What lifestyle modifications should be addressed for this client?

❹ What client teaching should the nurse provide?

❺ What are the expected outcomes for this client?

For suggested responses, see page 641.

Posttest

1 A client is prescribed verapamil (Isoptin) to manage his hypertension. The nurse should instruct the client that verapamil will have which of the following effects on the body?

(1) Lower blood pressure
(2) Lower blood pressure and heart rate
(3) Increase urinary output
(4) Increase heart rate

2 Phenazopyridine (Pyridium) is prescribed to a client with dysuria. The client asks the nurse about the side effects of this medication. The nurse should inform the client to expect which of the following urine characteristics?

(1) Decrease in volume
(2) Foul in odor
(3) Increased in volume
(4) Orange/red in color

3 A client's blood pressure (BP) continues to drop despite IV fluids. Intravenous dopamine is ordered. The client asks the nurse about the possible benefits of this medication. The nurse responds to the client based on the understanding that dopamine treats shock by:

(1) Blocking AV node conduction.
(2) Causing vasoconstriction and increasing systemic BP.
(3) Decreasing rate of myocardial contraction.
(4) Promoting diuresis.

4 The client being seen in an ambulatory clinic has hypertension. During assessment, the client mentions that she will stop taking her antihypertensive medications as soon as her blood pressure is under control. In developing a medication teaching plan, the nurse includes which of the following instructions?

(1) "In order to maintain control of your blood pressure, the medication must be continued indefinitely."
(2) "Only the physician can answer this question."
(3) "The medication will probably be stopped after your blood pressure is normal."
(4) "The medication will be decreased in time."

5 The home health nurse instructs the client about use of an antihypertensive medication. The client plans to take an over-the-counter (OTC) medication for his cold. The nurse should instruct the client to avoid which of the following OTC products while taking an antihypertensive?

(1) Acetaminophen
(2) Aspirin
(3) Pseudoephedrine
(4) Steroid creams

6 A client arrives in the emergency department after complaining of unrelieved edema in her legs. The client is taking spironolactone (Aldactone). The nurse determines that which of the following data indicates the need to hold the medication?

(1) Blood glucose level of 130
(2) Blood pressure of 120/70
(3) Pulse of 90
(4) Potassium of 6.0 mEq/L

7 The nurse is preparing to administer a dose of cyclosporine by IV administration. Which of the following items should the nurse make available at the bedside during administration of this medication?

(1) A suction catheter
(2) Oral airway
(3) Latex-free cart
(4) Epinephrine

8 The nurse taking care of a client with uncomplicated hypertension anticipates seeing which of the following medication classification prescribed for controlling the disorder?

(1) Diuretics and beta blockers
(2) Diuretics and angiotensin converting enzyme (ACE) inhibitors
(3) Calcium channel blockers and ACE inhibitors
(4) Calcium channel blockers and beta blockers

9 The nurse is providing discharge instructions to a client receiving sulfisoxazole (Gantrisin). Which of the following is included in the plan of care for instructions?

(1) Call physician if the urine turns dark brown.
(2) Maintain a high fluid intake.
(3) Restrict fluid intake.
(4) Decrease the dosage when symptoms are improving.

10 The nurse would make it a priority to assess for first dose syncope when administering a dose of which class of antihypertensive medications?

(1) Angiotensin-converting enzyme (ACE) inhibitors
(2) Alpha blockers
(3) Beta blockers
(4) Calcium channel blockers

See pages 500–501 for Answers and Rationales.

Answers and Rationales

Pretest

1 Answer: 1 Rationale: A client taking a diuretic such as furosemide should self administer the medication in the morning to allow for diuresis throughout the day. This will help to prevent nocturia, which could cause disruption to the client's nightly sleep pattern. The timeframe in option 2 is not as early as option 1, while options 3 and 4 clearly increase the risk of nocturia.
Cognitive Level: Analysis
Nursing Process: Implementation; *Test Plan:* PHYS

2 Answer: 2 Rationale: The National Institutes of Health (NIH) Committee has defined hypertension as a systolic pressure of 140 or higher and diastolic of 90 or higher when two or more blood pressure measurements are averaged on two or more subsequent visits. Options 1, 3, and 4 are incorrect.
Cognitive Level: Application
Nursing Process: Implementation; *Test Plan:* PHYS

3 Answer: 4 Rationale: Losartan is an angiotensin II antagonist that inhibits the conversion of angiotensin I to angiotensin II, resulting in vasodilation and nor-

malizing blood pressure. The client should be assessed for dizziness, cough, and diarrhea while taking this medication.
Cognitive Level: Application
Nursing Process: Assessment; *Test Plan:* PHYS

4 **Answer: 2**. *Rationale:* Dry, persistent, tickling, and nonproductive cough is a common side effect of angiotensin converting enzyme (ACE) inhibitors.
Cognitive Level: Analysis
Nursing Process: Analysis; *Test Plan:* PHYS

5 **Answer: 4** *Rationale:* Beta blockers inhibit cardiac beta 1 receptors but also may affect beta 2 receptors in bronchial and vascular smooth muscle causing bronchoconstriction. Therefore, the client with COPD should avoid taking beta blockers. Options 1, 2, and 3 are incorrect.
Cognitive Level: Application
Nursing Process: Implementation; *Test Plan:* PHYS

6 **Answer: 2** *Rationale:* Indipamide (Lozol) is a thiazide diuretic. Its hypertensive effect may be caused by direct arteriolar vasodilation and decreased total peripheral resistance. Lozol may cause hypokalemia. Signs and symptoms of hypokalemia include muscle weakness and leg cramps. Electrolytes, particularly potassium, need to be evaluated. The other options are irrelevant.
Cognitive Level: Analysis
Nursing Process: Planning; *Test Plan:* PHYS

7 **Answer: 1** *Rationale:* Thiazide diuretics decrease the effect of antigout medication by increasing hypersensitivity to allopurinol. Hyperuricemia is a side effect of thiazide diuretics. Option 3 is not the best answer because with a diabetic neuropathy, although clients may experience pain and burning sensation in the lower extremities as well as signs of infection, there is no mention of diabetes history in the above question.
Cognitive Level: Analysis
Nursing Process: Analysis; *Test Plan:* PHYS

8 **Answer: 4** *Rationale:* Oxybutynin (Ditropan) is an antispasmodics medication used for urinary tract problems. It produces anticholinergic side effects such as dry mouth, constipation, urinary hesitancy, and decreased gastroenteritis motility. Periodic interruptions in therapy are recommended to assess continued need for this medication.
Cognitive Level: Application
Nursing Process: Implementation; *Test Plan:* PHYS

9 **Answer: 2** *Rationale:* Urinalysis and urine dipstick should be performed to assess for the presence of

blood cells and bacteria in the urine. Infection should be established before instituting pharmacologic therapy. Clients with urinary problems should be encouraged to increase fluid intake, but it is not the most important intervention at this time.
Cognitive Level: Application
Nursing Process: Implementation; *Test Plan:* PHYS

10 **Answer: 2** *Rationale:* Proscar is an androgen inhibitor used to treat benign prostatic hyperplasia (BPH). Pregnant or women of childbearing age should not be exposed to semen fluid of a male taking finasteride (Proscar). Proscar is teratogenic and may produce fetal abnormalities. Options 1, 3, and 4 are incorrect.
Cognitive Level: Application
Nursing Process: Implementation; *Test Plan:* PHYS

Posttest

1 **Answer: 2** *Rationale:* Verapamil is a calcium channel blocker that decreases blood pressure and heart rate. Option 1 is incomplete. Calcium channel blockers have no effect on urinary output (option 3). Option 4 is an opposite effect to this medication.
Cognitive Level: Application
Nursing Process: Implementation; *Test Plan:* PHYS

2 **Answer: 4** *Rationale:* Phenazopyridine is a urinary analgesic with a local anesthetic effect on the urinary tract mucosa. This medication relieves pain during urinary tract infection. It causes the urine to have an orange/red color. It has no effect on volume of urine. Foul odor to the urine may be caused by urinary tract infection.
Cognitive Level: Application
Nursing Process: Implementation; *Test Plan:* PHYS

3 **Answer: 2** *Rationale:* Dopamine acts on the alpha/beta adrenergic receptors resulting in vasoconstriction, increasing systemic BP, and increasing force and rate of myocardial contraction. Options 1, 3, and 4 are incorrect.
Cognitive Level: Application
Nursing Process: Implementation; *Test Plan:* PHYS

4 **Answer: 1** *Rationale:* Emphasis should be placed on the client's adherence to the plan of treatment to avoid serious consequences of noncompliance. The complications of high blood pressure include stroke, cardiac failure, and chronic renal failure.
Cognitive Level: Analysis
Nursing Process: Implementation; *Test Plan:* PHYS

5 **Answer: 3** *Rationale:* Some clients will experience an increased blood pressure with OTC cold preparations such as pseudoephedrine due to vasoconstriction. Therefore, they should avoid taking these medications with an antihypertensive. Options 1, 2, and 4 are incorrect.
Cognitive Level: Application
Nursing Process: Assessment; *Test Plan:* PHYS

6 **Answer: 4** *Rationale:* Aldactone is a potassium-sparing diuretic that increases sodium excretion and decreases potassium secretion in the distal convoluted tubule. Potassium levels greater than 5.5 mEq/L are contraindicated with spironolactone due to increased risk of hyperkalemia. The other options are describing normal conditions.
Cognitive Level: Analysis
Nursing Process: Assessment; *Test Plan:* PHYS

7 **Answer: 4** *Rationale:* Epinephrine and oxygen should be available at the bedside because of the risk of anaphylaxis during administration. An oral airway and suction catheter are not the priority items.
Cognitive Level: Application
Nursing Process: Planning; *Test Plan:* PHYS

8 **Answer: 1** *Rationale:* The Joint National Committee VI treatment algorithm recommends diuretics and beta blockers as the preferred agents for uncomplicated hypertension as they lower morbidity and mortality. ACE inhibitors, calcium channel blockers, alpha and beta blockers, and angiotension II antagonists are also acceptable as monotherapy.
Cognitive Level: Application
Nursing Process: Planning; *Test Plan:* PHYS

9 **Answer: 2** *Rationale:* Each dose of this medication should be administered with a full glass of water, and the client should be encouraged to maintain a high fluid intake. The medication is more soluble in alkaline urine. Option 4 is incorrect, and the client should not discontinue or decrease the dosage without consulting with physician.
Cognitive Level: Application
Nursing Process: Planning; *Test Plan:* PHYS

10 **Answer: 2** *Rationale:* Alpha blockers may cause first-dose syncope within 30 minutes to 1 hour after the first dose. The effect is transient and maybe diminished by administering the medication at bedtime.
Cognitive Level: Application
Nursing Process: Assessment; *Test Plan:* PHYS

References

Abrams, A. (2004). *Clinical drug therapy: Rationales for nursing practice* (7th ed.). Philadelphia: Lippincott, Williams, & Wilkins, pp. 797–831.

Aschenbrenner, D., Cleveland, L., & Venable, S. (2002). *Drug therapy in nursing*. Philadelphia: Lippincott, Williams, & Wilkins, pp.492–552.

Karch, A. (2003). *Focus on pharmacology* (2nd ed.). Philadelphia: Lippincott, Williams, & Wilkins, pp. 690–716.

Lehne, R. (2003). *Pharmacology for nursing care* (5th ed.). St. Louis, MO: Mosby, Inc., pp. 413–426, 469–490.

Lemone, P., & Burke, K. (2003). *Medical-surgical nursing: Critical thinking in client care.* (3rd ed.) Upper Saddle River, NJ: Prentice-Hall, pp. 127–1206.

McKenry, L., & Salerno, G. (2003). *Mosby's pharmacology in nursing* (21st ed.). St. Louis, MO: Mosby, Inc., pp. 668–698.

Pearson, L. (2001). *Nurse practitioner's drug handbook.* (3rd ed.). Springhouse, PA: Springhouse Corporation, pp. 87–1017.

Pentosan. (2001, July 12). http://www.nursespdr.com.

Youngkin, E., Swain, K., Kissinger, J., & Israel, D. (1999). *Pharmacotherapeutics: A primary care clinical guide.* Stamford, CT: Appleton & Lange, pp. 312–1478.

Reproductive System Medications

OBJECTIVES

▪ Describe general goals of therapy when administering medications associated with the reproductive system.

▪ Discuss side effects and adverse effects of estrogens, progestins, and androgens.

▪ Describe nursing considerations related to medications used to treat erectile dysfunction.

▪ Discuss effects of oxytocin (Pitocin) on the uterus.

▪ Identify indications, contraindications, side effects, and adverse reactions of ergonovine (Ergotrate) and methylergonovine (Methergine).

▪ Identify action and use for ritodrine (Yutopar).

▪ Identify indications, contraindications, side effects, and adverse reactions of magnesium sulfate.

▪ Describe specific nursing considerations when administering magnesium sulfate.

▪ List significant client education points related to reproductive system medications.

[Media Link]

Use the CD-ROM enclosed with this text, or log onto the address given to access the free, interactive Companion Website created for this series. The CD-ROM and Companion Website accompanying this book offer additional practice opportunities and information—NCLEX Review, Case Studies, Glossary, In Depth with NCLEX, and more.

www.prenhall.com/hogan

REVIEW AT A GLANCE

anabolic steroid *an androgen with anabolic properties, rarely prescribed but often abused by athletes to increase muscle mass*

androgen *a medication that induces or increases male hormone-like effects*

cryptorchidism *a congenital condition characterized by failure of the testis to descend into the scrotum*

hepatotoxic *toxic to the liver*

Homan's sign *calf pain on dorsiflexion of the foot often caused by deep vein thrombosis*

hypogonadism *underdevelopment of the gonads*

priapism *painful penile erection that does not spontaneously subside*

Pretest

1 The physician has written an order for sildenafil (Viagra). The client asks about the dosage of this medication. Which of the following items is included in the nurse's response?

(1) The smallest possible dose to achieve erection is utilized.
(2) The dose is started high and worked down until erection is not achieved.
(3) Almost every man uses 50 mg, so that is what the doctor prescribes.
(4) Higher doses create longer erections, so it is up to the client which dose is ordered.

2 The nurse is preparing the pregnant client to have her labor augmented with oxytocin (Pitocin). Further teaching is needed when the client states: "This medication will:

(1) Work with the hormones that my body is producing that make contractions."
(2) Cause my uterus to contract harder and more often."
(3) Create one long continuous contraction until the baby is born."
(4) Be given through my IV a little bit at the time."

3 The client with preterm labor is being administered magnesium sulfate (generic) intravenously. Which of the following client manifestations is an expected effect of this medication?

(1) Decreased deep tendon reflexes
(2) Decreased respiratory rate
(3) Nervousness and tremors
(4) Nausea and diarrhea

4 The nurse is teaching a client about clomiphene (Clomid). The nurse explains to the client that this medication is indicated for treatment of which of the following health problems?

(1) Infertility
(2) Hypogonadism
(3) Postpartum hemorrhage
(4) Hormone replacement therapy

5 The client taking Ortho Tri-Cyclen combination oral contraceptives calls the clinic reporting that she has forgotten her pills for the last 2 days. Which of the following suggestions would the nurse provide to the client?

(1) "Take 2 pills today and tomorrow, and use a backup method for the rest of the cycle."
(2) "Take 2 pills today, and then one each day until the pill pack is finished."
(3) "Take 1 pill each day until all the pills are gone, and use a backup method for the rest of the cycle."
(4) "Stop taking the pills and use condoms until the next mense, then restart a new pill pack."

6 For which of the following clients would you expect the physician to prescribe ritodrine (Yutopar)?

(1) A client at 27 weeks gestation with regular uterine contractions
(2) A client at 41 weeks gestation with irregular uterine contractions
(3) A client who delivered at 40 weeks gestation having postpartum hemorrhage
(4) A client at 38 weeks gestation with hypertension and seizures

7 The hypertensive client is experiencing a post-partum hemorrhage. Which medication would you expect the certified nurse-midwife to prescribe?

(1) Ergonovine (Ergotrate)
(2) Methylergonovine (Methergine)
(3) Oxytocin (Pitocin)
(4) Carboprost tromethamine (Hemabate)

8 The client with infertility will be starting menotropin (Humegon) and human chorionic go-nadotropin (Chorex) injections this cycle. During instruction regarding medication administration, the client asks why she needs to have the Chorex, and not just the menotropin (Humegon). The nurse's response would include that Chorex:

(1) Facilitates release of the mature follicle from the ovary.
(2) Matures the follicle so an ovum is ready to be re-leased.
(3) Prevents more than 1 or 2 ova from being released.
(4) Prepares the lining of the uterus for the fertilized egg.

9 A 16-year-old male client has been prescribed testosterone cypionate (Andonate) to treat hypo-gonadism. He asks: "Why do I need these hor-mones anyway?" Which of the following would be the best response by the nurse?

(1) "Testosterone is necessary to prevent your muscles from atrophying."
(2) "This medication is a form of testosterone. Your doc-tor can best explain it to you."
(3) "Testosterone prevents your body from becoming feminine-looking."
(4) "This medication will replace the testosterone that your body is not producing."

10 The client has been prescribed danocrine (Dana-zol) for treatment of endometriosis. The nurse determines that the instruction on taking this medication has been successful when the client states:

(1) "This medication is taken by mouth twice daily."
(2) "I'll need to take this medication for the rest of my life."
(3) "I'll be giving myself injections weekly with this med-ication."
(4) "This medication is worn as a patch on my ab-domen."

See pages 529–530 for Answers and Rationales.

I. Estrogens

A. Action and use

1. Hormone replacement therapy (HRT) after spontaneous or surgically induced menopause

2. Relieves symptoms of menopause such as hot flashes, night sweats, sleep dis-turbances, and vaginal dryness; protects against coronary heart disease and os-teoporosis

3. Used to treat female **hypogonadism**, a condition characterized by underdevel-opment of the gonads

4. Adjunctive therapy for osteoporosis (oral or transdermal forms only)

5. Used in men to decrease the progression of prostate carcinoma

B. Common medications (Table 13-1)

C. Administration considerations

1. Report symptoms of menopause to provider for dosage adjustment

Table 13-1	Generic Name/Trade Name	Route	Usual Adult Dose	Nursing Implications
Common Estrogens	Estradiol (Alora, Climara, Estraderm, Vivelle)	Transdermal	0.5 mg/day	Teach when and where to reapply new patch
	Fem Patch	Transdermal	0.025 mg/day	Replace patch q 7 days
	Estrace	Intravaginal	1–2 g, 1 to 3 times weekly	Place cream deep into vagina; avoid douching
	Estring	Intravaginal	2 gm every 90 days	Place ring near cervix, check placement periodically
	Estradiol hemihydrate (Vagifem)	Intravaginal	25 μg twice/wk	Place cream deep into vagina
	Estradiol, Micronized (Estrace)	Oral	0.5–2.0 mg/day	Take daily or cyclically
	Conjugated estrogens, equine (Premarin)	Oral	0.625 mg/day	Take daily or cyclically; may not be accepted by vegans
	Conjugated estrogens, synthetic (Cenestin)	Oral	0.625–1.25 mg/day	Take daily or cyclically
	Estropipate (Ogen, Ortho-Est)	Oral	0.625 mg/day	Take daily or cyclically
	Esterified estrogens (Estratab Menest)	Oral	0.3–1.25 mg/day	Take daily or cyclically

2. Dose should be given with food to reduce nausea

3. Intravenous (IV) estrogen is given slowly by direct IV injection at a rate of 5 mg/min

4. Rapid IV injection may cause skin flushing

5. Estradiol transdermal should be applied to clean, dry area on the trunk of the body (including buttocks and abdomen)

6. Replace patch according to schedule

7. Cream form of the medication should be applied deeply into vagina, to assist in retention

8. Intravaginal ring (Estring) should be placed near cervix and checked for placement periodically

D. Contraindications

1. Current undiagnosed vaginal bleeding

2. History of breast cancer

3. Cautious use in smokers

4. Cautious use in women with history of deep vein thrombosis (DVT) or thrombophlebitis

5. Use cautiously with severe renal or hepatic disease

E. Significant drug interactions

1. May create need to increase doses of warfarin, oral hypoglycemic agents, or insulin

2. Barbiturates and rifampin may decrease effectiveness of estrogens

F. Significant food interactions: none reported

G. Significant laboratory studies

1. May increase levels of high density lipoproteins (HDL), phospholipids, and triglycerides in blood

2. May decrease low density lipoprotein (LDL) and total cholesterol levels

3. May increase bone density

H. Side effects

1. Increased skin pigmentation when exposed to sunlight

2. Weight gain and fluid retention

3. Nausea (oral forms)

4. Change in libido and increased breast tenderness

5. Headaches, moodiness, and hypertension

I. Adverse effects/toxicity

1. May increase risk of breast cancer

2. Endometrial cancer risk increases if uterus is intact and there is no concurrent progestin use

J. Nursing considerations

1. Assess blood pressure (BP) prior to and periodically during use

2. Monthly self breast exams and annual mammograms are recommended

3. In clients with breast cancer and bone metastasis, severe hypercalcemia (greater than 15 mg/dL) may be caused by estradiol therapy

4. Nausea frequently occurs in the morning, but disappears after 1 or 2 weeks of treatment

K. Client education

1. Teach client the correct dosage and amount and route of administration, including how often to change transdermal patches

2. Advise client to take medication with food if nausea occurs, usually at beginning of therapy

3. Inform client that cigarette smoking increases risk of thrombus formation

4. Advise client to report signs of fluid retention (edema, weight gain)

5. Inform client that when taken cyclically, vaginal bleeding will likely occur during the week each month when the estrogen is withheld

6. Instruct client to remain lying down for 30 minutes after administration of vaginal creams

7. Instruct client to place cream deep into vagina, avoid douching, and wash applicator with warm, soapy water after use

8. Advise client to use panty liners or mini-pads, but avoid use of tampons

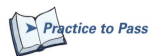

Practice to Pass

The client has been started on estradiol (Estrace), and asks how to use this medication. How do you respond?

9. Instruct client to report positive **Homan's sign**, which is calf pain on dorsi-flexion of the foot, possibly caused by formation of clots in the vein

10. Caution client that risk of blood clot formation is high with use of morning-after pill; teach signs of thrombophlebitis such as tenderness, swelling, redness in extremity, and pain

11. Instruct client to take medications exactly as prescribed

II. Progestins

A. Action and use

1. Cause the endometrium to change from proliferative to secretory in the latter half of the menstrual cycle in preparation for implantation of an embryo

2. Decrease mid-cycle bleeding in peri- and post-menopausal women or in women with dysfunctional uterine bleeding

3. Used to treat post-menopausal syndrome

4. Used to treat amenorrhea, breast cancer, and renal cancer

B. Common medications (Table 13-2 and Table 13-3)

C. Administration considerations

1. Must be discontinued immediately if pregnancy is suspected

2. Intramuscular (IM) injection should be given deeply; injection site may be irritated

3. Oral capsules contain peanut oil; they should not be given to clients with allergy to peanuts

D. Contraindications

1. Pregnancy

2. Cautious use with current or past history of depression

E. Significant drug interactions: decreased effectiveness when taken concomitantly with anti-epileptic medications

F. Significant food interactions: none reported

G. Significant laboratory studies

1. Increased LDL

2. Decreased HDL

3. Abnormal liver function tests

4. May affect coagulation, thyroid, and endocrine function

Table 13-2	Generic/Trade Name	Route	Usual Adult Dose
Common Progestins	Medroxyprogesterone acetate (Provera, Cycrin)	Oral	5 or 10 mg on days 1–12
	Norethindrone acetate (Aygestin)	Oral	0.35–2.5 mg on days 1–12
	Progesterone (Micronized, Prometrium)	Oral	200 mg on days 1–12

Table 13-3	Generic/Trade Name	Route	Usual Adult Dose	Notes
Common Estrogen-progestin Hormone Replacement Medications	Conjugated estrogens, equine/ medroxyprogesterone acetate (Prempro)	Oral	0.625/2.5 mg daily	Obtained from urine of mares
	Ethinyl estradiol/ norethindrone acetate (Femhrt)	Oral	5 μg/1 mg daily	
	Estradiol/norgestimate (Ortho-Prefest)	Oral	1.0/0.09 mg	Cycle of 3 days on and 3 days off
	Estradiol/norethindrone (CombiPatch)	Transdermal	0.05/0.14 mg daily	

H. Side effects

   1. Depression

   2. Male-pattern baldness

   3. Increased or decreased libido

   4. Insomnia and somnolence

   5. Fluid retention

I. Adverse effects/toxicity

   1. Change in menstrual flow, amenorrhea, and breast changes

   2. Edema

   3. Cholestatic jaundice

J. Nursing considerations

   1. Prior to administration in clients with current or history of depression, make certain a plan is in place to deal with worsening or recurrent depressive symptoms

   2. A thorough physical examination should be done with special attention to pelvic organs, breasts, and hepatic function

   3. A Pap test should be done prior to initiation of therapy and every 6 to 12 months while client is taking the medication

   4. Monitor vital signs, including blood pressure (BP)

   5. Monitor intake and output (I & O)

K. Client education

   1. Instruct client how to use medication and the timing of use

   2. Warn client about possible side effects; ascertain client knows which symptoms to report, such as sudden severe headache, vomiting, dizziness, fainting, pain in calves, acute chest pain, and dyspnea

   3. Inform post-menopausal women of possibility of resumption of cyclical vaginal bleeding

4. Instruct client to monitor BP and I & O

5. Caution client to avoid exposure to ultraviolet (UV) light

6. Instruct diabetic clients to monitor the glucose levels closely

7. Instruct client to take medication with food if GI upset occurs

III. Androgens

A. Action and use

1. **Androgens** are steroids that stimulate the action of endogenous hormones

2. Used primarily to treat male androgen (testosterone) deficiency in men with delayed puberty, hypogonadism, oligospermia, **cryptorchidism** (a congenital condition characterized by failure of the testis to descend into the scrotum), or orchiectomy

3. Used for hormone replacement therapy in women who experience decreased energy and libido

4. Used to suppress tumor growth in androgen-sensitive breast cancer

5. Danazol (Danocrine) is used to treat endometriosis and fibrocystic breast disease in women

B. Common medications (Table 13-4)

C. Administration considerations

1. Medically indicated androgen use will often result in virilization and side effects must be monitored closely

2. Buccal tablets should not be chewed or swallowed

3. Testoderm should be applied to scrotal skin; dry shave the area

4. Androderm should be applied to non-scrotal skin; apply to clean dry area of back, abdomen, upper arms, or thighs

Table 13-4

Common Androgens

Generic Name	Trade Name	Route
Testosterone base	Andro, Histerone, Malogen, Testamone, Tesaqua, Testoject	IM q 2–3 days, PO QD, or buccal QD
Testosterone cypionate	Andro-Cyp, Andronate, depAndro, Depotest, Depo-Testosterone, Duratest, T-Cyprionate, Testa-C, Testred, Testoject LA, Virilon IM	IM q 2–4 weeks
Testosterone enanthate	Andro LA, Andropository, Andryl, Delatest, Delatestryl, Everone, Malogex, Testone LA, Testrin-PA	IM q 2–4 weeks
Testosterone propionate	Malogen, Testex	IM q 2–4 weeks
Testosterone	Androgel	Apply 1 packet to upper arms, shoulders, or abdomen each day
Testosterone transdermal	Androderm, Testoderm	Two 5-mg patches on arm, back, abdomen, or thigh; one 6-mg patch to scrotum
Danazol	Danocrine	PO in 2 divided doses

5. Use very cautiously in children because of the bone maturation effects

6. Can reduce blood glucose levels, thus reducing insulin requirements in the diabetic client

7. IM preparations may crystallize at low temperatures, therefore the vial may need warming and shaking to re-dissolve the crystals

D. Contraindications

1. Pregnancy and lactation

2. Congestive heart failure (CHF), renal and liver failure

3. Enlarged prostate

E. Significant drug interactions

1. Increased action of warfarin, can cause bleeding

2. Increased action of oral hypoglycemic agents, insulin, and glucocorticoids

3. Additive **hepatotoxicity** (toxic to liver) when administered with other hepatotoxic medications

4. Increase the effect of imipramine (increased paranoid symptoms)

F. Significant food interactions: none reported

G. Significant laboratory studies

1. Complete blood count (CBC): hemoglobin (Hgb) and hematocrit (Hct) will increase in women

2. Decrease in HDL and increase in LDL levels

H. Side effects

1. In both genders are dose-related, including lowered voice, edema, acne, change in libido, increased facial hair growth, and increase in aggressive tendencies

2. In male: gynecomastia, oligospermia, impotence, decreased ejaculatory volume, and urinary urgency

3. In female: menstrual irregularities, enlarged clitoris, breast size decrease, male pattern baldness, deepening of voice, and increase in oiliness of skin

I. Adverse effects/toxicity

1. Androgens will increase male sex characteristics in pre-pubertal boys; x-ray examination of the epiphyseal growth plate must be done every 6 months in pre-pububescent boys

2. **Priapism** (painful penile erection) may also occur

3. Polycythemia may develop

J. Nursing considerations

1. Assess client for edema, weight gain, and any changes in skin

2. Assess lung and heart sounds

3. Assess client for signs of liver dysfunction

4. Evaluate client for signs of depression

5. Assess client for the presence of secondary sexual characteristics

K. Client education

1. Instruct client to apply transdermal patches to shaved skin

2. Advise client to weigh herself/himself twice weekly and report increased weight

3. Instruct client to notify provider if fluid retention develops

4. Explain to client the signs of virilization

5. Advise women to use a nonhormonal contraceptive while on therapy

6. Instruct client to take medication with meals or a snack

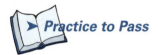

► Practice to Pass

A 16-year-old male client with hypogonadism is starting testosterone enanthate (Andropository) therapy. You are developing a plan of care for this client. What information should be included in the plan regarding the effects of this medication?

IV. Anabolic Steroids

A. Action and use: developed to replace androgens

B. Common medications (Table 13-5)

C. Administration considerations

1. **Anabolic steroids** are androgens with anabolic properties and are rarely prescribed, but are commonly abused by athletes in an attempt to enhance performance

2. Medically indicated androgen use will often result in virilization, and side effects must be monitored

D. Contraindications

1. During pregnancy and lactation

2. Contraindicated with CHF, renal and liver failure, and enlarged prostate

E. Significant drug interactions

1. Increased action of warfarin, oral hypoglycemic agents, insulin, and glucocorticoids

2. Additive hepatotoxicity when administered with other hepatoxic medications

F. Significant food interactions: none reported

G. Significant laboratory studies

1. May cause increase in serum aspartate aminotransferase (AST)

2. May increase bilirubin level

3. May suppress clotting factors II, V, VII, and X

Table 13-5	Generic	Trade Name	Route
Common Anabolic Steroids	Nandrolone	Durabolin, Deca-Durabolin	IM
	Oxandrolone	Oxandrin	IM
	Oxymetholone	Androl-50	IM
	Stanazolol	Winstrol	IM

4. Hgb and Hct will increase in female

5. HDL level will decrease and LDL level will increase

H. Side effects

1. In both genders: lowered voice, edema, acne, change in libido, increased facial hair growth, and increase in aggressive tendencies

2. In male: gynecomastia, oligospermia, impotence, and decreased ejaculatory volume

3. In female: menstrual irregularities, enlarged clitoris, decreased breast size, male pattern baldness; voice changes and hair growth patterns are not reversible after discontinuation of use

I. Adverse effects/toxicity

1. Hepatotoxicity, especially when used with other hepatoxic effects

2. Abusers of anabolic steroids often share needles, increasing the incidence of hepatitis B and C and HIV transmission

J. Nursing considerations

1. Assess client athletes from junior high through adulthood (especially football players, bodybuilders, weightlifters, sprinters, and endurance sport participants) for anabolic steroid abuse

2. Assess client for edema, weight gain, and skin changes

3. Assess lung and heart sounds

4. Assess clients for signs of liver dysfunction

5. Evaluate clients for signs of depression

6. Assess client for the presence of secondary sexual characteristics

K. Client education

1. Educate client on the risks of using anabolic steroids if they admit to using medication that has been obtained illegally

2. Educate client about the risks of sharing needles

3. Instruct client about the risks of contamination when using non–U.S.-manufactured or veterinary-quality substances

4. Inform client to notify physician of using these medications

V. Medications for Erectile Dysfunction

A. Actions and use

1. Enhance normal erectile response to sexual stimuli through inhibition of phosphodiesterase type 5 (PDE5)

2. Increase corpus cavernosus arterial inflow and decrease venous outflow, resulting in erection

3. Used for erectile dysfunction

B. Common medications (Table 13-6)

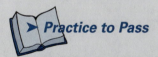

Practice to Pass

A client has admitted to using illegally obtained anabolic steroids IM with his athletic teammates for the past 2 years. How would you explain to the client the laboratory studies that the physician will likely order, and why they are needed?

	Generic Name	Trade Name	Usual Adult Dose	Route
Table 13-6 **Common Medications for Erectile Dysfunction**	Sildenafil	Viagra	25, 50, or 100 mg 1 hour prior to intercourse	PO
	Papaverine plus phentolamine	Cerespan, Genabid, Pavabid, Pavacot, Pavagen, Pavarine, Pavased, Pavatine, Pavatym, Paverolan	0.1 ml	Intrapenile injection
	Alprostadil (Prostaglandin E1)	Caverject (injectable); Muse (transurethral pellets)	5–40 µg intra- cavernosum injection; 125, 250, 500, or 1000 µg transurethral pellet	Intrapenile injection or transurethral

C. Administration considerations

1. Sildenafil (Viagra) should not be used more than once per day

2. Alprostadil (Caverject) should not be used more than once per 24 hours and up to 3 times per week

3. Alprostadil: reconstitute using 1 mL of diluent of bacteriostatic or sterile water

4. Alprostadil (Muse) should not be used more than twice in 24 hours

D. Contraindications

1. Contraindicated in clients with cardiovascular diseases, MI, cerebrovascular accident (CVA), or dysrhythmias within 6 months

2. Clients with CHF and unstable angina

3. With use of nitroglycerine or other nitrates

4. Hypertension (BP greater than 170/110) or hypotension (BP less than 90/50)

E. Significant drug interactions

1. Life-threatening hypotension can occur with concurrent use of nitroglycerine or nitroprusside

2. Increased adverse effects with antidepressants

3. Alprostadil increases risk of bleeding if used concurrently with warfarin

F. Significant food interactions: none reported

G. Significant laboratory studies: none reported

H. Side effects

1. Ecchymosis and painless fibrotic nodules in the corpus cavernosus may occur with injections

2. With transurethral administration: a dull penile pain, prolonged erection (4 to 6 hours)

3. Sildenafil: headache, blurred vision, flushing, dyspepsia, and nasal congestion

I. Adverse effects/toxicity

1. Priapism may occur and must be treated as a medical emergency

    2. Upper respiratory infection and urinary tract infection (UTI)

    3. Urethral bleeding

    4. Increased motor activity

J. Nursing considerations

    1. Obtain a thorough medical history of clients experiencing erectile dysfunction, especially history of cardiovascular disease

    2. Obtain accurate history of onset of the problem to assess for possible psychological cause since not all cases of sexual dysfunction are truly erectile dysfunction

    3. Sildenafil (Viagra) is the most prescribed medication in the United States, and has been presented as a panacea for all sexual problems in the population

    4. Sildenafil is usually taken 1 hour prior to sexual activity

K. Client education

    1. Instruct client how to inject the medication into the corpus cavernosum using a 3/8-inch, 27- or 28-gauge needle 1-mL syringe

    2. Instruct client to insert transurethral pellets with a plastic introducer about 1½ inches into the urethra

    3. Educate client on maximum use of the medication in a 24-hour time block and in each week

    4. Instruct client to take Viagra 1 hour prior to sexual activity

    5. Advise client taking Viagra to report chest pain or palpitations immediately

    6. Inform client that eating a high-fat meal before taking sildenafil may cause drug to take longer to work

    7. Advise client not to take these medications with concurrent use of drugs containing nitrates

VI. Contraceptives

A. Action and use

    1. Decrease the incidence of ovulation to prevent conception

    2. Thin the endometrial lining of the uterus, decreasing the incidence of implantation if fertilization takes place

    3. Decrease fallopian tube ciliary peristalsis, which decreases the likelihood of an ovum meeting a sperm

    4. Thicken cervical mucus, preventing sperm from penetrating into the uterine cavity

    5. Used as a birth control

B. Common medications (Table 13-7)

C. Administration considerations

    1. If an adolescent has not yet attained maximum growth, estrogen may cause the epiphyseal plates to close

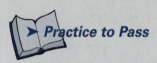

▶ *Practice to Pass*

The client has been experiencing erectile dysfunction. He asks if sildenafil (Viagra) is the only medication that can be used to treat his condition. How do you answer?

Type	Estrogen	Progestin	Brand name	Usual Adult Dose
Table 13-7 **Common Contraceptives**				
Combination orals	Ethinyl estradiol, mestranol	Norethindrone, ethynodiol acetate, levonorgestrel, desogestrel, norgestrel, norgestimate	Triphasil, Tri-Cyclen, Tri-Norinyl, Desogen, Demulen, Ovrette, Mircette, LoEstrin, Ovcon, Nordette	Estrogen: 10–50 μg; progestin: 0.05–1.5 mg
Progestin-only orals	N/A	Norethindrone	Micronor, Nor-QD	0.35 mg
Combination injectable	Estradiol cypionate	Medroxyprogesterone acetate	Lunelle	Estrogen: 5.0 mg Progestin: 25 mg
Progestin-only injectable	N/A	Medroxyprogesterone acetate	Depo-Provera	150 mg IM Q 85–90 days
Progestin-only intradermal	N/A	Levonorgestrel	Norplant	216 mg divided equally in 6 silastic tubes

2. Estrogen may decrease milk supply

3. Smokers older than 35 years of age are recommended to either quit smoking or use another method of birth control due to increased risk of deep vein thrombosis (DVT)

4. Dosing schedule is usually based on a 28-day menstrual cycle

D. **Contraindications:** estrogen-containing methods are contraindicated in female with a history of CVA, DVT, and with known or suspected breast, ovarian, or endometrial cancer

E. **Significant drug interactions**

1. Progestin efficacy decreases in presence of anti-epileptic medications

2. Most antibiotics such as ampicillin, isoniazid, nitrofurantoin, rifampin, penicillin V, sulfonamides, and tetracyclines will decrease effectiveness of contraceptives

3. Increased effects of benzodiazepines, beta blockers, caffeine, corticosteroids, and theophylline occur

F. **Significant food interactions:** none reported

G. **Significant laboratory studies**

1. Progestin other than desogestrel increases total cholesterol and LDL

2. Desogestrel decreases total cholesterol and increases HDL

3. Thyroid stimulating hormone (TSH) will become slightly elevated while on combination oral contraceptives (OCT)

H. **Side effects**

1. Estrogen-containing methods: cyclical weight gain, increased skin pigmentation, breast enlargement and tenderness, and irritability

2. Progestin-containing methods: decreased libido, depression, acne, and male pattern hair loss

3. The symptoms of possible complications of combination OCT form the acronym ACHES: **A**bdominal pain (liver tumor formation), **C**hest pain, **H**eadache, and **E**ye problems (embolus), and **S**evere leg pain (thrombophlebitis)

I. **Adverse effects/toxicity**

1. Spotting, change in menstrual flow, amenorrhea

2. Nausea, vomiting, abdominal cramps, bloating

3. Headaches, depression, edema

J. **Nursing considerations**

1. No one hormonal contraceptive method works best for all females

2. Finding the right combination and dosage of hormones may occur by trial-and-error

3. Encourage smokers to quit because of increased risk of DVT, especially after age 35

4. Monitor for signs and symptoms of thrombophlebitis (calf pain, possible redness and warmth and possible edema in affected leg)

K. **Client education**

1. Instruct client to take OCT exactly as directed

2. Instruct client about the methods of using different OCTs

a. Combination orals: instruct client to take 1 pill daily at the same time each day; the last 5 to 7 days of the pills are inert; the client might experience withdrawal bleeding during the last 5 to 7 days

b. Progestin-only orals: instruct client to take 1 pill each day at exactly the same time; each pill is a medicated pill; there is no week off hormones; bleeding will be irregular or may not occur

c. Medroxyprogesterone acetate (Depo Provera): bleeding will be irregular until the second or third dose is given; after the third dose, most females develop amenorrhea

3. Advise client not to miss doses

4. Instruct client to follow schedule below for missed dose

a. If 1 dose is missed, take 2 tablets the next day

b. If 2 doses are missed, take 2 tablets as soon as remembered with the next pill or take 2 tablets daily for the next 2 days; use a back-up method such as condom for the rest of the pill pack

c. If 3 doses are missed, begin a new compact of tablets starting on day one of the cycle after the last pill was taken; use a back-up contraceptive method

5. Instruct client to report prolonged vaginal bleeding or amenorrhea

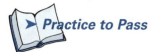

Practice to Pass

The client is considering beginning combination oral contraceptive pills. What questions do you need to ask as part of her medical history?

6. Advise client to wait at least 3 months before becoming pregnant after stopping the OCT

7. Advise client to conduct breast self-examination

VII. Fertility Medications

A. Action and use

1. Used when an infertility workup determines that the cause of an inability to conceive after 12 months of unprotected intercourse is due to lack of ovulation

2. Will stimulate ovulation or follicular maturation

B. Common medications (Table 13-8)

C. Administration considerations

1. Ovulation induction agents are expensive and can cost over $1,000 per cycle

2. Multifetal pregnancy will occur in 12 to 20 percent of cases, mostly twins

3. Clients should start with smaller doses, and then increasing dosages will be used if the cycle does not achieve ovulation

D. Contraindications

1. Inability to keep track of the dosing schedule

2. Lack of access to emergency medical care

3. Primary ovarian failure

4. Hepatic dysfunction

E. Significant drug interactions: none reported

F. Significant food interactions: none reported

G. Significant laboratory studies: none reported

H. Side effects

Table 13-8	Generic name	Trade Name	Mechanism of Action	Usual Adult Dose/Timing in Cycle
Common Fertility Medications	Clomiphene	Clomid, Sereophene, Milophene	Promotes follicular maturation and ova release through stimulating production of FSH and LH	50 mg Q day × 5 days, PO, beginning on 5th day after mense begins
	Menotropins	Pergonal, Humegon	Promotes development of follicle	75 IU each FSH and LH or 150 IU each daily for 9–12 days, IM
	Follitropins	Metrodin, Gonal-F, Follistim	Stimulates follicle maturation	SC
	Gonadorelin	Factrel	Synthetic GnRH, promotes release of LH	100 mcg SC or IV during days 1 to 7 of menstrual cycle (if known)
	Human chorionic gonadotropin	A.P.L., Chorex, Gonic, Pregnyl	Promotes release of a mature ovum from follicle	5,000 to 10,000 USP units given 1 day after last follitropin or menotropin dose; 7–9 days after last clomiphene dose, IM

1. Ovarian hyperstimulation syndrome is more common in female with polycystic ovaries

2. Nausea and vomiting, constipation, bloating, abdominal pain

3. Transient blurring, diplopia, photophobia

4. Vasomotor flushes, breast discomfort

5. Headache, fatigue, dizziness, vertigo

I. Adverse effects/toxicity

1. Ovarian enlargement resulting in lower abdominal or pelvic pressure or pain

2. Tenderness or infection of injection site

3. Heavy menses, exacerbation of endometriosis

4. Mental depression

5. Insomnia

J. Nursing considerations

1. Make certain that the client understands the potential for multi-fetal pregnancy

2. Full diagnostic measures are important if abnormal bleeding occurs

3. Client should have an ophthalmic examination at regular intervals if clomiphene is prescribed more than 1 year

4. Client with pelvic pain should be assessed carefully

K. Client education

1. Instruct client in the different techniques of administering medication

2. Advise client to take the medication at same time every day

3. Instruct client about the side effects and the importance of reporting them

4. Explain to client that if there is a response, ovulation usually occurs 4 to 10 days after last day of treatment

5. Inform client that the incidence of multiple births is increased as high as 6 times normal

6. Instruct client to report yellowing of eyes, light-colored stools, and itchy skin promptly

7. Outline the treatment regimen including probable office visits for ultrasound examination of the ovaries

8. Explain that client should have intercourse at least every other day beginning on the fifth day after the last dose of clomiphene (Clomid), or the day prior to hormone chorionic gonadotropin (HCG) administration and 3 days following

9. Explain to client that if a dose is missed:

   a. Take medication as soon as possible

b. If not remembered until time for next dose, double the dose, then resume regular dosing schedule

c. If more than one dose is missed, notify the physician

VIII. Medications for Labor and Delivery

A. Oxytocics

1. Action and use

   a. Initiate or improve uterine contraction at term

   b. Facilitate involution in the treatment or prevention of postpartum hemorrhage

   c. Used to stimulate letdown reflex in nursing mother and relieve pain from breast engorgement

2. Common medications (Table 13-9)

3. Administration considerations

   a. Only oxytocin (Pitocin) is Food and Drug Administration (FDA) approved for use during labor

   b. Methylergonovine (Methergine) is used only for post-partum control of excessive bleeding and hemorrhage

   c. Oxytocin should never be administered by more than one route at a time

   d. Diluted IV oxytocin solution should be administered continuously

   e. Pitocin IV preparation: for inducing labor, 10 unit (1 mL) of Pitocin in 1 liter of D_5W or normal saline (NS) to give 10 mU/mL; for postpartum bleeding, 10 to 40 units in 1 liter the same solution to give 10 to 40 mU/mL

   f. The nurse should have a clear understanding of when medication is to be administered in relation to delivery

4. Contraindications

   a. Methergonovine is contraindicated with hypertension and should be avoided, if possible, in clients planning to breast-feed, as they inhibit lactation

   b. Contraindicated in unfavorable fetal position or presentations that are undeliverable

   c. Fetal distress in which delivery is not imminent

Table 13-9	Generic/Trade Name	Mechanism of Action	Usual Adult Dose and Route
Common Oxytocic Medications	Oxytocin (Pitocin)	Tonic contractions	Induction: 10 or 20 units in 1 liter of IV fluid, titrate via pump to achieve appropriate uterine activity. Postpartum: 10–20 units in IV bag or IM; also intranasal spray to promote milk ejection reflex (let-down)
	Methylergonovine (Methergine)	Clonic contractions	Used postpartum only; 0.2 mg IM or q 6 hr PO up to 6 doses

       d. Prematurity, placenta previa

       e. Previous surgery of uterus or cervix including cesarean section

  5. Significant drug interactions: pitocin/vasoconstrictors may cause severe hypertension

  6. Significant food interactions: none reported

  7. Significant laboratory studies: pitocin intrapartum increases unconjugated fetal bilirubin

  8. Side effects

       a. Methylergonovine (Methergine): significant increase in systolic and diastolic BP

       b. In fetus: bradycardia or other dysrhythmias, hypoxia, intracranial hemorrhage, trauma from too rapid propulsion through pelvis

       c. In mother: nausea and vomiting, postpartum hemorrhage, pelvic hematoma

       d. All oxytocics will cause uterine cramping when administered postpartum

NCLEX!

  9. Adverse effects/toxicity

       a. Uterine tetany leading to fetal demise

       b. Uterine rupture has been documented with overdose

       c. Newborns exposed to oxytocin in utero have higher incidence of hyperbilirubinemia

  10. Nursing considerations

NCLEX!

       a. Antepartum and intrapartum: monitor uterine contraction pattern, fetal heart rate (FHR), and BP

NCLEX!

       b. Postpartum: monitor lochia and BP

       c. Massage the injection site after deep injection of oxytocin into deltoid muscle to assist quick absorption

       d. Obtain baseline tracing of uterine contraction and FHR prior to medication

NCLEX!

       e. Increase IV dosage of oxytocin only after assessing contraction, FHR, maternal BP and heart rate

NCLEX!

       f. Do not increase rate of Pitocin once the desired contraction pattern is achieved (contraction frequency of 2 to 3 minutes lasting 60 seconds)

NCLEX!

       g. Oxytocin should be discontinued if contraction frequency is less than 2 minutes or duration is more than 90 seconds

  11. Client education

       a. Explain to client the indication for administration

       b. Prepare client for route of administration and possible side effects

NCLEX!

       c. Instruct client to report sudden headache

B. Ergot alkaloids

1. Action and use

    a. Used to control postpartum hemorrhage

    b. Cause clonic contractions

2. Common medication: ergonovine (Ergotrate), 0.2 mg IV over 60 seconds only in emergency, more commonly given IM

3. Administration considerations: causes rebound uterine relaxation

4. Contraindications

    a. Contraindicated in hypersensitivity to ergot medication

    b. Cautious use with hypertension, unstable angina, recent myocardial infarction

5. Significant drug interactions: none reported

6. Significant food interactions: none reported

7. Significant laboratory studies: none reported

8. Side effects

    a. Significant increase in systolic and diastolic BP

    b. Uterine cramping

    c. Decreased milk production

9. Adverse effects/toxicity

    a. Hypertension

    b. Ergotism or overdose: nausea, vomiting, weakness, muscle pain, insensitivity to cold, paresthesia of extremities

10. Nursing considerations: closely monitor lochia and blood pressure after administration

11. Client education

    a. Explain indication for administration to client

    b. Prepare client for route of administration and possible side effects, such as cramping

    c. Instruct client to report increased blood loss, increased temperature, or foul-smelling lochia

    d. Instruct client to perform pad count to monitor bleeding

    e. Instruct client not to smoke because of increased/additive vasoconstriction with ergonovine use

C. Prostaglandins

1. Action and use

    a. To terminate pregnancy from twelfth week through second trimester

    b. Dinoprostone (Prepidil, Cervidil) has FDA approval only for cervical ripening prior to labor induction

Table 13-10	Category	Generic/Trade Name	Dose and Route	Indications for Use
Common Prostaglandins	Prostaglandin E2	Dinoprostone (Prepidil, Cervidil)	Prepidil intracervical gel: 0.5 mg Cervidil vaginal insert: 10 mg	Ripening of cervix prior to induction of labor
	Prostaglandin F2	Carboprost tromethamine (Hemabate)	Hemabate: 250 μg IM, may repeat at 15 to 90 minute intervals as needed up to 2 mg total dose	Postpartum hemorrhage

c. Carboprost tromethamine (Hemabate) has FDA approval only for control of postpartum bleeding

2. Common medications (Table 13-10)

3. Administration considerations

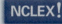

a. Client should remain in supine position for 10 minutes after administration of dinoprostone

b. Before dinoprostone, client should receive antiemetic and antidiarrheal medications

4. Contraindications

a. Use with caution in hypertension and with history of asthma

b. Use of dinoprastone during labor has been documented to cause uterine rupture and fetal demise

c. Acute pelvic inflammatory disease

d. History of pelvic surgery

5. Significant drug interactions: none reported

6. Significant food interactions: none reported

7. Significant laboratory studies: none reported

8. Side effects

a. Diarrhea, nausea, vomiting, possible increase in BP

b. Uterine cramping

c. Tension headache

d. Flushing, cardiac dyshythmias

9. Adverse effects/toxicity

    a. Hypertension

    b. Uterine tetany may develop with pre-labor or intrapartum administration

    c. Uterine rupture

NCLEX!

10. Nursing considerations

    a. Prenatal: follow manufacturer's instructions for placement of medication; client must remain recumbent for up to 20 to 30 minutes after administration, and have fetal monitoring during this time

    b. Postpartum: monitor lochia and BP, be prepared for client to develop diarrhea

11. Client education

    a. Prenatal: client should report long or continuous contractions, as uterine tetany may develop; client should count fetal movement as an indicator of fetal well-being

    b. Postpartum: prepare client for route of administration and possible side effects

D. Uterine Relaxants

1. Action and use

    a. Inhibit contractions and therefore arrest labor for at least 48 hours so that corticosteroids (β-methasone) can be given to facilitate fetal lung maturity

    b. Used for cessation of contractions to allow intrauterine fetal resuscitation when uterine hyperstimulation is present

    c. Used to delay delivery in preterm labor

2. Common medications (Table 13-11)

Table 13-11

Common Uterine Relaxant Medications

Generic/Trade Name	Category	Usual Adult Dose	Notes
Terbutaline sulfate (Brethine)	β-adrenergic	SC: 0.25 mg q 20 min up to 3 doses IV: 10 to 80 μg/min PO: 2.5 mg q 4–6 hr	Not FDA-approved for preterm labor but most commonly used medication
Ritodrine (Yutopar)	β-adrenergic	IV: initially 100 μg/min, increase by 50 μg/min q 10 min to max 350 μg/min PO: 10 mg q 2 hr for 24 hours, then 10–20 mg q 4–6 hr	FDA-approved for preterm labor, increased incidence of pulmonary edema
Nifedipine (Procardia)	Calcium channel blocker	PO: 10 mg q 20 min for 2–3 doses; max 40 mg in 1 hr	Not FDA-approved for preterm labor but commonly used; may cause oligohydramnios
Indomethacin (Indocin)	NSAID	50 mg loading dose rectally, followed by 25 mg PO Q 6 hr for 2–3 days	Not FDA-approved for preterm labor but used as 3rd line; increased risk of fetal complications

3. Administration considerations

    a. Medication is started at lowest possible dose and increased as indicated in table until contractions cease

    b. Be certain about recommended dose

    c. If GI symptoms occur, advise client to take the medications with food

    d. Dilute IV terbutaline by adding each 5 mg to 1,000 mL D_5W or NS to yield a concentration of 5 µg/mL

    e. Infuse the medication via microdrip and infusion pump

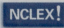

4. Contraindications

    a. Known fetal anomaly incompatible with life

    b. β-adrenergics contraindicated in presence of pulmonary edema

    c. Cautious use if cervix is dilated greater than 5 cm or if gestational age is less than 20 or greater than 36 weeks

    d. Severe hypertension and coronary artery disease (CAD)

5. Significant drug interaction: increased incidence of pulmonary edema when used concurrently with corticosteroids (β-methasone) for fetal lung maturity acceleration

6. Significant food interactions: caffeine will increase side effects of β-adrenergics

7. Significant laboratory studies: β-adrenergics will cause hyperglycemia, worse with concomitant corticosteroid use

8. Side effects

    a. β-adrenergics: maternal and fetal tachycardia, palpitations, tremors, jitteriness, and anxiety

    b. May cause or exacerbate constipation

    c. Nausea and vomiting

9. Adverse effects/toxicity

    a. β-adrenergics: pulmonary edema

    b. Nifedipine (Procardia) and indomethacin (Indocin) can cause oligohydramnios

    c. Indomethacin (Indocin) can cause premature closure of the ductus arteriosis leading to fetal death

10. Nursing considerations

    a. β-adrenergics: if client continues on to deliver after receiving uterine relaxant medications, be prepared with oxytocic for treatment of post-partum hemorrhage

    b. Monitor vital signs and I & O

       c. Nifedipine (Procardia): avoid grapefruit juice during administration (interferes with effect)

       d. Use indomethacin for a short period of time (2 to 3 days)

       e. If mother uses terbutaline during pregnancy, monitor the neonate for hypoglycemia

    11. Client education

       a. Educate client as to possible side effects and coping strategies

       b. Instruct client about use and dose of oral medications and importance of taking them on time

       c. Nifedipine (Procardia): encourage client change position slowly due to possible orthostatic hypotension

       d. Instruct client on how to self-monitor pulse

       e. Advise client to consult physician prior to taking over-the-counter (OTC) medications

  E. Magnesium sulfate

    1. Action and use

       a. When given parenterally, it acts as central nervous system (CNS) depressant and also depresses smooth, skeletal, and cardiac muscle function

       b. Used to arrest preterm labor and to prevent or to treat seizures with preeclampsia and eclampsia

    2. Administration considerations

       a. It is used in conjunction with β-adrenergics, which increases risk of pulmonary edema

       b. A 4-gram loading dose is often utilized, which must be given over 20 to 30 minutes via infusion pump

    3. Contraindications

       a. Preterm labor

       b. Fetal anomaly incompatible with life

       c. Pulmonary edema or CHF

       d. Anuria, renal failure

       e. Organic CNS disease

    4. Significant drug interactions: none reported

    5. Significant food interactions: none reported

    6. Significant laboratory studies: none reported

    7. Side effects

       a. Flushed warm feeling, drowsiness

       b. Decreased deep tendon reflexes

       c. Decreased hand grasp strength

        d. Fluid and electrolyte imbalance, hyponatremia

        e. Nausea and vomiting

   8. Adverse effects/toxicity

        a. Lack of deep tendon reflexes and/or hand grasp

        b. Respiratory depression leading to respiratory arrest

   9. Nursing considerations

        a. Check patellar reflex prior to dose

        b. Monitor hand grasps, deep tendon reflexes, respiratory rate, and serum levels

        c. IV infusion flow rate is generally adjusted to maintain urine flow of at least 30 to 50 mL/h, monitor I & O carefully

        d. Monitor IV site closely to avoid extravasation

        e. Monitor vital signs

        f. Take accurate daily weight

   10. Client education

        a. Educate client about side effects of medication

        b. Advise client to report signs of pre-eclampsia including headache, epigastric pain, and visual disturbance

        c. Instruct family to report any signs of confusion

Case Study

The pregnant client with pre-eclampsia has been scheduled to have labor induced after cervical ripening. The client is planning to breast-feed her infant.

❶ What medications can be used for cervical ripening, and how are they administered?

❷ How will the labor be induced physiologically?

❸ The client delivered 5 minutes ago and is now experiencing a postpartum hemorrhage. What medication(s) would you anticipate the physician ordering for administration at this time?

❹ The client has seized. What medication should you prepare to administer?

❺ A few days postpartum, the client asks what hormonal methods of contraception she can use. How do you answer her question?

For suggested responses, see page 641.

Posttest

1 The client asks why her oral contraceptive Desogen contains both desogestrel and ethinyl estradiol. Which of the following responses would be best?

(1) "Desogestrel is a weak estrogen and progestin combination that requires additional estrogen to work."
(2) "Together the hormones prevent the ovum from maturing and the sperm from penetrating through the cervical mucus."
(3) "Estrogens alone would prevent pregnancy, but progestins are added so that spotting doesn't occur."
(4) "Taking each hormone separately would prevent most pregnancies, but the combination is more effective."

2 The nurse preparing to conduct medication teaching would question an order for sildenafil (Viagra) when the client has which of the following conditions?

(1) History of type II diabetes and peripheral vascular disease
(2) Myocardial infarction (MI) 4 years ago
(3) Congestive heart failure (CHF)
(4) Benign prostatic hyperplasia

3 The client is to begin clomiphene (Clomid) for treatment of infertility. You conclude that the client needs additional teaching on this medication when she states:

(1) "This medication will help make me ovulate."
(2) "I'll take this medicine orally for 5 days this month."
(3) "I'll be giving myself shots 5 days out of the month."
(4) "If this medication doesn't work, there are others to try."

4 Which client is most likely to have testosterone transdermal (Androderm) prescribed for his condition?

(1) A 45-year-old with status/postbilateral vasectomy
(2) A 17-year-old with status/postcryptorchidism repair
(3) A 23-year-old with status/postvaricocele repair
(4) A 32-year-old with status/postbilateral orchiectomy

5 The client is being prepared to have labor induced with oxytocin (Pitocin). Medication teaching has been effective when the client states:

(1) "I'll take this medication by mouth to make my uterus contract."
(2) "This medication will be given to me as an IM injection."
(3) "Pitocin is a synthetic version of a hormone my body produces naturally."
(4) "A large dose of this medication will be given to me in my IV line."

6 For which of the following clients would the nurse anticipate the physician ordering ergonovine (Ergotrate)?

(1) A client with untreated chronic hypertension
(2) A breast-feeding mother whose baby was delivered by forceps
(3) A bottle-feeding mother who is a carrier for Hepatitis C
(4) A normotensive mother with postpartum hemorrhage

7 A female client taking Demulen, a combination oral contraceptive pill, calls with sudden onset of blurred vision. The nurse's best response would be to ask her to:

(1) Come in to see the physician now.
(2) Make an appointment to see the physician tomorrow.
(3) See an ophthalmologist as soon as possible.
(4) Have her call back after taking a nap.

8 The client in preterm labor has just received 2.5 mg terbutaline sulfate (Brethine) SC. Which statement would the client be most likely to make?

(1) "My heart seems to be beating really slowly."
(2) "My arms and legs feel so heavy and thick."
(3) "This medication makes me feel so sleepy."
(4) "My hands are so shaky I can't write."

9 For which of the following clients would the nurse question an order for testosterone enanthate (Delatestryl)?

(1) A 16-year-old with moderate acne
(2) A 32-year-old with liver disease
(3) A 66-year-old with melanoma
(4) A 25-year-old with testicular cancer

10 The client is to receive dinoprostone (Prepidil) for cervical ripening prior to induction of labor. For the administration of this medication, the client should be placed in which of the following positions?

See pages 530–531 for Answers and Rationales.

(1) On her left side
(2) On her right side
(3) On her back with knees bent and apart
(4) On her hands and knees

Answers and Rationales

Pretest

1 **Answer: 1** *Rationale:* Dosing of all medication is started small and increased if needed to minimize the risks of side effects. Viagra should be taken approximately 1 hour prior to sexual activity. Option 3 is incorrect because Viagra comes at three different doses: 25, 50, and 100 mg. Option 2 is incorrect because the smallest dose is utilized, while option 4 is incorrect because the client does not titrate the dose at will.
Cognitive Level: Application
Nursing Process: Implementation; *Test Plan:* PHYS

2 **Answer: 3** *Rationale:* Oxytocin (Pitocin) used for labor induction augments the endogenous oxytocin. It is administered as a dilute solution of 10 or 20 units in 1 liter IV fluid via infusion pump, with a goal of increasing the frequency and intensity of contractions. Options 1, 2, and 4 are correct statements, indicating that the client understands these aspects of medication action.
Cognitive Level: Application
Nursing Process: Evaluation; *Test Plan:* PHYS

3 **Answer: 1** *Rationale:* Magnesium sulfate when given parenterally acts as a central nervous system (CNS) depressant and also depressant of smooth, skeletal, and cardiac muscle function. The side effects of this medication when taken IV are drowsiness, flushing, heaviness in the limbs, and decreased deep tendon reflexes. Option 2 is incorrect because a decreased respiratory rate is a sign of magnesium toxicity. Option 3 is incorrect because these are signs of CNS excitability. Option 4 is incorrect as well because this is the side effect of magnesium sulfate when taken orally.
Cognitive Level: Application
Nursing Process: Assessment; *Test Plan:* PHYS

4 **Answer: 1** *Rationale:* Clomiphene (Clomid) stimulates the production of lotein hormone (LH) and follicle stimulating hormone (FSH), and therefore increases ovulation in women with anovulatory infertility. Clomiphene is not used to treat hypogonadism (option 2), post partum hemorrhage (option 3) or as hormone replacement therapy (option 4).
Cognitive Level: Application
Nursing Process: Assessment; *Test Plan:* PHYS

5 **Answer: 1** *Rationale:* When 2 pills are missed, the client should "catch up" by taking 2 pills per day for 2 days and then one pill until finishing the pill pack. This will keep her cycle controlled and will minimize the chance of mid-cycle bleeding. However, the client could ovulate when missing 2 or more pills. Thus a backup method such as condoms should be utilized for the rest of the cycle.
Cognitive Level: Application
Nursing Process: Planning; *Test Plan:* HPM

6 **Answer: 1** *Rationale:* Ritodrine (Yutopar) is a beta-adrenergic medication utilized for tocolysis in the treatment of preterm labor. It stimulates beta 2 receptors in uterine smooth muscle, reducing intensity and frequency of uterine contractions and lengthening gestation period. Options 2 and 4 are incorrect because the clients do not require medication with a tocolytic effect. Option 3 is incorrect because ritodrine is not used for postpartum hemorrhage.
Cognitive Level: Application
Nursing Process: Planning; *Test Plan:* PHYS

7 **Answer: 3** *Rationale:* Oxytocin (Pitocin) is used to control postpartum hemorrhage and promotion of postpartum uterine involution. It causes the least increase in blood pressure of all of these oxytoxic medications, and therefore, by considering the history of the client, would be used first in this case.
Cognitive Level: Analysis
Nursing Process: Planning; *Test Plan:* PHYS

8 **Answer: 1** *Rationale:* Human chorionic gonadotropin (Chorex) serves to release the matured ovum from the follicle, which has matured by the action of the menotropin or Humegon (option 2).

Chorex does not limit the number of ova released (option 3) or prepare the uterine lining for the fertilized egg (option 4).
Cognitive Level: Application
Nursing Process: Implementation; *Test Plan:* PHYS

9 **Answer: 4** *Rationale:* Testosterone is responsible for development of male sex organs and the secondary sex characteristics, and facilitates growth of bone and muscle. In cases of hypogonadism, too little testosterone is naturally produced, and supplementation may be required. The responses in options 1 and 3 do not identify the purpose of this medication for a 16-year-old. The response in option 2 is incomplete and does not address the client's learning need.
Cognitive Level: Analysis
Nursing Process: Implementation; *Test Plan:* PHYS

10 **Answer: 1** *Rationale:* Danocrine (Danazol) is an androgen used in the treatment of endometriosis. It is taken orally B.I.D. for several months. Option 2 is incorrect because the medication is given for 3 to 6 months; therapy may be extended to 9 months if necessary. It is important to know that regimen cannot be repeated. Danazol is only given orally (options 3 and 4).
Cognitive Level: Application
Nursing Process: Evaluation; *Test Plan:* PHYS

Post Test

1 **Answer: 2** *Rationale:* Progestins thicken cervical mucus to prevent sperm penetration, while estrogen administration prevents the luteinizing hormone (LH) surge that stimulates ova maturation. Option 1 is incorrect because additional estrogen is not needed. Option 3 is incorrect because taking estrogens alone would not prevent pregnancy. Option 4 is incorrect because the contraceptive is made as a combination product without the option of taking them separately.
Cognitive Level: Application
Nursing Process: Implementation; *Test Plan:* PHYS

2 **Answer: 3** *Rationale:* Sildenafil is a medication used for erectile dysfunction among male population. It is contraindicated if the client has had MI, cerebrovascular accident (CVA), or life-threatening dysrhythmia in the past six months, or if the client has hypotension, hypertension, unstable angina, or CHF.
Cognitive Level: Application
Nursing Process: Planning, *Test Plan:* PHYS

3 **Answer: 3** *Rationale:* Clomiphene (Clomid) induces ovulation through stimulation of luteinizing

hormone (LH) and follicular stimulating hormone (FSH). It is taken orally in 50 mg dosage for five days each month, beginning on day 5 of the menstrual cycle. Options 1, 2, and 4 are incorrect because they are factually correct, which means the client understands medication teaching.
Cognitive Level: Application
Nursing Process: Evaluation; *Test Plan:* PHYS

4 **Answer: 4** *Rationale:* Androderm will replace the testosterone that should be produced by the testes. This therapy is utilized when the testes have been removed to maintain libido, sexual functioning, and secondary male characteristics. The clients in options 1, 2, and 3 do not require additional testosterone.
Cognitive Level: Application
Nursing Process: Planning; *Test Plan:* PHYS

5 **Answer: 3** *Rationale:* Oxytocin (Pitocin) is administered by diluting 10 or 20 units in 1 L of IV fluid, and administering small amounts (not large, as in option 4) via infusion pump. The synthetic oxytocin supplements the endogenous oxytocin, and uterine contractions result. The medication is not given by mouth (option 1) or IM (option 2).
Cognitive Level: Application
Nursing Process: Evaluation; *Test Plan:* PHYS

6 **Answer: 4** *Rationale:* Ergonovine (Ergotrate) causes uterine contractions, and is indicated for use only in normotensive postpartum women. This medication causes an increase in blood pressure, so option 1 is incorrect. The clients described in options 2 and 3 are not presenting any signs and symptoms of bleeding, thus using this medication would be irrelevant.
Cognitive Level: Analysis
Nursing Process: Assessment; *Test Plan:* PHYS

7 **Answer: 1** *Rationale:* The symptoms of possible complications of combination oral contraceptives form the acronym ACHES: **A**bdominal pain, **C**hest pain, **H**eadache, **E**ye problems, and **S**evere leg pain (calf or thigh). The complications indicated by these symptoms are: **A**bdominal pain—liver tumor formation; **C**hest pain, **H**eadache and **E**ye problems—embolus; **S**evere leg pain—thrombophlebitis. Sudden onset of blurred vision may indicate blood clot formation and subsequent pressure on the optic nerves.
Cognitive Level: Application
Nursing Process: Implementation; *Test Plan:* PHYS

8 **Answer: 4** *Rationale:* Terbutaline sulfate (Brethine) is a smooth muscle relaxant, and therefore used to

treat both bronchospasm as well as premature labor. A beta-adrenergic, the medication causes side effects of increased heart rate with a sensation of the heart beating harder, palpitations, muscle tremors, and nervousness. The symptoms in options 1, 2, and 3 are the opposite of those caused by terbutaline.
Cognitive Level: Analysis
Nursing Process: Assessment; *Test Plan:* PHYS

9 **Answer: 2** *Rationale:* Testosterone preparations are contraindicated with pre-existing liver disease. Acne (option 1), melanoma (option 3), and testicular cancer (option 4) are not contraindications for use of this medication.
Cognitive Level: Application
Nursing Process: Planning; *Test Plan:* PHYS

10 **Answer: 3** *Rationale:* Prepidil is a form of prostaglandin E2, and is used for cervical ripening. The gel is inserted around the cervix either through a speculum or sterile vaginal exam. Positioning the client on her back with knees up and apart will facilitate administration of the gel.
Cognitive Level: Application
Nursing Process: Planning; *Test Plan:* PHYS

References

Abrams, A. (2004). *Clinical drug therapy: Rationales for nursing practice* (7th ed.). Philadelphia: Lippincott, pp. 409–424, 965–980.

Deglin, J. & Vallerand, A. (2003). *Davis's drug guide for nurses* (9th ed.). Philadelphia: F.A. Davis, pp. 261–1332.

Grimes, D. (2001). FDA approves combined monthly injectable contraceptive. *In the Contraception Report:* 12 (3). Totowa, NJ: Emron.

Karch, A. (2003). *Focus on nursing pharmacology* (2nd ed.). Philadelphia: Lippincott, Williams & Wilkins, pp. 522–540.

Lehne, R. (2004). *Pharmacology for nursing care* (5th ed.). Philadelphia: W.B. Saunders, pp. 669–1165.

Lowdermilk, D., Perry, S., & Boback, I. (2000). *Maternity and women's health care* (7th ed.). St. Louis, MO: Mosby, Inc., pp. 131–134.

Matteson, P. (2001). *Women's health during the childbearing years: A community-based approach.* St. Louis, MO: Mosby, Inc., pp. 191–561.

McKenry, L. & SaLerno, G. (2003). *Mosby's pharmacology in nursing* (21st ed, revised reprint). St. Louis, MO: Mosby, pp. 889–926.

McKinney, E., Ashwill, J., Murray, S., James, S., Gorrie, T., & Droske, S. (2000). *Maternal child nursing.* Philadelphia, W.B. Saunders.

Olds, S., London, M., & Ladewig, P. (2000). *Maternal newborn nursing* (6th ed.). Upper Saddle River, NJ: Prentice-Hall, Inc., pp. 659–983.

Wilson, B., Shannon, M. & Stang, C. (2003). *Nurse's drug guide 2003.* Upper Saddle River, NJ: Prentice-Hall, pp. 228–1245.

Sherwen, L., Scoloveno, M., & Weingarten, C. (2003). *Maternity nursing: care of the childbearing family* (4th ed.). Stamford, CT: Appleton & Lange, pp. 277–983.

CHAPTER 14

Respiratory System Medications

Caron Martin, MSN, RN

CHAPTER OUTLINE

Bronchodilators
Inhaled Corticosteroids
Inhaled Nonsteroidals
Leukotriene Modifiers

Antihistamines
Medications to Control Bronchial
   Secretions
Oxygen

OBJECTIVES

▌ Describe general goals of therapy when administering respiratory system medications.

▌ Discuss action, contraindications, side effects, and adverse/toxic effects of bronchodilators.

▌ Identify client teaching points related to the administration of inhaled respiratory medications.

▌ Identify nursing considerations related to the administration of intravenous bronchodilators.

▌ Discuss nursing considerations when administering antihistamines, decongestants, expectorants, antitussives, and mucolytics.

▌ Identify signs and symptoms of oxygen toxicity.

▌ Describe nursing considerations related to the administration of oxygen.

▌ Identify client education points related to safety and home care use of oxygen.

▌ List significant client education points related to respiratory system medications.

 [Media Link]

Use the CD-ROM enclosed with this text, or log onto the address given to access the free, interactive Companion Website created for this series. The CD-ROM and Companion Website accompanying this book offer additional practice opportunities and information—NCLEX Review, Case Studies, Glossary, In Depth with NCLEX, and more.

www.prenhall.com/hogan

REVIEW AT A GLANCE

acute asthma attack *bronchospasm with shortness of breath, wheezing, and cough*

adrenergic agonist *medication that has the same effects as that of the sympathetic nervous system*

anticholinergic *effect caused by blockade of acetylcholine receptors that inhibits the transmission of parasympathetic nervous system impulses*

antihistamine *a medication used to treat allergic symptoms that competes with histamine for receptor sites so that the action of histamine is blocked; the result is to inhibit smooth muscle contraction, decrease capillary permeability, decrease salivation and tear formation, and inhibit vascular permeability and edema formation*

antitussive *a medication that aids in quieting a nonproductive, ineffective cough*

atelectasis *incomplete lung expansion or collapse of the alveoli*

catecholamine *an agent released from the adrenal medulla in response to stimulation of the sympathetic nervous system*

decongestant *medication that relieves nasal stuffiness by shrinking swollen nasal mucous membranes*

expectorant *a medication used to aid clients with sputum production during cough*

histamine *substance released from mast cells and basophils in response to stimuli, such as in allergic reactions or cellular injury; the effects of histamine include bronchoconstriction*

hypoxemia *deficiency of oxygen in the arterial blood*

hypoxia *a state in which insufficient oxygen is available to meet the needs of body cells and tissues*

inhaler *device used for administration of a medication by inhalation*

interleukin *plasma protein that increases during the inflammatory process*

lacrimal *a term referring to glands or ducts involved with secretion of tears*

leukotrienes *substances released when the client is exposed to an allergen and experiences an allergic response; they cause inflammation, bronchoconstriction, and mucus production*

mast cell *type of cell involved in hypersensitivity reactions; they are found in several places but many are in the skin, nasal region, and lungs; they contain histamine, kinins, chemotactic factors, leukotrienes, prostaglandins and thromboxanes; irritants or allergens cause breakdown of mast cells, causing release of bronchoconstrictive and inflammatory substances, resulting in airway edema, bronchospasm, and excess mucus production*

mucolytic *a medication that is administered by inhalation to thin respiratory secretions*

nebulizer *a device used for inhalation medications that produces a fine spray or mist*

neutrophils *white blood cells that increase in concentration in response to inflammation or infection*

noncatecholamine *not of the sympathetic nervous system*

opioid *narcotic agent that acts on the central nervous system to change (reduce) pain perception*

parotitis *inflammation of the salivary or parotid glands*

rhinitis *inflammation of the mucous membrane of the nose*

status asthmaticus *severe asthma that cannot be controlled with typical medications; symptoms of asthma are present in spite of treatment efforts*

sympathomimetic *medication that mimics the effect of the sympathetic nervous system*

xanthines *medications that lead to bronchodilation by inhibiting the enzyme phosphodiesterase (PDE) and thereby increasing cyclic adenosine monophosphate*

Pretest

1 The nurse who administers albuterol (Proventil) to a client with symptoms of an acute asthma attack anticipates which of the following intended effects?

(1) Dilation of the airway
(2) Elevation of the heart rate
(3) Constriction of the airway
(4) Slowing of the heart rate

2 The nurse should question an order for epinephrine (Primatene) in the treatment of acute bronchitis when the client has which of the following diseases?

(1) Asthma
(2) Coronary artery disease
(3) Hypotension
(4) Bradycardia

3 Which item should the nurse plan to omit from the meal tray of the client being treated with theophylline (Theo-Dur)?

(1) Peas
(2) Beans
(3) Milk
(4) Coffee

4 The nurse is assessing a client with chronic obstructive pulmonary disease (COPD) who is being treated with beclomethasone dipropionate (Beclovent) via oral inhaler. Which client manifestation would the nurse conclude is a side effect of this medication?

(1) Moist mucous membranes
(2) Decrease in the audible wheezes
(3) Oral fungal infection
(4) Decreased respiratory rate

5 A client on the inpatient unit is having an acute asthma attack. Which of the medications from the medication sheet would the nurse administer?

(1) Aminophylline (Truphylline)
(2) Bitolterol (Tornalate)
(3) Triamcinolone acetonide (Azmacort)
(4) Cromolyn (Intal)

6 The nurse is evaluating the effectiveness of client teaching about home medication administration. Which statement by the client indicates that more teaching is needed related to zafirlukast (Accolate)?

(1) "I will take the drug a few weeks before I expect to notice an improvement in my symptoms."
(2) "I will use this medication when I have the symptoms of an acute asthma attack."
(3) "I will increase my fluid intake while I am taking this medication."
(4) "I will plan to take my medicine one hour before meals."

7 Which statement would the nurse include when giving a client instructions about loratadine (Claritin)?

(1) "This medication will make you drowsy."
(2) "It will take this medication a few hours before it takes effect."
(3) "This medication will help in an acute asthma attack."
(4) "Be sure to take this medication on an empty stomach."

8 In which circumstance should the nurse inform the client to stop taking oral phenylephrine (Neo-Synephrine)?

(1) After three days of continuous use
(2) If the client develops hypertension or tachycardia
(3) If the client develops a dry irritated oral cavity
(4) If the client develops rebound congestion

9 The nurse correctly teaches the client about which potential side effect of guaifenesin (Robitussin)?

(1) Gastric irritation
(2) Hypertension
(3) Hypotension
(4) Urinary retention

10 The nurse is caring for a client with acute bronchitis who is using a non-rebreather mask. The nurse notices that the flaps on the sides of the mask are off. Which action is appropriate?

(1) Allow the client to continue to use this mask as it appears to be functional.
(2) Change the client to a nasal cannula.
(3) Replace the non-rebreather mask with a new one.
(4) Call the physician.

See page 572 for Answers and Rationales.

I. Bronchodilators

A. Beta-adrenergics

1. Action and use

   a. Act as sympathetic nervous system (SNS) **adrenergic agonists**; raise intracellular levels of cAMP (cyclic adenosine monophosphate), which dilates constricted bronchi and bronchioles by relaxing smooth muscle

   b. Medications that lead to bronchodilation stimulate beta 2 adrenergic receptors in the smooth muscle of the bronchi and bronchioles

c. Medications can have alpha, beta 1 or beta 2 activity; beta 1 adrenergic receptors increase heart rate and force of myocardial contraction

d. Used during an **acute asthma attack**, which is characterized as bronchospasm with shortness of breath and wheezing, for quick airway dilation; used also for emphysema, acute and chronic bronchitis, and relief of bronchospasm; alpha adrenergic stimulators can act as a decongestant due to constriction of blood vessels in the nasal cavity

e. Beta adrenergic agents can be classified as **catecholamines** released from the adrenal medulla in response to stimulation of SNS or **noncatecholamines**, which are not released by SNS; all beta adrenergic agents stimulate beta 2 receptors; catecholamines affect both alpha and beta receptors and cause cardiovascular effects

2. Common medications (Table 14-1)

a. Selective beta 2 agonists are the preferred drugs for bronchial smooth muscle dilation as they produce fewer cardiac side effects

b. Albuterol (Proventil, Ventolin, Proventil Repetabs, Volmax): predominately a beta 2 stimulator; given PO or by inhalation; it is not as likely to cause cardiac side effects and is used for prevention and treatment of bronchoconstriction

c. Ipratroprium bromide (Atrovent): has **anticholinergic** effect or sympathetic nervous system effect; given by inhalation

d. Bitolterol (Tornalate): beta 2 stimulant; given by inhalation; it is not as likely to cause cardiac side effects

e. Levalbuterol (Xopenex): short-acting beta 2 agonist used for prevention and treatment of bronchoconstriction; it is given by nebulizer and is not as likely to cause cardiac side effects

f. Ephedrine: alpha and beta stimulant and therefore causes nasal decongestion; given PO, IM, IV, or SC

g. Epinephrine (Adrenalin, Primatene, Bronkaid, Bronitin, Medihaler-Epi): alpha and beta stimulant; given SC, IM, or by inhalation; epinephrine has beta 1 adrenergic action causing increased heart rate and increased force of myocardial contraction

h. Ethylnorepinephrine (Bronkephrine): alpha and beta stimulant, given IM or SC

i. Isoetharine (Arm-a-Med Isoetharine): beta 1 and beta 2 stimulant; given by inhalation

j. Isoproterenol (Isuprel, Medihaler-Iso); beta 1 and beta 2 stimulant; given IV, sublingual, or by inhalation; used for short acting bronchodilation effect but also has cardiac stimulant effects

k. Metaproterenol (Alupent, Metaprel): beta 2 stimulant; given PO or by inhalation; causes cardiac and CNS stimulation in higher doses

l. Pirbuterol (Maxair): beta 2 stimulant; given by inhalation; short acting beta 2 agonist used for prevention and treatment of bronchoconstriction; not as likely to cause cardiac side effects

	Generic/ Trade Name	Usual Adult Dose	Side Effects	Nursing Implications
Table 14-1 **Common Beta Adrenergic Agents**	Albuterol (Proventil)	Oral 2–4 mg T.I.D. or Q.I.D.	Nervousness, restlessness, tremors, headache, insomnia, chest pain, angina, palpitations, hypertension, hypokalemia, hyperglycemia	Assess breath sounds prior to and during administration; administer oral medications with meals; allow at least one minute between doses of inhaled medication
	Ipratroprium Bromide (Atrovent)	2 inhalations Q.I.D. at no less than 4 hours intervals (max. 12 inhalations in 24 hours)	Blurred vision, acute eye pain, bitter taste, dry oropharyngeal membranes, hoarseness, cough, nasal dryness, urinary retention, headache	Auscultate lungs before and after inhalation; instruct client to close eyes while activating inhaler; should not be used for emergency treatment; is an anticholinergic agent
	Bitolterol (Tornalate)	2 inhalations q 8 hours	Absence of the cardiovascular side effects of some beta adrenergic agents because this drug is specific for the beta 2 receptor sites	This drug is a short-acting beta adrenergic agent and the most typical dosing schedule is PRN for treatment of symptoms or as prophylaxis for dyspnea prior to exercise
	Isoproterenol (Isuprel)	1–2 inhalations Q.I.D.	Angina, hypertension, nervousness, paradoxical bronchospasm, restlessness, tachycardia, tremor	Not used frequently because of the potential for cardiac stimulation, but when used is given by inhalation
	Levalbuterol (Xopenex)	0.63–1.25 mg T.I.D. by nebulizer	Increased cough, dyspepsia, hyperglycemia, anxiety, dizziness, headache	Given by nebulizer; client should contact physician before taking OTC medications; instruct client in proper use of nebulizer
	Metaproterenol (Alupent)	1–3 inhalations Q.I.D.	Nervousness, anxiety, tremors, headache, insomnia, angina, dysrhythmias, hypertension	Observe for paradoxical bronchospasm (wheezing); observe client for rebound bronchospasm and drug tolerance
	Salmeterol (Serevent)	2 inhalations q 12 hr	Headache, nervousness, tachycardia, muscle cramps, trembling, diarrhea	May cause hypokalemia; instruct client on use of inhaler; used for acute attack
	Terbutaline (Brethine)	2.5–5 mg PO q 6–8 hrs 2 inhalations q 4–6 hrs	Angina, dysrhythmias, hypertension, nausea, vomiting, hyperglycemia, tachycardia	Administer orally with meals to decrease gastric irritation; teach client to rinse mouth to prevent drying

m. Salmeterol (Serevent): beta 2 stimulant; given by inhalation; used very commonly because of the 12-hour duration of action; used for prophylaxis of acute bronchoconstriction

n. Terbutaline (Brethine): beta 2 adrenergic agonist; long-acting bronchodilator; administered PO, SC, or by inhalation

o. Ipratroprium bromide/albuterol sulfate (Combivent): combination product

3. Administration considerations

   a. May see adverse effects with albuterol, bitolterol, levalbuterol, and pirbuterol if used too frequently because they lose beta 2 specific actions at larger doses (so beta 1 receptors are stimulated and the result can be elevated heart rate, nausea, anxiety, palpitations, and tremors)

   b. Epinephrine, ephedrine, and ethylnorepinephrine can be used as a nasal decongestant due to the alpha stimulation

   c. Use with caution in young children and monitor for tremors, restlessness, hallucinations, dizziness, palpitations, tachycardia, and gastrointestinal (GI) difficulties

   d. Epinephrine is given subcutaneously for bronchoconstriction; effects are usually seen in 5 minutes and may last up to 4 hours

   e. Salmeterol is not used in an acute asthma attack because of the slow onset of action (20 minutes); not to be dosed more often than every twelve hours due to the 12-hour duration of action

4. Contraindications

   a. Albuterol is contraindicated in clients with hypersensitivity to the drug as well as those with tachyarrhythmias and severe coronary artery disease

   b. Contraindicated with hypersensitivity to **sympathomimetics**, which mimic the effect of SNS

   c. Sympathomimetics are used with caution in clients with cardiovascular disease because of potential for increasing the myocardial oxygen demand

   d. Use caution in clients with hypertension, diabetes mellitus, seizures, and hypothyroidism

   e. Avoid use with monoamine oxidase (MAO) inhibitors and sympathomimetics

   f. Children under 12 should not use inhalations of albuterol, bitolterol, metaproterenol, and terbutaline

   g. Avoid use of extended-release albuterol in children under the age of 12

   h. Catecholamines should not be used in clients with tachydysrhythmias

5. Significant drug interactions

   a. Concurrent use of MAO inhibitors may lead to hypertensive crisis

   b. Use with other sympathomimetics may cause additive adrenergic effects

   c. The action of beta agonists is antagonized by beta adrenergic blocking agents and therefore therapeutic effects may be minimized

   d. Potassium-losing diuretics may increase the risk of hypokalemia

   e. Cardiac glycoside toxicity may occur with concurrent use of cardiac glycosides and beta adrenergic agents, especially in the presence of hypokalemia

   f. These drugs can potentiate the therapeutic and adverse effects of other bronchodilators

g. Effects of sympathomimetics can be intensified by thyroid hormone, decongestants, and some antihistamines

6. Significant food interactions: none reported

7. Significant laboratory studies

   a. Sympathomimetics can stimulate liver production of glucose

   b. Sympathomimetics can exacerbate the symptoms of hyperthyroidism

8. Side effects

   a. When beta 1 receptors are stimulated, the client may experience nervousness, tremors, increased heart rate, and increased blood pressure

   b. With alpha and beta adrenergic stimulation, the client may experience insomnia, restlessness, anorexia, tremors, cardiac stimulation, and vascular headache

   c. With nonselective beta agonists, the client may experience cardiac stimulation, tremors, anginal pain, and vascular headache

   d. With beta 2 adrenergic agents, the client may experience hypotension, vascular headache, and tremors

   e. Muscle tremors are the most frequent side effect of terbutaline

   f. Additional side effects may include hypokalemia, hyperglycemia, nausea, vomiting, chest pain, and arrhythmias

   NCLEX!
   g. Paradoxic bronchospasm and urinary retention may also occur

9. Adverse effects/toxicity

   a. CV: tachyarrhythmias, chest pain

   b. CNS: restlessness, agitation, nervousness, and insomnia

10. Nursing considerations

    NCLEX!
    a. Monitor the elderly clients carefully

    NCLEX!
    b. Monitor vital signs, especially heart rate and blood pressure when administering beta agonists (because of the cardiovascular effects)

    NCLEX!
    c. Proper use of metered dose inhaler (MDI) is essential for maximum benefit (see Box 14-1 for client education about use and care of inhalers)

    d. Use appropriate diluent when giving medications

    NCLEX!
    e. Ask client about current medications (including over–the–counter or OTC and herbal products) and about any history of drug allergies

    f. At times, use of multiple drugs is effective and dosages of each can be reduced

    NCLEX!
    g. Note amount, color, and character of sputum

    h. Monitor baseline pulmonary function tests and periodically throughout drug therapy to determine effectiveness of therapy

    i. Administer oral medications with meals to decrease GI irritation

    j. Solutions may remain diluted for 24 to 48 hours

    k. Monitor blood glucose levels in diabetic clients

Box 14-1

Client Education About the Use and Care of Metered Dose Inhalers

The correct steps in administering medication with a metered-dose inhaler (MDI) are as follows:

- Insert the medication firmly into the inhaler.
- Remove the cap and hold the inhaler upright.
- Shake the inhaler for 3 to 5 seconds to ensure even mixing of medication in propellant.
- Tilt the head back slightly and hold the inhaler upright.
- Position the inhaler 1–2 inches away from the open mouth or attach it to a spacer/holding chamber. If a medicine chamber is used, seal the lips around the mouthpiece.
- Press on the inhaler while beginning to breathe in slowly through mouth.
- Breathe in slowly and deeply for 3 to 5 seconds.
- Hold the breath for 8 to 10 seconds as able to allow the medication to move down into airways.
- Wait 1 to 3 minutes as per product directions before the next inhalation if another inhalation is ordered.
- Rinse the mouth with water and blow the nose.
- Use mild soap and water to clean the mouthpiece. Allow to air dry.
- Store the inhaler at room temperature.

    l. Avoid intramuscular (IM) injections

  11. Client education

    a. Monitor blood glucose level closely in diabetic clients because some medications, especially epinephrine, may elevate blood glucose levels; an adjustment in maintenance doses of hypoglycemic agents may be indicated

    b. Contact physician prior to taking OTC medications to ensure there is no potential interaction

    c. Instruct client to report chest pain, palpitations, seizures, headaches, hallucinations, or blurred vision to physician

    d. Caution client not to take more than the prescribed dose because of the potential for hypertension, tachycardia, dysrhythmias, and angina

    e. Record PRN use of these drugs, noting the date, time, symptoms, and whether or not the symptoms subsided

    f. Instruct client regarding the proper use of inhaled preparations and have the client give a return demonstration

    g. Instruct client on the care of the nebulizer and/or the inhaler:

        1) Inhaler and nebulizer tubing and apparatus should be washed daily in warm water and dried

        2) White vinegar can be used to rinse the nebulizer tubing

        3) Clients should read and follow manufacturer's instructions about use, storage, and cleaning of equipment

    h. Wait 1 to 3 minutes (some references suggest 3 to 5 minutes) between inhalations of aerosol medications

    i. Caution client to avoid eye contact with inhaler spray

j. Teach client that the anticipated response to a nebulizer or inhalation treatment is absence of wheezing and dyspnea

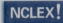

k. Teach client to take the medication exactly as ordered; dosages should not be doubled and frequency of doses should not be increased

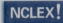

l. Instruct client to avoid contact with the allergen that tends to cause bronchoconstriction and avoid contact with smoke and other irritants, such as aerosol hair spray, perfumes, and cleaning products

m. Increase fluid intake if not contraindicated by other diseases

n. Teach clients early recognition of symptoms of respiratory difficulty (such as activity intolerance and waking at night with asthma symptoms) so that intervention can begin as soon as possible

o. Avoid caffeine as this may increase the nervousness and insomnia of bronchodilating drugs

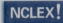

p. An inhaled bronchodilator is the treatment of choice in an acute asthma attack

q. Do not break, chew, or crush extended-release tablets

r. Nervousness and tremors may be experienced when a medication is newly administered but frequently decrease over time

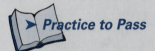

Practice to Pass

A client is admitted to the emergency department with inspiratory and expiratory wheezes, dusky color, and pulse oximetery of 88%. What is the appropriate action of the nurse in the emergency department?

B. Xanthines

1. Action and use

a. Xanthines act by inhibiting the enzyme phosphodiesterase (PDE), the enzyme that breaks down cAMP (cyclic adenosine monophosphate), and thereby increasing the amounts of cAMP; the result of the increased amounts of cAMP is bronchial dilation due to smooth muscle relaxation

b. Xanthines can also act by increasing catecholamine levels, inhibiting calcium ion movement into smooth muscle, inhibiting prostaglandin synthesis, and inhibiting the release of bronchoconstrictive substances from leukocytes and **mast cells** (which contain histamine, prostaglandins and thromboxanes)

c. These drugs cause bronchodilation and thereby increase the ability of the cilia to clear mucus from the airways

d. These medications are used to treat bronchoconstriction associated with COPD (diseases such as chronic bronchitis, asthma, and emphysema) and other chronic respiratory disorders

e. These drugs have a slow onset of action and therefore are utilized in the prevention of asthma attacks rather than the treatment of an acute attack; can be used during an asthma attack if it is mild to moderate

f. Can be used as an additional treatment in pulmonary edema by decreasing vascular permeability and paroxysmal nocturnal dyspnea (PND)

g. The medications are useful for symptom control of clients with asthma and reversible bronchospasm (may occur in clients with chronic bronchitis and emphysema)

NCLEX!

    h. Utilized in the treatment of **status asthmaticus,** which is characterized by severe asthma that can not be controlled with typical medications (use IV theophylline if client has not responded to the faster-acting beta agonist)

2. Common medications (Table 14-2)

    a. Theophylline (Bronkodyl, Elixophyllin, Slo-bid, Theo-Dur, Theo-24, Theo-bid, Quibron-T, Uniphyl): given orally; closely related to caffeine

    b. Aminophylline (Truphylline): parenteral form of theophylline; shorter acting than theophylline

    c. Dyphylline (Dilor)

    d. Oxtriphylline (Choledyl)

3. Administration considerations

NCLEX!

    a. Administer cautiously to the elderly because of potential for increased sensitivity

Table 14-2

Common Xanthines

Generic/ Trade Name	Usual Adult Dose	Side Effects	Nursing Implications
Theophylline (Theo-Dur, Bronkodyl)	PO/IV 5 mg/kg loading dose, then 0.4 mg/kg/hr for nonsmoker, 0.6 mg/kg/hr for smoker	Seizures Anxiety Headaches Insomnia Dysrhythmias Tachycardia Angina Palpitations Nausea	Additive cardiovascular and CNS effects may occur with sympathomimetics. Medications should be administered at scheduled intervals to maintain therapeutic blood levels. Administer oral preparations with food or water to decrease GI irritation. May be given one hour before or two hours after meals to increase the rate of absorption.
Aminophylline (Truphylline)	IV 6 mg/kg over 30 min. loading dose, then PO/IV 0.5 mg/kg/hr for smoker, 0.75 mg/kg/hr for nonsmoker	Vomiting Anorexia Cramps Tremors	IV aminophylline is stable after mixed for up to 24 hours. Client should be instructed to increase the intake of liquids to decrease the viscosity of respiratory secretions. Encourage client not to smoke as a change in dosage may be required with smoking. Teach the client not to eat or drink foods or fluids that contain caffeine as this will have an additive effect when taking xanthines.
Dyphylline (Dilor)	PO up to 15 mg/kg q 6 hrs IM, 250–500 mg q 6 hrs		Serum levels of the medications should be checked every 4 to 6 months. Assess client for and teach client signs and symptoms of toxicity (anorexia, nausea, vomiting, stomach cramps, diarrhea, confusion, headache, restlessness, flushing, increased urination, insomnia, tachycardia, arrhythmias, and seizures).
Oxtriphylline (Choledyl)	PO 4.7 mg/kg q 8 hrs		Teach the client to notify health care professional if signs/symptoms of toxicity develop. Drug levels should be carefully monitored as tachycardia, ventricular dysrhythmias, or seizures may be the first signs of drug toxicity.

    b. Administer xanthines cautiously to children over 6 months of age

    c. Monitor carefully blood levels and therapeutic response to the medication to avoid potential toxicity

    d. Xanthines exhibit a direct stimulating effect on the CNS, which may be enhanced in children

    e. Therapeutic range of theophylline is 10 to 20 mcg/mL

    f. Use correct diluent and proper time of administration when giving parenterally

    g. Use cautiously in clients with cardiovascular disorders

    h. Theophylline is metabolized in the liver; some excretion occurs via the kidneys

    i. Theophylline dosages should be based on lean body weight because it does not enter the adipose tissue

    j. Theophylline can enter breast milk and cross the placenta

    k. Children metabolize the drug faster than adults

    l. Theophylline metabolism is slowed by hepatic failure

    m. Aminophylline is administered at a rate no faster than 25 mg/min because of the potential for cardiovascular collapse

    n. Dosages are often started low and titrated up as needed for relief of symptoms

    o. Adults who smoke cigarettes and children metabolize these medications more quickly and therefore may need higher doses for therapeutic effects

    p. Theophylline levels may be increased in liver disease, congestive heart failure (CHF), and acute viral infections because of impaired metabolism

  4. Contraindications

    a. Avoid use when there is known hypersensitivity to xanthines

    b. Avoid use in clients with tachydysrhythmias

    c. Contraindicated in clients with a history of peptic ulcer disease and GI disorders including acute gastritis because of increased gastric acid secretion

    d. Use cautiously in clients with cardiovascular disorders

    e. Theophylline can cause seizures and is therefore not given to clients with seizure disorders unless the bronchospasm is unresponsive to other treatments

    f. Theophylline is contraindicated in clients with hyperthyroidism because it can exacerbate the disease

  5. Significant drug interactions

    a. Levels of xanthines increase if taken with allopurinol, cimetidine, erythromycin, flu vaccine, and oral contraceptives

    b. Sympathomimetics can intensify cardiac and CNS stimulation

    c. Metabolism of theophylline is increased with smoking

    d. Phenytoin, rifampin, barbiturates, carbamazepine, phenytoin, and phenobarbital increase the metabolism of theophylline

6. Significant food interactions: drinks and foods with caffeine

7. Significant laboratory studies

   a. Adverse effects are more severe with drug levels of 20 to 25 mcg/mL

   b. Adverse cardiac effects are more frequently seen with drug levels above 30 mcg/mL

   c. Seizures may be seen with drug levels above 40 mcg/mL

8. Side effects

   a. Nausea, vomiting, anorexia, and gastroesophageal reflux during sleep

   b. Sinus tachycardia, extra systole, palpitations, and ventricular dysrhythmias

   c. Hyperglycemia and transient increased urination

9. Adverse effects/toxicity

   a. CNS: tremors, dizziness, hallucinations, restlessness, agitation, headache, and insomnia

   b. GI: nausea and vomiting

   c. CV: palpitations, tachydysrhythmias, chest pain, and tachycardia

10. Nursing considerations

   a. Assess for toxicity; note symptoms of restlessness, insomnia, irritability, tremors, nausea, and vomiting

   b. Restlessness is a symptom of a toxic reaction; however, it could signal hypoxia, and the nurse should assess the client for this

   c. Monitor for adverse effects (tremors, restlessness, hallucinations, and dizziness) in all clients, especially in children

   d. Monitor for cardiovascular side effects of palpitations and tachycardia

   e. Carefully monitor clients with a history of cardiac disorder

   f. Do not crush or allow client to chew sustained-release forms

   g. Refrigerate suppository forms

   h. Utilize appropriate diluent when administering medications

   i. Ask client about current medications (including OTC and herbal products) and history of any allergies

   j. Children may exhibit hyperactive behavior with administration of theophylline because of CNS stimulation

11. Client education

   a. Do not chew or crush sustained-release forms (irritating to the gastric mucosa)

   b. Teach mechanism of action, usage, and side effects

   c. Do not omit or double-up on doses; take exactly as prescribed

   d. Suppository forms should be refrigerated

   e. Notify physician if suppositories cause rectal burning, itching, or irritation

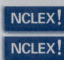

f. Notify physician if palpitations, nausea, vomiting, weakness, dizziness, chest pain, or convulsions occur

g. Monitor blood levels

h. Avoid use of caffeine as this could lead to an additive effect with xanthines

i. Avoid contact with the allergen that tends to cause the allergic response if possible; avoid contact with smoke and other respiratory irritants such as aerosol hair spray, perfumes, and cleaning products

j. Increase fluid intake if no contraindication with other disease process

k. Take medications even when there are no symptoms of asthma

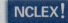

l. Inform physician prior to taking OTC medication

m. Take medications with food if GI symptoms develop

II. Inhaled Corticosteroids

A. Action and use

1. Exact mechanism of action is unknown; however, it is thought that inhaled corticosteroids stabilize the membranes of cells that release bronchoconstricting substances such as **histamine** and thereby decrease the release of these substances

2. Cell membranes of **neutrophils** (white blood cells that increase in concentration in response to inflammation) are stabilized and therefore inflammation-causing substances are not released; the result is decreased inflammation and bronchodilation

3. Reducing inflammation decreases mucosal edema and mucous secretions and thereby decreases bronchoconstriction

4. Inhaled corticosteroids may have a role in increasing responsiveness of bronchial smooth muscle to beta agonist drugs

5. These agents appear to be involved in the inhibition of the movement of fluid and protein into tissues as well as the inhibition of the production of prostaglandins, **leukotrienes** (substances released after exposure to an allergen) and **interleukins** (plasma proteins that increase during the inflammatory process)

6. These agents also promote the mobilization of mucus by increasing mucociliary action

7. Used in chronic asthma to decrease inflammation and therefore decrease airway obstruction and are used prophylactically, not during acute attack

8. Used to treat bronchospastic disorders when bronchodilators are not completely effective

9. Used to treat chronic bronchitis, COPD, and cystic fibrosis

B. Common medications (Table 14-3)

C. Administration considerations

1. Proper technique is essential when administering medications by inhalation route

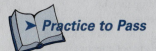

A client comes to the clinic with results of lab work that was drawn earlier that day. The theophylline level is 25 mcg/mL. The client has diabetes and his BUN is 52 mg/dL and creatinine level is 2.1 mg/dL. What actions should the nurse take?

Generic Trade Name	Usual Adult Dose	Side Effects	Nursing Implications
Beclomethasone dipropionate (Beclovent)	2 inhalations 2–4 times per day, 42 mcg per inhalation		Monitor respiratory status and lung sounds for the effectiveness of therapy When client changes from systemic to inhalation corticosteroids, assess for adrenal insufficiency
Budesonide (Pulmocort)	1–2 inhalations B.I.D., 200 mcg per inhalation	Headache, dyspepsia, gastroenteritis, back pain, flulike syndrome	May cause hyperglycemia Monitor growth in children Advise clients to take medications exactly as ordered
Flunisolide (AeroBid-M)	2 inhalations B.I.D. 250 mcg per inhalation		Teach client to use bronchodilator prior to corticosteroid when both are ordered to maximize effectiveness of drug therapy Teach client that corticosteroids are for the prophylaxis of asthma attack and are not effective in an acute attack
Fluticasone aerosol (Flovent)	88–440 mcg B.I.D.	Headache, agitation, depression, fatigue, insomnia, restlessness, nasal stuffiness, sinusitis, nausea, muscle soreness	Teach client to avoid smoking and known allergens Instruct the client on the proper use of the metered dose inhaler and nebulizer
Triamcinolone acetonide (Azmacort)	2 inhalations T.I.D. to Q.I.D. with inhalations at 100 mcg per inhalation	In general side effects for inhaled corticosteroids: Dysphonia Hoarseness Oropharyngeal fungal infections Bronchospasm Cough Wheezing Dry mouth Adrenal suppression with increased dose and long-term therapy Decreased growth in children	

2. Chemical structures of inhaled corticosteroids have been slightly altered so there is not as much systemic absorption and therefore less likelihood of systemic side effects

3. Beclomethasone has greater anti-inflammatory action and causes fewer side effects than dexamethasone

4. If client is also taking a systemic corticosteroid, the dose may need to be decreased with the addition of inhaled corticosteroids

5. Beclomethasone, flunisolide, and fluticasone are available as nasal solutions for the treatment of allergic rhinitis

6. Monitor for impaired bone growth in children receiving inhaled corticosteroids

D. Contraindications

1. Clients with known allergy

2. Clients with psychosis, fungal infection, acquired immunodeficiency syndrome (AIDS), tuberculosis, and idiopathic thrombocytopenia

3. Children under age of 2 years

4. Use cautiously in clients with diabetes, glaucoma, osteoporosis, ulcers, renal disease, CHF, myasthenia gravis, seizure disorders, inflammatory bowel disease, hypertension, thromboembolic disorders, or esophagitis

5. Use with caution in clients with infections due to potential for suppressed immune system

E. Significant drug interactions

1. There are relatively few drug interactions because these inhalers work locally rather than systemically

2. May need to adjust dose of antidiabetic agents secondary to potential for elevation of blood glucose levels when corticosteroids are administered orally

3. Rifampin, barbiturates, and phenytoin cause a decreased corticosteroid effect

F. Significant food interaction: none reported

G. Significant laboratory studies

1. There may be a decreased response to skin test antigens

2. Skin testing should be postponed if possible until after corticosteroid therapy

H. Side effects

1. Pharyngeal irritation and sore throat

2. Coughing

3. Dry mouth

4. Oral fungal infections

5. Sinusitis

I. Adverse effects/toxicity

1. Adrenocortical insufficiency, fluid and electrolyte disturbances, nervous system effects, and endocrine effects if absorbed systemically

2. Increased susceptibility to infection, dermatologic effects, and osteoporosis

3. Diarrhea, nausea, vomiting, and stomach upset

4. Headache, fever, dizziness, angioedema, rash, urticaria, and paradoxical bronchospasm

5. **Rhinitis** or inflammation of the mucous membranes of the nose, menstrual disturbances, and palpitations

J. Nursing considerations

NCLEX!

1. Ask client about current medications (including OTC and herbal products) and history of any allergies

2. Teach client about early signs of respiratory difficulty (such as activity intolerance and awakening with asthma symptoms)

3. Teach client to avoid allergens

4. Chronic use of inhaled corticosteroids can predispose the client to osteoporosis

NCLEX!

5. Rinse mouth after use of medication because oropharyngeal candidiasis and/or hoarseness can occur

6. Assess sputum color and viscosity for signs of infection

K. Client education

NCLEX!

1. Use the medications as prescribed; do not overuse

2. Keep equipment clean and in working order per manufacturer's guidelines

3. Rinse mouth after use of inhalation devices such as **inhaler** or **nebulizer**

4. Pediatric clients may need a physician's order to keep this inhaler with them at school

NCLEX!

5. Do not abruptly stop taking this medication; dose should be tapered slowly over a 2-week period under the direction of a physician

6. Wear a bracelet or necklace to identify self as utilizing a steroid

NCLEX!

7. Teach client about the symptoms of steroid use, including moon face, acne, increased fat pads, increased edema; the physician should be notified if these symptoms arise

8. Instruct client to report signs of decreased amounts of steroid levels including nausea, dyspnea, joint pain, weakness, and fatigue

NCLEX!

9. Report weight gain of more that 5 pounds in a week

10. Avoid contact with the allergen responsible for producing the allergic response if possible

11. Teach client about early recognition of respiratory difficulty so treatment can begin early

12. Drug should be taken at approximately the same time each day for maximal effectiveness

13. Inhaled corticosteroids are to be used as maintenance drugs and are ineffective in acute bronchospasm

III. Inhaled Nonsteroidals

A. Action and use

1. These agents stabilize mast cells so bronchoconstrictive and inflammatory substances are not released when stimulated with an allergen; therefore, inflammation is limited

2. Used to prevent and treat inflammation of the airways; decreasing inflammation decreases mucosal edema and mucous secretions and thereby decreases bronchoconstriction

3. Used for prophylaxis of acute asthma attacks

4. Used also for the prevention and treatment of allergic rhinitis

B. Common medications (Table 14-4)

1. Cromolyn (Intal): oral spray or nebulizer solution for oral inhalation; Nasalcrom is the nasal spray form of cromolyn

2. Nedocromil (Tilade): given by inhalation

C. Administration considerations

1. Reduction in the dose of bronchodilators and corticosteroids may be indicated with the use of these drugs

2. Use with caution in clients with impaired hepatic or renal function

3. Administer by inhalation

4. Nasal solution is used for prevention and treatment of allergic rhinitis

5. It may take 3 weeks of daily dosing to see therapeutic effects

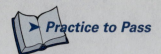

➤ Practice to Pass

A client is newly diagnosed with chronic obstructive pulmonary disease (COPD). The medications that are to be taken at home include albuterol (Proventil) and beclomethasone dipropionate (Beclovent). What client teaching is needed related to these medications?

Table 14-4				
Inhaled Nonsteroidal Medications	**Generic/Trade Name**	**Usual Adult Dose**	**Side Effects**	**Nursing Implications**
	Cromolyn (Intal)	Inhalation: 20 mg by inhalation or nebulizer solution or 2 sprays as aerosol B.I.D. Intranasal: one spray to each nostril T.I.D. to Q.I.D.	Headache Nasal irritation Sneezing Dry mouth Irritation of the throat and trachea Cough Unpleasant taste Toxic effects (rare):	Perform respiratory assessment to monitor effectiveness of therapy. When medication is used intranasally, assess for rhinitis (stuffiness, rhinorrhea). Dosages of other asthma medications may be reduced after 2 to 4 weeks of therapy with inhaled nonsteroidal medications. Client may require pretreatment with bronchodilator when using these inhalers. Do not use cloudy solution. Teach client to use medication exactly as prescribed.
	Nedocromil (Tilade)	Inhalation: 2 sprays B.I.D. to T.I.D. Dosages of each may be increased for prevention of bronchospasm	Bronchospasm Erythema Rash Urticaria Parotitis	Cromolyn can be administered 15 to 60 min prior to contact with known allergens to reduce the effects of the allergen. For intranasal use, instruct client to clear nasal passages prior to use and inhale medication through the nose.

D. Contraindications

1. Not to be used in acute bronchospasm or status asthmaticus

2. It is contraindicated in clients with a hypersensitivity

3. Use with caution in clients with impaired renal or hepatic function; lower dosages may be required

E. Significant drug interactions: none reported

F. Significant food interactions: none reported

G. Significant laboratory studies: none reported

H. Side effects (see Table 14-4)

I. Adverse effects/toxicity (see Table 14-4)

J. Nursing considerations

1. Ask client about current medications (including OTC and herbal products) and history of any allergies

2. Coronary artery disease (CAD) and/or dysrhythmias may be aggravated by the propellants in the aerosols; therefore, use with caution in clients with cardiac dysrhythmias

3. Pulmonary function testing may be ordered prior to administration of these medications

K. Client education

1. Take medications exactly as prescribed

2. Teach mechanism of action, usage, and side effects

3. Instruct client on proper use of inhaler to ensure maximal effectiveness of medication; teach use of spacer as appropriate

4. Record frequency and severity of asthma attacks

5. Inform client that it may take 2 to 4 weeks to see the results of the medication

6. Rinse mouth after taking medication to avoid dry mouth

7. Do not take during an acute attack as the symptoms may be aggravated

8. Bronchodilator should be taken optimally 20 to 30 minutes prior to taking cromolyn; see individual product literature; always wait a minimum of 3 to 5 minutes between inhalations

IV. Leukotriene Modifiers

A. Action and use

1. Leukotrienes are substances that are released when a client is suffering from an allergic response to an allergen

2. Leukotrienes cause inflammation, bronchoconstriction, and mucus production that leads to coughing, sneezing, and shortness of breath

3. Leukotriene modifiers work by blocking the action of leukotrienes by preventing them from attaching to receptors in circulating cells and cells in the lungs

4. Bronchoconstriction is prevented by inhibition of smooth muscle contraction of the bronchial airways

5. These medications are a newer class of asthma medications and provide relief of inflammatory symptoms of asthma; they are referred to as anti-inflammatory drugs

6. Leukotriene modifiers are used for prophylaxis and chronic treatment of asthma in adults and children over the age of 12; they are not used in managing an acute asthma attack

B. Common medications (Table 14-5)

1. Zileuton (Zyflo): inhibits the enzyme 5-lipoxygenase and therefore blocks production of leukotrienes; is given orally

2. Zafirlukast (Accolate): blocks specific leukotrienes called cystinyl leukotrienes that are thought to be mediators of asthma; inflammation in the lung is prevented; classified as a leukotriene receptor antagonist

3. Montelukast (Singulair): inhibits leukotriene receptors and is classified as a leukotriene receptor antagonist; is given orally

C. Administration considerations

1. They are used in adults and children 12 and over

2. It may take a week before therapeutic effects are seen

3. They have localized effects in the lungs

4. They are used alone or in combination with corticosteroids

5. Zafirlukast cannot be taken during lactation as it is excreted in breast milk

Table 14-5 Leukotriene Modifiers	Generic/Trade Name	Usual Adult Dose	Side Effects	Nursing Implications
	Zileuton (Zyflo)	600 mg PO, Q.I.D.	Fatigue Headache Weakness	Caution client that it takes about a week to see improvement in symptoms. Assess respiratory status to evaluate the effectiveness of therapy.
	Zafirlukast (Accolate)	20 mg PO, B.I.D.	Nasal congestion Otitis in children Dyspepsia Nausea	Monitor liver function tests for elevated AST and ALT levels. Singulair should be administered in the evening.
	Montelukast (Singulair)	10 mg PO, QD Children should take 5 mg QD	Increased liver enzymes Rash Fever Dizziness Diarrhea Abdominal pain Back pain Myalgia	Instruct client to take medication exactly as ordered. Advise client that these medications are for prophylaxis of asthma and are not effective for treatment of an acute attack.

6. Montelukast and zafirlukast are taken orally, metabolized in the liver and excreted in the feces

7. Zileuton is metabolized by the liver and excreted in the urine

8. Monitor hepatic aminotransferase enzymes when administering zileuton; discontinue the medication if levels elevate to five times the norm or if liver dysfunction develops

D. Contraindications

1. Zileuton is contraindicated in clients with liver disease and with elevations of transaminase (3 times the norm)

2. All are contraindicated in clients with hypersensitivity

E. Significant drug interactions

1. Theophylline, warfarin, and propranolol levels increase when administered with zileuton

2. Warfarin, tolbutamide, phenytoin, and carbamazepine levels increase when administered with zafirlukast

3. Decreased levels of zafirlukast are seen with concurrent administration of erythromycin

4. Increased levels of zafirlukast are seen with concurrent administration of aspirin

5. Phenobarbital and dilantin may decrease available montelukast due to initiation of hepatic metabolism

F. Significant food interaction: none reported

G. Significant laboratory studies

1. Monitor serum theophylline levels if used concurrently due to decreased theophylline clearance when taking zileuton

2. Monitor prothrombin time (PT) or international normalized ratio (INR) when client on zafirlukast or zileuton and warfarin as PT/INR may be elevated

H. Side effects

1. Headaches may occur with all drugs

2. Zileuton may also cause dyspepsia, nausea, dizziness, and insomnia

3. Zafirlukast may cause nausea and diarrhea

I. Adverse effects/toxicity

1. Limited information is available for zileuton because the drug is relatively new

2. Hepatotoxicity (zileuton)

J. Nursing considerations

1. Be sure the drug is prescribed for chronic, not acute, treatment of asthma

2. Monitor liver function tests

3. Ask client about current medications (including OTC and herbal products) and history of any allergies

4. Monitor liver enzymes during zileuton therapy and discontinue the medication if they reach 5 times the normal value or if liver dysfunction develops

K. Client education

1. Inform client that the drugs may take a week before therapeutic effects are seen

2. Teach client the mechanism of action, usage, and potential side effects

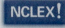

3. Liver function studies may be needed

4. Drugs help prevent some of the symptoms of asthma; they are not intended to be used for acute attacks

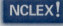

5. Take the medications exactly as prescribed

6. Avoid contact with the specific allergen if possible

7. Increase fluid intake if not contraindicated because of other disease processes

8. Take zafirlukast 1 hour before or 2 hours after meals

9. Montelukast and zileuton may be taken with or without food

V. Antihistamines

A. Action and use

1. The action of these drugs is to block or inhibit the action of histamine

   a. They work best early in the response as they do not displace histamine from the receptors

   b. **Antihistamines** compete with histamine for receptor sites so that the action of histamine can be blocked; thus, they do not prevent histamine release or reduce the amount released

2. Antihistamines reduce the effects of histamine (vasodilation, contraction of smooth muscles, increased GI and respiratory secretions, increased capillary permeability, increased heart rate and CNS transmission); therefore, antihistamines inhibit smooth muscle contraction (respiratory system, blood vessels, and GI tract), decrease capillary permeability, decrease salivation and tear formation and inhibit vascular permeability and edema formation

3. Antihistamines cause bronchial smooth muscle relaxation

4. They reduce bronchial, salivary, gastric, nasal, and **lacrimal** (tear) secretions

5. Antihistamines reduce itching (urticaria)

6. Antihistamines are used to treat allergies, allergic rhinitis (hay fever), allergic conjunctivitis, allergic contact dermatitis, vertigo, motion sickness, insomnia, allergic reactions, and cough; they are also used to treat the symptoms of sneezing and runny nose of the common cold

7. Used in the treatment of anaphylactic shock

8. Can be used as prevention or treatment for allergic reactions to medications

B. Common medications (Table 14-6)

1. Nonsedating antihistamines include loratadine (Claritin), cetirizine (Zyrtec), and fexofenadine (Allegra)

Table 14-6	Generic/Trade Name	Usual Adult Dose	Side Effects	Nursing Implications
Antihistamines	Second Generation or Non-sedating antihistamines:		Confusion Drowsiness (rare) Paradoxical excitement	Assess client for signs/symptoms of allergy to monitor effectiveness of medication. Increase fluid intake to 2 L daily to decrease viscosity of secretions.
	Loratadine (Claritin)	10 mg daily	Blurred vision Dry mouth	May cause false negative result on skin testing for allergies.
	Cetirizine (Zyrtec)	5–10 mg daily	GI upset Photosensitivity Rash	Administer QD dose prior to meals. Caution client to use sunscreen as client may be more prone to sunburn.
	Fexofenadine (Allegra)	60 mg B.I.D.	Weight gain Dizziness Drowsiness Fatigue Pharyngitis	Advise client not to drink alcohol or take other CNS depressants while taking these medications. Rinse mouth and use hard sugarless candy to relieve dry mouth.
	Astemizole (Hismanal)	10 mg QD		Contact physician if client has dizziness, fainting, or rapid heart rate. Advise client to take medication as ordered and to contact physician before taking other OTC medications.
	Selected first generation or traditional antihistamines:		Drowsiness Paradoxical excitement especially in children	Assess client for drowsiness or dizziness especially during the first few days of therapy. Encourage fluid intake up to 2 to 3 L daily. Teach client to use hard sugarless candy to relieve dry mouth.
	Diphenhy-dramine (Benadryl)	25–50 mg every 6–8 hr	Dry mouth Changes in vision Difficulty with urination	Give antihistamines prior to contact with allergens if possible.
	Chlorphenira-mine (Chlor-Trimeton)	4 mg every 4–6 hr up to 24 mg daily	Constipation Sedation Dizziness	Teach client not to operate heavy machinery or participate in other hazardous activity while taking these medications.
	Hydroxyzine (Vistaril)	25 mg every 4–6 hr	Syncope Muscular weakness Unsteady gait	Taking the medications at bedtime will eliminate problems with drowsiness.
	Meclizine (Antivert)	25–100 mg/d in divided doses	Insomnia	
	Azatadine (Optimine)	1–2 mg B.I.D.		

a. Cetirizine is a metabolite of hydroxyzine but causes less drowsiness

b. These second generation antihistamines cause less sedation than the first generation antihistamines

c. They are selective for the peripheral H1 receptors and do not cross the blood-brain barrier

d. Second-generation medications have a rapid onset of action after oral administration

2. Traditional antihistamines have sedative effects because they work peripherally as well as centrally; first generation H1 receptor antagonists bind to central and peripheral H1 receptors and can cause CNS depression (drowsiness or sedation) or stimulation (anxiety or agitation)

   a. CNS stimulation is more likely to occur in high doses and especially in children

   b. These drugs also have anticholinergic effects such as dry mouth, urinary retention, constipation, and blurred vision

   c. These drugs include diphenhydramine (Benadryl), brompheniramine (Dimetane), chlorpheniramine (Chlor-Trimeton), dimenhydrinate (Dramamine), doxylamine (Unisom), meclizine (Antivert or Bonine), azatadine (Optimine), phenindamine (Nolahist), tripelennamine (PBZ), azelastine (Astelin), clemastine (Tavist), cyproheptadine (Periactin), dexchlorpheniramine (Polaramine), hydroxyzine (Vistaril, Atarax), and promethazine (Phenergan)

C. Administration considerations

1. Antihistamines treat the symptoms but not the cause of the problem

2. Antihistamines may cause drowsiness

3. Antihistamines should not be used for treatment of an acute asthma attack or lower respiratory disorder

4. Most antihistamines are tolerated better when taken with meals

5. Bropheniramine, chlorpheniramine, and diphenhydramine are all available over the counter

6. Hydroxyzine is effective with pruritis

7. Most antihistamines are metabolized by the liver

8. Azelastine is topically applied to the nasal mucosa and action peaks in 2 to 3 hours; it does not tend to cause drowsiness but does leave an unpleasant taste in the mouth

NCLEX!

9. Hydroxyzine and promethazine cause profound drowsiness; diphenhydramine has a high incidence of drowsiness and anticholinergic effects

NCLEX!

10. Antihistamines may be used as a premedication prior to the administration of blood products to decrease the likelihood of allergic reactions

11. Oral antihistamines act in 15 to 60 minutes and last 4 to 6 hours; sustained-release medications last 8 to 12 hours

12. A rapid acting agent should be used with an acute allergic reaction

13. Longer-acting agents give more consistent relief with chronic allergic conditions

D. Contraindications

NCLEX!

1. Hypersensitivity

2. Astemizole should be used with caution in clients with liver dysfunction because of the potential for elevation in blood levels and potential cardiac malfunction

3. Loratadine is contraindicated in acute asthma treatment and in conditions affecting the lower respiratory tract

4. Diphenhydramine should not be given to nursing mothers or clients with conditions of the lower respiratory tract

5. Antihistamines should be used cautiously if clients have a history of increased intraocular pressure, cardiac or renal disease, hypertension, bronchial asthma, stenosing peptic ulcer disease, prostatic hyperplasia, convulsive disorders, or during pregnancy

6. Promethazine should not be used in children with hepatic disease, Reye's syndrome, history of sleep apnea, or family history of sudden infant death syndrome (SIDS)

7. Diphenhydramine is not recommended for use with infants or for children with chickenpox or flu-like infections

E. Significant drug interactions

1. Astemizole should not be used concurrently with erythromycin, ketoconazole, or itraconazole as this can lead to cardiac arrest and ventricular dysrhythmias

2. Anticholinergic effects are more pronounced if taken with tricyclic antidepressants, antipsychotic agents and some antiparkinson agents

3. Ethyl alcohol, anti-anxiety agents, tricyclic antidepressants, antipsychotic agents, opioid analgesics, sedative hypnotics, and MAO inhibitors increase the effects of first-generation antihistamines

4. Loratadine blood levels are increased when taken with azithromycin, clarithromycin, erythromycin, fluconazole, itraconazole, ketoconazole, miconazole, and cimetidine

F. Significant food interactions

1. Licorice and Claritin should not be taken together because of potential prolongation of the QT interval

2. Coffee and tea may reduce drowsiness caused by these medications

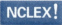 **G. Significant laboratory studies:** antihistamines can mask positive skin test results

H. Side effects

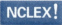 1. Drowsiness is the main side effect; however, children can experience paradoxical excitement with antihistamines

NCLEX!

2. Anticholinergic side effects include dry mouth and nose, changes in vision, difficulty urinating and constipation

3. CNS: sedation from drowsiness to deep sleep, dizziness, syncope, muscular weakness, unsteady gait, paradoxical excitement (especially in the older adult), restlessness, insomnia, and nervousness

4. GI: anorexia, nausea, vomiting, diarrhea, constipation, and jaundice

5. Urinary retention, impotence, vertigo, visual disturbances, blurred vision, tinnitus, hypotension, syncope, and headache

I. Adverse effects/toxicity

NCLEX!

1. Seizures can result from CNS effects

NCLEX!

2. Dysrhythmias, palpitations, and cardiac arrest

3. Aranulocytosis, hemolytic anemia, leukopenia, thrombocytopenia, and pancytopenia

NCLEX!

4. Overdose in children can cause hallucinations, convulsions, and death

J. Nursing considerations

NCLEX!

1. Ask client about current medications (including OTC and herbal products) and history of any allergies

2. Cetirizine, loratadine, and fexofenadine may be used in children over the age of 6

3. Assist client to determine factors that precipitate allergic reactions and to identify symptoms caused by allergens

NCLEX!

4. Assess client for drowsiness and dizziness especially during the first few days of therapy

5. Encourage fluid intake of 2000 to 3000 mL/day unless contraindicated by another condition

6. Give antihistamines prior to contact with allergen if possible

7. Administer medications at bedtime to help with the side effect of drowsiness

8. Administer intramuscular antihistamines deeply into large muscles

9. Intravenous injection should be over a few minutes

K. Client education

1. Take medications exactly as prescribed

2. Teach client potential side effects

3. Teach client action of the medication and potential drug interactions, and to check the labels of OTC medications for potential drug interactions

4. Avoid contact with the allergen responsible for the reaction if possible; if unable, take medication prior to exposure

5. Do not crush or chew sustained-release tablets

6. Do not take more than one medication at a time

7. Do not operate heavy machinery or participate in other hazardous activities while taking this type of medication

8. Do not use alcohol or other CNS depressants while taking this type of medication

9. Contact the physician if excessive sedation, confusion, or hypotension occur

10. Use hard sugarless candy to relieve dry mouth

11. Antihistamines may dry and thicken respiratory tract secretions and make them difficult to expectorate

12. Take with meals to decrease stomach upset

13. Take Claritin on an empty stomach to increase absorption

14. Avoid prolonged exposure to sunlight due to potential for sunburn

15. Take medication at bedtime to reduce drowsiness, which should become less significant after repeated doses

16. Do not take antihistamines for 72 hours prior to allergen skin testing to reduce likelihood of false negative results

VI. Medications to Control Bronchial Secretions

A. Nasal decongestants

1. Action and use

   a. **Decongestants** relieve nasal stuffiness by shrinking swollen nasal mucous membranes

   b. Adrenergic agents (sympathomimetics) do this by vasoconstriction, decreasing blood flow to the nasal mucosa and thereby reducing swelling

   c. Nasal steroids act as anti-inflammatory agents by suppressing the inflammatory response

   d. Used to relieve nasal congestion and nasal discharge caused by acute or chronic rhinitis (common cold), sinusitis, hay fever, and other allergies

   e. May be used to decrease local blood flow prior to nasal surgery

   f. May be used to aid visualization of nasal mucosa during diagnostic exams because of the effect of decreasing blood flow

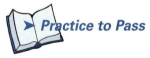

Practice to Pass

A 22-year-old college student comes to the university clinic because of problems with allergies. He is started on fexofenadine (Allegra). What teaching should the nurse in the clinic initiate?

2. Common medications (Table 14-7)

3. Administration considerations

    a. Nasal decongestants can be applied topically (with sprays or drops) or can be administered orally

    b. Sustained use of topical decongestants (longer than 3 days or in excessive amounts) can cause rebound congestion; therefore, oral agents should be used if needed for longer than 3 days

    c. Topical decongestants are potent decongestants with prompt onset of action

    d. Topical decongestants are preferred if the client has cardiovascular disease because of the decreased likelihood of cardiovascular side effects

4. Contraindications

    a. Avoid use when client has known hypersensitivity

    b. Adrenergic agents are contraindicated in clients with hypertension and CAD

    c. Clients with nasal mucosal infection should not take nasal steroids

    d. Decongestants should not be taken during pregnancy or lactation

    e. Contraindicated in clients taking tricyclic antidepressants or MAO inhibitors

    f. Use cautiously in clients with cardiac dysrhythmias, hyperthyroidism, diabetes mellitus, glaucoma, prostatic hypertrophy, and insomnia

5. Significant drug interactions

    a. Possible increased toxicity with sympathomimetics

    b. Possible increased sympathetic effect when given concurrently with MAO inhibitors (i.e., severe hypertensive crisis)

    c. Beta blockers decrease the effects of decongestants

    d. Concurrent use with digitalis agents can cause dysrhythmias

    e. Decongestants decrease effectiveness of antihypertensive agents

    f. Increased effect of nasal decongestants is seen with use of cocaine, digoxin, general anesthetics, antihistamines, epinephrine, ergot alkaloids, methylphenidate, MAO inhibitors, thyroid preparations and xanthines

6. Significant food interactions: none reported

7. Significant laboratory studies: none significant

8. Side effects

    a. Local nasal mucosal irritation and dryness

    b. Rarely nervousness, insomnia, palpitations, and tremor

    c. Rebound congestion is common

9. Adverse effects/toxicity

    a. If a topical decongestant is absorbed, it can cause cardiovascular disturbances such as hypertension and tachycardia

    b. CNS disturbances can occur if topical decongestant is absorbed and these include headache, nervousness, dizziness, confusion, delirium, and insomnia

Table 14-7	Generic/Trade Name	Usual Adult Dose	Side Effects	Nursing Implications
Nasal Decongestants	Phenylephrine (Neo-Synephrine)	2–3 sprays or drops in each nostril q 3–4 hr	Irritation of the nasal mucosa Dryness of the nasal mucosa Nervousness	May see increased toxicity with the administration of adrenergic decongestants and sympathomimetic agents. Beta blockers can decrease the effects of decongestants.
	Pseudoephedrine (Sudafed)	60 mg every 4–6 hr	Insomnia Palpitations Tremors	Antihypertensive medications can have decreased effectiveness when administered with decongestants.
	Ephedrine (Vicks Vatronol)	1 spray in each nostril no more frequently than every 4 hours	Rebound congestion Hypertension Tachycardia Headache	When a decongestant is to be administered for longer than three days, an oral agent is the treatment of choice. Nasal sprays can cause rebound congestion if used for longer than three days.
	Naphazoline (Privine)	1–2 drops or sprays in each nostril	Nervousness Dizziness Confusion Delirium	Cautious administration is needed with the elderly due to the potential for other medical conditions.
	Oxymetazoline (Afrin)	2–3 sprays or drops in each nostril B.I.D.	Insomnia Muscle tremors Nausea Vomiting	Teach client to take medications as directed. Teach client to consult the physician if side effects develop.
	Tetrahydrozoline (Tyzine)	2–4 drops in each nostril q 3–4 hr	Appetite loss Urinary retention	Smoking should be avoided as this decreases ciliary action and increases secretions.
	Xylometazoline (Otrivin)	2–3 drops or sprays in each nostril q 8–10 hr		Fluid intake should be increased to 2–3 L per day to liquefy secretions. Infants may be able to nurse better if a nasal solution is applied prior to feeding when the infant is suffering from congestion. Eating and drinking should be avoided after the administration of topical medications for at least 30 minutes.

      c. Muscle tremors, nausea, vomiting, appetite loss, and urinary retention

   10. Nursing considerations

      a. Ask client about current medications (including OTC and herbal products) and history of any allergies

      b. Assess client for other medical history to determine potential for possible side effects; older adults with significant cardiac disease should avoid nasal decongestants because they are at high risk for hypertension, dysrhythmias, nervousness, and insomnia

      c. For administration of nose drops, have the client lie down or sit with neck hyperextended to instill the medication

      d. Medication droppers should be washed after each use to prevent contamination

      e. Client should sit and squeeze nasal spray container once and avoid touching nares with spray dispenser; tip of dispenser should be rinsed after each use

      f. Observe client for decrease in nasal congestion

      g. Observe for tachycardia, hypertension and cardiac dysrhythmias; also observe for rebound nasal congestion, chronic rhinitis, and ulceration of the nasal mucosa

   11. Client education

      a. Take medications exactly as prescribed

      b. Teach client potential side effects, especially palpitations, insomnia, restlessness, and nervousness

      c. Do not use alcohol or other CNS depressants while taking this medication

      d. Do not operate heavy machinery while taking this medication

      e. Avoid use of caffeine while taking this medication as it can cause nervousness, tremors, and insomnia

      f. Avoid smoking because it increases secretions and decreases ciliary action

      g. Avoid exposure to crowds to minimize the spread of disease

      h. Fluid intake should be increased to 2000 to 3000 mL per day unless contraindicated by another medical condition

      i. Nasal congestion in infants can decrease ability to suck effectively; application of a nasal solution prior to feeding can increase infant's ability to feed

      j. Avoid eating or drinking for 30 minutes after medication administration

      k. Practice good hand washing

      l. Rinse droppers and spray bottles after each use to avoid contamination

B. Expectorants

   1. Action and use

      a. **Expectorants** increase fluid flow in the respiratory tract and reduce viscosity of secretions to aid in removal of secretions by cough reflex and ciliary action

b. They are used for relief of nonproductive cough associated with the common cold, bronchitis, laryngitis, and influenza; they also thin secretions

c. Guaifenesin (glyceryl guaiacolate) (Robitussin, Guiatuss, Humibid, and others): most common oral expectorant

2. Common medications (Table 14-8)

3. Administration considerations

a. Use with caution in the elderly or debilitated clients

b. Use with caution in clients with asthma and respiratory insufficiency

c. Not used as commonly as in the past because of questionable effectiveness

4. Contraindications: iodide expectorants are contraindicated in clients with thyroid problems because of the potential for altered thyroid function

5. Significant drug interactions: iodinated products may produce hypothyroid effects when given with lithium

6. Significant food interactions: none significant

7. Significant laboratory studies: guaifenesin may interfere with results of color tests for 5-hydroxyindoleacetic acid and vanillylmandelic acid

8. Side effects

a. Nausea, vomiting, and gastric irritation

b. Rash

9. Adverse effects/toxicity

a. CNS: dizziness and headache

b. GI: nausea and vomiting

c. Skin: rash

10. Nursing considerations: ask client about current medications (including OTC and herbal products) and history of any allergies

Table 14-8 Expectorants	Generic/Trade Name	Usual Adult Dose	Side Effects	Nursing Implications
	Guaifenesin (Robitussin)	200–400 mg q 4 hrs (dose should be cut in half for children)	Dizziness Headache Nausea Diarrhea Stomach pain Vomiting	Assess respiratory status to evaluate effectiveness of medication. Increase fluid intake to assist with liquefying secretions. Sustained release tablets should not be crushed or chewed.
	Potassium iodide (Pima syrup)	300–650 mg B.I.D. or T.I.D. after meals	Rash Urticaria	Instruct client on effective coughing. Avoid driving due to the potential for dizziness. Contact health care professional if cough persists longer than one week.
	Terpin hydrate elixir	85–170 mg T.I.D. to Q.I.D.		

Respiratory System Medications **563**

11. Client education

    a. Take medications exactly as prescribed

    b. Be aware of potential side effects

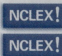

    c. Do not operate heavy machinery while taking this medication

    d. Do not use alcohol or other CNS depressants while taking this medication

    e. Report a fever or cough to physician if it lasts longer than a week

    f. Increase fluid intake if not contraindicated by other disease processes

    g. Avoid smoking as this increases secretions and decreases ciliary action

    h. Avoid drinking fluids for 30 minutes after taking this medication

    i. Take iodide preparations with fruit juice or milk to decrease the bitter taste

C. Antitussives

1. Action and use

    a. **Opioid** (narcotic) and nonopioid **antitussives** suppress the cough reflex by directly affecting the cough center; nonopioid antitussives do this without the CNS suppression of the opioid antitussives

    b. Peripherally acting agents (glycerin, ammonium chloride) have local anesthetic effects to decrease irritation of the pharyngeal mucosa; they are available in gargles, lozenges, and syrups; lozenges increase saliva flow and therefore suppress the cough

    c. They are used to stop a nonproductive cough or a dry, hacking, and nonproductive cough that interferes with rest and sleep

2. Common medications (Table 14-9)

3. Administration considerations

    a. There is a potential for addiction and CNS and respiratory depression with opioid antitussives

    b. Most antitussives are given in a liquid form or as oral tablets

    c. Antitussives in syrup form may soothe irritated mucosa in the pharynx

    d. Dextromethorphan is preferred over codeine as it provides desired effect without use of opioids; dextromethorphan is available in many OTC products and does not require a prescription

4. Contraindications

    a. Dextromethorphan is contraindicated if client has asthma, emphysema, or consistent headaches

    b. Hypersensitivity

    c. Codeine preparations are contraindicated in clients with respiratory depression, increased intracranial pressure, severe liver or renal disease, hypothyroidism, adrenal insufficiency, or seizure disorders

    d. Cautious use of non-opioid agents is recommended for clients with seizure disorders, hypotension, glaucoma, and prostatic hyperplasia

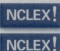

Table 14-9	Generic/Trade Name	Usual Adult Dose	Side Effects	Nursing Implications
Antitussive Medications	Nonopioid antitussives:		Dizziness Headache Drowsiness	Assess for inability to cough effectively from too much cough suppression. Assess for side effects.
	Benzonatate (Tessalon Perles)	100 mg TID up to 600 mg/day	Sedation Nausea & vomiting Constipation	Cough may be a useful diagnostic tool and protective for the client, therefore, antitussives should be used only for an
	Dextro-methorphan (Robitussin DM, others)	10–30 mg every 4–8 hr up to 120 mg/day	Nasal congestion Dry mouth Urinary retention	irritating, nonproductive, ineffective cough. Teach client not to operate heavy machinery while taking this medication.
	Opioid antitussives:		Can exhibit the above side effects in addition to:	The significant difference in the nursing implications for the opioid antitussives is the potential for respiratory depres-
	Dimetane-DC, Tussar SF, Novahistine DH, Robitussin AC	10–30 mg every 4–8 hr	Hypotension Bradycardia Respiratory depression	sion and drug dependence. These medications should be used with caution especially in the elderly client.

5. Significant drug interactions

   a. Opioid antitussives may potentiate the action of sedating drugs such as anesthetic agents, tranquilizers, hypnotics, alcohol, MAO inhibitors, and tricyclic antidepressants

   b. Dextromethorphan should not be given with MAO inhibitors

   c. Avoid use of dextromethorphan with selegiline because of risk of confusion, coma, and hyperpyrexia

   d. Medications that increase antitussive effects of codeine include CNS depressants such as alcohol, anti-anxiety agents, barbiturates, and sedative hypnotics

6. Significant food interactions: use of parsley and dextromethorphan can produce serotonin syndrome

7. Significant laboratory studies: none significant

8. Side effects

   a. Dizziness, headache, drowsiness or sedation, nausea, vomiting, constipation, pruritus, nasal congestion, dry mouth, blurred vision, and sweating

   b. Dependence and respiratory depression with codeine

   c. Dry mouth, palpitations, thickened respiratory mucus, anorexia, urinary retention or frequency, diarrhea, photosensitivity, and dysuria with non-opioids

    d. Nasal congestion and burning of the eyes with benzonatate

  9. Adverse effects/toxicity

NCLEX!

    a. Opioid agents: hypotension, bradycardia, and respiratory depression

    b. CNS: dizziness, headache, and sedation

    c. GI: nausea, constipation, and GI upset

  10. Nursing considerations

NCLEX!

    a. Ask client about current medications (including OTC and herbal products) and history of any allergies

    b. Assess for inability to cough effectively from excessive cough suppression

    c. Observe for listed side effects and potential drug dependence

    d. Cough may be a useful diagnostic tool and protective measure for the client; therefore, antitussives should be used only cautiously for irritating, nonproductive and ineffective cough

  11. Client education

NCLEX!

    a. Take medication exactly as prescribed

    b. Be aware of potential side effects

    c. Do not operate heavy machinery while using these types of medications

    d. Avoid alcohol and other CNS depressants while taking these medications

    e. Notify physician if client has a cough that lasts longer than a week, a persistent headache, fever, or rash

    f. Do not drink liquids for 30 to 35 minutes after taking a chewable tablet or a lozenge

    g. Avoid smoking because it increases secretions and decreases ciliary action

    h. For excessive respiratory secretions, teach client coughing, deep breathing, and benefits of ambulation

    i. Liquefy secretions with increased oral intake up to 2000 to 3000 mL/day unless contraindicated

D. Mucolytics

  1. Action and use

    a. Mucolytics are administered by inhalation to liquefy (thin) mucus in the respiratory tract

    b. They are used with sinusitis and the common cold

    c. Aid in the removal of viscous secretions

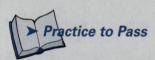

➤ Practice to Pass

An 80-year-old client is admitted to the hospital. She is lethargic with a respiratory rate of 8 per minute and cyanosis around the lips. When questioning the daughter, she tells the nurse that her mother has had a nonproductive cough for about 2 weeks and has been taking Dimetane-DC. What are the appropriate nursing actions?

Table 14-10	**Generic/Trade Name**	**Usual Adult Dose**	**Side Effects**	**Nursing Implications**
Mucolytic Medications	Sodium chloride solution by nebulization Acetylcysteine (Mucomyst) (nebulizer)	Mucomyst Nebulization, 1–10 mL of 20% solution every 2–4 h	Oral irritation Sore throat Cough Nausea Vomiting Headaches Bronchospasm	Determine current medications and allergies. Usually given with bronchodilators as may cause bronchospasm. Be prepared to suction client if cough is ineffective. Rinse mouth after therapy to avoid oropharyngeal irritation.
	Dornase alfa (rhDNAse; Pulmozyme) (a proteolytic enzyme) (for clients with cystic fibrosis only)	2.5 mg daily via nebulizer (adults and children age 5 and older)		Discard unused medication after four days. Increase fluid intake to thin secretions. Teach client to avoid smoking as this increases secretions and decreases ciliary action.

d. An oral form of acetylcysteine (Mucomyst) can be used to treat acetaminophen overdose

2. Common medications (Table 14-10)

3. Administration considerations

   a. Not used as commonly anymore because of questionable effectiveness

   b. These drugs are nebulized using a face mask or a mouth piece; can be instilled into a tracheostomy

   c. Acetylcysteine is effective one minute after inhalation; maximal effect is in 5 to 10 minutes

   d. Acetylcysteine is effective immediately after direct instillation

4. Contraindications

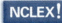

   a. Use with caution for asthmatic clients

   b. Proteolytic enzymes are contraindicated in asthmatic clients due to allergy potential

   c. Contraindicated in client with hypersensitivity to these agents

5. Significant drug interactions

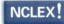

   a. Activated charcoal limits the effectiveness of acetylcysteine

   b. Mucomyst is incompatible with tetracyclines, erythromycin, lactobionate, amphotericin B, and ampicillin sodium

    6. Significant food interactions: none significant

    7. Significant laboratory studies: none significant

    8. Side effects

        a. Oral irritation and sore throat

        b. Cough

        c. Nausea and vomiting

        d. Headaches

    9. Adverse effects/toxicity: bronchospasm

  10. Nursing considerations

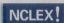

        a. Ask client about current medications (including OTC and herbal products) and history of any allergies

        b. Administer medications as prescribed

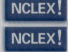

        c. May cause bronchospasm and are usually given with bronchodilators

        d. Suction client if cough is ineffective

        e. Rinse mouth after therapy to decrease oropharyngeal irritation

        f. Discard unused medication after four days

  11. Client education

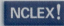

        a. Take medication exactly as prescribed

        b. Be aware of potential side effects

        c. Increase fluid intake unless contraindicated by other disease processes

        d. Avoid smoking as this increases secretions and decreases ciliary action

VII. Oxygen

A. Indications

    1. **Hypoxia,** deficiency of oxygen (O_2) in the cells and tissues, and **hypoxemia,** deficiency of O_2 in the arterial blood, are indications for the use of supplemental oxygen

    2. Some conditions in which O_2 therapy is indicated include conditions associated with decreased arterial PO_2 levels (pulmonary edema), decreased cardiac output (myocardial infarction), decreased blood oxygen-carrying capacity (anemia), and increased O_2 demand (sepsis, sustained fever)

B. Types of delivery systems

    1. Nasal cannula (nasal prongs): the most common form of O_2 delivery

    a. Two prongs go into the nostrils and tubing attaches to the oxygen source and the flowmeter

    b. Client can eat and talk with a nasal cannula

    c. Oxygen can be administered at a rate ranging from 1 L/min to 6 L/min

    d. Dryness of mucous membranes can occur

2. Nasal catheter: inserted into the throat through a nostril and should be changed to the other nostril every 8 hours; not used frequently because of client discomfort; gastric distention sometimes occurs

3. Oxymizer: a nasal cannula with a reservoir that can deliver higher concentrations of O_2 than a regular cannula without the use of a mask; delivers approximately twice the amount of O_2 of a regular cannula

4. Face mask: a mask that fits over the client's mouth and nose

    a. Simple face mask: flow rate is 5 to 10 L/min with O_2 delivery capabilities of 40 to 60%

    b. Partial rebreather mask: consists of a face mask with a reservoir bag; some of the air client exhales goes into the reservoir bag and is mixed with 100% O_2 for the next inhalation; this system permits the conservation of O_2 and can deliver 70 to 90% O_2 at rates of 6 to 15 L/min

    c. Non-rebreather mask: delivers the highest concentration of O_2 by mask; no exhaled air goes into the reservoir bag; the reservoir bag contains O_2, which client breathes in with inspiration; exhaled air goes out through the side vents and can deliver 60 to 100% O_2 at flow rates of 6 to 15 L/min

    d. Venturi mask: the percentage of O_2 to be administered is adjusted by a dial at the end of the mask; amount of air pulled into the system varies with the needed amount of O_2 gives precise oxygen concentrations

C. Oxygen toxicity

1. Lung tissue can be damaged from prolonged exposure to high O_2 concentrations; the exact amount of O_2 and length of time required to cause O_2 toxicity varies with different clients depending on the degree of underlying lung disease; some sources say that lung damage can occur with O_2 delivery of greater than 50% for longer than 24 to 48 hours

2. Atelectasis or alveolar collapse can result with O_2 administration at rates of 60% for more than 36 hours or 90% for more than 6 hours

3. Adult respiratory distress syndrome (ARDS) can result from breathing 80 to 100% oxygen for longer than 24 hours

4. Symptoms of O_2 toxicity begin as a nonproductive cough, substernal chest pain, gastrointestinal upset, and dyspnea; as it worsens, the client develops decreased vital capacity, decreased lung compliance, and hypoxemia; atelectasis, pulmonary edema, and pulmonary hemorrhage can result if the problem is not reversed

5. Oxygen should be weaned as soon as possible and according to the client's SaO_2 level

D. Administration and nursing considerations

1. Oxygen therapy can be anxiety-provoking; provide sufficient explanation and allow client to express anxieties

2. Flow rate is measured in liters per minute; it is a measure of the amount of O_2 delivered but is not completely accurate, because there is loss of O_2 content with leaking and mixing with room air

3. Oxygen analyzers are available to measure the amount of O_2 the client inhales, and this is recommended every 4 hours to provide precise measurement of the percentage of O_2 client is receiving

4. Clients with COPD should not receive O_2 at high percentages because higher levels of O_2 in the bloodstream can cause hypoventilation; a COPD client's drive to breathe is from low levels of O_2 tension; a client with COPD can usually tolerate a rate of up to 2 L/min by nasal cannula

5. Check O_2 delivery system frequently to ensure proper functioning

6. Oxygen should be humidified when the client is receiving the O_2 at a rate higher than 2 L/min

7. A face mask should fit the client's face to avoid unnecessary leakage of O_2; if the mask is too snug, skin irritation can occur

8. Masks can be replaced with a nasal cannula during mealtime with a physician's order

9. The reservoir bag on a partial rebreather should deflate slightly with inspiration

10. Provide reassurance if client becomes claustrophobic

11. The flaps on the side of the nonrebreather mask should be open during expiration and closed during inhalation

12. Monitor SaO_2 with pulse oximeter during oxygen administration; with physician order, O_2 may be titrated to achieve the desired SaO_2 level

13. Assess for signs and symptoms of hypoxia and respiratory distress; also assess for changes in vital signs and color changes

14. Monitor arterial blood gases (ABGs) per physician order

15. Normal arterial O_2 levels decrease with age

16. Provide oral care for client comfort because of the potential for drying of mucous membranes

17. Identify clients at high risk for the development of O_2 toxicity

E. Client education

1. Prepare client for the noise that occurs with the flow of O_2

NCLEX!

NCLEX!

NCLEX!

NCLEX!

2. Avoid open flames with O_2 administration due to the flammable nature of O_2

3. Ensure there are not frayed electrical cords near the O_2 so there is no chance of a spark causing combustion

4. Smoking is prohibited when O_2 therapy is being utilized

5. Inform client that O_2 delivery can cause dryness of the mouth and nasal mucosa

6. Remove O_2 when client uses an electric razor

7. Continue O_2 therapy at home as prescribed by physician

8. Keep O_2 tank in the holder and away from direct sunlight to reduce effects of heat

9. Instruct client signs of hypoxia and to report them to physician

---

Case Study

R. C. is a 14-year-old girl with newly diagnosed asthma. She will be using albuterol (Ventolin) and beclomethasone (Beclovent) inhalers. You are the nurse working in the doctor's office where R. C. comes for her check-ups.

❶ What teaching does R. C. need about albuterol?

❷ What teaching does R. C. need about beclomethasone?

❸ What developmental issues related to a newly diagnosed illness should you anticipate, and how will you respond?

❹ What are the anticipated effects and the side effects of the medications?

❺ What assessment will you do when R. C. comes for office visits to assess how she is dealing with her disease and its treatment?

For suggested responses, see pages 641–642.

Posttest

1 A 6-year-old child with asthma is being treated with metaproterenol (Alupent). The mother informs the nurse that she has been using the medication more frequently lately because the child's symptoms have worsened. For what potential side effects should the nurse monitor the client?

(1) Nervousness and tachycardia
(2) Lethargy and bradycardia
(3) Decreased blood pressure and dizziness
(4) Increased blood pressure and fatigue

2 The nurse is teaching a client about salmeterol (Serevent) that is to be used at home. Which statement indicates that the client has understood the teaching?

(1) "I will use this medication every 6 hours."
(2) "I will take a dose of this medicine when I notice I am wheezing."
(3) "I know this medicine commonly causes increased heart rate."
(4) "This medicine is to keep me from having an attack, not to stop one that has started."

3 A client takes oxtriphylline (Choledyl) for chronic obstructive pulmonary disease (COPD). Which explanation by the nurse correctly teaches the client the rationale for taking this medication?

(1) "The medicine increases your heart rate to help with blood flow."
(2) "The medicine helps your heart beat stronger and get more blood to the lungs."
(3) "The medicine is used to dilate your airways and make it easier for you to breathe."
(4) "The medicine thins the secretions in your lungs and makes it easier for you to cough."

4 A client is to be started on theophylline (Theo-Dur). The nurse should plan to consult the physician about changing the order if the client has which of the following conditions?

(1) Hypothyroidism
(2) Bradycardia
(3) Hyperthyroidism
(4) Sick sinus syndrome

5 A client is admitted to the hospital with an exacerbation of chronic obstructive pulmonary disease (COPD). Triamcinolone acetomide (Azmacort) is one of the home medications. Dexamethasone (Decadron) is added intravenously in the hospital. The nurse should anticipate which of the following because of interaction of these two medications?

(1) An increase in the Azmacort
(2) A higher dose of Decadron
(3) An increase in the symptoms with administration of the two drugs
(4) A smaller dose of Azmacort and/or Decadron

6 The nurse should question an order for fluticasone aerosol (Flovent) when a client has which condition?

(1) Acquired immunodeficiency syndrome (AIDS)
(2) Asthma
(3) Coronary artery disease (CAD)
(4) Chronic obstructive pulmonary disease (COPD)

7 Which statement by the client indicates teaching has been effective about the administration of nedocromil (Tilade)?

(1) "I will take this medication only during an acute attack."
(2) "I may have to increase my dose of beclomethasone (Beclovent) after I start taking this medication."
(3) "I will take this medication daily regardless of whether or not I experience symptoms."
(4) "I should see therapeutic effects of this medication as soon as I begin taking it."

8 A nurse is doing an admission history on a client who takes zileuton (Zyflo). Which manifestation noted during the initial assessment would the nurse conclude is most likely a side effect of the medication?

(1) Lethargy
(2) Constipation
(3) Headaches
(4) Diarrhea

9 An 80-year-old client who complains of nausea is given promethazine (Phenergan) 12.5 mg intravenously. Which safety measure should the nurse institute?

(1) Provide the client with no-skid slippers for ambulation.
(2) Show the client the emergency cord in the bathroom and give instructions for use.
(3) Put a chair next to the client's bed to make it easier for her to get herself out of bed.
(4) Keep the client in bed with the side rails up.

10 The nurse informs the client that oxymetazoline (Afrin) should not be utilized if the client has which of the following conditions?

(1) Hypotension
(2) Hypertension
(3) Hypothyroidism
(4) Emphysema

See page 573 for Answers and Rationales.

Answers and Rationales

Pretest

1 **Answer: 1** *Rationale:* The symptoms of an acute asthma attack are related to constriction of the airway. The medication is a beta-adrenergic agent administered to dilate the airway. Option 2 is a side effect of the medication but is not the intended effect. Options 3 and 4 are incorrect because bradycardia and bronchoconstriction are the opposites of the expected side effect and intended effect, respectively.
Cognitive Level: Application
Nursing Process: Evaluation; *Test Plan:* PHYS

2 **Answer: 2** *Rationale:* Adrenergic agents are contraindicated for clients with cardiovascular disease because of the potential to increase myocardial oxygen demand. Epinephrine would raise the heart rate and blood pressure but may decrease oxygenation of the myocardium for the client with cardiovascular disease. Asthma (option 1), hypotension (option 3) and bradycardia (option 4) are not contraindications for use of epinephrine (Primatene).
Cognitive Level: Analysis
Nursing Process: Planning; *Test Plan:* SECE

3 **Answer: 4** *Rationale:* Caffeine in coffee or tea can have an additive effect with theophylline, and therefore coffee should be eliminated from the meal tray. Peas (option 1), beans (option 2), and milk (option 3) are not problematic because they do not contain caffeine.
Cognitive Level: Application
Nursing Process: Planning; *Test Plan:* PHYS

4 **Answer: 3** *Rationale:* A potential side effect of an inhaled corticosteroid is oral fungal infection. It would be therapeutic to have a decrease in audible wheezes (option 1). Inhaled corticosteroids can cause dry mouth (option 2) and with less respiratory effort from effective therapy, the nurse should anticipate a decreased respiratory rate (option 4).
Cognitive Level Analysis
Nursing Process Assessment; *Test Plan:* PHYS

5 **Answer: 2** *Rationale:* Bitolterol is an adrenergic bronchodilator that is effective to provide bronchodilation in an acute asthma attack. Aminophylline (option 1) is a xanthine, triamcinolone (option 3) is an inhaled corticosteroid, and cromolyn (option 4) is an inhaled nonsteroidal. All three of these agents can be used with asthma; however, they are not effective during an acute attack.
Cognitive Level: Analysis
Nursing Process: Analysis; *Test Plan:* PHYS

6 **Answer: 2** *Rationale:* Zafirlukast is a leukotriene modifier. This is a newer class of medications for the prophylaxis and chronic treatment of asthma. Because they are not to be used during an acute attack, this response indicates that the client needs more teaching. Fluid intake should increase to liquefy secretions and assist the client with expectoration. This medication should be taken one hour before meals or two hours after meals. It does take a few weeks of medication administration for the client to begin to see positive results.
Cognitive Level: Analysis
Nursing Process: Evaluation; *Test Plan:* PHYS

7 **Answer: 4** *Rationale:* Claritin should be taken on an empty stomach to increase absorption. It is a second-generation antihistamine and does not cause drowsiness like the first-generation medications (option 1). It has a rapid onset of action (option 2) and is not effective in an acute asthma attack (option 3).
Cognitive Level: Application
Nursing Process: Implementation; *Test Plan:* PHYS

8 **Answer: 2** *Rationale:* Cardiovascular side effects are possible with the administration of decongestants. If the client develops these symptoms, the medication should be discontinued and the physician notified. Oral agents should be used for long-term therapy (option 1). Rebound congestion (option 4) is more likely with nasal spray decongestants. Often, decongestants cause a dry mouth (option 3), but the client should use hard sugarless candy rather than discontinue the medication.
Cognitive Level: Application
Nursing Process: Implementation; *Test Plan:* PHYS

9 **Answer: 1** *Rationale:* Guaifenesin is an expectorant. Potential side effects are nausea, vomiting, gastric irritation, rash, dizziness, and headache. It does not cause hypertension (option 2), hypotension (option 3), or urinary retention (option 4).
Cognitive Level: Application
Nursing Process: Implementation; *Test Plan:* PHYS

10 **Answer: 3** *Rationale:* A non-rebreather mask should have flaps on the sides that are open during expiration and closed on inspiration. The idea is for the client to breathe in oxygen and not the expired carbon dioxide. If the flaps are missing, the client needs a new mask. The nurse should not change the oxygen order (option 2) and it is unnecessary to call the physician (option 4).
Cognitive Level: Application
Nursing Process: Implementation; *Test Plan:* PHYS

Posttest

1 **Answer: 1** *Rationale:* Potential side effects with this medication are stimulation of the central nervous system (CNS) and the cardiovascular (CV) system. Metaproterenol is a beta 2 stimulant and these effects are not as likely, but with increased doses, they may occur, especially in a 6-year-old child. Lethargy and bradycardia (option 2), decreased blood pressure (option 3), and fatigue (option 4) are not consistent with either CNS or CV stimulation.
Cognitive Level: Application
Nursing Process: Assessment; *Test Plan:* PHYS

2 **Answer: 4** *Rationale* Use of salmeterol is prophylactic, not for an acute attack. Salmeterol is predominately a beta 2 stimulant and therefore does not frequently cause tachycardia (option 3). It takes 20 minutes for onset of action and is used for prophylaxis, not treatment of acute attack (option 2). It is dosed every 12 hours because of a 12-hour duration of action (option 1).
Cognitive Level: Application
Nursing Process: Evaluation; *Test Plan:* PHYS

3 **Answer: 3** *Rationale:* Oxtriphylline is a xanthine bronchodilator, and the mechanism of action is to increase the amount of cyclic adenosine monophosphate (cAMP), which leads to bronchial dilation because of relaxation of smooth muscle. Xanthines can increase heart rate and force of myocardial contraction, but that is not the rationale for the administration of the medication.
Cognitive Level: Application
Nursing Process: Evaluation; *Test Plan:* PHYS

4 **Answer: 3** *Rationale:* Theophylline is contraindicated in clients with hyperthyroidism as the disease can be exacerbated. It is also contraindicated in clients with tachydysrhythmias. Options 2 and 4 result in low heart rates and are therefore incorrect.
Cognitive Level: Analysis
Nursing Process: Planning, *Test Plan:* PHYS

5 **Answer: 4** *Rationale:* When both an inhaled and systemic corticosteroid are used, a decrease in the dose of one or the other medication may be appropriate due to the additive effect of local and systemic corticosteroids. Options 1 and 2 are incorrect because they indicate increased doses, while option 3 is incorrect because the symptoms should decrease rather than increase.
Cognitive Level: Application
Nursing Process: Analysis; *Test Plan:* PHYS

6 **Answer: 1** *Rationale:* Administration of corticosteroids such as fluticasone suppresses the immune system and the administration of these drugs is contraindicated in clients with suppressed immune systems (as in AIDS). Fluticasone may be helpful with asthma (option 2) and COPD (option 4). It is not contraindicated with CAD (option 3), although it may be used cautiously because of possible fluid retention.
Cognitive Level: Analysis
Nursing Process: Analysis; *Test Plan:* PHYS

7 **Answer: 3** *Rationale:* Necrodomil should be used as ordered even if no symptoms are noted. This medication is used for the prophylaxis of asthma, not during an acute attack (option 1). It is possible that a decreased amount of bronchodilator and/or inhaled corticosteroid may be needed after starting this medication (not increased as in option 2), but this is not certain. It can take 3 weeks of daily dosing prior to seeing therapeutic effects (option 4).
Cognitive Level: Application
Nursing Process: Evaluation; *Test Plan:* PHYS

8 **Answer: 3** *Rationale:* Zileuton is a leukotriene modifier that blocks production of leukotriene and thereby reduces inflammation. Side effects of zileuton include headaches, dyspepsia, nausea, dizziness, and insomnia. They do not include lethargy (option 1), constipation (option 2), or diarrhea (option 4), although zafirkulast, another leukotriene modifier, may cause nausea and diarrhea.
Cognitive Level: Application
Nursing Process: Assessment; *Test Plan:* PHYS

9 **Answer: 4** *Rationale:* Promethazine is a traditional antihistamine that causes profound drowsiness because it works centrally as well as peripherally. It can cause central nervous system depression or stimulation. The client should be kept in bed with the side rails up until the effects of the drug wear off to promote client safety. The effects are heightened by the client's age. The actions in options 1, 2, and 3 provide a lower margin of safety for the client.
Cognitive Level: Analysis
Nursing Process: Implementation; *Test Plan:* SECE

10 **Answer: 2** *Rationale:* Afrin is a topical decongestant and an adrenergic agent that promotes nasal decongestion by vasoconstriction. Adrenergic decongestants are contraindicated for the client with hypertension and coronary artery disease. Contraindications do not include hypotension (option 1), hypothyroidism (option 3), or emphysema (option 4).
Cognitive Level: Application
Nursing Process: Implementation; *Test Plan:* PHYS

References

Abrams, A. (2004). *Clinical drug therapy: Rationales for nursing practice* (7th ed.). Philadelphia: Lippincott, Williams and Wilkins, pp. 255–740.

Ball, J., & Bindler, R. (2003). *Pediatric nursing: Caring for children* (3rd ed.). Stamford, CT: Appleton and Lange, pp. 406–455.

Deglin, J., & Vallerand, A. (2003). *Davis's drug guide for nurses* (9th ed.). Philadelphia, PA: F. A. Davis, pp. 839–841.

Elkin, M., Perry, A., & Potter, P. (2000). *Nursing interventions and clinical skills* (2nd ed.). St. Louis, MO: Mosby, Inc., pp. 727–734.

Kozier, B., Erb, G., Berman, A., & Burke, K. (2003). *Fundamentals of nursing: Concepts, process, and practice* (7th ed.). Upper Saddle River, NJ: Prentice-Hall, Inc., pp. 1248–1282.

Lehne, R. (2004). *Pharmacology for nursing care* (5th ed.). St. Louis, MO: Mosby, pp. 796–819.

LeMone, P., & Burke, K. (2003). *Medical surgical nursing: Critical thinking in client care* (3rd ed.). Upper Saddle River, NJ: Prentice-Hall, Inc., pp. 1325–1508.

Lilley, L., & Aucker, R. (2002). *Pharmacology and the nursing process* (3rd ed.). St. Louis, MO: Mosby, Inc., pp. 456–491.

McKenry, L. & Salerno, G. (2003). *Mosby's pharmacology in nursing* (21st ed. revised reprint). St. Louis, MO: Mosby, pp. 703–746.

Phipps, W. (1999). "*Management of persons with problems of the lower airway.*" In W. Phipps, J. Sands, & J. Marek (Eds.). *Medical surgical nursing: Concepts and clinical action.* St. Louis, MO: Mosby, Inc., pp. 922–1004.

Phipps, W. (1999). "*Management of persons with problems of the upper airway.*" In W. Phipps, J. Sands, & J. Marek (Eds.). *Medical surgical nursing: Concepts and clinical action.* St. Louis, MO: Mosby, Inc., pp. 865–867.

Smeltzer, S., & Bare, B. (2003). *Textbook of medical-surgical nursing* (10th ed.). Philadelphia: Lippincott, William & Wilkins, pp. 464.

Tierney, L., McPhee, S., & Papadakis, M. (2002). *2002 Current medical diagnosis & treatment* (41st ed.). New York: The McGraw-Hill Companies, Inc., pp. 1641–1642.

CHAPTER 15

Visual and Auditory Medications

Joseann Helmes DeWitt, RN, MSN, C, CLNC

OBJECTIVES

▌ Describe general goals of therapy when administering visual or auditory medications.

▌ Describe actions and uses of mydriatic, miotic, and cycloplegic medications.

▌ Discuss the mechanism of action of medications used to treat glaucoma.

▌ Describe drug-induced ototoxicity.

▌ Identify medications that cause ototoxicity.

▌ Identify correct procedures for administering visual and auditory medications.

▌ List significant client education points related to administering visual or auditory medications.

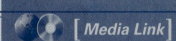

[Media Link]

Use the CD-ROM enclosed with this text, or log onto the address given to access the free, interactive Companion Website created for this series. The CD-ROM and Companion Website accompanying this book offer additional practice opportunities and information—NCLEX Review, Case Studies, Glossary, In Depth with NCLEX, and more.

www.prenhall.com/hogan

REVIEW AT A GLANCE

aqueous humor *fluid formed by the ciliary body; contained in the anterior and posterior chambers of the eye; bathes and feeds posterior surface of the cornea, lens, and iris*

cerumen *substance secreted by the glands at the outer third of the ear canal; if accumulated, may cause obstruction of the ear canal; also called "ear wax"*

cornea *protective anterior covering of the eye; normally is transparent and allows light to enter*

cycloplegia *paralysis of ciliary muscle*

external ear *the outer ear (pinna) and the external auditory canal*

intraocular pressure *pressure within the eye*

keratitis *inflammation of the cornea; usually caused by trauma, microorganisms, or immune-mediated responses*

miosis *constriction of pupils caused by contraction of the sphincter muscle alone or in combination with relaxation of the dilator muscle*

mydriasis *dilation of pupils caused by contraction of dilator muscle and relaxation of the sphincter muscle*

narrow-angle glaucoma *an acute form of glaucoma characterized by increased intraocular pressure caused by an impairment in the rate of outflow of aqueous humor, also called angle-closure or closed angle glaucoma*

open-angle glaucoma *a chronic form of glaucoma that leads to a change in the appearance of the optic disk and results in visual loss as the cup of the disk becomes enlarged; increased intraocular pressure may or may not be associated with this*

disorder; open-angle glaucoma is the most common type of glaucoma

photophobia *intolerance to light*

systemic absorption *entry of drug into the body and circulating fluids*

tonometry *a measurement of tension, such as intraocular tension or pressure; used to detect glaucoma*

tympanic membrane *the thin partition of transparent tissue between the external auditory canal and the middle ear*

uveitis *an intraocular inflammatory disorder; may involve the iris, ciliary body, choroids, retina, or cornea*

vertigo *the sensation of moving around in space or spinning, also called "dizziness"*

Pretest

1 Which of the following is the priority in nursing management of the client prior to administering the first dose of an ophthalmic medication?

(1) Assessing the client's understanding of purpose of medication
(2) Assessing the client's eye and vision status
(3) Assessing the client's history of hypersensitivity to medications
(4) Assessing the client's understanding of the action of the medication

2 Which of the following techniques performed by the client demonstrates an understanding of appropriate administration of ophthalmic medications?

(1) Pulls lower lid down and instills medication directly onto the eye.
(2) Pulls lower lid down and instills medication into conjunctival sac.
(3) Pulls lower lid up and instills medication directly onto the eye.
(4) Pulls lower lid up and instills medication into conjunctival sac.

3 The external ear canal of a client with an ear infection is obstructed with edema. Which of the following techniques do you instruct the client to use regarding medication administration?

(1) Insert a gauze ear wick and apply medication to wick.
(2) Wait until swelling subsides before instilling medication.
(3) Request a change in the route of medication.
(4) Insert the dropper past the edematous canal.

4 A client with open-angle glaucoma is being treated with oral acetazolamide (Diamox). Which of the following statements made by the client indicates a need for further teaching?

(1) "I can take the medication with milk."
(2) "I should take the medication in the morning."
(3) "I can mix the medication with alcohol."
(4) "I can crush the tablet and mix it in juice."

5 A client being treated with dorzolamide (Trusopt) as treatment for glaucoma asks for an explanation on how the medication will affect the disease. The nurse's response includes which of the following information about the actions of the medication?

(1) The medication decreases production of aqueous humor.
(2) The medication causes pupil constriction.
(3) The medication increases the production of aqueous humor.
(4) The medication increases the outflow of aqueous humor.

6 A client is describing symptoms experienced since beginning pilocarpine (Isopto Carpine) for treatment of glaucoma. The nurse concludes that which of the following symptoms indicates a side effect from systemic absorption?

(1) Dry mouth
(2) Hypertension
(3) Exacerbation of asthma
(4) Constipation

7 The nurse concludes that an adult client understands proper otic medication administration after observing the client use which of the following techniques for administering an otic solution?

(1) The client pulls the pinna down and back before administering the medication.
(2) The client pulls the pinna up and back before administering the medication.
(3) The client places the dropper into the ear canal before administering the medication.
(4) The client tilts the head towards the affected side before administering the medication.

8 The nurse determines that a client with newly diagnosed glaucoma understands the purpose for the prescribed ophthalmic beta-blocker when which of the following statements is made?

(1) "The medication is given to reduce my intraocular pressure."
(2) "I can stop the medication once my intraocular pressure is normal."
(3) "The medication is given to increase my intraocular pressure."
(4) "This medication is the only treatment available for glaucoma."

9 As a nurse working in an outpatient surgical clinic, which of the following preoperative medications should be questioned for a client with a history of glaucoma?

(1) Atropine (generic)
(2) Diphenhydramine (Benadryl)
(3) Hydroxyzine (Vistaril)
(4) Promethazine (Phenergan)

10 A client who has begun taking brinzolamide (Azopt) indicates understanding of medication instructions when making which of the following statements?

(1) "I will reduce my daily fluid intake."
(2) "I will consume 2 liters of fluid daily."
(3) "I will consume a diet high in sodium."
(4) "I will consume a diet low in potassium."

See pages 600–601 for Answers and Rationales.

I. Medications to Treat Glaucoma

A. Beta-blockers (beta-adrenergic antagonists)

1. Action and use

   a. Decrease production of **aqueous humor** (fluid formed by the ciliary body in the eye)

   b. Reduce **intraocular pressure** (pressure within the eye) in **open-angle glaucoma** (a change in the appearance of the optic disk resulting in visual loss)

        c. Exact mechanism of action is unknown

        d. The most commonly used class of drugs used in management of chronic, primary open-angle glaucoma

   2. Common medications (Table 15-1)

   3. Administration considerations

        a. Available in ophthalmic solution and ophthalmic suspension

        b. Drugs cross placenta, enter breast milk

        c. Use nasolacrimal occlusion to minimize **systemic absorption** (entry of drug into the body and circulating fluids)

        d. Use cautiously in clients with renal failure, diabetes, asthma, and chronic obstructive pulmonary disease (COPD)

        e. Administer with caution to clients receiving cardiovascular agents such as antihypertensives and antiarrhythmics

        f. May mask symptoms of hyperthyroidism

        g. Drug may be β_1 selective (cardiac), β_2 selective (pulmonary), or both β_1 and β_2 selective

        h. Because it is β_1 selective, betaxolol (Betoptic) is usually the drug of choice for clients with pulmonary disease

   4. Contraindications

        a. Hypersensitivity

        b. Sinus bradycardia or second- or third-degree heart block

        c. Cardiogenic shock or congestive heart failure (CHF)

   5. Significant drug interactions

        a. The beta-blocking agents may be absorbed systemically; review the client's current medications to avoid drug–drug interactions; most drug interactions occur as result of systemic absorption

        b. Systemic absorption of ophthalmic beta-blockers increase the effects of insulin, verapamil, prazosin, clonidine, and nonsteroidal anti-inflammatory drugs (NSAIDs)

Table 15-1	Drug Name	Usual Adult Dosage
Beta-Adrenergic Blocking Agents for Ophthalmic Use	Betaxolol (Betoptic)	1 drop of 0.5% solution twice daily or 1 drop of 0.25% suspension twice daily
	Carteolol (Ocupress)	1 drop of 1% solution twice daily
	Levobunolol (Betagan)	1 drop of 0.25% solution once or twice daily or 1 drop of 0.5% solution twice daily
	Metipranolol (OptiPranolol)	1 drop of 0.3% solution twice daily
	Timolol (Timoptic)	1 drop of 0.25% or 0.5% solution once or twice daily

    c. Adverse cardiovascular effects may occur when beta-adrenergic blockers are used in combination with other cardiovascular agents such as antihypertensives and antidysrhythmics

    d. Use of these agents with ophthalmic epinephrine may decrease effectiveness

6. Significant food interactions: none reported

7. Significant laboratory studies: if systemic absorption occurs, glucose or insulin tolerance tests may be affected

8. Side effects

    a. Primarily local reactions: eye irritation, burning, stinging

    b. Rare occurrences of allergic reaction, eye inflammation, **photophobia** (intolerance to light), burning, stinging, pruritis, blurred vision, and rashes

9. Adverse effects/toxicity

    a. Systemic adverse reactions or toxicity affecting the cardiovascular system include bradycardia or tachycardia, CHF, dysrhythmias, hypotension, and edema of lower extremities

    b. Systemic adverse reactions or toxicity affecting respiratory system include wheezing, cough, exacerbation of asthma, and bronchospasm

    c. Systemic adverse reactions or toxicity affecting the central nervous system (CNS) include weakness, ataxia, confusion, and depression

    d. Systemic adverse reactions or toxicity affecting the gastrointestinal (GI) symptom include nausea and vomiting

10. Nursing considerations

    a. Obtain baseline vital signs and neurologic status

    b. Obtain baseline vision and intraocular pressure data

    c. Assess for cardiovascular disease, renal failure, diabetes, lactation, or thyrotoxicosis

    d. Assess for signs and symptoms of hypersensitivity such as burning, itching, redness, and swelling occurring after medication administration

11. Client education

    a. Instruct client with diabetes mellitus that beta-blocking agents may mask symptoms of hypoglycemia

    b. Inform health care provider if surgery is being considered; gradual withdrawal of beta-blocking agent 48 hours before surgery may be required (withdrawal is controversial)

    c. Encourage client to have routine eye examinations and measurement of intraocular pressure

    d. Do not stop medication unless instructed to do so by the health care provider

    e. Report symptoms of breathing difficulty, swelling of extremities, slow heart rate

NCLEX!

NCLEX!

NCLEX!

Box 15-1

Administration of Ophthalmic Medications

Instillation of Eyedrops

- Wash hands
- Cleanse exudates from eye(s) if necessary
- Tilt client's head toward the side of the affected eye
- Gently pull lower eyelid down, have client look up (this forms a "sac")
- Instill drops in the sac formed by lower lid, *not* onto the eye
- Unless specifically indicated otherwise, apply gentle pressure for 30 seconds to 1 minute over the inner canthus next to the nose. This prevents absorption through the tear duct and drainage of the medication
- Unless specifically indicated otherwise, the client should close the eye(s) gently. Avoid squeezing the eye(s) tightly as this forces the medication out

Instillation of Eye Ointment

- Follow the same procedure for instillation of eyedrops except that the ointment is expressed directly into the conjunctival sac from the inner canthus to the outer canthus
- Unless specifically indicated otherwise, the client should close the eye(s) and gently massage the eye(s) to distribute the medication

Note: To avoid contamination and risk of infection, do not touch the dropper or tube to the eye, eyelashes, or any other surface.
Note: Remove contact lenses before instilling ophthalmic medications.

NCLEX!

    f. Instruct client to wear dark glasses and to avoid bright light if photophobia is present

    g. Refer to Box 15-1 for administration of ophthalmic medications

B. Adrenergic medications (adrenergic agonists)

    1. Action and use

        a. Decrease production of aqueous humor

        b. Decrease intraocular pressure

        c. Exact mechanism of action is unknown

        d. Used in management of open-angle glaucoma, often in combination with other drugs

        e. Used in management of glaucoma secondary to **uveitis** (intraocular inflammatory disorder)

        f. Used to produce **mydriasis** (pupil dilation) for ocular examination

        g. Used to produce local hemostasis during eye surgery to control bleeding

    2. Common medications (Table 15-2)

    3. Administration considerations

        a. If epinephrine hydrochloride (Epifrin, Glaucon) is used in conjunction with miotics, instill miotic first

        b. Drugs cross placenta, enter breast milk

Table 15-2	Drug Name	Usual Adult Dosage
Adrenergic Agonist Agents for Ophthalmic Use	Dipivefrin (Propine)	1 drop every 12 hours
	Epinephrine hydrochloride (Epifrin, Glaucon)	1 drop of 0.5–2% solution once or twice daily
	Hydroxyamphetamine (Paredrine)	For dilation: 1 or 2 drops of 1% solution
	Naphazoline (Allerest, Vaso Clear)	OTC: 1 drop of 0.012–0.03% up to four times daily
		RX: 1 drop of 0.1% every 3 to 4 hours as necessary
	Oxymetazoline (OcuClear)	OTC: 1 drop of 0.025% every 6 hours as needed
	Phenylephrine (Neo-Synephrine)	OTC: 1 or 2 drops of 0.12% solution up to 4 times daily as necessary
		RX: 1 drop of 2.5% or 10% solution daily
	Tetrahydrozoline (Murine Plus, Visine)	OTC: 1 or 2 drops of 0.05% solution up to 4 times a day

   c. Do not administer ophthalmic solution that contains precipitates or has turned brown

4. Contraindications

   a. Not for treatment of narrow-angle glaucoma or abraded **cornea** (protective anterior covering of the eye) because pupil dilation will further restrict ocular fluid outflow, precipitating an acute attack of glaucoma

   b. Hypersensitivity to epinephrine and phenylephrine

5. Significant drug interactions

   a. Significant drug interactions are related to systemic absorption of adrenergic agonists

   b. Systemic absorption of adrenergic agonists interfere with actions of beta-blocking agents and some antihypertensive agents

   c. Phenylephrine should not be administered to clients taking monoamine oxide inhibitors (MAOIs)

6. Significant food interactions: none reported

7. Significant laboratory studies: none reported

8. Side effects

   a. Local reactions include eye pain and stinging on initial instillation

   b. CNS side effects include headache, blurred vision, brow ache, photophobia, and difficulty with night vision

   c. Rebound **miosis** (constriction of pupils) may occur with phenylephrine

   d. Elderly clients with cardiac disease may experience blood pressure (BP) elevations with phenylephrine

9. Adverse effects/toxicity: systemic adverse effects are unusual, but may occur especially in clients with cardiovascular disease; symptoms include confusion, tachycardia, hypertension, diaphoresis, and tremors

10. Nursing considerations

   a. Obtain history of allergies or hypersensitivity to specific agents

   b. Obtain baseline vital signs

   c. Obtain baseline vision and intraocular pressure data

   d. Assess cardiac, respiratory, and renal function routinely

 11. Client education

   a. Inform client that drugs may discolor contact lenses

   b. Do not blink for at least 30 seconds after instilling medication

   c. Report a decrease in visual acuity, floating spots, sensitivity to light, eye redness, or headache to health care provider

   d. Refer to Box 15-1 for administration of ophthalmic medications

C. Cholinergic agents (miotics, cholinesterase inhibitors)

 1. Action and use

   a. Increase outflow of aqueous humor, decrease resistance to aqueous flow

   b. Produce miosis

   c. Used in treatment of open-angle and angle-closure glaucoma

   d. Used to facilitate miosis before ophthalmic examination or after ophthalmic surgery

   e. Generally used for clients who fail to respond to first line agents (beta-blockers)

 2. Common medications (Table 15-3)

 3. Administration considerations

   a. Drug crosses placenta, enters breast milk

   b. Do not administer ophthalmic solution that contains precipitates or has turned brown

   c. Pilocarpine can be stored at room temperature

 4. Contraindications

   a. Acute iritis

   b. Conditions in which pupillary constriction is not desirable

 5. Significant drug interactions: concurrent use with beta-adrenergic blocking agents may increase risk of cardiovascular reactions

 6. Significant food interactions: none reported

Table 15-3	Drug Name	Usual Adult Dosage
Cholinergic Agents for Ophthalmic Use	Carbachol (Carboptic)	1 drop of 0.75–3% solution 3 times daily
	Pilocarpine (Isopto Carpine, Pilocar)	1 drop of 0.25–4% solution up to 4 times daily
	Pilocarpine ocular therapeutic system (Ocusert Pilo-20, Ocusert Pilo-40)	As prescribed by health care provider

7. Significant laboratory studies: none reported

8. Side effects

    a. Visual blurring, myopia, irritation, brow pain, and headache

    b. Systemic reactions include abdominal pain, bronchoconstriction, diarrhea, hypotension, nausea, vomiting, diuresis, diaphoresis, exacerbation of asthma

9. Adverse effects/toxicity

    a. Toxic effects produce ataxia, confusion, seizures, coma, respiratory failure, hypotension, and death

    b. Prolonged use of cholinergics may lead to retinal detachments, obstruction of tear drainage, and cataracts

    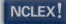

    c. Acute toxicity is reversible by the intravenous (IV) administration of atropine, an anticholinergic agent that is the antidote

10. Nursing considerations

    a. Obtain baseline vital signs and neurologic status

    b. Obtain baseline vision and intraocular pressure data

    c. Assess for cardiovascular disease, renal failure, diabetes, lactation, or thyrotoxicosis

    d. Assess for signs and symptoms of hypersensitivity such as burning, itching, redness, and swelling occurring after medication administration

11. Client education

    a. Difficulty adjusting quickly to changes in illumination may occur as a result of miosis

    b. Refer to Box 15-1 for administration of ophthalmic medications

D. **Carbonic anhydrase inhibitors**

1. Action and use

    a. Are nonbacteriostatic sulfonamides that lower intraocular pressure by decreasing the aqueous production

    b. Exact mechanism of action is unknown

    c. Oral carbonic anhydrase inhibitors are used to treat open-angle, secondary, and angle-closure glaucoma

    d. Ophthalmic carbonic anhydrase inhibitors are used to treat open-angle glaucoma and ocular hypertension

    e. Commonly used preoperatively in intraocular surgery

2. Common medications (Table 15-4)

3. Administration considerations

    a. Oral acetazolamide (Diamox) is administered for maintenance

    b. Intravenous route is used preoperatively or to rapidly reduce increased intraocular pressure

Table 15-4	Drug Name	Usual Adult Dosage	Route
Carbonic Anhydrase Inhibitor Agents	Acetazolamide (Diamox)	Capsules: 500 mg PO twice daily	Oral
		Tablets: 250 mg PO 1 to 4 times daily	Oral
		IV: 500 mg intravenously	Intravenous
	Brinzolamide (Azopt)	1 drop three times daily	Ophthalmic
	Dichlorphenamide (Daranide)	100–200 mg PO initially, followed by 100 mg every 12 hours; maintenance dosage of 25–50 mg 1 to 3 times daily	Oral
	Dorzolamide (Trusopt)	1 drop of 2% solution 3 times daily	Ophthalmic
	Methazolamide (Neptazane)	50–100 mg 2 or 3 times daily	Oral

    c. Give oral form with food or milk to decrease GI side effects

    d. May crush tablets and suspend in liquid

    e. Do not use alcohol or glycerin in administration of drug

    f. To minimize nocturia, schedule doses early in day

    g. Administer with caution to clients with adrenocortical insufficiency

4. Contraindications

    a. Hypersensitivity to antibacterial sulfonamides

    b. Chronic noncongestive angle-closure glaucoma

    c. Hyponatremia, hypokalemia, or other electrolyte imbalances

    d. Hepatic or renal dysfunction

5. Significant drug interactions

    a. Interference with renal excretion of quinidine, salicylates, lithium

    b. Carbonic anhydrase inhibitors decrease excretion of amphetamines, mecamylamine (Inversine), and quinidine, which could result in prolonged duration of drug actions

6. Significant food interactions: none reported

7. Significant laboratory studies

    a. False-positive results in tests for urinary protein

    b. Monitor sodium, potassium, bicarbonate levels for imbalances

8. Side effects

    a. Oral agents: anorexia, diarrhea, diuresis, nausea, vomiting, lethargy, weakness, weight loss, metallic bitter taste, and paresthesia of fingers, hands and toes

    b. Topical agents: topical allergic reaction, photosensitivity, superficial **keratitis** (inflammation of the cornea)

9. Adverse effects/toxicity

    a. Stevens-Johnson syndrome with acetazolamide (Diamox)

   b. Bone marrow depression with acetazolamide

   c. Acidosis

   d. Blood dyscrasias

   e. Hypokalemia

10. Nursing considerations

   a. Potential exacerbation of renal stones; monitor renal function

   b. Monitor for fluid volume depletion related to diuresis

   c. Monitor intake and output (I & O), skin turgor, mucous membranes, and weight

   d. Monitor urinalysis, complete blood cell count (CBC), electrolytes

11. Client education

   a. Unless contraindicated, encourage a diet high in potassium and low in sodium

   b. Unless contraindicated, encourage a fluid intake of at least 2 liters per day to decrease the risk of renal stones

   c. Instruct client to report changes in urine color, rashes, fever

   d. Refer to Box 15-1 for administration of ophthalmic medications

E. Sympathomimetic agents

1. Action and use

   a. Lower intraocular pressure by decreasing aqueous humor production and increasing its outflow

   b. Mechanism of action is unknown

   c. Used in management of open-angle glaucoma

2. Common medications

   a. Dipivefrin (Propine): 1 drop of 0.1% to 0.2% solution once or twice daily to affected eye(s)

   b. Epinephrine: 1 drop of 0.1% to 2% solution once or twice daily

3. Administration considerations

   a. Administer with caution to clients with cardiovascular disease, hypertension, asthma, diabetes mellitus, hyperthyroidism, and parkinsonism

   b. Onset of action for epinephrine is 1 hour; peak effect occurs in 4 to 8 hours

   c. Onset of action for dipivefrin (Propine) is 30 minutes; peak effect in 1 hour

   d. Assess for sensitivity to sulfites

   e. Avoid concurrent use with MAO inhibitors

4. Contraindications

   a. **Narrow-angle glaucoma** (increased intraocular pressure resulting from impairment in the rate of aqueous humor flow)

   b. Predisposition to narrow-angle glaucoma

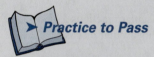

Practice to Pass

A client with open-angle glaucoma is having the medication regimen changed to acetazolamide (Diamox). What important teaching and information do you provide to the client?

5. Significant drug interactions

   a. Ophthalmic beta-blockers

   b. Digitalis

   c. MAO inhibitors

6. Significant food interactions: none reported

7. Significant laboratory studies: none reported

8. Side effects

   a. Local: brow pain, burning, eye irritation, headache, watering eyes, stinging, photophobia

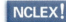

   b. Systemic: hypertension, diaphoresis, tachycardia, palpitation, tremors, light-headedness

9. Adverse effects/toxicity

   a. Tachycardia or hypertension

   b. Systemic absorption may result in adverse cardiovascular reactions and adverse CNS reactions, especially in clients with cardiovascular disease

10. Nursing considerations

   a. Assess vital signs

   b. Obtain baseline intraocular pressure and vision data

   c. Maintain pressure on lacrimal sac for 1 to 2 minutes after instillation of drug to minimize systemic absorption

   d. Obtain heart rate and blood pressure periodically to detect systemic effects

11. Client education

   a. Prolonged use of epinephrine may result in pigment deposits in the conjunctiva

   b. Discuss use of contact lenses with prescriber; use may or may not be permitted

   c. Report symptoms of increased heart rate, heart palpitations, or elevated BP to health care provider

   d. Refer to Box 15-1 for administration of ophthalmic medications

F. Prostaglandin agonist

1. Action and use

   a. Increases aqueous humor outflow

   b. Used in management of open-angle glaucoma and ocular hypertension

2. Common medication: latanoprost (Xalatan), 1 drop in affected eye every evening

3. Administration considerations

   a. Administer 5 minutes apart from other antiglaucoma ophthalmic medications

   b. If pilocarpine (Isopto Carpine) is included in drug regimen, it should be administered 1 hour after administration of prostaglandin agonist

   c. May be used in conjunction with other agents to lower intraocular pressure

4. Contraindications: hypersensitivity to latanoprost or benzalkonium

5. Significant drug interactions: none reported

6. Significant food interactions: none reported

7. Significant laboratory studies: none reported

8. Side effects

    a. Blurred vision, photophobia, burning, stinging, and itching

    b. Longer, thicker, darker eyelashes

9. Adverse effects/toxicity

    a. Conjunctival hyperemia

    b. Increasing iris pigmentation

10. Nursing considerations

    a. Assess for hypersensitivity to latanoprost or benzalkonium chloride

    b. Assess for burning, itching, stinging after initial administration of medication

11. Client education

    a. Drug may cause an increase in iris pigmentation

    b. Do not exceed once-a-day dose

    c. Remove contact lenses before use and for 15 minutes after instillation of medication

    d. Report symptoms of burning, itching, stinging after administration to health care provider

    e. Refer to Box 15-1 for administration of ophthalmic medications

II. Mydriatics and Cycloplegics

A. Anticholinergics

1. Action and use

    a. Produce mydriasis

    b. Produce **cycloplegia** (paralysis of the ciliary muscle)

    c. Used in treatment of ocular pain secondary to inflammatory disorders such as uveitis and keratitis

    d. Used for relaxation of ciliary muscle to improve measurement of refractive errors

    e. Used preoperatively and postoperatively for intraocular surgery

2. Common medications (Table 15-5)

3. Administration considerations

    a. Use with caution in clients with primary glaucoma

    b. Use with caution in clients with predisposition to angle-closure glaucoma

    c. Apply ointment several hours before vision examination

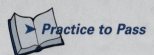

Practice to Pass

A client receiving pilocarpine (Isopto Carpine) ophthalmic solution for glaucoma is prescribed latanoprost (Xalatan) for concurrent therapy with the pilocarpine. What teaching and information do you provide to this client?

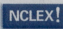
NCLEX!

NCLEX!

NCLEX!

Table 15-5	Drug Name	Usual Adult Dosage
Mydriatic and Cycloplegic Agents for Ophthalmic Use	Atropine sulfate	1 drop of 1% solution
	Cyclopentolate hydrochloride (Cyclogyl)	1 drop of 0.5–2% solution
	Homatropine hydrobromide	1 drop of 2–5% solution
	Scopolamine hydrobromide	1 drop of 0.25% solution
	Tropicamide (Mydriacyl)	1 drop of 1% solution
	Cyclopentolate and phenylephrine (Cyclomydril)	1 drop in each eye every 5 to 10 minutes as needed; do not exceed 3 doses
	Scopolamine and phenylephrine (Murocoll-2)	For mydriasis: 1 to 2 drops in eye, may repeat in 5 minutes if necessary
	Torpicamide and hydroxyamphetamine (Paremyd)	1 to 2 drops into conjunctival sac

   d. Compress lacrimal duct during administration and for 2 to 3 minutes after administration

4. Contraindications

   a. Severe systemic reactions to atropine

   b. Hypersensitivity to anticholinergic drugs

5. Significant drug interactions: results from systemic absorption; decreases effectiveness of phenothiazines and haloperidol

6. Significant food interactions: none reported

7. Significant laboratory studies: none reported

8. Side effects

   a. Local: blurred vision, photophobia, allergic lid reactions

   b. Systemic: confusion, delirium, drowsiness, dry mouth, flushing, and tachycardia

9. Adverse effects/toxicity

   a. Hallucinations, tachycardia, slurred speech, psychiatric and behavioral problems, fever, respiratory depression, coma

   b. Acute glaucoma can be precipitated by pupillary dilation; if not recognized and treated, acute glaucoma can result in blindness

   c. Dry mouth and tachycardia may be symptoms of scopolamine toxicity

10. Nursing considerations

    a. Obtain baseline intraocular pressure and vision status data

    b. Combination drugs produce greater mydriasis

    c. Systemic side effects are more pronounced in infants and children with blond hair and blue eyes

    d. Monitor for tachycardia, confusion, slurred speech, dry mouth, dry skin, weakness, drowsiness

11. Client education

    a. Mydriasis may last from 3 days (scopolamine) to 12 days (atropine)

b. Inform client that blurred vision may occur

c. Wear dark sunglasses and avoid bright light for photophobia

d. Intraocular pressure and vision should be monitored over the course of the therapy

e. Withhold the medication if experiencing tachycardia or dry mouth (symptoms of toxicity)

f. Instruct client to use sugarless hard candy to combat dry mouth

g. Report symptoms of tachycardia and dry mouth to health care provider

h. Refer to Box 15-1 for administration of ophthalmic medications

B. Adrenergics: refer to Section I-B Medications to Treat Glaucoma

III. Anti-inflammatory and Anti-infective Medications for the Eye

A. Nonsteroidal anti-inflammatory drugs (NSAIDs)

1. Action and use

  a. Flurbiprofen (Ocufen) and suprofen (Profenal) are used to inhibit intraoperative miosis

  b. Diclofenac (Voltaren) is used to treat postoperative inflammation after cataract extractions

  c. Ketorolac (Acular) is used to treat conjunctivitis and seasonal allergic ophthalmic pruritis

2. Common medications (Table 15-6)

3. Administration considerations

  a. Systemic effect may be produced if absorbed

  b. NSAIDs have the potential to cause increased bleeding; therefore, clients with increased bleeding tendencies should be monitored closely

4. Contraindications

  a. Sensitivity to aspirin or phenylacetic acid derivatives

  b. Sensitivity to systemic NSAIDs

5. Significant drug interactions: none reported

6. Significant food interactions: none reported

Table 15-6	Drug Name	Usual Adult Dosage
Nonsteroidal Anti-inflammatory Agents for Ophthalmic Use	Diclofenac (Voltaren)	1 drop of 0.1% solution 4 times a day for up to 6 weeks
	Flurbiprofen (Ocufen)	1 drop of 0.03% solution every 30 minutes beginning 2 hours prior to surgery (4 drops total)
	Ketorolac (Acular)	1 drop of 0.5% solution 4 times daily
	Suprofen (Profenal)	2 drops of 1% solution given 3 hours, 2 hours, and 1 hour before surgery; or 2 drops every 4 hours while awake 1 day prior to surgery

7. Significant laboratory studies: potential to cause increased bleeding; monitor CBC and coagulation studies

8. Side effects: local—transient burning or stinging on application, itching, allergic reaction, pain, and redness

9. Adverse effects/toxicity: bleeding

10. Nursing considerations: assess for hypersensitivity symptoms such as burning, itching, redness, and swelling occurring after administration of medication

11. Client education

   a. Inform client that NSAIDs may potentiate bleeding in clients with known bleeding tendencies

   b. Refer to Box 15-1 for administration of ophthalmic medications

B. **Antibacterial, antifungal, and antiviral agents**

1. Action and use

   a. Antibacterial agents are indicated in the management of bacterial infections such as conjunctivitis, blepharitis, keratitis, uveitis, and hordeolum (sty)

   b. Antifungal agents are indicated in the management of fungal blepharitis, conjunctivitis, and keratitis

   c. Antiviral agents are indicated in the management of herpes simplex virus keratitis and herpes simplex virus keratoconjunctivitis

2. Common medications (Table 15-7)

3. Administration considerations

   a. If indicated, obtain culture specimen from eye(s) before administering first dose of medication

   b. Remove exudates from eyes before administering medication

4. Contraindications: hypersensitivity

5. Significant drug interactions

   a. Paraaminobenzoic acid (PABA) reduces the action of sulfonamides (sulfacetamide sodium)

   b. Ophthalmic anesthetics should not be administered within 30 minutes of sulfonamides (sulfacetamide sodium)

   c. Sulfonamides are incompatible with thimerosol and silver preparations

6. Significant food interactions: none reported

7. Significant laboratory studies: monitor CBC count and coagulation studies in clients with potential for bleeding

8. Side effects

   a. Local: dermatitis, itching, stinging, swelling

   b. Systemic: chloramphenicol (Chloroptic) may cause blood dyscrasias

9. Adverse effects/toxicity

   a. Stevens-Johnson Syndrome, systemic lupus erythematosus (SLE) with sulfacetamide sodium

Table 15-7	Drug Name	Usual Adult Dosage
Antibacterial, Antifungal, and Antiviral Agents for Ophthalmic Use	*Antibacterial*	
	Bacitracin (Baciguent)	1 cm of ointment in conjunctival sac every 3 to 4 hours
	Chloramphenicol (Chloroptic)	Thin strip of 1% ointment in conjunctival sac every 3 hours or more as needed
	Ciprofloxacin ophthalmic solution (Ciloxan)	1 drop every 2 hours while awake for 48 hours, then every 4 hours while awake for 5 days
	Erythromycin (Ilotycin ophthalmic ointment)	Thin strip of ointment in conjunctival sac daily or up to 6 times daily as needed
	Gentamicin sulfate (Garamycin)	Thin strip of ointment in conjunctival sac 2 or 3 times daily; one drop of solution every 4 hours
	Norfloxacin ophthalmic solution (Chibroxin)	1 drop four times daily
	Ofloxacin (Ocuflox)	1 drop every 2 to 4 hours while awake for 2 days, then four times daily for up to 5 more days
	Polymyxin B sulfate	1 cm ointment in conjunctival sac every 3 to 4 hours
	Sulfacetamide sodium (Bleph-10 liquifilm, Isopto Cetamide, Sodium Sulamyd)	1 drop every 1 to 3 hours during day, and as prescribed during night hours
	Sulfisoxazole diolamine (Gantrisin)	1 drop every 1 to 3 hours during day, and as prescribed during night hours
	Tobramycin (Tobrex solution and ointment)	1 drop of solution every 4 hours; thin strip of ointment every 8 to 12 hours
	Antiviral	
	Idoxuridine (Stoxil, Herplex)	1 drop of solution every hour during waking hours and every 2 hours during the night
		Ointment is applied in thin strip every 4 hours during the waking hours for a total of 5 times daily
	Tirfluridine (Viroptic)	1 drop of 1% solution in conjunctival sac every 2 hours during waking hours; maximum daily dose is 9 drops
	Vidarabine (Vira-A)	Thin strip of ointment in conjunctival sac every 3 hours, 5 times daily
	Antifungal	
	Natamycin (Natacyn)	For fungal keratitis: 1 drop of 5% solution in the conjunctival sac every 1 to 2 hours for 3 or 4 days, then for 6 to 8 times daily
		For fungal blepharitis and conjunctivitis: 1 drop 4 to 6 times daily

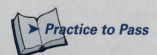

> **Practice to Pass**

A client with an eye infection has crusty drainage in and around the eye. Before administering the prescribed ophthalmic solution, what nursing measures do you implement?

      b. Blood dyscrasias with chloramphenicol

  10. Nursing considerations

      a. Monitor infected eye(s) for pain, drainage, redness, swelling

      b. Monitor for unusual bleeding or bruising with chloramphenicol

      c. Idoxuridine (Stoxil, Herplex) and trifluridine (Viroptic) should be stored in cool place or refrigerated

  11. Client education

      a. Inform health care provider of photosensitivity, redness, or swelling

      b. Inform health care provider of increased drainage, pain, or if no improvement seen within a few days

      c. Refer to Box 15-1 for administration of ophthalmic medications

C. Corticosteroids

1. Action and use: indicated for management of allergic and inflammatory ophthalmic disorders of the conjunctiva, cornea, and anterior segment of the eye

2. Common medications (Table 15-8)

3. Administration considerations

   a. Corticosteroids should be used for short-term treatment only

   b. Use with caution in clients with cataracts and chronic open-angle glaucoma

4. Contraindications: hypersensitivity and corneal abrasion

5. Significant drug interactions: corticosteroids may mask hypersensitivity reactions to other drugs

6. Significant food interactions: none reported

7. Significant laboratory studies: none reported

8. Side effects: local—stinging after application

9. Adverse effects/toxicity: visual disturbances, headache, and eye pain

10. Nursing considerations

   a. Corticosteroids may mask symptoms of infection and hypersensitivity reactions

   b. Corticosteroids may increase susceptibility to infection

11. Client education

   a. Instruct client to avoid use of contact lenses during and for the prescribed time after use of corticosteroid therapy

   b. Do not discontinue the medication without instructions from the prescriber

   c. Encourage client to have eye(s) examined for progress

   d. Refer to Box 15-1 for administration of ophthalmic medications

IV. Anesthetic Medications for the Eye

A. Action and use

1. Prevent initiation and transmission of nerve impulses

2. Used to prevent pain during procedures such as **tonometry** (measurement of intraocular tension, used to detect glaucoma), subconjunctival injections, removal of foreign bodies, and removal of sutures

Table 15-8	Drug Name	Usual Adult Dosage
Common Corticosteroid Agents for Ophthalmic Use	Dexamethasone (Maxidex, Decadron) Fluorometholone (FML S.O.P., FML) Hydrocortisone (Cortamed) Medrysone (HMS Liquifilm) Prednisolone (Pred-Forte, Predair-A)	For all medications: Give drops as prescribed, usually following a dose-frequency reduction schedule of every 3 hours, then every 6 hours, then three times daily, then twice daily, then once daily, then every other day

B. **Common medications**

1. Proparacaine hydrochloride (Alcaine, Ophthaine): 1 to 2 drops of 0.5% solution (single dose) to affected eye(s)

2. Tetracaine hydrochloride (Pontocaine): 1 to 2 drops of 0.5–1.0% solution (single dose) to affected eye(s)

C. **Administration considerations**

1. Rapid onset within 20 seconds, and duration is 15 to 20 minutes

2. Tetracaine hydrochloride can cause systemic toxicity

D. **Contraindications:** hypersensitivity

E. **Significant drug interactions:** tetracaine hydrochloride is compatible with mercury or silver salts

F. **Significant food interactions:** none reported

G. **Significant laboratory studies:** none reported

H. **Side effects:** proparacaine (Ophthaine, Ophthetic) causes allergic contact dermatitis, cycloplegia, conjunctival congestion, delayed corneal healing

I. **Adverse effects/toxicity**

1. CNS excitation symptoms: blurred vision, dizziness, nervousness, restlessness, trembling

2. CNS depression (follows CNS excitation): dyspnea, drowsiness, dysrhythmias

J. **Nursing considerations**

1. To protect cornea, apply eye patch until blink reflex has returned

2. Assess for hypersensitivity symptoms such as burning, itching, stinging

K. **Client education:** do not touch or rub the eye until anesthesia has worn off

V. **Auditory Medications**

A. **Antibiotics for the ear**

1. Action and use

a. Used in the management of infections of the **external ear** (external auditory canal surface)

b. Chloramphenicol (Chloromycetin Otic) is used in the treatment of infections caused by such organisms as *Enterobacter aerogenes, Escherichia coli, Haemophilus influenzae, Pseudomonas aeruginosa,* and other organisms.

2. Common medications

a. Chloramphenicol (Chloromycetin Otic): 2 or 3 drops instilled in ear canal every 6 to 8 hours

b. Gentamicin sulfate otic solution (Garamycin): 3 or 4 drops instilled in ear canal 3 times daily

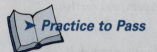

▶ *Practice to Pass*

A client is being discharged from the outpatient clinic after undergoing removal of a foreign body from the left eye. The clinician used proparacaine hydrochloride (Ophthaine) for the anesthetic agent. What discharge instructions and information do you provide to this client?

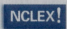

NCLEX!

NCLEX!

      c. Note: otic preparation of gentamicin sulfate has not been approved by the Food and Drug Administration (FDA); prescribers in the United States use the *ophthalmic* preparation for otic infections

  3. Administration considerations

      a. Unless contraindicated, warm ear drops by running medication bottle under warm water, immersing bottle in a cup of warm water, or by holding bottle in the hand or pocket for 30 minutes prior to administration

      b. Assess client's baseline hearing status

      c. Assess client for ear drainage, earache, erythema, pain, and **vertigo** (dizziness)

      d. Assess that the ear canal is clear and not impacted with **cerumen** (ear wax) before medication administration

      e. Assess for intact **tympanic membrane** (the thin membrane between the external auditory canal and middle ear)

  4. Contraindications

      a. Hypersensitivity

      b. Perforation of tympanic membrane

  5. Significant drug interactions: none reported

  6. Significant food interactions: none reported

  7. Significant laboratory studies: assess for blood dyscrasias with chloramphenicol

  8. Side effects

      a. Local: burning, rash, redness, swelling, blurred vision

      b. Systemic: hypersensitivity reaction

  9. Adverse effects/toxicity

      a. Hypersensitivity reaction

      b. Rare occurrence of systemic hematologic toxicity

  10. Nursing considerations

      a. Assess for signs of hypersensitivity such as burning, rash redness, and swelling after the administration of the medication

      b. Discontinue use if hypersensitivity reaction occurs

      c. Monitor auditory canal for drainage and pain

      d. Monitor for hearing disturbances

NCLEX!

NCLEX!

NCLEX!

NCLEX!

For instillation of eardrops in older children and adults:

- Assess the ear canal for cerumen or edema
- Tilt client's head toward the unaffected side
- Gently pull the pinna of the ear up and back
- Instill the eardrops—*do not* insert dropper into the ear canal
- Gently massage the area anterior to the ear to facilitate entry of the drops into the ear canal

For instillation of eardrops in children 3 years and younger:

- Assess the ear canal for cerumen or edema
- Tilt client's head toward the unaffected side
- Gently pull the pinna of the ear slightly down and back
- Instill the eardrops—*do not* insert dropper into the ear canal
- Gently massage the area anterior to the ear to facilitate entry of the drops into the ear canal

11. Client education

   NCLEX!

   a. Advise client to inform health care provider of increased pain, drainage, or no improvement in symptoms within a few days of treatment

   b. Refer to Box 15-2 for instillation of otic medications

B. **Corticosteroids**

   1. Action and use

      a. Used for antibacterial, antifungal, and anti-inflammatory effects

      b. Used for antipruritic and antiallergic effects

   2. Common medications (Refer to Table 15-9)

   3. Administration considerations

      a. Assess client's hearing status

      b. Assess client for ear drainage, earache, erythema, pain, and vertigo

      c. Assess that the ear canal is clear and not impacted with cerumen before medication administration

   NCLEX!

      d. Assess for intact tympanic membrane

      e. May be given in combination with antibiotics to treat infections of the external ear canal or mastoid cavity

Table 15-9

Corticosteroid Agents for Otic Use

Drug Name	Usual Adult Dosage
Betamethasone (Beenesol) Hydrocortisone (Cortamed) Dexamethasone (Decadron) Hydrocortisone with acetic acid (VoSol HC, Acetasol HC) Hydrocortisone with alcohol (EarSol-HC) Hydrocortisone with acetic acid and benzethonium (AA-HC Otic)	For all medications unless otherwise directed: Instill 3–4 drops 2 to 3 times daily, or saturate a cotton wick and insert into ear canal. Moisten wick every four to 6 hours with 3 to 5 drops of solution. Remove the wick after 24 hours and use prescribed amount of drops 3 to 4 times daily.

   4. Contraindications

      a. Hypersensitivity to sulfites

      b. Perforation of tympanic membrane

   5. Significant drug interactions: none reported

   6. Significant food interactions: none reported

   7. Significant laboratory studies: none reported

   8. Side effects: corticosteroids may mask infection or exacerbate an existing infection

   9. Adverse effects/toxicity: corticosteroids may mask infection or exacerbate an existing infection

   10. Nursing considerations: assess for hypersensitivity after administration of medication

   11. Client education

      a. Hearing should be monitored during duration of treatment

      b. Inform health care provider of new onset of ear drainage, heat, fever, odor, or pain

      c. Inform health care provider if no improvement is seen within a few days of treatment

      d. Refer to Box 15-2 for administration of otic medications

C. Other medications (over-the-counter medications)

   1. Action and use

      a. Acetic acid (alcohol, glycerin, or propylene glycol) is used after swimming or bathing to restore normal acid pH to the ear canal

      b. Glycerin, mineral oil, and olive oil are used as emollients for relief of itching and burning in the ear

      c. Propylene glycol enhances antibacterial effects and acidity of acetic acid

      d. Carbamide peroxide is an antibacterial agent used to help remove accumulated cerumen

   2. Common medications (refer to Table 15-10)

   3. Administration considerations: generally considered safe and effective

   4. Contraindications: hypersensitivity; otherwise generally considered safe

   5. Significant drug interactions: none reported

   6. Significant food interactions: none reported

   7. Significant laboratory studies: none reported

   8. Side effects: generally considered safe without side effects

   9. Adverse effects/toxicity: generally considered safe without side effects

   10. Nursing considerations: assess for hypersensitivity

Table 15-10	Drug Name	Usual Adult Dosage
Common Over-the-Counter (OTC) Agents for Otic Use	Boric acid and isopropyl alcohol (Aurocaine 2)	Follow package directions
	Carbamide peroxide (Auro Ear Drops)	Follow package directions
	Carbamide peroxide and glycerin (Dent's Ear Wax Drops, E.R.O. Ear drops, Ear Wax Removal System)	Follow package directions
	Hydrocortisone, propylene glycol, alcohol, benzyl benzoate (Earsol-HC Drops)	Instill 3–4 drops 2 to 3 times daily, or saturate a cotton wick and insert into ear canal. Moisten wick every 4 to 6 hours with 3 to 5 drops of solution. Remove the wick after 24 hours and use prescribed amount of drops 3 to 4 times daily.
	Isopropyl alcohol (Aurocaine 2)	Follow package directions
	Isopropyl alcohol in glycerin (Swim-Ear Drops)	Follow package directions

11. Client education

    a. Advise client to seek evaluation by health care provider if symptoms do not improve within several days

    b. Advise client to inform health care provider if adverse reactions occur or if symptoms worsen

    c. Refer to Box 15-2 for administration of otic medications

D. Medications that cause ototoxicity

    1. Analgesics

        a. Aspirin and other salicylates

        b. NSAIDs

    2. Antibiotics

        a. Aminoglycosides

        b. Clarithromycin

        c. Erythromycin

        d. Vancomycin

    3. Antineoplastic Agents

        a. Cisplatin

        b. Mechlorethamine

    4. Loop diuretics

        a. Bumetanide (Bumex)

        b. Ethacrynic acid (Edecrin)

        c. Furosemide (Lasix)

NCLEX!

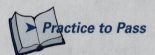

Practice to Pass

A client returns to the clinic complaining that the medication prescribed for an ear infection "runs right back out of my ear." What assessment and instructions do you provide for this client?

Case Study

A client with newly diagnosed open-angle glaucoma is prescribed betaxolol (Betoptic). The client also has a history of pulmonary disease.

❶ How does the nurse explain glaucoma and the purpose of the medication to this client?

❷ The client expresses concern about the new medication and the possible interference with the treatment and course of the preexisting pulmonary disease. What information should be provided to the client?

❸ What information does the client need regarding the side effects and signs and symptoms of hypersensitivity to betaxolol (Betoptic)?

❹ What instructions does the nurse provide specifically related to the potential side effect of photophobia?

❺ What instructions does the client need regarding proper administration of ophthalmic medications?

For suggested responses, see page 642.

Posttest

1 A client being treated with carteolol (Ocupress) has type 1 diabetes. What specific teaching instructions related to the medication and diabetes does the nurse provide to this client?

(1) "There are no special considerations for diabetic clients receiving Ocupress."
(2) "Beta-blocking agents may mask signs and symptoms of hypoglycemia."
(3) "Do not administer the medication if glucose is greater than 200."
(4) "Beta-blocking agents increase the risk of hyperglycemia."

2 A client indicates an understanding of instructions about self-administration of the prescribed otic solution when which of the following statements is made?

(1) "I run the bottle of medication under cool running water before administering the medication."
(2) "I run the bottle of medication under warm running water before administering the medication."
(3) "I warm the bottle of medication in the microwave before administering the medication."
(4) "I warm the bottle of medication in my hand for 5 minutes before administering the medication."

3 A client with a history of pulmonary disease is being treated with betaxolol (Betoptic). After the nurse has provided instructions and information about the medication, the client asks, "how can eye drops affect my lungs?" The nurse's explanation includes which of the following?

(1) The medication does not have any effects on the pulmonary system.
(2) The client is only at risk if the prescribed ophthalmic medication is cardioselective ($Beta_1$).
(3) The client is only at risk if the prescribed ophthalmic medication is given at the same time as the oral medications taken for pulmonary disease.
(4) If the ophthalmic medication is systemically absorbed, it can have the same systemic effects as other beta-blocking agents.

4 A client telephones the outpatient clinic and complains of severe ear pain that ceased suddenly and now the ear is draining. The client has otic antibiotics remaining from a previous ear infection 2 months ago and wants to know if it is safe to use the medication. The nurse's response is based on which of the following?

(1) The client should be referred to a health care provider, and should not use any medications until the ear is evaluated.
(2) Since the client has recently been treated with otic antibiotics for an ear infection, the medication would be safe to use.
(3) The client should begin using the antibiotic and seek evaluation if no improvement is seen within 2 days.
(4) The shelf life of otic medications is 3 months, therefore the medication would be safe to use.

5 The nurse evaluates that a client is demonstrating appropriate technique for using ophthalmic medication when the client does which of the following?

(1) Cleanses crust from the eye by wiping from the outer canthus inward with a cotton ball
(2) Cleanses crust from the eye by wiping from the inner canthus outward with a cotton ball
(3) Cleanses crust from the eye by wiping from the outer canthus inward with a cotton swab
(4) Cleanses crust from the eye by wiping from the inner canthus outward with a cotton swab

6 A client prescribed gentamicin sulfate (Garamycin) for an ear infection telephones the clinic and states that the medication bottle indicates "for ophthalmic use" and refuses to use the medication. Your response to the client is based on which of the following?

(1) An error is likely in the dispensing of the medication since the clinician is treating an otic infection.
(2) It is an accepted and safe practice in the United States for clinicians to prescribe ophthalmic Garamycin for otic use.
(3) An error was likely committed by the clinician in prescribing the medication.
(4) The client requires further teaching on proper medication administration.

7 A client with a history of cardiovascular disease is admitted to the nursing unit with bradycardia and hypotension. The nurse suspects that these symptoms may be adverse effects of which of the following medications recently started as therapy for glaucoma?

(1) Carteolol (Ocupress)
(2) Acetazolamide (Diamox)
(3) Dorzolamide (Trusopt)
(4) Latanoprost (Xalatan)

8 A client is receiving an ophthalmic anesthetic agent preoperatively for removal of sutures. Priority nursing care includes which of the following?

(1) Measures to protect the airway
(2) Measures to reduce hypersensitivity
(3) Measures to control body temperature
(4) Measures to protect the eye

9 A client with narrow-angle glaucoma informs the nurse of an outpatient colonoscopy scheduled for later in the week. The client understands subsequent teaching when which of the following statements are made?

(1) "I will inform my doctor and the nursing staff of my glaucoma and the medication I am taking."
(2) "I will stop taking my medication 2 days before the colonoscopy."
(3) "I will stop taking my medication 1 day before the colonoscopy."
(4) "My glaucoma is not a factor when having outpatient procedures done."

10 Which action taken by the client indicates an understanding of instructions for administration of dipivefrin (Propine)?

(1) The client maintains pressure on the lacrimal sac for 1 to 2 minutes after instillation of medication.
(2) The client avoids lacrimal pressure after instillation of medication.
(3) The client instills medication directly onto the eye.
(4) The client maintains pressure on lacrimal sac for 30 seconds after instillation of medication.

See pages 601–602 for Answers and Rationales.

Answers and Rationales

Pretest

1 Answer: 3 *Rationale:* Assessment of allergies and reactions to medications is essential when administering a new medication. Hypersensitivity responses can occur with ophthalmic medications, and severe adverse reactions may occur with hypersensitivity to the medication because it is systemically absorbed. Options 1, 2, and 4 are important to the nursing management of the client; however, avoiding reactions to the medication is the priority.
Cognitive Level: Application
Nursing Process: Assessment; *Test Plan:* PHYS

2 Answer: 2 *Rationale:* Correct technique for administration of ophthalmic medications includes pulling the lower eyelid down and instilling medication into the conjunctival sac. Options 1, 3, and 4 each contain information that is either partially or totally incorrect.
Cognitive Level: Analysis
Nursing Process: Evaluation; *Test Plan:* HPM

3 Answer: 1 *Rationale:* For an external ear canal obstructed with edema, a gauze wick is inserted past the edematous segment. The medication is then applied to the outside wick, allowing the medication to be absorbed along the path of the wick. Option 2 delays treatment. Option 3 is unnecessary, and option 4 is a hazardous activity that could cause damage to the client's ear.
Cognitive Level: Application
Nursing Process: Implementation; *Test Plan:* PHYS

4 Answer: 3 *Rationale:* Acetazolamide should not be mixed with alcohol or glycerin. To minimize gastrointestinal distress, the client may take the medication with milk or may crush it and mix it with juice. Acetazolamide is taken in the morning to avoid nocturnal diuresis.
Cognitive Level: Analysis
Nursing Process: Evaluation; *Test Plan:* PHYS

5 Answer: 1 *Rationale:* Carbonic anhydrase inhibitor agents such as dorzolamide decrease aqueous production by approximately one-half of baseline, thereby lowering intraocular pressure. Dorzolamide does not cause pupil constriction (option 2), increase aqueous humor production (option 3) or increase outflow of aqueous humor (option 4).
Cognitive Level: Application
Nursing Process: Implementation; *Test Plan:* PHYS

6 Answer: 3 *Rationale:* Precipitation of an asthmatic attack is a systemic side effect of pilocarpine. Other side effects include salivation, hypotension, diarrhea, nausea, and vomiting. Dry mouth (option 1), hypertension (option 2) and constipation (option 4) are opposites of known side effects.
Cognitive Level: Analysis
Nursing Process: Analysis; *Test Plan:* PHYS

7 Answer: 2 *Rationale:* The adult client pulls the pinna up and back for administration of otic solutions. The pinna is pulled down in the child (option 1). Droppers should never be inserted into the ear canal (option 3), and the head should be tilted toward the unaffected side (option 4).
Cognitive Level: Analysis
Nursing Process: Evaluation; *Test Plan:* PHYS

8 Answer: 1 *Rationale:* Ophthalmic beta-blockers are administered to reduce intraocular pressure (not increase it as in option 3) by decreasing production of aqueous humor. The medication must be continued as lifelong therapy to maintain a stable intraocular pressure (option 2). Some glaucoma may be surgically treated (option 4).
Cognitive Level: Application
Nursing Process: Evaluation; *Test Plan:* PHYS

9 Answer: 1 *Rationale:* Atropine, an anticholinergic agent, can precipitate acute glaucoma as a result of pupillary dilation; therefore, clients with preexisting

glaucoma or a predisposition to acute glaucoma should not receive atropine. There are no contraindications for diphenhydramine, hydroxyzine, or promethazine in the client with glaucoma.
Cognitive Level: Analysis
Nursing Process: Planning; *Test Plan:* SECE

10 **Answer: 2** *Rationale:* Carbonic anhydrase inhibitors such as brinzolamide may exacerbate the potential for renal calculi. Increasing fluid intake to 2 liters per day may reduce this risk. Diet recommendations include increasing potassium and reducing sodium.
Cognitive Level: Analysis
Nursing Process: Evaluation; *Test Plan:* PHYS

Posttest

1 **Answer: 2** *Rationale:* Beta-blocking agents may mask symptoms of hypoglycemia such as tachycardia and tremors. There is no indication to check serum glucose level before administering medication (option 3); however, the client should be aware of the medication's potential to mask symptoms of hypoglycemia (options 1 and 4).
Cognitive Level: Application
Nursing Process: Implementation; *Test Plan:* PHYS

2 **Answer: 2** *Rationale:* Warming eardrops (if not contraindicated) makes administration of the medication more comfortable. Warming can be achieved by running the bottle under warm water (not cool, as in option 1), placing the bottle of medication in a cup of warm water, or by carrying in the hand or pocket for 30 minutes (option 4). The medication should *never* be warmed in the microwave (option 3), serious injury to ear canal and tympanic membrane may occur.
Cognitive Level: Analysis
Nursing Process: Evaluation; *Test Plan:* SECE

3 **Answer: 4** *Rationale:* Clients with pulmonary disease are generally prescribed Betoptic for glaucoma because it is Beta$_1$ selective (cardioselective). However, the client must still be monitored for pulmonary side effects and respiratory difficulties that may occur with systemic absorption. The explanations in options 1, 2, and 3 do not address this effect.
Cognitive Level: Application
Nursing Process: Implementation; *Test Plan:* PHYS

4 **Answer: 1** *Rationale:* The symptoms the client reports may indicate a ruptured tympanic membrane. The ear canal and tympanic membrane should always

be evaluated before instilling otic medications, making options 2, 3, and 4 incorrect.
Cognitive Level: Application
Nursing Process: Implementation; *Test Plan:* PHYS

5 **Answer: 2** *Rationale:* Crust from eyes is cleansed using cotton balls wiping from the inner canthus to the outer canthus. Swabs (options 3 and 4) should not be used as damage to eye could occur. Option 1 represents incorrect technique.
Cognitive Level: Analysis
Nursing Process: Evaluation; *Test Plan:* PHYS

6 **Answer: 2** *Rationale* Otic Garamycin is not approved for use in the United States. It is a safe and accepted practice for clinicians to prescribed ophthalmic Garamycin for otic use. The client should be informed of this practice. Options 1 and 3 are incorrect because no error was made. Option 4 is incorrect because the client has not indicated inadequate knowledge of medication administration.
Cognitive Level: Analysis
Nursing Process: Implementation; *Test Plan:* PHYS

7 **Answer: 1** *Rationale:* Carteolol is a beta-blocking agent with side effects of hypotension and bradycardia if systemically absorbed. The other medications, acetazolamide and dorzolamide, carbonic anhydrase inhibitors, and latanoprost, a prostaglandin, do not affect heart rate and blood pressure.
Cognitive Level: Analysis
Nursing Process: Analysis; *Test Plan:* PHYS

8 **Answer: 4** *Rationale:* The blink reflex is lost when ophthalmic anesthetic agents are used, therefore the eye is at risk for injury. Priority is given to protecting the cornea from irritants, debris, and rubbing. Generally, an eye patch is applied for protection. Since the medication is local and the client is not anesthetized, the airway not compromised (option 1) and the body temperature should remain at pre-procedure reading (option 3). Clients are assessed for allergies or past hypersensitivity reactions (option 2) before the medication is administered.
Cognitive Level: Analysis
Nursing Process: Planning; *Test Plan:* SECE

9 **Answer: 1** *Rationale:* Atropine sulfate is commonly used preoperatively in outpatient procedures such as a colonoscopy. The client needs to alert the staff about the diagnosis of glaucoma, since the use of atropine

is contraindicated in narrow-angle glaucoma because it could precipitate acute glaucoma.
Cognitive Level Analysis
Nursing Process: Evaluation; *Test Plan:* SECE

10 **Answer: 1** *Rationale:* Maintaining pressure on the lacrimal sac for 1 to 2 minutes is recommended for

dipivefrin to minimize systemic absorption of the medication. Eye drops are instilled into the conjunctival sac, never directly onto the eye.
Cognitive Level: Analysis
Nursing Process: Evaluation; *Test Plan:* PHYS

References

Abrams, A. (2004). *Clinical drug therapy: Rationales for nursing practice* (7th ed.). Philadelphia: Lippincott Williams & Wilkins, pp. 935–948.

Aschenbrenner, O., Cleveland, L., & Venable, S. (2002). *Drug therapy in nursing.* Philadelphia: Lippincott Williams & Wilkins, p. 1124.

Deglin, J. D. & Vallerand, A. H. (2003). *Davis's drug guide for nurses* (9th ed.). Philadelphia: Lippincott.

Karch, A. M. (2003). *Focus on pharmacology* (2nd ed.). Philadelphia: Lippincott Williams & Wilkins, pp. 842–845.

Kee, J., & Hayes, E. (2003). *Pharmacology: A nursing process approach* (4th ed.). Philadelphia: Saunders, pp. 684–699.

Kozier, B., Erb, G., Berman, A. J., & Burke, K. (2003). *Fundamentals of nursing: Concepts, process, and practice* (7th ed.). Upper Saddle River, NJ: Prentice Hall, Inc.

Lehne, R. (2004). *Pharmacology for nursing care* (5th ed.). St. Louis, MO: Mosby, pp. 1098–1106, 1121–1126.

LeMone, P., & Burke, K. M. (2003). *Medical-surgical nursing: Critical thinking in client care* (3rd ed.). Upper Saddle River, NJ: Prentice Hall, Inc.

McKenry, L. M. & Salerno, E. (2003). *Pharmacology in Nursing* (21st ed. revised reprint.). St. Louis: Mosby, pp. 790–810, 814–818.

CHAPTER 16

Herbal Agents

Donna Polverini, RN, MS

CHAPTER OUTLINE

Overview of Phytomedicines   Specific Phytomedicines   Nursing Management

OBJECTIVES

- Define the terms commonly associated with the use of herbs as supplements.
- Describe the general goals of therapy when administering specific herbal supplements.
- Describe the uses and dosages of various herbs used as supplements.
- Identify the cautions associated with the use of specific herbal supplements, including adverse effects, contraindications, and drug interactions.
- List the key client teaching points related to the use of herbs as supplements.

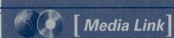

[Media Link]

Use the CD-ROM enclosed with this text, or log onto the address given to access the free, interactive Companion Website created for this series. The CD-ROM and Companion Website accompanying this book offer additional practice opportunities and information—NCLEX Review, Case Studies, Glossary, In Depth with NCLEX, and more.

www.prenhall.com/hogan

REVIEW AT A GLANCE

bulk *unpackaged, loose body of the plant used for tea or decoction*

decoction *liquid form of the herb brewed from the seeds, bark, and root; the herb is covered with boiling water, covered, boiled, and simmered; it is then strained and water added for consumption*

extract *a solution or preparation containing the active ingredient of the herb made by pressing the herb and then soaking it in alcohol or water, which is al-* *lowed to evaporate; usually, it is put in a small amount of water for use*

phytomedicine *therapeutic agents or preparations made or derived from plants or plant parts*

phytotherapy *the science of using plant-based medicines to treat illness*

standardization *the act of conforming to a basis of comparison in size, weight, quality, strength, or the like*

tea *a liquid preparation using fresh or dried herb; boiling water is poured over the herb and allowed to steep for a period of time*

tincture *liquid extracts of the herb most often alcohol-based, used internally or externally, taken in drops in small amount of juice or water; glycerin-based extracts are available when alcohol should be avoided*

Pretest

1 The client asks the nurse about a magazine advertisement related to the use of ginger for the treatment of arthritis. The nurse focuses client education on which of the following?

(1) The client's ability to accurately assess the reliability of information sources
(2) The author of the article
(3) The type of magazine in which the advertisement was found
(4) The client's level of education

2 A female client taking feverfew for the prevention of migraine headaches reports to the nurse that she thinks she may be pregnant. Based on knowledge of feverfew, what would be the nurse's priority action?

(1) Instruct the client to discontinue use of the feverfew.
(2) Instruct the client to have a pregnancy test performed.
(3) Arrange for the client to see her health care provider.
(4) Instruct the client to reduce the dosage of the feverfew.

3 A male client taking valerian root as a sleep aid demonstrates safe administration of the herb when he states that the herb:

(1) May be taken safely with lorazepam (Ativan) in small doses.
(2) Should have the active ingredient valepotriate removed from the extract.
(3) May be used safely in children over the age of 5
(4) Is not effective in the capsule form.

4 A client taking saw palmetto to treat symptoms of benign prostatic hyperplasia (BPH) complains of diarrhea. Based on knowledge of this herb, the nurse concludes that the diarrhea is most likely related to which of the following?

(1) The form of the herb extract
(2) Client history of allergy
(3) The age of the client
(4) The dose of the herb

5 A 50-year-old female client presents to the health clinic with complaints of hot flashes and night sweats. After determining that the symptoms are not related to any underlying disease process, the nurse supports client use of which of the following phytomedicines?

(1) Echinacea
(2) Black cohosh
(3) Bilberry
(4) Valerian root

6 The client is taking garlic on a daily basis. Which of the following statements made by the client demonstrates understanding of its use?

(1) "The effectiveness of garlic is based on scientific research."
(2) "Garlic may be used safely with ginger."
(3) "There are no remedies for the bad breath caused by the garlic."
(4) "I can take garlic safely with over-the-counter medications."

7 Which of the following statements made by the nurse is most appropriate when providing client education regarding the use of hawthorn?

(1) "You may use hawthorn for acute episodes of chest pain or angina."
(2) "Hawthorn will not affect your heart rate."
(3) "You should not take hawthorn while taking captopril (Capoten)."
(4) "Hawthorn is known to produce the same effects as verapamil (Calan)."

8 A client has been taking nutrition bars containing Korean ginseng for the past 2 weeks to increase concentration and stamina. Based on knowledge of the herb, the nurse instructs the client to do which of the following?

(1) Avoid operating machinery or driving a car while taking the nutrition bar.
(2) Avoid this form of the herb, which is known to increase adverse effects.
(3) Avoid use of the nutrition bar with coffee, tea, or cola.
(4) Continue use of the nutrition bar daily as desired.

9 A client taking St. John's wort in capsule form to treat mild depression for the past week complains of it ineffectiveness. Which of the following statements made by the nurse is most appropriate?

(1) "You may need to switch to another form of the herb."
(2) "You should take the herb at night."
(3) "It may take several weeks for the therapy to be effective."
(4) "St. John's wort may not be effective for your type of depression."

10 In evaluating the effectiveness of saw palmetto for the treatment of benign prostatic hyperplasia (BPH), the nurse would be least likely to focus on which of the following assessments?

(1) Residual volume
(2) Size of the prostate
(3) Urinary frequency
(4) Dysuria

See pages 623–624 for Answers and Rationales.

I. Overview of Phytomedicines

A. General information

1. The Food and Drug Administration (FDA) classification of herbs is as dietary supplements

2. Other than phytomedicines, names for herbal therapies also include botanicals, nutraceuticals, and dietary supplements

3. Herbal supplements are not substitutes for conventional medicine

4. Doses of herbs are not yet standardized in many countries other than Germany; dosage of herbs is according to product literature, although in most cases a research-based safe dose is yet to be determined

5. Most herbs, except ginger, are contraindicated during pregnancy and lactation

B. Popularity

1. They are increasing in popularity in the Western world

2. This may be partially the result of the Western culture move toward a "back-to-nature" mentality

C. Frequency of use

1. More than 28 million Americans report taking one or more herbal supplements

2. Primary users tend to be college-educated women between the ages of 35 and 49

II. Specific Phytomedicines

A. Bilberry (*Vaccinium myrtillus,* European blueberry, huckleberry, whortleberry*)*

1. Description

   a. Relative of blueberry and cranberry

   b. Shrub with small, sweet black berries

   c. Active ingredients: anthocyanoside (antioxidant bioflavonoid), pectin (soluble fiber)

   d. Stabilizes collagen activity

   e. Prevents production and release of compounds that promote inflammation, such as histamine and prostaglandins

   f. Relaxes smooth muscle in vasculature

   g. Inhibits platelet aggregation

   h. Reduces permeability and strengthens capillary wall membrane

2. Uses

   a. Most commonly used for treatment of simple diarrhea

   b. Prevention and treatment of eye disorders: diabetic retinopathy, night blindness, macular degeneration, glaucoma, cataracts

   c. Diabetes mellitus

   d. Antioxidant

   e. Possible treatment of varicose veins, hemorrhoids

3. Dosage

   a. Dosage varies considerably

   b. Standardization should contain 25% anthocyanoside

   c. 240–480 mg of the standardized extract BID or TID

   d. 20–60 g of the dried fruit QD

4. Cautions

   a. May increase coagulation time

   b. May interfere with iron absorption when taken internally

   c. Use cautiously with acetylsalicylic acid (aspirin), anticoagulants, vitamin E, fish oils, feverfew, garlic, ginger, ginkgo

   d. Contraindicated in pregnancy and lactation

   e. Avoid long-term large doses, doses over 1.5 g/kg/day may be fatal, doses over 480 mg/day may be dangerous

B. Black cohosh (*Cimicifuga racemosa*, black snakeroot, bugroot, rattleweed, rattleroot, squawroot, cimifuga)

NCLEX!

1. Description

   a. Active ingredients: triperpenoid glycosides, isoflavenones, aglycones

   b. Binds to estrogen receptors

   c. Inhibits luteinizing hormone

   d. Apparent estrogen-like activity

2. Uses

   a. Primarily used for treatment of premenstrual syndrome (PMS) and post-menopausal symptoms

   b. Promotes labor of pregnancy

   c. Decreases blood pressure

   d. Treatment of snake bites

   e. Recommended uses by herbalists: dysmenorrhea, rheumatism, antispasmodic, astringent, diuretic, expectorant, sedative

3. Dosage

   a. Research-based safe dosage yet to be determined

   b. 40 mg qd

   c. Possible stimulation of estrogen synthesis with 8 mg/day for 8 weeks

4. Cautions

   a. Contraindicated use with antihypertensives

   b. May cause bradycardia, hypotension, joint pain

   c. Contraindicated in lactation

   d. Use in pregnancy only when birth is imminent to promote labor

C. **Echinacea** (*Echinacea purpurea,* snake root, purple or American cone flower, sampson root black sampson, hedgehog, survey root)

   1. Description

      a. Member of daisy family with 9 species

      b. Active ingredients: polysaccharides, alkylamides, flavonoids, caffeic acid derivatives (echinacosides), essential oils and others

      c. Available in capsule, tablet, candle, glycerite, hydroalcoholic extract, fresh-pressed juice, lollipop, lozenge, tea, and tincture forms

      d. Activates T lymphocytes and intensifies phagocytosis of macrophages

      e. Stimulates tumor necrosis factor, interferon and interleukin

      f. Nonspecific stimulation of immune system

      g. Stabilizes hyaluronic acid (a component of connective tissue) to protect cells and connective tissue from microorganism invasion and attack from free radicals

      h. Inhibits lipoxygenase to reduce inflammation

2. Uses

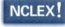
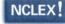

   a. Most common: prevention or reduction of symptoms of cold/influenza

   b. Boost immune system and increase body's resistance to infection, particularly upper respiratory and urinary infection

   c. Treatment of herpes simplex and Candida infection

   d. Topically: improve wound healing, antioxidant protection from ultraviolet A and B light rays

3. Dosage

   a. Standardized preparation should contain 3.5% echinaside

   b. Available in capsule of powdered herb, expressed juice, tincture, water/alcohol based formula, fluid extract, solid extract, lozenge forms

   c. Dosage dependent on formula potency; varies according to source consulted

   d. Typically supplied in 380-mg capsules: 1 to 3 capsules TID at mealtime with water

   e. Regime should consist of 8 weeks on and 1 week off to reduce decreased effects with continued use

NCLEX!

NCLEX!

4. Cautions

   a. Not to be used in presence of autoimmune disease (e.g. HIV/AIDS, collagen disease, multiple sclerosis, tuberculosis), severe illness or allergy to sunflower or daisy family

   b. Not to be used with immunosuppressants (e.g. corticosteroids or cyclosporine)

   c. Prolonged use (longer than 8 week cycle) may cause hepatotoxicity and suppression of immune system

   d. Not to be used with other hepatotoxicants (e.g. anabolic steroids, amiodarone, methotrexate, ketoconazole)

   e. May influence fertility by spermatazoa enzyme interference

   f. Many tinctures contain large amounts of alcohol

   g. Contraindicated in alcoholism, children, pregnancy, and lactation

   h. Adverse effects: allergic reaction and anaphylaxis

D. **Feverfew** *(Tanacetum parthenium,* bachelor's button, febrifuge plant, feather few, feather foil)

1. Description

   a. Short, bushy perennial; member of daisy family with yellow flowers and yellow-green leaves resembling chamomile

   b. Active ingredients: sesquiterpene lactones, especially parthenolide, essential oils

NCLEX!

   c. Suppresses secretion of granules in platelets and neutrophils to inhibit platelet aggregation

   d. May suppress production of prostaglandins (thromboxane, leukotriene)

   e. Inhibits release of serotonin

2. Uses

   a. Principle use: prevention of recurrent migraine headaches, treatment of arthritis

   b. Relief of menstrual pain

   c. Asthma

   d. Dermatitis, psoriasis

   e. Antipyretic (promotes diaphoresis)

3. Dosage

   a. Dosage varies according to source consulted

   b. Standardized preparation should contain 0.2% parthenolide

   c. Available in freeze-dried leaf, dried plant part, capsules, infusion

   d. Supplied in 380 mg capsules containing pure leaf and 250 mg capsules of leaf extract

   e. Most sources recommend anywhere from 50 to 125 mg of the dried herb taken with or after meals to reduce GI colic

   f. Migraine: 0.25 to 0.5 mg to prevent attack; 1 to 2 g to control attack

   g. May chew one fresh or frozen leaf/day to obtain dose, but may cause mouth sores or gastric distress

   h. Infusion: ½ to 1 tsp of herb in 1 cup boiling water, steep for 5 to 10 minutes, 2 cups qd

4. Cautions

   a. Long-term studies not done

   b. Contraindicated in pregnancy, lactation, and under the age of 2

   c. Cross allergy to ragweed

   d. Adverse effects: allergic reaction, lip and tongue swelling, mouth ulcers, abdominal colic, palpitations, increased menstrual flow

   e. Sudden withdrawal may cause post feverfew syndrome (muscles aches, pain and stiffness); taper off to discontinue

   f. Other proven (conventional) remedies for relief of migraine should be used first

   g. May interfere with blood clotting mechanism; not to be used with anticoagulants such as aspirin, warfarin (Coumadin), bilberry, garlic, ginger, ginkgo

   h. Feverfew is known to cause rebound headaches

E. **Garlic** (*Allium sativum,* stinking root or rose, nectar of the gods, camphor of the poor, poor man's treacle, rustic treacle)

1. Description

   a. Empirical support for effectiveness and use; most widely researched herb

   b. Active ingredients: (23 constituents), allicin (odorless, sulfur-containing amino acid), ajoene

   c. Should be crushed or bruised to effectively convert various enzymes, protein, lipids, amino acids and other ingredients to active ingredient, allicin

   d. Allicin and ajoene not found in dried garlic, but may be present if dried at low temperatures or taken in enteric-coated tablets

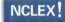

   e. Inhibits platelet aggregation

   f. Well-documented research shows that it inhibits metabolism of cholesterol, reduction of cholesterol

   g. Increases bile acid secretion

2. Uses

   a. Principle use: reduce cholesterol (decreases triglycerides, low-density lipoproteins, increases high-density lipoproteins)

   b. Principle use: treatment of mild hypertension

   c. Reduce risk of stroke

   d. Antibacterial, antiviral, antifungal

   e. Anticancer properties

   f. Lay use: antihelmintic, antispasmodic, diuretic, carminative (relieves flatulence, digestant, expectorant, topical antibiotic

3. Dosage

   a. Available in dried powder, fresh bulb, tablets (allicin total potential), tablets (garlic extract), antiseptic oil, fresh extract, freeze-dried garlic powder, garlic oil (essential oil)

   b. Commercial preparation not standardized; should deliver minimum of 10 mg aliin daily or 5,000 mcg of total allicin potential

   c. A high dose of garlic can lead to GI problems

4. Cautions

   a. Avoid large amounts of garlic with ASA (aspirin) or anticoagulants, such warfarin (Coumadin), or other herbs affecting coagulation (bilberry, feverfew, ginger, ginkgo)

   b. May potentiate diabetes drugs

   c. Adverse effects: contact dermatitis, vertigo, garlic breath, hypothyroidism, GI irritation, nausea and vomiting with large doses

   d. Enteric-coated tablets containing powdered form may reduce bad breath, but are not as potent as raw garlic

   e. Contraindicated in pregnancy, GI (peptic ulcer and GERD) and bleeding disorders

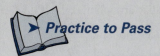

Practice to Pass

Name three types of phytomedicines that are contraindicated in the client with a history of hemorrhagic stroke.

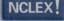

f. Chronic use may lower hemoglobin levels

g. When used to decrease cholesterol levels, plan should be monitored by the health care provider

F. Ginger *(Zingiber officinal,* Jamaica ginger, African ginger, Cochin ginger, black ginger, race ginger)

1. Description

   a. Green-purple flower resembling the orchid

   b. Active ingredient: sesquiterpenes, aromatic ketones (gingerols) and volatile oils

   c. Inhibits thromboxane production to enhance effects of anticoagulation

   d. Inhibits leukotrienes and prostaglandins to produce anti-inflammatory and analgesic effect

2. Usage

   a. Principle use: antiemetic, improve appetite, treatment of motion sickness, vertigo

   b. Diuretic, digestion aid, dyspepsia

   c. Anti-inflammatory in treatment of rheumatoid arthritis and osteoarthritis

   d. Relief of muscle pain

   e. Antitumor, antioxidant, antimicrobial

3. Dosage

   a. Dosage depends on use—consensus varies

   b. Available in capsules, liquid, powder extract, root, chewable tablets, tea, candied form

   c. Most commonly available in 500 mg capsules of powdered form

   d. Antiemetic: 500 to 1,000 mg in four divided doses/day of powdered ginger

   e. Dyspepsia, diuretic, vertigo: 2 to 4 g/day in divided doses or 2 cups tea with 1 tsp fresh ginger root each or 15 tsp powdered ginger or two 1-inch squares of candied ginger that may be repeated every 4 hours as needed

   f. Antiemetic: 1 to 2 g in 2 divided doses

   g. Motion sickness: 1 g 30 minutes before travelling and 0.5 to 1.0 g every 4 hours as needed during trip; (most effective when regimen started several days before travelling)

4. Cautions

   a. Adverse effects: headache, anxiety, insomnia, elevated blood pressure, tachycardia, asthma attach, postmenopausal bleeding

   b. Contraindicated in postoperative nausea caused by increased risk of bleeding

   c. Not to be used concomitantly with bilberry, feverfew, garlic, ginkgo, or other anticoagulants such as ASA (aspirin) or warfarin (Coumadin)

    d. Severe overdose: possible CNS depression and cardiac arrhythmias

    e. Excess of 6 g/day results in gastric irritation and ulcer formation

    f. Conflicting data related to safe use during pregnancy; (relatively safe according to FDA) contraindicated in treatment of hyperemesis gravidarum

G. Ginkgo (*Ginkgo biloba,* EGB 761, GBE, GBX, Tebonin, Tebofortan, Ginkogink)

  1. Description

    a. Active ingredients: flavone glycosides, flavonoids, terpene lactones (such as ginkgolides and bilobalide)

    b. Ginkgo biloba extract referred to as GBE

    c. Flavinoids act as antioxidants by destroying lipid layer of cell membrane

    d. Flavone glycosides produce mild platelet aggregation

    e. Ginkgolides antagonize platelet-activating factor to decrease coagulation

    f. Bilobalide increases cerebral circulation to improve tissue perfusion and increase memory

    g. Protects brain from effects of hypoxia

  2. Uses

    a. Cerebral vascular insufficiency and symptomatic relief of organic brain dysfunction to improve short-term memory loss

    b. Peripheral vascular disease (e.g., Raynaud's Disease, intermittent claudication), varicosities

    c. Senile macular degeneration

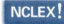

    d. Treatment of age-related mental decline related to short-term memory loss, poor concentration

    e. Treatment of depression-related cognitive disorders

    f. Treatment of depression in older adults particularly that are related to chronic cerebrovascular deficiency not responding to standard drug therapy

    g. Tinnitus, vertigo

    h. Improvement of symptoms of early-stage senility of Alzheimer's type

  3. Dosage

    a. Standardization should contain 24% flavonoids and 6% terpenes

    b. Available in capsule or tablet form containing 40 mg GBE, nutrition bars, sublingual sprays, tablets, concentrated alcohol extract of fresh leaf

    c. Treatment of vascular disorders, tinnitus or vertigo: 120 to 160 mg/day in 2 or 3 divided doses

    d. Treatment of dementia: 120 to 140 mg/day in 2 or 3 divided doses

  4. Cautions

    a. Effects may not be apparent for 4 to 8 weeks

b. Not to be used concomitantly with bilberry, feverfew, garlic, ginger or other anticoagulants, such as ASA (aspirin) or warfarin (Coumadin)

c. Avoid use of unprocessed ginkgo leaves that contain allergens related to urushiol, the chemical responsible for the itch in poison ivy

d. Crude, dried leaf or tea may not contain sufficient active ingredients to be effective

e. Large doses my cause restlessness, headache, nausea, vomiting, diarrhea

f. Edible solid form sold in Oriental shops should be kept out of reach of children as seeds may cause seizures

g. Avoid use in pregnancy, lactation, children

H. Ginseng, Korean (*Panax ginseng,* American ginseng, Panaschinseng)

1. Description

   a. Active ingredients: Triterpenoid saponin glycosides (ginsenosides, panaxosides)

   b. Possible effect on pituitary gland with action similar to corticosteroids

   c. Improves glycosylated hemoglobin (HbA1c) and aminoterminalpropeptide (PIIINP) concentrations

   d. Hypertensive effect with low doses, hypotensive effect with higher doses

   e. Improves serum cholesterol and triglyceride levels

2. Uses

   a. Most common: counteract effects of physical and mental fatigue

   b. Improve stamina and concentration in healthy individuals

   c. Treatment of chronic hepatotoxicity related to alcohol and drug ingestion

   d. Improve body's ability to resist stress and disease, increase vitality

   e. Regulation of blood pressure

   f. Improve psychomotor performance (attention, auditory reaction time)

   g. Reduce serum cholesterol and triglyceride levels

   h. Regulation of blood glucose levels in type II diabetes

   i. Aphrodisiac

3. Dosage

   a. Depends on species and strength

   b. Confirmation of standards varies according to source

   c. Available in capsule, extract, root powder, tea, cream, eye gel, nutrition bar, oil, bulk

   d. Little consensus on dosing with wide variations, but universal acceptance of ginseng-free period; dosing should be spaced at intervals, e.g. 2 to 3 weeks on, 12 weeks off

   e. 0.5 to 1.0 g in 2 divided doses for 2 to 3 weeks, 1 to 2 weeks off

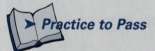

➤ Practice to Pass

A college student asks the nurse about the use of gingko biloba during exam week to enhance performance on exams. What client education is necessary?

    f. Best taken in morning, 2 hours before meal, not less than 2 hours after meal

  4. Cautions

    a. Most side effects reported related to excessive/inappropriate use

    b. Avoid concomitant use with stimulants, e.g. coffee, tea, cola

    c. May potentiate MAOI actions

    d. Adverse effects: insomnia, palpitations, pruritus

I. Ginseng, Siberian (*Eleutherococcus senticosus,* five fingers, tartar root, Western ginseng, seng and sang, Asian ginseng, Jintsam)

  1. Description

    a. Active ingredients: eutherosides

    b. Pharmacologic actions not well understood

    c. Elevates lymphocyte count (T cells), boosts immune system

  2. Uses

    a. Enhance physical and mental performance under stress

    b. Improve athletic performance

    c. Increase oxygen metabolism, work capacity and exhaustion time in variety of illnesses (e.g. atherosclerosis, diabetes, chronic bronchitis)

    d. Stimulate WBC production in clients undergoing antineoplastic therapy

  3. Dosage

    a. Little consensus on dosing with wide variations, but general consensus on ginseng-free period of 2 to 3 weeks every 4 to 8 weeks

    b. 0.6 to 3 g qd

  4. Cautions

    a. Adverse reactions: hypertension, tachycardia, insomnia and irritability

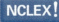

    b. Contraindicated in pregnancy, lactation, premenopausal women, hypertension, CNS stimulants or antipsychotic medications

J. Hawthorn (*Crataegus oxyacantha,* Mayblossom, Maybush, whitehorn, LI 132)

  1. Description

    a. Small to medium tree of several species; leaves, flowers, berries (fruit) are used in standardized extracts

    b. Active ingredients: flavonoids, primarily procyanidins and proanthocyanidins

    c. Acts as antioxidant that decreases damage by free radicals to cardiovascular system by increasing levels of vitamin C intracellularly

    d. Increases coronary and myocardial circulation

    e. Decreases peripheral vascular resistance to decrease blood pressure

    f. Increases strength of myocardial contraction (positive inotropic effect) and decreases heart rate (negative chronotropic effect)

    g. Angiotensin-converting enzyme (ACE) activity that prevents the conversion of angiotensin I to angiotensin II, a potent vasoconstrictor

    h. Decreases total plasma cholesterol and low-density lipoprotein (LDL) levels

    i. Improves cardiac function in chronic angina clients and those with early congestive heart failure

NCLEX!

2. Uses

    a. Treatment of mild hypertension

    b. Treatment of athero- and arteriosclerosis

    c. Treatment (prevention) of chronic angina: not intended for acute angina

    d. Treatment of early congestive heart failure

3. Dosage

    a. Standardized preparation should contain 18.75% oligomeric procyanidins and 2.2% flavenoids

    b. Available in extract, berry capsule, leaf capsule, extended-release capsule, dried fruit, tincture

    c. Dried fruit: 0.2 to 1.0 g tid

    d. Liquid extract (1:1 in 25% alcohol): 0.5 to 1/0 mL tid

    e. Tincture (1:5 in 45% alcohol): 1 to 2 mL tid or 20 to 40 drops tid

4. Cautions

NCLEX!

    a. Contraindicated with concomitant use of prescription antihypertensives or nitrates

    b. Supervision of health care provider necessary for those with existing cardiac disease

    c. May interfere with digoxin pharmacodynamics and monitoring

    d. Adverse effects: nausea, fatigue, perspiration and cutaneous eruption of the hands, increased CNS depression and sedation

    e. Contraindicated in pregnancy and lactation

NCLEX!

K. Milk thistle (*Silbyum marianum,* Mary thistle, Marian thistle, Lady's thistle, Holy thistle, silymarin, the "liver herb")

1. Description

    a. Tall plant, prickly leaves, milky sap, member of daisy family

    b. Active ingredients: silymarin and its component silybinin to act as hepatoprotectant

    c. Promotes glutathione production, a powerful endogenous antioxidant

    d. Binds to hepatocyte membrane and block uptake of toxins into liver cell

e. Stimulates nucleolar polymerase A activity to promote new liver cell growth

f. Stimulates regeneration of liver by stimulating protein synthesis

g. Inhibits action of leukotriene by Kupffer cells

h. Binds to site on liver cell membrane, blocking availability for attack from phalloidine, the toxin in death cap mushroom

i. Stabilizes liver cell membrane by decreasing turnover rate of phospholipids

2. Uses

a. Reduces hepatotoxicity related to psychoactive drugs such as phenothiazines

b. Adjunct therapy in liver inflammation related to cirrhosis, hepatitis, and fatty infiltrate related to alcohol or other toxins

c. Treatment of overdose of death cap mushroom

3. Dosage

a. Available in capsule, tablet, extract, and 200 mg concentrated seed extract equal to 140 mg silymarin

b. 140 mg tid (dosage varies according to source)

c. Standardization should contain at least 70 to 80% silymarin

4. Cautions

a. Insoluble in water, not to be taken in tea form

b. Avoid alcohol-based extract in decompensated cirrhosis

c. Cross allergy to ragweed

d. Adverse effects: loose stools, diarrhea in high doses

e. Contraindicated in pregnancy and lactation

f. Close monitoring by health care provider in presence of active liver disease

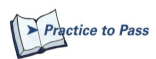

► Practice to Pass

What phytomedicine is known as the liver herb? Why?

L. **Saw palmetto** (*Serenoa repens,* sabal, American dwarf palm tree, LSESR)

1. Description

a. Shrub-like palm tree with red–brown-black berries

b. Active ingredients: saturated and unsaturated fatty acids and sterols from berries (liposterolic acid)

c. Reduces action of 5-alpha-reductase enzyme that converts testosterone to dehydrotestosterone (DHT) in aging (effects similar to finasteride [Proscar] with fewer side effects)

d. No effect on prostatic-specific antigen

e. May reverse testicular and mammary gland atrophy

f. May increase sperm production and increase sexual vigor

2. Uses

     a. Demonstrated effects through research: symptomatic treatment of benign prostatic hyperplasia (BPH)

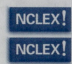

     b. Helps initiate urine stream, decreases urinary frequency, residual volumes, nocturia, dysuria; unclear whether actual prostatic size is reduced

     c. Lay uses: treatment of asthma, bronchitis, treatment of gynecomastia

3. Dosage

     a. Standardized extract should contain 85 to 95% fatty acids and sterols

     b. Mild to moderate BPH: 160-mg standardized liposterolic acid twice/day with meals to decrease GI distress OR 1 to 2 g fresh berry decoction OR 0.5 to 1.0 g dried berry po tid

4. Cautions

     a. Long-term use with approximately 6 weeks for initial effects

     b. Insoluble in water, not to be taken in tea form

     c. Adverse effects: nausea, abdominal pain, hypertension, headache, diarrhea with large doses

NCLEX!

     d. May interfere with Fe absorption

NCLEX!

     e. Supervision by health care provider necessary for diagnosed BPH

M. St. John's wort (*Hypericum perforatum,* amber, goat weed, touch-and-heal, Johnswort, witch's herb, klamath weed, chassediable, devil's scourge)

1. Description

     a. Yellow perennial flower with red pigmented leaves containing small black dots

     b. Active ingredient: hypericin from red pigment leaves, pseudohypericin and flavonoids, tannin and others

     c. Inhibits reuptake of serotonin

     d. Low monoamine oxidase inhibitor (MAOI)

     e. Actions not well determined or understood

     f. Effects comparable to imipramine (Tofranil)

     g. Produces fewer side effects than prescription antidepressants

2. Uses

NCLEX!

     a. Treatment of mild to moderate depression

b. Not intended for treatment of suicidal ideation, psychotic behavior or severe depression

c. Possible antibacterial, antiviral, wound healing properties

3. Dosage

a. Standardization should contain 0.14 to 0.3% hypericin

b. Available in capsule, sublingual, dried plant, oil, tea, liquid tincture, topical cream

c. Depression: capsules—300 mg tid; tincture—40 to 80 drops tid; tea—1 to 2 cups A.M. and P.M. with 1 to 2 heaping tsp dried herb per cup (steeped for 10 minutes); therapy should continue for 4 to 6 weeks

4. Cautions

a. Not to be used concomitantly with prescription antidepressants, especially selective serotonin reuptake inhibitors (SSRI) or monoamine oxidase inhibitors (MAOI) or foods containing tyramine (such as aged cheese, smoked meats, liver, figs, dried or cured fish, yeast, beer, Chianti wine)

b. Not to be used concomitantly with opioids, amphetamines, OTC cold and flu preparations

c. May inhibit absorption of iron

d. Adverse effects (may continue for 2 to 4 weeks): GI distress, emotional vulnerability, fatigue, pruritus, weight gain, headache, dizziness, restlessness

e. May cause photosensitivity; avoid sun exposure, especially if fair skinned

f. May decrease digoxin levels

g. Contraindicated in pregnancy, lactation and children

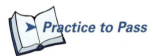

Practice to Pass

What are some other names used to identify St. John's wort?

N. **Valerian root** (*valerian officinalis,* wild valerian, garden heliotrope, setwall, capon's tail, all-heal, Amantilla, Baldrian wurzel, benedicta)

1. Description

a. Tall perennial with hollow stem, leaves and white or red flowers

b. Active ingredients: valepotriates and susquiterpine derivatives, valeric acid, valeranone and others

c. Binds weakly to gammaaminobutyric acid (GABA) receptor sites to decrease CNS activity, causing sedation with decreased side effects

d. Action similar to benzodiazepines, but non-addicting, non dependence, no morning hangover

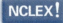

2. Uses

a. Sedative, reduction of anxiety

b. Treatment of insomnia

       c. Adjunct therapy for benzodiazepine withdrawal

       d. Possible antispasmodic

  3. Dosage

       a. Standardization should contain minimum of 0.5 to 0.8 valerenic acid or 0.8% valeric acid; tincture should contain 2% essential oils

       b. Available in capsule, tablet tincture, tea

       c. Composition and purity vary widely

       d. Insomnia: 150 to 500 mg of root extract ½ hour before bedtime or as tea with 1 tsp dried root per cup; repeat dose 2 to 3 times if needed

       e. Anxiety: 200 to 300 mg each A.M.

  4. Cautions

       a. Valepotriate (which may be carcinogenic) should be removed from final product

       b. Not to be used concomitantly with other sedative/hypnotics, anxiolytics or antidepressants

       c. May be used safely while operating machinery or car, although CNS effects should be monitored

       d. Sedation not increased with alcohol use, although caution should be exercised

       e. Adverse effects: headache, mild, temporary upset stomach

       f. Adverse effects with overdose or long term use (overdose with 2.5 g): excitability, insomnia, cardiac dysfunction, blurred vision, hepatotoxicity, severe headache, morning headache, nausea

       g. May cause hepatotoxicity; monitor liver function and avoid use in hepatic dysfunction

       h. Extract contains 40 to 60% alcohol; avoid use with alcoholism

       i. Contraindicated in pregnancy and lactation

III. Nursing Management

  A. General assessment

    1. Physical exam

       a. Vital signs, height, weight, lung sounds

       b. Depending on herb, liver and kidney function status

    2. History

       a. Age

       b. Comorbid diseases

       c. Allergies, including food and others

       d. Use of prescription, over-the-counter medications, and phytomedicines, all to be entered into the client's chart

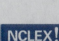

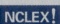

    e. Cultural beliefs that may be related to race or ethnicity

    f. Pregnancy (or potential) and lactation

B. Principles of herbal administration

  1. General use

NCLEX!

    a. Not intended for acute illness episodes or long-term therapy

    b. Appropriate as adjunct to conventional Western therapies

NCLEX!

    c. Therapeutic effectiveness is slower than prescription medications; may take as long as several weeks, depending on the herb

    d. Many herbs available in multiple forms, including teas, extracts, tinctures, capsules/tablets containing powdered or freeze dried forms of the herb

    e. Most herbs possess multiple uses, such as skin wash, gargle, compress, lotion, and eye bath

    f. They are not intended to replace healthy lifestyle

NCLEX!

    g. Safe use in pregnancy and lactation is either contraindicated or unknown and may dry up breast milk during lactation

    h. Although they may be effective in children, phytomedicines should be avoided in acute, sudden onset illness

NCLEX!

    i. Many interact with other herbs, food and prescription medications

  2. Government regulation

    a. Dietary Supplement Health and Education Act (DSHEA) of 1994 defines herbs as dietary supplements

    b. Not defined as medicines, herbs cannot make therapeutic claims, only how they affect structure and function of the human body

NCLEX!

    c. Food and Drug Administration (FDA) does not regulate use of the phytomedicines in the United States but approves certain ones for their action on the body (how they affect structure and function)

    d. FDA does not monitor herbs for their quality, composition or preparation

    e. Formulations vary in their potency and recommended dosage with frequent lack of consensus on dosing

    f. The National Center for Complementary and Alternative Medicine (NCCAM), under the National Institute of Health (NIH), is the main research component in the government on phytomedicine

3. Safety, labeling and purity

    a. Container labels must carry a disclaimer stating the FDA does not evaluate the product for treating, curing or preventing disease

    b. Labels should contain specific directions for dosing and use

    c. Only the standardized extract, when available, should be used

    d. Not all phytomedicines have empirical support for their safety and efficacy

    e. Much of the research and standardization originates in Europe, where use of phytomedicine is popular, particularly in Germany

    f. Many herbs contain toxic substances (e.g. arnica, belladonna, hemlock, lily of the valley and sassafras)

    g. Health care providers should report all adverse effects of phytomedicines to the FDA

C. Client education

1. Instruct the client to obtain a complete history and physical before starting any therapy with herbs

2. Instruct client that phytomedicines are not effective for or to be used for acute illness or episodes

3. Instruct client that phytomedicines take longer to work than prescription medications, usually weeks

4. Instruct the client to report use of all herbs to health care provider

5. Recommend client start with one herb at a time, at lower than recommended doses and closely monitor response

6. Instruct client to know particular use, dosing, and safe administration of each herb and to take only as directed

7. Teach client that herbs may cause allergic reactions and adverse effects; in the event of such, the client should discontinue the herb and report symptoms to the health care provider

8. Instruct client to become familiar with all herb/herb, herb/drug and herb/food interactions

9. Instruct client to purchase herbs from a reputable source and be aware of where and how the herb was processed

10. Instruct client to purchase standardized form of herbs, if possible

11. Teach client that "natural" or "all natural" does not equate with safety or efficacy of the herb

12. Instruct client to become familiar with many various names by which particular herbs are identified

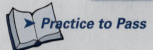

Practice to Pass

The client asks the nurse about safe use of phytomedicines. What should the nurse tell the client regarding what to look for on the container label?

NCLEX!

NCLEX!

NCLEX!

NCLEX!

NCLEX!

13. Instruct clients to avoid use of phytomedicines in pregnancy (potential for pregnancy), lactation and in children

14. Teach client to accurately assess advertising claims; provide reputable sources of information, including the following websites:

- American Botanical Council: http://herbalgram.org/abcmission.html

- Herb Research Foundation: http//www.herbs.herbs.org

- NCCAM: http://nccam.nih.gov

Case Study

A 30-year-old female visits the physician's office with complaints of migraine headaches. Vital signs reveal BP 118/76, pulse 82, respirations 18. She denies any allergies to medications. She states her neighbor takes feverfew with good results for relief of her headaches.

❶ What other assessment data is necessary for the nurse to gather related to the possible use of the feverfew?

❷ What client teaching should be done regarding the dosage of feverfew?

❸ What are the pharmacologic actions of feverfew?

❹ What client teaching is needed regarding discontinuation of the feverfew?

❺ What over-the-counter (OTC) medications or herbs should the client be instructed to avoid?

For suggested responses, see page 643.

Posttest

1 Which of the following statements made by the client taking saw palmetto indicates a need for further teaching?

(1) "I will take saw palmetto in the morning as a tea."
(2) "I will take the herb with meals or food."
(3) "Large amounts of the herb may cause diarrhea."
(4) "It may take as long as 6 to 8 weeks before effects of the therapy may be noticed."

2 Use of hawthorn to treat hypertension is similar in action to which of the following medications?

(1) Furosemide (Lasix)
(2) Capoten (Captopril)
(3) Hydralazine (Apresoline)
(4) Amlodipine (Norvasc)

3 A client using phytomedicines is able to demonstrate safe and effective use when the client makes which of the following statements?

(1) "Phytomedicines may be used effectively for sudden and acute illness."
(2) "The FDA regulates the medicinal use of herbs only when taken as directed,"
(3) "It is important to know the use of each particular herb in order to determine the appropriate dose."
(4) "Large doses of phytomedicines are safe since they are natural substances."

4 A client taking ginkgo biloba complains of itchy skin. Which of the following statements made by the nurse is most appropriate?

(1) "Tell me what form of ginkgo you have been using."
(2) "This reaction is common and should disappear in a few days."
(3) "It is important to avoid the sun while taking gingko."
(4) "Discontinue use of the ginkgo until the symptoms disappear."

5 The client taking St. John's wort should be instructed to avoid which of the following activities?

(1) Bowling
(2) Sunbathing
(3) Yoga
(4) Weightlifting

6 The client asks the nurse about the purpose of taking valerian root. Which of the following uses would be least appropriate?

(1) Relief of insomnia
(2) Relief of muscle spasms
(3) Reduction of anxiety
(4) Treatment of hypertension

7 The nurse supports use of bilberry in which of the following clients?

(1) The client taking iron pills for the treatment of anemia
(2) The client taking warfarin (Coumadin) for the treatment of thrombophlebitis
(3) The client taking Vitamin E to improve the immune system
(4) The client taking estrogen for the treatment of premenstrual syndrome

8 The nurse instructs the client taking valerian root to avoid the use of which of the following medications?

(1) ASA (aspirin)
(2) Codeine
(3) Clonidine (Catapres)
(4) Alprazolam (Xanax)

9 The nurse suggests that a client diagnosed with increased intraocular pressure may benefit from which of the following phytomedicines?

(1) Black cohosh
(2) Valerian root
(3) Saw palmetto
(4) Bilberry

10 The nurse would recommend ginger to treat which of the following complaints by the client?

(1) Nausea and vomiting
(2) Varicose veins
(3) Cold and flu symptoms
(4) Fatigue

See page 625 for Answers and Rationales.

Answers and Rationales

Pretest

1 Answer: 1 *Rationale:* The focus of the education should be on the client's ability to assess the reliability of the information source. Although all of the other options are also correct, option 1 is a global response and takes into consideration all of the other options.
Cognitive Level: Analysis
Nursing Process: Assessment; *Test Plan:* HPM

2 Answer: 1 *Rationale:* Feverfew has not been proven safe for use in pregnancy and lactation. It is important for the client to discontinue use of the feverfew immediately until the pregnancy has been verified. Client education should also include that those who may possibly become pregnant should avoid the use of any herbs. Therefore, first the client should be instructed to discontinue use of the feverfew and then have a pregnancy test performed. Option 3 is incorrect be-

cause the client would need to see the health care provider only if she is pregnant. Option 4 is incorrect because the dosage of the feverfew is not relevant.
Cognitive Level: Analysis
Nursing Process: Implementation; *Test Plan:* HPM

3 **Answer: 2** *Rationale:* The active ingredient valepotriate may be carcinogenic and should be removed from the form of the herb. Option 1 is incorrect as lorazepam (Ativan) and valerian root exhibit similar actions and may not be taken together safely. Option 3 is incorrect as the herb has not been proven safe in children, regardless of age. Option 4 is incorrect as the form of the herb is irrelevant to its effectiveness.
Cognitive Level: Application
Nursing Process: Evaluation; *Test Plan:* HPM

4 **Answer: 4** *Rationale:* Saw palmetto taken in doses greater than the recommended 160 mg standardized liposterolic acid BID may produce diarrhea. This side effect is not related to the form of the extract or the client's age (options 3 and 4). Allergy to ragweed is not related to the use of saw palmetto (option 2).
Cognitive Level: Analysis
Nursing Process: Assessment; *Test Plan:* PHYS

5 **Answer: 2** *Rationale:* One of the major uses of black cohosh is in the treatment of postmenopausal symptoms, which include hot flashes and night sweats. Black cohosh is also used to promote labor in pregnancy, to reduce blood pressure and cholesterol levels and is used in the treatment of poisonous snake bites. The other options identify incorrect herbs for treatment of the symptoms listed.
Cognitive Level: Application
Nursing Process: Analysis; *Test Plan:* PHYS

6 **Answer: 1** *Rationale:* The effectiveness of garlic is based on scientific evidence and clinical trials. Garlic has the ability to affect bleeding times and should not be taken with other herbs that have the same action, making option 2 incorrect. Option 3 is incorrect because garlic may be taken in enteric-coated tablets of garlic powder, which is effective in reducing bad breath although this form may not be as potent as raw garlic. Option 4 is incorrect because garlic should not be used with over-the-counter medications such as ASA (Aspirin) or ibuprofen (Motrin) that may also affect bleeding times.
Cognitive Level: Analysis
Nursing Process: Evaluation; *Test Plan:* HPM

7 **Answer: 3** *Rationale:* Hawthorn should be avoided with concomitant use of prescription antihypertensive

medications, such as captopril (Capoten), an ACE inhibitor. Hawthorn is similar in action to the ACE inhibitors and works to reduce blood pressure by blocking the conversion of Angiotensin I to Angiotensin II, which is a potent vasoconstrictor. Option 1 is incorrect because hawthorn is only effective in the treatment of chronic stable angina. As with any phytotherapy, use should be restricted to chronic, self-limiting conditions and not for acute episodes. Option 2 is incorrect as hawthorn has a negative chronotropic effect to decrease heart rate. Option 4 is incorrect as verapamil (Calan) is a calcium channel blocker and works to decrease blood pressure by blocking the influx of calcium ions across the cardiac and arterial muscle cell membrane.
Cognitive Level: Analysis
Nursing Process: Implementation; *Test Plan:* PHYS

8 **Answer: 3** *Rationale:* Korean ginseng should not be used in combination with coffee, tea, or colas. Option 1 is incorrect as there is no evidence that the herb affects the ability to drive a car or operate machinery (no known CNS effects). Option 2 is incorrect as the form of the herb is not related the adverse effects. Option 4 is incorrect as there are specific precautions with the use of Korean ginseng; for example, a ginseng-free period is recommended, usually 2–3 weeks on and 1–2 weeks off.
Cognitive Level: Application
Nursing Process: Implementation; *Test Plan:* HPM

9 **Answer: 3** *Rationale:* St. John's wort may take several weeks before the effects are evident. (All phytomedicines are slower to work than prescribed medications.) The form of the herb is not related to its effectiveness, making option 1 incorrect. St. John's wort in capsule form should be taken TID, making option 2 incorrect. Option 4 is incorrect as St. John's wort is appropriate for the treatment of mild to moderate depression.
Cognitive Level: Analysis
Nursing Process: Implementation; *Test Plan:* HPM

10 **Answer: 2** *Rationale:* There is conflicting evidence that saw palmetto will actually reduce the size of the prostate. Clinical evidence supports the use of the herb to reduce symptoms of residual volume (option 1), urinary frequency (option 3) and dysuria (option 4), common symptoms of the disorder.
Cognitive Level: Application
Nursing Process: Evaluation; *Test Plan:* PHYS

Posttest

1 **Answer: 1** *Rationale:* Saw palmetto should be avoided in tea form as it is insoluble in water. The other options are true statements and therefore do not require further teaching.
Cognitive Level: Analysis
Nursing Process: Evaluation; *Test Plan:* PHYS

2 **Answer: 2** *Rationale:* Hawthorn is similar in action to ACE inhibitors. They prevent the conversion of angiotensin I to angiotensin II, a potent vasoconstrictor. The other answers are incorrect. Furosemide (Lasix) is a loop diuretic (option 1); hydralazine (Apresoline) is a direct-acting peripheral vasodilator (option 3); amlodipine (Norvasc) is a calcium channel blocker (option 4).
Cognitive Level: Comprehension
Nursing Process: Analysis; *Test Plan:* PHYS

3 **Answer: 3** *Rationale:* Many herbs may be used for different reasons. The dosage of some herbs depends on its specific use. Option 1 is incorrect as acute and sudden illness should not be treated with phytotherapy. Option 2 is incorrect as the FDA does not evaluate phytomedicines for the treatment, cure or prevention of disease, but how they affect the structure and function of the human body. Although not regulated in the United States by the FDA, most are regulated by the Dietary Supplement and Health Education Act of 1994 as dietary supplements. Option 4 is incorrect as many side effects and adverse reactions may occur with improper dosing and the words "natural" or "all natural" can be misleading.
Cognitive Level: Analysis
Nursing Process: Evaluation; *Test Plan:* HPM

4 **Answer: 1** *Rationale:* Unprocessed ginkgo leaves should be avoided as they contain ginkgolic acids, which are potent allergens, related to the substance uroshiol, which is the chemical responsible for the itch in poison ivy. Option 2 is incorrect as the symptoms will continue with continued use of the unprocessed leaves. Option 3 is incorrect as photosensitivity is not related to the use of ginkgo in any form. Option 4 is incorrect as relief of symptoms may be obtained from discontinuing use but will only reoccur if use of the unprocessed leaves is resumed.
Cognitive Level: Analysis
Nursing Process: Implementation; *Test Plan:* PHYS

5 **Answer: 2** *Rationale:* One of the side effects of St. John's wort is photosensitivity requiring the client to avoid direct exposure to sunlight, especially if fair-skinned. The other options are incorrect and not relevant.
Cognitive Level: Application
Nursing Process: Planning; *Test Plan:* HPM

6 **Answer: 4** *Rationale:* Valerian root is used as a sedative, to reduce anxiety, treat insomnia and relieve muscle spasms. It is also used as adjunct therapy for the withdrawal of benzodiazepines, as it has similar action to this class of medications without the addiction or dependence. Valerian root has not been known to have any effect on blood pressure, making option 4 incorrect
Cognitive Level: Application
Nursing Process: Implementation; *Test Plan:* HPM

7 **Answer: 3** *Rationale:* There are no known contraindications for the use of bilberry in conjunction with estrogen, although clients should always inform the health care provider when planning to utilize phytomedications. Bilberry may interfere with iron absorption when taken internally, making option 1 incorrect. Option 2 is incorrect as bilberry may increase coagulation time and should be avoided with the use of anticoagulants such as warfarin (Coumadin). Since vitamin E can antagonize vitamin K, it plays a peripheral role in blood clotting and should be avoided with concomitant use of bilberry, making option 3 incorrect.
Cognitive Level: Analysis
Nursing Process: Analysis; *Test Plan:* PHYS

8 **Answer: 4** *Rationale:* Alprazolam (Xanax) is a short- to intermediate-acting benzodiazepine. Concomitant use of this drug with valerian root should be avoided since their actions are similar and the herb may potentiate the action of the alprazolam (Xanax). The other options are incorrect.
Cognitive Level: Application
Nursing Process: Implementation; *Test Plan:* HPM

9 **Answer: 4** *Rationale:* Increased intraocular pressure is symptomatic of glaucoma. Bilberry is useful in the treatment of this and other eye disorders, such as diabetic retinopathy, night blindness, macular degeneration, and cataracts. The other options are incorrect.
Cognitive Level: Application
Nursing Process: Implementation; *Test Plan:* HPM

10 **Answer: 1** *Rationale:* The most common use of ginger is the relief of nausea and vomiting. It is also useful in the treatment of motion sickness and as an anti-inflammatory in osteoarthritis and rheumatoid arthritis. The other options are incorrect.
Cognitive Level: Application
Nursing Process: Implementation; *Test Plan:* PHYS

References

Aschenbrenner, D. S., Cleveland, L. W., & Venable, S. J. (2002). Lifestyle, diet, and habits: Nutritional considerations. In *Drug therapy in nursing* (pp. 131–156). Philadelphia: Lippincott, Williams & Wilkins.

Bello, C., & West, D. (2001). Using herbal therapy wisely. [Electronic version]. *Clinical Letter for NPs,* 5(1), 1–7.

Blake, S. (1999). *Alternative remedies.* [Computer Software]. St. Louis: Mosby.

Complementary and Alternative Medicine at the NIH. (2002, Summer). NCCAM plays key role in integrative medicine task force. *NCCAM Newsletter,* IX(2). Retrieved from http://nccam.nih.gov./news/newsletter/

Fetrow, C. W., & Avila, J. R. (2001). *Professional's handbook of complementary & alternative medicines.* (2nd ed.). Springhouse, PA: Springhouse.

Freeman, L. W. (2000). Herbs as medical intervention. In Freeman, L. W. & Lawlis, G. F. (Eds.). *Mosby's complementary & alternative medicine* (pp. 388–423). St. Louis, MO: Mosby.

Ignatavicius, F., & Workman, M. L. (2002). *Medical-surgical nursing: Critical thinking for collaborative care (4th ed.).* Philadelphia: W. B. Saunders.

Kee, J. & Hayes, E. (2003). *Pharmacology: A nursing process approach* (4th ed.). Philadelphia: Saunders, pp. 143–155.

Lehne, R. (2004). *Pharmacology for nursing care* (5th ed.). St. Louis, MO: Mosby, pp. 1137–1147.

McKency, L. & Salerno, G. (2003). *Mosby's pharmacology in nursing* (21st ed. revised reprint). St. Louis, MO: Mosby, pp. 232–246.

Miller, C. A. (1998). How safe are herbs? *Geriatric Nursing,* 19, 163–164.

O Neill, C. K., Avila, J. R., & Fetrow, C. W. (1999). Herbal medicines: Getting beyond the hype. *Nursing, 29,* 58–61.

Vogelzang, J. L. (2001). What you need to know about dietary supplements. *Home Healthcare Nurse, 19,* 50–52.

Wilson, B. B., Shannon, M. T., & Stang, C. L. (2003). *Nurse's Drug Guide.* Upper Saddle, NJ: Prentice Hall.

Appendix A

➤ Practice to Pass Suggested Answers

Chapter 1

Page 6: *Suggested Answer*—The pregnant client is advised to avoid all medications during the pregnancy. Since she reports these discomforts occasional in frequency, the nurse may recommend some nonpharmacologic remedies for the headaches and backaches, such as taking a rest period or lying down during the day, or application of ice to the forehead or back.

Page 12: *Suggested Answer*—Most medications depend on a functioning renal system for excretion from the body. For a client with chronic renal failure, the priority considerations are related to appropriate dosing with the drug and for careful assessment of the client for toxic effects of the drug. The drug regimen for clients with chronic renal failure is often complex; the nurse will review with the client the prescribed drugs and the schedule for administration. If the client is being treated with hemodialysis for chronic renal failure, the nurse will review with the client what drugs are taken takes before and after the dialysis treatment.

Page 13: *Suggested Answer*—The correct volume to administer morphine sulfate 15 mg in this example is 0.6 mL. The problem can be set up this way: 25 mg:1 mL = 15 mg: x mL.

$$25x = 15, x = 15 \div 25, x = 0.6 \text{ mL}.$$

The nurse doing a drug calculation will review the answer and note that, if 25 mg is contained in 1 mL, then 15 mg will be contained in a volume less than 1 mL, in this case 0.6 mL. The nurse enhances client safety through accurate dosing by performing a "common sense" check at the end of each drug calculation.

Page 16: *Suggested Answer*—The intravenous (IV) route has no barriers to absorption of medication because it bypasses the gastrointestinal tract and does not need to be absorbed from muscle or subcutaneous tissue. Because it enters the bloodstream directly, it reaches the target tissues quickly and provides the most rapid action for analgesia or any other drug effect.

Page 19: *Suggested Answer*—There are several strategies the nurse can use in this situation:

- Do the teaching using short, simple sentences and provide a demonstration where possible.
- Use an interpreter or, if unavailable, ask a member of client's family to interpret.
- Search online or using other resources to find drug information materials in the client's language.
- Develop a diagram of the drug schedule that uses pictures and numbers.
- Observe the client for cues that signal lack of effective communication during the teaching session.

Chapter 2

Page 47: *Suggested Answer*—Peak and trough laboratory findings guide dosage and dosing schedule for certain drugs such as vancomycin (Vancocin). Changes will be prescribed based on these findings and the clinical manifestations of the client. Apparently the trough level was low and so the dosing schedule was increased from every eight hours to every six hours. The dosage may also have been increased. If the trough is low, the therapeutic drug level is not being maintained which could limit the drug's therapeutic effectiveness and allow microorganisms to replicate causing continuation or exacerbation of the infection. Explain the rationale for the change to the client. Ask for clarification of what the client means by "tied down," and facilitate the client's exploration of possible options to not being "tied down." Client compliance is necessary for effective outcomes.

Page 53: *Suggested Answer*—Assess number and characteristics of stools, abdominal cramping, if there is newly developed fever, and length of time on antibiotic therapy. If pseudomembranous colitis is suspected, arrange for a stool specimen for culture and sensitivity for *Clostridium difficile*. If specimen is positive for *C. difficile,* collaborate with the prescriber about discontinuing the antibiotic, initiating therapy with vancomycin po or IV or with metronidazole (Flagyl) to treat the pseudomonas colitis, and issues related to maintaining fluid and electrolyte balance. If the diarrhea is mild, the antibiotic may be continued. An absorbent anti-diarrheal as Kaolin and Pectin (Kao-tin) may be prescribed. Monitoring hydration status and potassium level will be important. Provide for good hygiene.

Page 62: *Suggested Answer*—Take tetracycline on an empty stomach with a full glass of water. Take one hour before and two hours after meals, ingestion of milk or milk products, or antacids that would interfere with the efficacy of the drug. If the client is taking oral contraceptives, advise the client to use an alternative method of contraception during therapy and for one month after discontinuation of the tetracycline as the drug will interfere with effectiveness of oral contraceptives. Breakthrough bleeding may occur as well. Report severe side effects and clinical manifestations of Candida infection. Avoid direct sunlight and ultraviolet lights including tanning beds because of risk for photosensitivity. If in the sun, advise client to wear long sleeves, long-legged pants, hat, and sunglasses. Sunscreen and sunblocks may be used, but may not prevent a photosensitivity reaction. Teach the client to store tetracycline in a tightly covered container protected from moisture and light, i.e., not in the medicine cabinet in the bathroom. Keep health care appointments for follow-up exams and tests.

Page 76: *Suggested Answer*—Explain to the client that taking the acyclovir before symptoms occur better enables the antiviral drug to be effective in reducing the viral load and preventing complications. The drug's efficacy is best when the virus is residing in the body's cells and before the virus is released from the cell. The drug's effectiveness will diminish over time, but its effectiveness is optimized with early introduction as evidenced by persons with HIV not becoming symptomatic for longer periods of time. There are other antiviral agents available that are used in combination for future needs and to retard development of drug resistance. Offer to arrange for the client to discuss the treatment strategy with the prescriber if concerns persist.

Page 78: *Suggested Answer*—Xerostomia is dryness of the mouth. Amantadine (Symmetrel), an antiviral, is also an anticholinergic agent that can cause dryness of mucous membranes, such as in the mouth. Oral care is important for comfort and also to protect the integrity of the oral cavity that harbors pathogenic

microorganisms. Frequent mouth rinses with water or warm saline solution can be refreshing and cleansing. Avoid hydrogen peroxide and commercial mouthwashes that contain alcohol because both can contribute further to dryness of the mouth. Sucking on hard candy may stimulate secretion of saliva, and there are artificial saliva products available. Keep the client hydrated.

Page 84: *Suggested Answer*—Determine first what the client means by "stuff" (the drug, the central line, or some other concern) and what is the client's understanding of "the bad things that can happen." As would be appropriate based on the information gleaned from the client, reaffirm the purpose of the therapy and explain what is done to minimize the risks or possible deleterious effects. For example, explain that premedication is provided to mitigate adverse reactions of the Amphotericin B, including antiemetic, antihistamine, and antipyretic agents. Analgesics are available if needed to maintain comfort as well. The client will also be hydrated before, during, and after the antifungal administration that will facilitate removal of toxins. Allow the client to verbalize concerns. Offer to arrange for the client to discuss concerns further with the physician if necessary. The client may prefer not to be alone so arrange for someone (family, friend, pastoral care, volunteer) to be with the client during the drug administration, if possible. Prudent nursing interventions can help this acutely ill client through a difficult time of treatment.

Chapter 3

Page 107: *Suggested Answer*—Three measures to prevent renal toxicity secondary to cisplatin administration include:

1. Assessment of BUN and creatinine before administration and periodically during treatment
2. Provide adequate intravenous or oral hydration (1000–1500 mL in 6 to 8 h) before administration
3. Administer mannitol (Osmitrol) or furosemide (Lasix) to promote diuresis

Page 109: *Suggested Answer*—

1. Promote oral hygiene before meals and at bedtime with fluorinated toothpaste, a soft toothbrush, and dilute baking soda rinse.
2. Assess oral cavity daily and report any redness, irritation, or white patches observed (monilia).
3. Educate the client to report soreness at the first sign of irritation.

Page 115: *Suggested Answer*—

1. Ensure that IV site was not started more than 48 h before administration.
2. Assess IV site for any redness or irritation, and restart if present.
3. Assess blood return and ensure that the vein is easily accessible and full.
4. Remove dressing from the site to provide clear access during administration.

5. Ensure IV site is not positioned in the area of a joint (with underlying tendons and nerves nearby) or on the dorsal side of the hand.

Page 118: *Suggested Answer—*

1. Assess client's usual bowel history prior to administration.
2. Provide a high-fiber diet.
3. Obtain an order for stool softeners at least twice daily.
4. Auscultate abdomen Q shift for bowel sounds.
5. Assess bowel movements Q shift.
6. Obtain an order for laxatives if the client has not had a bowel movement after 48 hours of administration.

Page 127: *Suggested Answer—*

1. Take oral temperature at the same time every day and report to MD if ≥ 101° F.
2. Maintain oral hygiene before meals and at bedtime.
3. Avoid eating raw fruits and vegetables.
4. Avoid proximity to fresh flowers or plants.
5. Refrain from emptying boxes filled with kitty litter, or fish tanks/aquariums.
6. Avoid large crowds and young children, and those with known infections.

Chapter 4

Page 153: *Suggested Answer—*A client who has been placed on anticoagulation therapy must understand that this treatment regimen will require close follow-up and long-term monitoring. The client must understand that the anticoagulant medication will make the client more susceptible to bleeding. Safety instructions must be given to the client to prevent bleeding episodes, such as using soft toothbrushes, electric razors, and avoiding trauma. The client must also be made aware of potential drug and food interactions. Compliance with the treatment regimen is an important process towards realizing the client's health goals. Both verbal and written instruction should be given to the client to enhance understanding and provide a reference past-discharge.

Page 156: *Suggested Answer—*Low-dose aspirin (ASA) therapy is used as a "blood thinner" for its antiplatelet effect. The dosage used is normally one baby ASA or 81 mg per day. If the client takes the normal adult dose of grains X or 650-mg q 4 to 6 hours, they will be taking medication to treat fever, aches and pains. Taking too much ASA can lead to potential health consequences such as ASA toxicity. Gastrointestinal hemorrhage can occur with the prolonged use of ASA at high doses. The client can always be referred back to the physician for further clarification in writing of the required dosage.

Page 159: *Suggested Answer—*Nursing interventions aimed at preventing or reducing the likelihood of increased bleeding would include: (1) minimizing the number of injections, (2) coordinating lab draws to avoid increased risk, (3) applying pressure after venipuncture and lab draws, (4) maintain aseptic technique and limit (if possible) the number of invasive procedures, (5) taking vital signs (using automatic blood pressure cuffs) and (6) continued assessment for possible bleeding sources (internal, retroperitoneal, intracranial, and gastrointestinal). The nurse must monitor the client closely and keep in close communication with the physician.

Page 163: *Suggested Answer—*It is important to know how long the topical agent has been in contact with the client's skin because there can be potential for skin damage upon removal of the agent. If the area is dry, then the nurse should irrigate the area gently with normal saline to minimize tissue irritation. Consult the physician and or pharmacist regarding removal and/or application procedures.

Page 175: *Suggested Answer—*Since anemia is a broad category and is sometimes a symptom of an illness as well as a disease entity, it is hard to make a general statement that medication by itself will restore adequate blood cell levels to correct anemia. Medication in conjunction with adequate dietary sources is a very effective treatment plan. However, if one is not sure of the underlying cause for the anemia, this may not be enough to restore blood levels. It would be important to verify the type of anemia that the client has to fully explore the answer. Clients who have vitamin B_{12}, folic acid, and iron-deficiency anemias can be treated successfully with combination diet and medication therapy in order to restore adequate blood cell levels.

Page 183: *Suggested Answer—*Cholesterol-lowering medications should be taken at night because the body normally performs the function of cholesterol synthesis at that time. If the body were normally undergoing that function, using the medication at that time would increase its biological effect and efficiency.

Chapter 5

Page 197: *Suggested Answer—*OTC diet pills contain many unknown chemicals that might interact with Transderm-Nitro, an antianginal medication and this could put the client at risk for additional cardiac problems. The client should be praised for wanting to lose the weight, but advise her to contact the physician prior to taking OTC medications.

Page 201: *Suggested Answer—*Your client may be experiencing an adverse reaction to the beta-adrenergic blocking medication. The beta 2 receptors in the lungs are probably being affected. Evaluate the vital signs, check the pulse oximetry, and notify the physician. Be prepared to take further actions as ordered to relieve the client's symptoms and increase gas exchange.

Page 204: *Suggested Answer—*Assess the vital signs including heart rate, BP, respiration and mental status. Evaluate whether the client is experiencing any chest pain. The Cardizem drip is a calcium channel blocker and may be causing a second-degree, Mobitz I (Wenckebach) heart block. Reduce the rate of the Cardizem drip by half and notify the physician. Do not leave the client alone.

Page 207: *Suggested Answer—*Turn off the infusion pump, remove the tubing but maintain a patent IV site with a saline lock or a NS infusion directly into the site. *Do not use the tubing* *containing the Nipride.* The client is experiencing profound hypotension with compensatory tachycardia from the Nipride drip. Notify the physician urgently. Assess the client's vital signs including mental status, HR, and BP. Maintain an airway, IV site, and monitor the client continuously.

Page 211: *Suggested Answer*—The client may be experiencing digitalis toxicity. Assess vital signs including mental status, heart rate, and blood pressure. Discuss the need to obtain a digoxin level and potassium with the physician. If necessary, draw the venous blood sample and send to the laboratory. Ask the client if he or she is taking other medications that might have interacted with digoxin.

Chapter 6

Page 235: *Suggested Answer*—Rhinitis or upper respiratory infection may decrease the effectiveness of this therapy. The information should be passed on to the prescribing physician. The client should be advised to contact the nurse again if there is any increase in urine output.

Page 236: *Suggested Answer*—Clients should weight themselves daily. The are advised to notify the nurse if there is a weekly gain of more than 5 pounds since mineralcorticoids can alter fluid and electrolyte balance. Since this client has gained 5½ lb in 2 days, the nurse should assess vital signs, edema, lung sounds, and skin to gather additional data related to fluid overload. Once the nurse has a comprehensive picture, the information should be reported to the prescriber.

Page 240: *Suggested Answer*—The nurse should encourage this action and should explain to the client the importance of wearing a Medic-Alert identification. If the client should become ill or injured, the information about the client's health contained in this identification will have an impact on treatment. The most common side effects of glucocorticoid therapy are mental status changes including affect, mood, behavior, aggression and depression. Clients taking glucocorticoids should be advised to wear some sort of personal identification in the event that they become mentally incapacited and cannot care for themselves temporarily.

Page 243: *Suggested Answer*—Increased effects of anticoagulant therapy can result when taken with thyroid medications. The nurse should monitor the client's prothrombin time (PT) or international normalized ratio (INR) to determine whether the warfarin is being maintained in an appropriate dosage range.

Page 246: *Suggested Answer*—Digitalis toxicity and increased risk of dysrhythmias may result when these two drugs are taken together. Thus, the nurse should monitor serum digoxin levels and look for early signs of digoxin toxicity such as anorexia and nausea. The nurse should also observe the cardiac monitor (if in use) for dysrhythmias, or look for an irregular pulse or change in pulse rate of a client who does not have a cardiac monitor in place.

Page 252: *Suggested Answer*—A musculoskeletal assessment needs to be performed including inspection and gentle palpation of the vertebral column, particularly the lower thoracic and lumbar vertebrae. Back pain along with restriction of spinal move-

ment and tenderness could be related to one or more compression fractures. Fractures in the distal end of the radius and the upper third of the femur may also occur.

Page 254: *Suggested Answer*—Insulin not in use should be refrigerated. Temperatures less than 36°F or greater than 86F need to be avoided and all insulin should be kept away from direct heat and light. A slight loss of potency may occur if the bottle has been in use for more than 30 days, even when the expiration date has not been passed. Therefore, a spare bottle of insulin should always be available.

Page 256: *Suggested Answer*—The client's health care provider needs to be notified. Also, the blood glucose level needs to be monitored at least every four hours and the urine tested for ketones if the blood glucose level is greater than 240 mg/dl. Also, regularly prescribed insulin or oral hypoglycemics need to be taken and instructions must be given to drink 8 to 12 ounces of sugar-free liquids every hour.

Page 260: *Suggested Answer*—The nurse needs to assess the client's financial status and initiate an immediate social service referral to determine what resources may be available. The American Diabetes Association (ADA) has a toll-free phone number (800-232-3472 in the United States) and will refer a diabetic client to the appropriate agencies or resources. The American Association of Diabetic Educators (800 TEAM-UP-4) can also refer a diabetic client to a certified diabetes educator in the client's own area.

Chapter 7

Page 268: *Suggested Answer*—Cisapride has been withheld by the Food and Drug Administration because of drug interactions that may lead to prolonged QT intervals and ventricular tachycardia.

Page 272: *Suggested Answer*—The client should contact a healthcare provider if diarrhea lasts longer than 2 days, which will allow the healthcare provider to rule out any infectious or colonic disorder.

Page 276: *Suggested Answer*—Activated charcoal should be given to counteract the effects of ipecac syrup. This may be administered orally as a flavored drink to disguise the taste, or it may be administered via a nasogastric tube.

Page 287: *Suggested Answer*—Misoprostol (Cytotec) can cause miscarriages. This information is vital for the pregnant client to be aware of so that the client can make informed decisions about whether or not to take this medication.

Page 288: *Suggested Answer*—The nurse should assess swallowing ability. Certain proton pump inhibitors must be swallowed whole while others may be opened and sprinkled on applesauce.

Chapter 8

Page 305: *Suggested Answer*—The nurse should assess the client for signs of hypersensitivity, which include any of the following: rash, urticaria, edema, and difficulty breathing. Hypersensitivity reaction is a medical emergency and must be assessed for and treated promptly.

Page 306: *Suggested Answer*—The nurse should assess the following three items:

1. Obtain a complete blood count (CBC) with differential and platelet count prior to the administration of colony stimulating factors.
2. Assess CBC and platelet count following the administration of medication. Report a neutrophil count of 20,000/mm³ to physician.
3. If CBC, particularly hemotocrit, is rising rapidly (74% in two weeks) assess carefully for hypertension and seizure activity.

Page 310: *Suggested Answer*—The following items should be considered when determining learning objectives for a client who will be receiving immunosuppressant agents.

1. Educate regarding the prevention of infection (e.g., avoid overcrowded areas or people with known infections, take in adequate nutrition, maintain good hygiene practices).
2. Educate regarding all laboratory studies that should be conducted, such as CBC, platelet count, renal and studies of liver function.
3. Educate about supportive care for flu-like symptoms.
4. Educate about action, side effects, and nursing implications of medications being administered.

Page 313: *Suggested Answer*—The following items should be incorporated into client teaching during an outbreak of hepatitis A:

1. Hepatitis A is transmitted by fecal-oral route.
2. Instruct on proper hygiene and sanitation.
3. Instruct on proper food preparation.
4. Hepatitis A transmission occurs from person-person contact and has been noted in areas with overcrowding, such as schools or day care centers.

Page 317: *Suggested Answer*—The following nursing interventions are should be implemented to relieve flu-like symptoms caused by medications used to treat multiple sclerosis:

1. Administer acetaminophen (Tylenol) for relief of pain or fever.
2. Provide adequate fluid intake to support fluid volume deficit.
3. Assess intake and output every 8 hours.
4. Provide adequate rest to promote healing.
5. Assess vital signs every 4 hours and administer antipyretic agents for temperature over 101°F.

Chapter 9

Page 335: *Suggested Answer*—Assess the "diaper rash" before presenting a teaching plan. Take a history of the rash, the infant's usual foods, and the usual skin care the infant is now receiving. There can be several reasons for diaper rash, e.g., it might be caused by remaining in diaper to long or by over-ingestion of a food to which the child is sensitive or it might caused by some

topical agent the mother is using at present. It also might be caused by a substance being used elsewhere, such as at a child care center. Sensitizers could be in soap, "baby wipes," topical powders, ointments, and even the diapers. Thus, the first step is to eliminate any food that is being used and any topical substance that is being used that seem likely to be sensitizers. The interventions aimed at restoring intact skin should be as simple as possible. There are skin protectants that might be helpful, such as A and D medicated diaper rash ointment or Balmex ointment. However, these are unlikely to be helpful if the culprit is a food (step one). Directions for any topical preparation should be closely followed (e.g., "thicker is not better"). Exposure of the skin to air for 15 minutes four times a day can be helpful in drying out a rash. If the steps are followed and there is no improvement after 7 days, a healthcare provider should be seen, since it could be a different problem, such as a fungal infection.

Page 336: *Suggested Answer*—The client might try Capsin, a topical analgesic lotion containing capsaicin in concentrations of 0.02% or 0.075%. The active ingredient is derived from capsicum oleoresin, which is found in a number of common chili pepper plant species. It can help manage minor pain associated with arthritis, sprains, strains, and simple backaches.

The precise mechanism of action is not fully known. However, capsaicin is believed to work by depleting the supply of the neurotransmitter substance P resulting in a reduction of pain perception. An initial burning sensation may occur after application, but generally will subside after continued use. It is applied to affected areas three to four times daily; if applied less often optimum pain relief may not occur and the burning sensation may persist.

It is for external use only and contact with eyes, mucous membranes, broken or irritated skin should be avoided. It should not be bandaged. If symptoms persist or worsen after 7 days of continued use, the healthcare provider should be consulted.

Page 337: *Suggested Answer*—Erythema (sunburn) is a familiar acute result of ultraviolet B overexposure, typically beginning 2 to 8 hours after irradiation and peaking at 24 to 36 hours. The lighter the complexion, the more severe the risk of sunburn. After severe overexposure, desquamation (peeling) occurs, reflecting changes in keratinocyte proliferation. There is a clear relationship in humans between the incidence of skin cancer and such variables as skin color, geographic latitude, and history of occupational and leisure-time exposure to sunlight.

The cousin needs advice on a photoprotection program. Sunscreens are a key ingredient in such a program and should be applied ½ hour before exposure. Probably a strong sunscreen with a SPF of 15 or above would be advisable in this situation. Reapplication may be advisable after swimming or sweating. A broad-brimmed hat shields the face, neck, and ears. Planning to do outdoor activities early in the morning (before 10 a.m.) or late in the afternoon (after 3 p.m.) is a simple form of photoprotection.

Page 344: *Suggested Answer*—A typical client with head lice (pediculosis capitis) has few, if any, easily observable signs of infestation. The child may complain of itching around the ears and over the sides of the neck, but these changes occur so gradually that clients frequently give them little attention.

Nits represent eggs cemented to the side of hairs, and they cannot be removed easily. Lice are spread from human to human by direct physical contact and through fomites.

A shampoo with lindane 1% (Kwell), permethrin (Elimite cream, Nix liquid) or pyrethrin and piperonyl butoxide combination (Rid shampoo) would be used to treat pediculosis capitis. Kwell is the least desirable product for children because of risk of seizures. In this case, even if no nits are identified in the child's hair it would not be wrong to use the shampoo as directed for the child. A nit comb is usually packaged with the shampoo and is used to contribute to the removal of nits from the hair.

All potentially contaminated articles of clothing, bedding, and personal hygiene products need to be disinfected. For head lice, the focus would be brushes, combs, hats, scarves, and coats. Items can be treated with rubbing alcohol or placed in home dishwasher. Towels, sheets, pillowcases, and bedding should be laundered in hot water. For items that are difficult to clean, freezing works well. It is not necessary to fumigate the house to rid the client of head lice.

Page 347: *Suggested Answer*—The client should use a topical product that contains salicylic acid to treat the wart. The product should be used as per its directions. General hygiene measures for the foot should also be discussed. This would include proper washing and drying of feet, wearing clean socks that are changed daily, and making sure to wear shoes (rather than go barefoot). If the wart does not heal within the time specified on the product directions, further treatment should be sought.

Chapter 10

Page 362: *Suggested Answer*—Discontinue the PCA, call a physician stat, and be prepared to give an antihistamine or epinephrine for an allergic reaction.

Page 367: *Suggested Answer*—The client is probably experiencing acetaminophen toxicity because of taking acetaminophen (Tylenol) as well as cold medication with acetaminophen in it. Acetaminophen is toxic to the liver and should not be taken in doses exceeding 4 grams per 24 hours.

Page 375: *Suggested Answer*—The tube feeding usually needs to be turned off for 30 minutes to one hour prior to the medication administration and for 1–2 hours afterward. A nurse who has questions about the effects of a change in rate can also consult the agency pharmacist.

Page 384: *Suggested Answer*—Because of the multiple medication profile, medications such as antihypertensives and antidiabetic medications, including insulin, may need adjustment.

Page 391: *Suggested Answer*—Opioids, especially meperidine (Demerol), should not be administered because of possible fatal interaction between these medications.

Chapter 11

Page 414: *Suggested Answer*—Neuroleptic malignant syndrome (NMS) is a potentially fatal reaction to antipsychotic drugs. At one time it was thought to occur in about 1 percent of the clients taking antipsychotics with an accompanying mortality rate of up to 30 percent. Increased awareness and vigilance by nurses and others has significantly reduced both morbidity and mortality rates. It occurs most often when high-potency antipsychotic drugs are prescribed. Haloperidol (Haldol) is frequently cited as the causative neuroleptic. Onset is from 3 to 9 days after initiation of an antipsychotic. It is manifested by muscular rigidity, tremors, impaired ventilation, muteness, altered consciousness, and autonomic hyperactivity. The cardinal symptom is high body temperature. Temperatures as high as 108°F (42.2°C) have been reported. More likely temperatures are 101°F to 103°F. Dantrolene (Dantrium) and bromocriptine (Parlodel) are the drugs of choice for treating NMS and should be continued for 8 to 12 days after improvement. Antipsychotics should not be reinstituted for at least 2 weeks after complete resolution of NMS symptoms.

Page 424: *Suggested Answer*—Sexual dysfunction (e.g., anorgasmia, delayed ejaculation, decreased libido) is common, occurring in about 70 percent of men and women. Other common reactions include nausea (21 percent), headache (20 percent) and manifestations of CNS stimulation, including nervousness (15 percent), insomnia (14 percent), and anxiety (10 percent). Dizziness, fatigue, and anorexia associated with weight loss are also seen in clients taking fluoxetine (Prozac).

Page 430: *Suggested Answer*—The medication regime should include that lithium should be taken exactly as prescribed even if feeling "well." Other important points are as follows:

* If a dose is missed, take as soon as remembered unless within 2 hours of next dose (6 hours if extended release).
* Medication may cause dizziness or drowsiness—do not drive or perform activities that require alertness or precision until response to medication is known.
* Low sodium levels may predispose client to toxicity-need to drink 2000 to 3000 mL of fluid each day and eat a diet with consistent and moderate sodium intake.
* Avoid excessive amounts of coffee, tea, and cola because of diuretic effect.
* Avoid activities that cause excess sodium loss—especially summer sun, hot weather, saunas, and exertion.
* Notify healthcare professional of fever, vomiting and diarrhea.
* Advise client that weight gain may occur—review principles of low-calorie diet.
* Instruct client to discuss any OTC medication with healthcare professional before taking.
* Advise client to use contraception—notify healthcare professional if pregnancy suspected.
* Review side effects and symptoms of toxicity with client.
* Instruct client to stop medications and report signs of toxicity to healthcare professionals promptly.

- Explain to clients with cardiovascular disease or who are over 40 years of age about the need for ECG evaluation before and periodically during therapy. Always report fainting, irregular pulse, or difficulty breathing immediately.

Page 440: *Suggested Answer*—Common side effects of Ativan include daytime sedation, ataxia, dizziness, headache, blurred vision, hypotension, tremors, and slurred speech.

Page 449: *Suggested Answer*—The primary nursing priority for this client is maintaining physiological stability during the withdrawal phase. Other important priorities include to promote client safety, provide appropriate referral and followup, and to encourage client to participate in the intervention process and become familiar with self-help, rehabilitation, and aftercare.

Chapter 12

Page 460: *Suggested Answer*—Tinnitus, hearing impairment, deafness, vertigo or sense of fullness in the ears.

Page 468: *Suggested Answer*—Avoid potassium-containing agents or salts, anticholinergics, potassium-sparing diuretics, ace inhibitors.

Page 470: *Suggested Answer*—Modifiable factors for hypertension include increased sodium intake, obesity, excess alcohol consumption, decreased potassium intake, smoking, and sedentary lifestyle.

Page 470: *Suggested Answer*—Routine labs include BUN and creatinine, electrolytes, liver function tests, WBC, and differential.

Page 473: *Suggested Answer*—If the client is taking a medication with a potassium-sparing effect, salt substitutes, which are high in potassium, should be avoided. Otherwise, the client could develop hyperkalemia, which can cause cardiac dysrhythmias as well as other manifestations.

Chapter 13

Page 508: *Suggested Answer*—

1. Squeeze the prescribed amount of cream into the applicator, and insert the cream deep into the vagina 1 to 3 times per week as directed.
2. Do not douche.
3. Remain recumbent for at least 30 minutes, and preferably use at bedtime to retain medication for a longer time.

Page 512: *Suggested Answer*—

1. Secondary sex characteristics such as pubic, axillary, chest, and facial hair, deepening voice, and enlargement of the testes and penis will begin to develop.
2. Testosterone can cause premature closure of the epiphyseal plates with subsequent loss of potential adult height, therefore the physician may be ordering wrist X-rays every 6 months to monitor for this condition.

3. Acne may develop.
4. Libido may increase.

Page 513: *Suggested Answer*—

1. Liver function studies to determine if hepatotoxicity has occurred.
2. HIV and hepatitis B and C panels because of to needle sharing.

Page 515: *Suggested Answer*—Other medications can be used, such as papaverine with phentolamine (Cerespan) and alprostadil (Muse). However, sildenafil (Viagra) is the only oral medication. Viagra is also contraindicated with hypertension, recent myocardial infarction (MI) or cerebrovascular accident (CVA), and other cardiovascular diseases.

Page 518: *Suggested Answer*—

1. Has she ever had a deep vein thrombus (DVT), embolus, myocardial infarction (MI), or cerebrovascular accident (CVA)?
2. Is she taking any other medications, especially antibiotics and anticonvulsants?
3. When was her last mense? Could she be pregnant at this time?

Chapter 14

Page 541: *Suggested Answer*—This client appears to be suffering from bronchoconstriction as evidenced by wheezing and the dusky color. The pulse oximeter reading of 88 percent is too low. The client's color also indicates a low oxygen level. Appropriate actions by the nurse include administration of oxygen with continuous pulse oximetry to evaluate the effects of the oxygen. Since we do not know this client's history, starting oxygen at 2 L/min via nasal cannula is appropriate in case there is a history of chronic obstructive pulmonary disease. Further actions include obtaining an order for a bronchodilator and administration of the medication. Obtaining a nursing history and keeping the client on bed rest to conserve energy are also appropriate nursing interventions.

Page 545: *Suggested Answer*—This client has a theophylline level of 25 mg/dL, which is too high. More data is needed to determine the reason for the increased level. Dosage should be checked to be sure that the client is taking the medication as prescribed. Theophylline doses should be based on lean body weight as it does not enter the adipose tissue, and therefore the proper dose should be calculated and adjusted accordingly. The reason for the elevated BUN and creatinine should be explored. Some theophylline is excreted via the kidneys and if there is renal disease, that could be part of the reason for the increased theophylline level. A liver profile will likely be ordered as theophylline is metabolized via the liver. The age of this client is not mentioned, but the nurse should consider the client's age and understand there is potential for increased sensitivity to theophylline in the elderly client and dosages may need to be decreased. The nurse should monitor the client for toxic effects of theophylline due to the elevated level. These include seizures, tachycardia, tremors, dizziness, hallucinations, restlessness, agitation, headaches, insomnia, nausea, vomiting, tachyarrhythmias, and chest pain. Adverse cardiac effects are not usually seen until the theophylline level exceeds 30 mg/dL. Seizure activity is not usually seen until levels exceed 40 mg/dL.

Page 548: *Suggested Answer*—The client needs to know the therapeutic action of theses medications. Proventil is given to dilate the constricted airways. Proventil can be used for the prevention and the treatment of acute bronchoconstrictive attacks. Of the two medications listed, Proventil is the one that can be taken in the event of an acute attack, as Beclovent is preventative. The difficulty with ventilation should improve with the administration of these agents and if it does not, the client should seek medical attention. Beclovent is an inhaled corticosteroid and is administered to decrease inflammation in the airways. Reassure the client that inhaled corticosteroids are not as likely to cause systemic side effects as corticosteroids that are administered orally. In addition to the action of the medications and the anticipated effects, the client should also be informed of potential side effects of the medications. Side effects of albuterol include hypotension, headaches, tremors, decreased potassium levels, increased blood glucose, nausea, vomiting, chest pain, irregular heart rhythm, restlessness, agitation, and insomnia. Side effects of beclomethasone include pharyngeal irritation, coughing, dry mouth, oral fungal infections, sore throat, and sinusitis. The client may also experience diarrhea, nausea, and vomiting. The nurse should utilize wording that the client understands and not give too much information in the first session. This client is newly diagnosed and may not hear all that is said due to the anxiety caused by a new diagnosis. Remember each client should be treated as an individual and some need and can assimilate more information than others. The basic information that is needed in this case is the way the medications work, how they are to be administered, signs that the medication is working properly or not working properly, and the potential side effects of the medication. Additional information can be given at a later date or as indicated by the individualized needs of the client.

Page 558: *Suggested Answer*—Fexofenadine (Allegra) is an antihistamine. The action of the medication is to block the action of histamine by competing with histamine for receptor sites and therefore decreasing the response of the client to histamine. This medication should ease breathing and decrease allergic secretions. The medication is used prophylactically to decrease allergic reactions and should be taken regularly, not during an acute allergic attack. Fexofenadine (Allegra) is a nonsedating antihistamine and has a rapid onset after oral administration. This medication is to treat the symptoms, but the cause of the allergic reaction should be avoided when possible. Fexofenadine (Allegra) may be tolerated better if taken with meals. Some of the side effects can include drowsiness, dry mouth, visual changes, constipation, and difficulty with urination. The client may also experience nausea, vomiting, diarrhea, dizziness, syncope, muscular weakness, unsteady gait, restlessness, and nervousness. Fluid intake should be increased to decrease the potential dry mouth ef-

fect and also to thin respiratory secretions and therefore ease expectoration. The medication should be taken exactly as prescribed. The physician should be contacted prior to taking any over-the-counter (OTC) medications. Alcohol and other central nervous system depressants should be avoided while on this medication. Hard sugarless candy may help if the client has a problem with dry mouth. Prolonged exposure to the sun can cause sunburn.

Page 565: *Suggested Answer*—Dimetane-DC is an opioid antitussive medication. There is a potential for respiratory depression with these medications. The client is 80, which makes her more at risk because of potential for the effects of medications to intensify in the elderly. She may have decreased renal function and not be able to excrete the medication as readily. The client is definitely in respiratory difficulty as evidenced by a respiratory rate of 5 per minute and cyanosis. The client is also lethargic which may be because of the narcotic but also could be related to decreased oxygenation and increased CO_2 levels. The client should be started on oxygen and oxygen saturation should be measured continuously. Respiratory effort should be monitored. Arterial blood gases should be drawn, and a work-up should be done to determine the cause of the cough. No more antitussive agents should be administered. The client will likely have an chest x-ray and be admitted to the hospital for possible intubation and mechanical ventilation. Education of the daughter and the client (when she is more responsive) should be initiated to discuss the adverse effects of opioid antitussive medications. Assessment of the underlying reason for the cough (such as respiratory disease) is important. Two weeks is an excessive time period for the administration of antitussive medications. Teaching is indicated to correct this as well. The client should be assessed for liver, renal, thyroid, and adrenal diseases as any of these can intensify the effects of opioid antitussive medications. The nurse should also obtain a history as to the concurrent use of central nervous system depressants such as alcohol and anti-anxiety agents, as these can intensify the effects of opioid antitussive medications.

Chapter 15

Page 585: *Suggested Answer*—Oral acetazolamide may cause gastrointestinal (GI) side effects such as anorexia, nausea, vomiting, and weight loss. To reduce risk of GI side effects, the client should take the medication with food or milk. Since acetazolamide also causes diuresis, instruct the client to take medication early in the day to avoid nocturia. Acetazolamide may also exacerbate renal stones. Unless contraindicated, the client should be instructed to consume at least 2000 mL of fluid per day and consume a diet high in potassium and low in sodium. The client should also maintain follow-up visits to monitor for fluid and electrolyte imbalances.

Page 587: *Suggested Answer*—Instruct the client to administer pilocarpine 1 hour after the administration of latanoprost. Inform client of side effects such as blurred vision, photophobia, burning, stinging, and itching. Latanoprost may also cause an increase in iris pigmentation. The client should remove contact lenses before use, and for 15 minutes after instillation of the medication.

Page 591: *Suggested Answer*—The eye is cleansed of crust and drainage before the administration of ophthalmic medications. To properly clean the eye, use a cotton ball moistened with sterile normal saline or other prescribed solution. Wipe the eye from the inner canthus towards the outer canthus. To avoid contamination of the other eye, use a separate cotton ball for each eye. The eyelid and eyelashes are cleansed.

Page 593: *Suggested Answer*—Proparacaine hydrochloride temporarily causes a loss of the blink reflex due to the effects of anesthesia. To protect the cornea, an eye patch is applied until the blink reflex returns. Instruct the client to avoid touching or rubbing the eye until the anesthesia has worn off. Because the client had a foreign body removed, instructions also include reporting drainage, severe irritation, delayed healing, or any other symptoms that may indicate an infection.

Page 597: *Suggested Answer*—Initially, an examination of the client's ear canal is done to determine the presence of cerumen or edema, which would prevent the flow of medication into the canal. If cerumen is present, it is removed by the clinician. If edema is present, a wick may be inserted to allow absorption of the medication. If the ear canal is clear, evaluate the client's administration technique. Instruct the client to pull the pinna up and back, tilt head toward the unaffected side or lie on the side with the affected ear up. After the medication is instilled, allow time for the medication to flow into the ear canal by remaining in the position for 2 to 3 minutes.

Chapter 16

Page 611: *Suggested Answer*—Three types of phytomedicines that are contraindicated in the client with a history of hemorrhagic stroke are bilberry, feverfew, and garlic (also ginkgo and ginger). Since a hemorrhagic stroke is caused by a bleed, any medication or herb (such as these) that prolongs coagulation time should be avoided.

Page 613: *Suggested Answer*—Ginkgo is recommended for age-related mental decline. By increasing cerebral circulation, it is believed to improve short-term memory and concentration. New evidence suggests effective use in the treatment of Alzheimer's and dementia. The appropriate phytotherapy for this client would be American ginseng, which will help the client (student) improve concentration, stamina, and increase the body's ability to resist stress.

Page 616: *Suggested Answer*—Milk thistle is known as the liver herb. It has been shown to protect hepatocytes from toxins and enhances regeneration of the liver cells. It has also been shown to be effective in reducing hepatotoxicity with concomitant use of psychoactive drugs such as phenothiazines and in treating overdose of the death cap mushroom.

Page 618: *Suggested Answer*—Some other names used to identify St. Johns' wort are amber goatweed, Johnswort, klamanthweed, God's wonder plant, touch-and-heal, witch's herb, chassediable, and devil's scourge. Since many of the herbs are identified by several names, including the English common, brand name, or foreign translation, it is important to be familiar with these names to help the client identify them appropriately.

Page 621: *Suggested Answer*—The ability to assess labeling of the container is necessary for safe and effective use of phytotherapy. Read the label for the specific, intended use. Also, the client should read the label for dosage, placing more trust in phytomedicines that contain a standardized form of the herb. The dosage should be clear and include length of therapy required for expected results. The client should also read the label to determine where the herb was manufactured. Although some European herbs are highly regulated and standardized, caution should be taken with those herbs manufactured or purchased outside of the United States, which may be contaminated. The letters "USP" (United States Pharmacopoeia) demonstrate standards were followed in its manufacture and that the herb has an approved use by the FDA. If use of the herb has not been approved by the FDA, the label should at least read "NF" (National Formulary), meaning that the manufacturer has at least followed the same standards of quality and purity.

➤ *Case Study Suggested Answers*

Chapter 1

1. The nurse will assess this client's ability to read the medication labels accurately since the client has diminished vision; the nurse is also concerned with client's ability to accurately draw up the prescribed dose of Humulin since the insulin syringe calibrations are small. Assessment of the client's short-term memory in relation to the medication regimen is also indicated. The client may forget to take ordered medications or may take the medication and then forget and take the dose again. The nurse plans ahead to make these assessments in a way that is sensitive to the older client's feelings about age-related changes.

2. During this home visit, the nurse will gather data on the client's current blood pressure, blood glucose level, and the client's report of pain in knees. These data will provide information on the effects of the drug regimen.

3. Based on the nurse's assessment of the client's ability to be accurate and to comply with the drug regimen, the nurse may suggest measures to assist the client with medication management:

   - Use of a drug dosing box that can be prepared weekly and serves to remind client of time of dose for each day
   - One week's doses of insulin can be prepared and placed in refrigerator with labels for each day's use
   - Prepare a large-print label for the medication supply
   - A family member can be enlisted to assist the client with this activity, keeping track of the number of pills in the supply as a way of evaluating the client's use of the drug

4. The client's report of feeling dizzy should be carefully assessed in this client. Client safety during these episodes is of high priority. The nurse will listen to the client's description for information on the timing and circumstances of feeling "dizzy"; the drug lisinopril has a side effect of orthostatic hypotension, which may cause the symptom of dizziness when the client changes position especially from sitting to standing. The nurse will measure the client's blood pressure when the client is lying down and again when standing to note if there is significant difference in these values. The symptom of dizziness, especially associated with weakness and sweating, may occur if the client experiences hypoglycemia that may result from inadequate food intake and the dose of Humulin; the effects of Humulin last for 24 hours after injection and its peak effects occur at 4 to 12 hours after injection. The nurse will instruct the client to move positions slowly and to have an available source of sugar at hand to deal with onset of this symptom; the nurse may make a judgment to contact the physician to discuss this situation.

5. The nurse will plan to use printed educational materials for this client based on the following:
   - The client's interest in reading about the prescribed drug therapy
   - The client's reading level as compared to the reading level of the prepared materials
   - The print size of the prepared materials
   - The client's primary language

   The nurse will introduce the materials one at a time and spend time reviewing them with the client to prevent sensory and information overload.

Chapter 2

1. Assess allergies to previous penicillin therapy and to cephalosporins because there is cross-sensitivity between the two classes of antibiotics; occurrence of mild erythematous, maculopapular rash is not a hypersensitivity reaction but needs to be reported to the health care provider. Gastrointestinal side effects do not preclude the client from taking amoxicillin.

   Assess vital signs, especially temperature, to establish baseline febrile status to assess the immunological response, to determine if interventions are indicated for client's comfort, and to determine baseline for future evaluation of drug therapy effectiveness.

   Determine if the client is pregnant. Safe use during pregnancy has not been established although antibiotic therapy will probably be implemented. The risks for rheumatic heart disease and acute glomerulonephritis as sequelae to a "strep throat" infection is significant.

   Assess renal function since the drug is usually excreted through the kidneys; periodic assessment of BUN and creatinine would be indicated for prolonged therapy.

   If CBC results are available, leukocytosis with elevated neutrophils, bands, and stabs would be expected with this diagnosis of an acute bacterial infection.

   Assess concurrent medications that may interact, such as tetracycline may interfere with the anti-infective property of the amoxicillin, and probenecid (Benemid) delays excretion of the antibiotic and prolongs its effect.

2. Assess for improvement of clinical manifestations including fever, dysphagia, malaise, and inflamed, erythematous posterior oropharynx and tongue with white pustules. Improvement of signs and symptoms should be observed within 48 to 72 hours of antibiotic therapy. Identify negative results on re-culture of oropharynx and resolution of leukocytosis if respective laboratory findings available. No or minimal side effects occur.

3. Assess number and characteristics of stools. Pseudomembranous colitis is characterized by at least 4 to 6 watery stools a day with blood and/or mucus, a newly developed fever, abdominal cramping. If pseudomembranous colitis is suspected, arrange for culture and sensitivity on a stool specimen. If positive, collaborate with the physician regarding discontinuation of the antibiotic and initiation of

vancomycin (Vancocin) or metronidazole (Flagyl) to treat the colitis.

If the diarrhea is mild, yogurt or buttermilk can be added to the diet to counter eradication of the normal intestinal flora. An absorbent antidiarrheal agent as kaolin and pectin (Kao-tin) may be prescribed. In either case, ensure hydration and assess for hypokalemia, which often demonstrates nonspecific symptoms as muscle weakness, fatigue, anorexia, nausea, irritability, and depressed T wave.

4. The full course of antibiotic therapy must be completed in order to better ensure eradication of the pathogenic organisms, to prevent re-growth of organisms that can occur with premature discontinuation of the antibiotic, and to decrease the risk for drug resistance to develop.

   The antibiotic should be continued for at least 48 to 72 hours after clinical manifestations of the infection are resolved. Further, this client with a hemolytic streptococcal infection needs at least 10 days of antibiotic therapy to prevent complications such as acute glomerulonephritis and acute rheumatic fever.

   If the drug is not used and is kept available for future self-administration, the client may not be taking the correct type of anti-infective and/or the drug potency may be less.

   The two infectious sequelae that could occur are acute rheumatic fever and acute glomerulonephritis.

5. If the client is taking oral contraceptives, advise client that the antibiotic may interfere with the effectiveness of the oral contraceptive and an alternate method of contraception will need to be used during therapy with amoxicillin and for one month after treatment has been discontinued. Break-through bleeding may occur.

   Take medication around the clock at evenly spaced intervals without interrupting sleep, as possible. This schedule better ensures sustaining a therapeutic drug level.

   If a dose is missed, take as soon as remembered, but do not double-dose at the next administration time. Report side effects such as rash, urticaria, wheezing, and GI adverse effects that are severe such as nausea, vomiting, and diarrhea. May take with food to minimize gastrointestinal distress. Practice good hygiene including washing hands frequently, disposing of tissues properly, not sharing eating utensils. Encourage fluid intake of at least eight glasses a day. Explain rationale for completing full course of treatment and for follow-up.

Chapter 3

1. The most important nursing diagnoses include the following:
   - Risk for infection related to intravenous administration of antineoplastic agents and resulting myelosuppression.
   - Risk for decreased cardiac output related to administration of a cardiotoxic chemotherapeutic agent.
   - Risk for injury: hemorrhage related to intravenous administration of antineoplastic agents and resulting myelosuppression.
   - Risk for imbalanced nutrition: less than body requirements related to intravenous administration of antineoplastic agents, which cause excessive nausea and vomiting.
   - Knowledge deficit related to the side effects of chemotherapy
   - Risk for altered oral mucous membranes related to intravenous administration of antineoplastic agents
   - Risk for impaired tissue integrity related to the administration of an intravenous vesicant chemotherapeutic agent

   The nursing diagnoses are listed in priority from the most life-threatening to the least. Since the development of infection is the most life-threatening, it is listed first. Adriamycin can cause cardiomyopathy and is therefore listed second. All of the agents can cause myelosuppression, therefore the risk for development of thrombocytopenia needs to be assessed. Excessive nausea and vomiting can cause nutritional alteration. Although knowledge deficit is an actual problem, the potential problems that precede it are more life-threatening should they occur. Methotrexate and 5-FU commonly cause altered mucous membranes, which can also promote nutritional alterations. While extravasation of a vesicant is a potential problem, it is listed last since it is rare.

2. The following are important diagnostic/assessment values that need to be obtained before initiating the chemotherapy:
   - Ejection fraction from the muga scan. If less than 50 percent, the physician should be notified before administration of Adriamycin.
   - Liver function studies (LFS) and CBC. If LFS are elevated, the physician should be notified for potential dosage reduction. The WBC and differential should be assessed to ensure the absolute granulocyte count (AGC) is $\geq 1500/mm^3$.
   - Obtain ultrasound of the liver and ensure no abnormality is found.
   - Client's vital signs, including weight, height, temperature, blood pressure and pulse.

3. A pre-treatment teaching plan for this client could include the following outlined elements:
   - Discuss chemotherapy agents prescribed
   - Discuss potential side effects and mechanisms of preventing
   - Nausea and vomiting
   - Stomatitis
   - Extravasation
   - Hemorrhagic cystitis
   - Sterility
   - Teach client to report burning or sting of chemotherapy upon administration
   - Teach client mechanisms to prevent infection
   - Teach oral care and demonstrate mixing of solutions

- Discuss contraceptive methods if appropriate
4. The orders that need further clarification with the physician are:
   - Loading dosage of Zofran exceeds the recommended dose of 20 mg.
   - The dose of 5-FU seems to be too low. Is it a transcription error?
   - Since this is the client's first dose of chemotherapy and he does not have a central venous line (CVC), does the MD intend on placing a temporary CVC such as a peripherally inserted central catheter (PICC) or triple-lumen catheter (TLC) for this treatment?
5. The following should be done to prepare the client for discharge from the hospital:
   - Reinforce continuation of oral hygiene after discharge.
   - Reinforce mechanisms to prevent infection.
   - Identify primary caregiver and/or financial resources to obtain one temporarily.
   - Teach anticipated nadir period, and signs and symptoms to report to the MD.

Chapter 4

1. A weight-based heparin therapy protocol is being used as it is the most effective method for achieving a therapeutic anticoagulation level in a short amount of time. Weight-based therapy helps individualize the dosage, client response, and therapeutic level. It takes into account individual requirements because the drug dosage is based on the client's weight. Many times, in adult clients, the dosage will be the same for all clients regardless of size and weight (e.g., antibiotic therapy). However, in most acute-care settings, it is important to go back to weight-based dosing to achieve a safe and therapeutic effect.
2. APTT would help to establish therapeutic blood levels of heparin administration. It would be important to obtain baseline CBC with differential, serum chemistry, and coagulation studies. In addition, labs should be done per protocol and the results trended to establish therapeutic levels. A doppler/vascular study may be necessary to evaluate the client's DVT.
3. The nurse can help to decrease C. W.'s anxiety by explaining why lab tests are necessary. It is important to offer the client information and emotional support to make the client feel a part of the health care team. It is important to spend time with the client and determine whether or not this anxiety is related to "frequent blood tests" or if there are any other underlying reasons that could be causing the client to be anxious.
4. It is important to give both verbal and written instructions for Coumadin therapy to the client before discharge. Referral to a dietician and continued follow-up will help to have the client feel that a health care team is available to supply necessary information and support. It would be important to include family members in the client teaching so that the client can meet therapeutic goals in a safe environment. It may be helpful to share with the client that many people are

on this medication on a long-term basis and live well within the guidelines without adverse effects.

Chapter 5

1. You would need several pieces of information before addressing discharge medications. What type of myocardial infarction (MI) did T. A. have?
   - Has the client been taking any medications?
   - Does the client the financial resources to comply with treatment?
   - Is the client interested in complying with treatment?
2. Assess vital signs including HR, B/P, and respiration to become familiar with client's baseline. Assess the client's baseline knowledge of the MI and long-term consequences so teaching can proceed from the level of understanding that the client currently has. Assess baseline knowledge of the role of each medication for the same reason. Ask the client about daily habits (getting up, eating, bedtime) as these will affect the teaching plan.
3. Teach the client as you assess the importance of each measurement. Instruct the client how to measure pulse and blood pressure. Discuss where the client could purchase a BP cuff. Discuss the importance of following the cardiac rehabilitation program if needed. Inform the client about available resources. Start teaching at least 24 hours before discharge. Do not wait until the client is dressed and ready to leave! After your initial assessment of the client's knowledge, use many resources to provide medication instructions. Use a written chart with specific names and doses of medications. Decide the best times of day for the client to take medication. When completed, make several copies. Attach one to the client's teaching record and give the remaining copies to the client.
4. Tell the client not to stop the medications because the client may experience worsening symptoms, including sudden hypertension (be certain to use language appropriate to the knowledge level of your client). This could lead to another MI or even stroke (CVA). Instruct the client to obtain enough medication before vacation because sometimes (depending on the location) a person might not be able to obtain the correct medication if a refill is needed.
5. Before discharge, sit down with the client and ask the client to tell you about the medications. Allow the client to look at the chart you have constructed together. This should not be a threatening time for the client. Encourage the client by reinforcing correct information, and fill in any missing information. Encourage her the client to ask questions and to call physician with any questions.

Chapter 6

1. Initially, clients diagnosed with diabetes feel a sense of powerlessness and loss of control. In most cases, their normal daily routines are altered and lifestyles become less flexible. Some clients may experience grief over the loss of

their former lifestyle and deny the existence of their diabetes. For many clients, a diagnosis of diabetes is difficult to cope with, and it becomes another major stress factor in their lives.

2. Successful client teaching depends upon how effectively the nurse has assessed the client's ability to learn and accept the teaching. The nurse must first determine if the client has a healthy and positive psychological attitude toward adapting to diabetes. If the client is ready and willing to accept diabetic teaching, then the nurse can provide successful educational experiences. The client's financial status also needs to be determined. Next the nurse needs to assess if the client is capable of learning diabetic teaching. To do this, the nurse must assess the client's educational and reading level. Educational material from The International Diabetic Center is developed at the second- and third-grade level. If the client is unable to read, then the nurse must develop appropriate strategies to present the information. Visual ability and the client's understanding of printed material are also necessary. A client's ability to conceptualize important concepts such as understanding adjustment of insulin dosages related to blood glucose monitoring is crucial to successful diabetic teaching. Other important data to assess are: manual dexterity and other physical limitations, visual acuity, availability of family or significant others to assist the client with learning, and client motivation to learn.

3. Key concepts to include during the first teaching session should focus on what the client does know about diabetes and its treatment and which diabetic issues are of most concern to the client. At this session, the nurse should also determine what the client hopes to get out of the teaching sessions and what the client wants to learn. Additional teaching sessions can then be structured on specific educational needs and those issues that are most important to the client.

4. Follow-up diabetic teaching resources may include: who to contact in the case of an emergency, case manager, personal physician, diabetic educator, social service, transportation, home care or public health agency referrals, and the American Diabetes Association.

5. Clients should be instructed to routinely follow up with their primary physician, dentist and eye care provider. Clients need to develop and review with the nurse their own individualized plan for follow-up medical care.

Chapter 7

1. The nurse should assess recent travel, food association, lactose intolerance, previous treatments, previous laxative use, normal bowel habits, and any similar symptoms in other household members.

2. The nurse should perform a full abdominal assessment, rectal examination, guaiac stool, assess for dehydration, and assess heart and lungs.

3. The following laboratory tests would be helpful: CBC, *H. pylori,* electrolytes, blood glucose, stool culture and sensitivity, and test stool for occult blood three times.

4. Dietary instructions by the nurse include to increase fluid intake, avoid dairy products and spicy, greasy foods. Also the client should avoid lactose and gluten products.

5. Possible etiologies of the client's symptoms are inflammatory bowel disease, irritable bowel syndrome, psychiatric disorder, or colonic neoplasm.

Chapter 8

1. The priority nursing diagnoses preoperatively include:
   - Risk for injury related to impaired clotting
   - Activity intolerance related to illness state and fatigue
   - Impaired tissue integrity related to edema
   - Ineffective family coping related to fear of the unknown
   - Pain related to liver enlargement
   - Knowledge deficit related to surgical experience
   - Excess fluid volume related to diminished liver function
   The most important nursing diagnoses postoperatively include:
   - Ineffective airway clearance related to pain and surgical incision
   - Pain related to surgical procedure
   - Fear related to life-threatening surgery
   - Disturbed body image related to extensive scarring
   - Deficient knowledge related to postoperative care, medication administration; and infection-related side effects of immunosuppressant medications.

2. It is important for the following laboratory studies to be assessed prior to and during the administration of the medications:
   - AST/ALT
   - Blood glucose
   - Blood urea nitrogen (BUN) and creatinine
   - Electrolytes: sodium, potassium, calcium, magnesium, and phosphorus
   - Complete blood count (CBC) and platelet count
   - Uric acid

3. The teaching plan for the client and family should include the following elements:
   - Discuss medications that have been prescribed by the physician.
   - Discuss potential side effects of medications.
   - Instruct the client and family on prevention of infection, since the goal of immunosuppressant therapy is to decrease the immune response and prevent rejection of the transplanted liver.
   - Instruct about pain relief measures.
   - Instruct on coping mechanisms to assist in preventing anxiety and depression.

4. Nursing interventions that should be implemented prior to discharge after portal vein repair include the following:
   - Instruct on signs and symptoms of bleeding, and to report any sign of bleeding to the physician.
   - Instruct on care of the incision site.
   - Instruct on prevention of infections.
   - Instruct on proper nutrition.

- Assess for signs and symptoms of liver failure.
- Assess AST/ALT periodically as available.
- Assess vital signs frequently.
- Instruct the client on turning, coughing, and deep breathing to prevent atelectasis.
- Provide pain relief measures.

5. SoluMedrol is administered following the portal vein repair to decrease the inflammation within the liver and diminish the likelihood of organ rejection.

Chapter 9

1. Dressing material (old linen, loose mesh bandage, soft gauze fluffs) can be applied to the legs and thoroughly wet with Burow's solution. Dressings should be kept moist for 20 minutes. These wet dressings will dry through evaporation. Wet dressings will cool inflamed skin. Local vasoconstriction will occur and will decrease the client's discomfort. Soaks can be used two to three times a day.

2. Topical steroids come in several strengths and forms. Side effects include atrophy, striae, folliculitis, hypopigmentation and hyperpigmentation, telangiectasia, perioral dermatitis, and perhaps even contact dermatitis. Most of these side effects are more likely with more potent agents. Lower-potency agents (non-fluorinated ones) should be used on the face, neck, and intertriginous areas such as axillae and groin. If stronger-potency agents are used under occlusion it can lead to adrenal suppression.

3. The two systemic drugs that are most likely to be ordered are hydroxyzine hydrochloride (Atarax) or diphenhydramine (Benadryl). Hydroxyzine has flexibility of dosage and low anticholinergic side effects. These drugs are H_1 antihistamines to decrease pruritus when it is histamine-related. The other ethods to reduce itching include use of topical corticosteroids to decrease inflammation, and hydration in the form of bland emollients and hydrating baths (oilated colloidal oatmeal bath [Aveeno]). For a severe rash in children, an oral steroid "burst" may be used to gain rapid control over symptoms.

4. The topical antihistamines are not recommended because of their potential for allergic sensitization. Topical doxepin (Zonalon) is available, but use over extensive areas can lead to drowsiness and anticholinergic side effects.

5. The usual duration of disease is about 10 to 14 days. The situation now is severe enough that a systemic steroid is required. There are a variety of products available, but prednisone is the oral medicine of choice. A single morning dose is usually therapeutic, increases adherence, and decreases steroid side effects. When oral corticosteroids are being discontinued, they need to be tapered slowly to prevent flare-up.

Chapter 10

1. Questions to ask the family upon arrival should include the following:

- When did the client have his last seizure?
- When did the client last take his seizure medication?
- What other medications is the client taking, both prescription and non-prescription?
- Is the client currently experiencing an unusual amount of stress?

2. Initial assessments should include level of conscious (LOC), mental status, and vital signs. These provide a baseline measurement of the client's neurological, cardiac, and respiratory status.

3. The priorities of care for the client while he is in the ED include to keep him seizure-free and explore why the client experienced the seizure.

4. The client education points that are of highest priority prior to discharge home include:
- Medication regimen including dose, schedule, side effects, adverse effects
- When to call physician
- The importance of always taking prescribed medication
- Health care followup needed to ensure therapeutic dosage levels

5. Medications or foods that could interfere with T. P.'s seizure medication include the following:
- Phenytoin: alcohol, antacids, antineoplastics, and antihistamines (note: the only foods that interfere with phenytoin are tube feedings, which do not apply to this client).
- Phenobarbital: theophylline, corticosteroids, and doxycycline

Chapter 11

1. Disulfiram (Antabuse) is taken by clients with alcoholism to help them refrain from drinking alcohol. This drug discourages drinking by causing severe adverse effects if alcohol is ingested. Disulfiram has no applications outside the treatment for alcoholism. It works in the following way:
- Disulfiram disrupts alcohol metabolism by causing irreversible inhibition of aldehyde dehydrogenase (the enzyme that converts acetaldehyde to acetic acid).
- Then, if alcohol is ingested, acetaldehyde will accumulate to toxic levels, producing unpleasant and potentially harmful effects.

2. Clients must be thoroughly informed about the potential hazards of treatment:
- Consumption of any alcohol can cause potentially hazardous or fatal effects.
- Teach clients orally and in writing to avoid all forms of alcohol, including alcohol in sauces, cough syrups, vanilla extract, etc.
- Inform client that disulfiram effects will persist for about 2 weeks after the last dose is taken—alcohol must not be taken during those 2 weeks.
- Encourage client to carry identification indicating this status.

---

3. The purpose for use of disulfiram is to help individuals avoid alcohol use until their recovery program is established and they are better able to avoid alcohol without the use of disulfiram.
4. Other treatment options available include 12-step recovery program meetings (Alcoholics Anonymous or other self-help programs), group therapy, aftercare groups, individual counseling if necessary, and group therapy if indicated.
5. Therapy may last for months or even years but should only be used with individuals who are healthy and motivated toward abstinence from alcohol.

Chapter 12

1. The additional subjective information include: smoking history; alcohol consumption history; family history for coronary heart disease and hypertension; history of cardiac or respiratory disorders or other chronic disease; work and activity levels; dietary habit and lifestyle and the presence of side effects.
2. Metoprolol is a cardioselective beta 1 antagonist that prevents stimulation of the beta receptors in the heart by epinephrine and norepinephrine. This medication blocks the sympathetic nervous system, especially the sympathetic to the heart, resulting in decreased heart rate and blood pressure. Common side effects include fatigue, dizziness, bradycardia, hypotension, and GI distress.
3. Lifestyle modifications include: dietary modifications, limit alcohol intake, stop smoking, increase activity and exercise, stress management techniques and weight loss if over weight, reduce sodium intake to no more than 100 mmol per day, maintain adequate intake of dietary potassium, reduce intake of dietary saturated fat and cholesterol for cardiovascular health.
4. Instruct the client to take blood pressure and pulse at the same time each day and report low and high readings; change position slowly to prevent dizziness; report side effects to provider; do not stop taking medication until discussed with provider; encourage lifestyle modifications; do not take OTC cold medications without consulting with the physician; limit alcohol intake; smoking cessation; dietary alternatives of low salt and low fat; stress reduction techniques. The nurse should also instruct client about the side effects of Lopressor.
5. Expected outcomes include:
   - Decreased blood pressure below 140/90
   - Maintaining a healthy life-style
   - Adopt a low-salt, low-fat diet
   - Develop a plan of regular exercise
   - Verbalize knowledge of hypertension disease process, related medications, and the importance of follow-up visits

Chapter 13

1. Dinoprostone is FDA-approved for cervical ripening prior to the induction of labor. Prepidil intracervical gel contains 0.5 mg of dinoprostone and is inserted into the cervix after direct visualization via speculum. Cervidil vaginal insert contains 10-mg dinoprostone, and one insert is placed into the posterior cul-de-sac, with the string protruding out of the vagina. The client should remain recumbent after administration.
2. Labor induction is accomplished by starting a peripheral IV, using either Y-tubing or piggy-backing into the main line, and infusing the oxytocin (Pitocin) solution via infusion pump. The oxytocin (Pitocin) solution is most commonly diluted as 10 units in 1 liter of IV fluid (although some practitioners will order 20 units in 1 liter.) The Pitocin is begun at 1 or 2 milliunits, and increased every 20 to 30 minutes until adequate contractions occur.
3. Because of the hypertension of preeclampsia, the oxytocin (Pitocin) solution infusion rate would be increased. If this did not control the hemorrhage, carboprost tromethamine (Hemabate) would be utilized, as it produces less increase in blood pressure than do either methylergonovine (Methergine) or ergonovine (Ergotrate).
4. Magnesium sulfate is most commonly used for the seizures of eclampsia. A 4- to 6-gram loading dose is given over 20 minutes, and then 1 to 2 grams per hour is usually run via IV infusion.
5. Breast-feeding women can use progestin-only preparations for contraception. This includes medroxyprogesterone acetate (Depo-Provera) IM, levonorgestrel intradermal implants (Norplant), or oral norethindrone (Micronor or Nor-QD).

Chapter 14

1. Albuterol is a beta adrenergic agent that is given orally or by inhalation and is used to treat and prevent bronchoconstriction. Albuterol will dilate constricted airways to ease breathing, and should be taken exactly as ordered. Beta 2 specific actions may be diminished at larger than prescribed doses. Therefore, the client may experience cardiac symptoms such as increased heart rate, and at larger doses, she may also experience nausea, anxiety, and tremors. The effects of this medication can be intensified by decongestants and some antihistamines. The physician should be notified prior to taking any OTC medications. Some clients experience hypotension and vascular headaches with albuterol. R. C. should have blood pressure and heart rate monitored regularly to ensure there are no cardiac side effects. She should be taught the proper use of an inhaler. She client should note the color, amount, and character of sputum. Oral doses of this medication should be taken with meals to decrease gastric upset. R. C. Should keep a record of when medications are taken and whether or not symptoms subside to determine the effectiveness of the medication. Inhalations of different medications should be taken at least one minute apart or longer depending on product literature. R. C. should avoid eye contact with the spray of an inhaled medication. Wheezing and dyspnea should decrease with

the administration of this medication. If this does not occur, the physician should be notified. R. C. should take the inhaler to school with her so that it can be taken as needed in the event of an acute asthmatic attack. R. C. should begin to note which allergens cause her difficulty and attempt to avoid them. Also, increased fluid intake will help liquefy any secretions and ease expectoration.

2. Beclomethasone is an inhaled corticosteroid that is thought to decrease the release of bronchoconstricting substances. Swelling in the airways is thought to diminish. This medication is to be used preventatively and not for an acute attack. R. C. should take the medication whether or not symptoms are present. Inhaled corticosteroids are not as likely to cause the typical systemic effects of corticosteroids because of the route of administration. Symptoms of a cold or the flu should be reported to the physician immediately due to the potential for suppression of the immune system. This is less likely with inhaled corticosteroids than with oral corticosteroids. Allergens should be identified and avoided. R. C. should be aware of symptoms and notice any increase or decrease. Difficulty should be reported to the physician. R. C. should be taught to note the amount, color and character of sputum. Increased fluid intake helps thin secretions and ease removal. Hard candy decreases difficulty with mouth dryness. She should wear a bracelet that identifies her as one who takes corticosteroids. The medication should be taken exactly as prescribed and not overused. The medication should not be stopped abruptly. The correct use of the inhaler should be taught as well as the need to rinse the mouth after inhalation of medication.

3. It is important for the nurse to understand the teenage client. Acceptance by the peer group as well as being similar to the peer group is very important to the 14-year-old. Exploration of ways the client can administer the needed medications without making her appear different from her peers would be beneficial. Another aspect to consider is that teenagers are normally healthy. Sickness in a teenager makes the young person different from the norm. Attempting to help R. C. incorporate the illness into her self-concept will aid in acceptance as well as compliance. The nurse should respond with compassionate understanding of the real issues faced by R. C. even if it seems insignificant to the health care worker. Assisting R. C. to determine ways that she can participate in the normal activities of a 14-year-old in spite of her illness will help with acceptance and compliance.

4. The anticipated effect of albuterol is to dilate the airway and ease breathing. With proper use of the medication, R. C. should experience less wheezing and dyspnea. Some of the side effects of albuterol are listed in the answer to question one. Additional side effects include tremors, hypokalemia, hyperglycemia, nausea, vomiting, chest pain, dysrhythmias, paradoxic bronchospasms, and urinary retention. The anticipated effect of beclomethasone is to decrease inflammation of the airway and therefore ease breathing. R. C. should no-

tice a decrease in the symptoms of dyspnea and wheezing. Potential side effects include pharyngeal irritation, coughing, dry mouth, oral fungal infections, sore throat, and sinusitis. Some clients experience diarrhea, nausea, vomiting, and stomach upset. Menstrual disturbances are possible and should be reported to the physician.

5. The nurse should assess respiratory function. She should talk to R. C. about the disease and assess her acceptance of the disease and the treatment. The nurse should determine whether or not medications are taken regularly and properly. It would be helpful to observe R. C. with self-administration of the inhaled medications to be sure her technique is appropriate. Determine whether or not R. C. is experiencing any side effects. Explore R.C.'s thoughts and feelings about the disease and its treatment, about the medications and whether or not the symptoms are controlled. Determine whether or not R. C. can participate in the activities that are important to her. Talk to her about whether or not she feels accepted by her friends and if she has any feelings about being different from her friends. This will give the nurse information about her acceptance of the disease and her tolerance not only of the disease, but of the treatment for the disease as well. Acceptance of the disease and its treatment will aide in compliance.

Chapter 15

1. Glaucoma is a disease of the eye characterized by an elevated intraocular pressure. The increase in intraocular pressure results from excessive production of aqueous humor or a decrease in the outflow of aqueous humor. Persistent high intraocular pressures may lead to blindness. The medication prescribed, Betoptic, is a beta-adrenergic blocking agent that decreases the production of aqueous humor, thereby reducing intraocular pressure.

2. Because of its ß selectivity, Betoptic is the drug of choice for clients with pulmonary disease. However beta-blocking agents are used cautiously in clients with pulmonary disease. The client should be monitored for cardiopulmonary complications.

3. Local side effects include burning, stinging, and eye irritation. Systemic absorption may lead to bradycardia, congestive heart failure, cardiac dysrhythmias, bronchospasm, insomnia, dizziness, vertigo, and gastrointestinal disturbances. The client should report these symptoms to the health care provider.

4. Photophobia may result from use of Betoptic. The client should wear dark sunglasses and avoid bright lights.

5. Instruct the client to wash hands, look up toward the ceiling, pull down the lower eyelid to form a sac, then to instill the medication into the sac. Instruct the client to avoid touching the eye, and to avoid touching the eyedropper to the eye or any other object. Instruct the client to use a nasolacrimal occulusion (press on the tear duct) to minimize systemic absorption.

Chapter 16

1. The nurse should assess the client for cross allergy to rag-weed, pregnancy (or potential for) or lactation. The client history and physical should be performed to assess for contraindications to the use of feverfew, such as bleeding disorders and the use of any anticoagulants or herbs that increase bleeding time, such as bilberry, ginger, garlic and ginkgo.

2. There is not consensus on the dosage of feverfew. Most sources recommend anywhere from 50 to 125 mg of the dried herb, which should be taken with or after meals to reduce GI colic. An accepted dose to prevent a migraine attack is 0.25 mg to 0.5 mg and 1 to 2 g to control a migraine attack.

3. Feverfew is effective in the prevention and treatment of recurrent migraine headaches by inhibiting the release of serotonin. It is believed that the activation of cerebral neurons containing serotonin (as well as norepinephrine) are responsible for the precipitation of a migraine headache.

4. Feverfew may cause post feverfew syndrome (muscle and joint pain, aching, and stiffness) when discontinued abruptly. To reduce the risk of these symptoms, the client should taper off the feverfew.

5. The client should be instructed to avoid any medications that have an anticoagulant effect, such as ASA (aspirin) and ibuprofen (Motrin). It is important to include education regarding accurate assessment of labels on other OTC medications, such as cold and influenza preparations that may contain these medications. Any other herbs that may play a role in blood clotting should be avoided, including bilberry, garlic, ginger and gingko.

Appendix B
Reference Tables

Common Abbreviations in Pharmacology

ac	before meals	mg	milligram
ACE	angiotensin converting enzyme	ml, mL	milliliter
ARB	angiotensin II receptor blocker	NSAID	nonsteroidal anti-inflammatory drug
ASA	acetylsalicylic acid (aspirin)	OD	right eye
bid	two times a day	OS	left eye
cc	cubic centimeter	OTC	over-the-counter
COX	cyclooxygenase	OU	both eyes
DMARD	disease modifying antirheumatic drug	pc	after meals
		PO	oral, by mouth
DPI	dry powder inhaler	PPD	purified protein derivative
gm (g)	gram	PR	per rectum
gr	grain	PRN	as needed
h, hr	hour	q	every
HRT	hormone replacement therapy	qd	every day
IM	intramuscular(ly)	qid	four times a day
IV	intravenous(ly)	qod	every other day
kg	kilogram	SC/SQ	subcutaneous(ly)
KVO	keep vein open	sl	sublingual
l, L	liter	stat	immediately
MAOI	monoamine oxidase inhibitor	tid	three times a day
MDI	metered dose inhaler		

Common Equivalents in Weights and Measures

Volume Equivalents		Mass Equivalents	
1 milliliter	= 0.034 fluid ounce	1 milligram	= 0.0154 grain (apothecary) = 1000 micrograms
1 liter	= 1000 milliliters = 33.8 fluid ounces = 2.11 pints = 1.06 quarts	1 gram	= 15.4 grains (apothecary) = 0.0322 ounce (apothecary) = 0.0353 ounce (avoirdupois)
1 cubic centimeter	= 1 milliliter	1 grain (apothecary)	= 64.8 milligrams = 0.0021 ounce (apothecary) = 0.0023 ounce (avoirdupois)
1 fluid ounce	= 29.6 milliliters = 2 tablespoons	1 ounce (apothecary)	= 3.1.1 grams
1 teaspoon	= 5 milliliters	1 ounce (avoirdupois)	= 28.4 grams
1 tablespoon	= 15 milliliters = 3 teaspoons	1 pound (avoirdupois)	= 454 grams = 0.454 kilogram = 16 ounces
1 cup	= 237 milliliters = 8 fluid ounces	1 kilogram	= 2.20 pounds (avoirdupois)
1 pint	= 473 milliliters = 16 fluid ounces = 2 cups		

Temperature Conversion

(Celsius degrees $\times$ 9/5) + 32 = Fahrenheit degrees

(Fahrenheit degrees − 32) $\times$ 5/9 = Celsius degrees

1 quart	= 946 milliliters = 32 fluid ounces = 2 pints
1 gallon	= 3785 milliliters = 128 fluid ounces = 4 quarts

Therapeutic Drug Levels

Generic & Sample Trade Names	Level in Conventional Units	Level in SI Units
acetaminophen (Tylenol)	0.2–0.6 mg/dL; toxic: > 5 mg/dL	13–40 micromoles/L
carbamazepine (Tegretol)	4–12 mcg/mL	375–900 nmol/L
digoxin (Lanoxin)	0.5–2.0 ng/mL	1.0–2.6 nmol/L
lidocaine (Xylocaine HCl)	1.5–6.0 mcg/mL	6–21 micromoles/L
lithium (Eskalith)	0.5–1.5 mEq/L	0.5–1.5 mmol/L
phenytoin (Dilantin)	10–20 mcg/mL	40–80 mcg/mL
procainamide (Pronestyl)	4–8 mcg/mL	17–40 micromoles/L
quinidine (Quinalgute)	2–6 mcg/mL	4.6–9.2 micromoles/L
salicylate (acetylsalicylic acid; Aspirin)	100–200 mg/L; toxic: >200mg/L	724–1448 micromoles/L; toxic: > 1450 micromoles/L
theophylline (Theo-Dur)	10–20 mcg/mL	55–110 micromoles/L
valproic acid (Depakene)	50–100 mcg/mL	350–700 micromoles/L
vancomycin (Vancocin)	30–40 mg/mL (peak); 5–10 mg/mL (trough)	20–40 mg/dL (peak); 5–10 (trough)

dL = deciliter; L = liter; mcg = microgram; mEq = milliequivalent; mg = milligram; mL = milliliter; ng = nanogram; nmol = nanomole

Selected Medication/Poison Toxicities and Antidotes

Substance at Toxic/Poisonous Level	Antidote
Acetaminophen (Tylenol)	acetylcysteine (Mucomyst)
Anticholinergics	physostigmine (Antilirium)
Benzodiazepines	flumazenil (Romazicon)
Calcium channel blockers	calcium chloride, calcium gluconate
Copper	penicillamine (Cuprimine)
Cyanide or nitrate	methylene blue (Urolene blue)
Digoxin (Lanoxin)	digoxin immune fab (Digibind)
Doxorubicin	dexrazoxane (Zinecard)
Heparin	protamine sulfate
Insulin	glucagon
Iron	deferoxamine (Desferal)
Isoniazid	pyridoxine (Nestrex)
Lead	succimer (Chemet)
Methotrexate	leucovorin calcium (Wellcovorin)
Nondepolarizing neuromuscular blockers	neostigmine (Prostigmin)
Opioids	naloxone (Narcan); nalfemene (Revex)
Warfarin sodium (Coumadin)	vitamin K (Aquamephyton)

Index

SINGLE PC LICENSE AGREEMENT AND LIMITED WARRANTY